Different **types of images:**
- Realistic and detailed anatomical illustrations for in-depth views
- Schematic illustrations to see functional relationships
- Photos of surface anatomy
- Orientation sketches
- Photographs of imaging processes

The figures

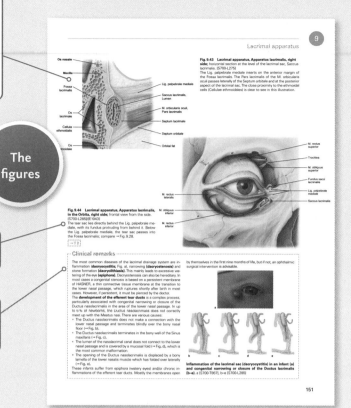

Detailed figure captions clarify the most important structures and topographical relationships.

The **illustrated Clinical remarks** feature shows a picture of the affected body area, which helps you to remember what you have learnt.

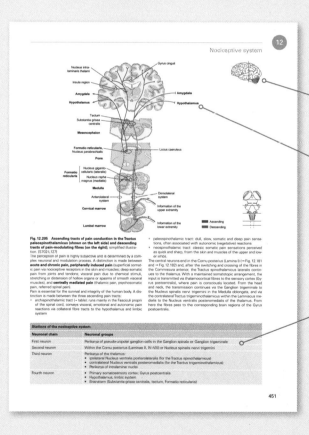

Orientation sketches give you the anatomical section depicted at a glance.

Learning tip: important structures are shown in **bold**.

Tables help to identify the relevant relationships.

Sample questions from the exam

Sample exam questions

To check that you are completely familiar with the content of this chapter, sample questions from an oral anatomy exam are listed here.

Sample questions from an **oral anatomy exam** are given at the end of each chapter to test your knowledge.

You will find these topics in the 17th edition

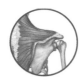
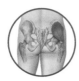

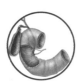

F. Paulsen, J. Waschke

Sobotta

Atlas of Anatomy

Translated by
T. Klonisch and S. Hombach-Klonisch

Friedrich Paulsen, Jens Waschke (eds.)

Sobotta

Atlas of Anatomy

Inner Organs

17th Edition

English version with Latin nomenclature

Translated by
T. Klonisch and S. Hombach-Klonisch,
Winnipeg, Canada

ELSEVIER

Original Publication
Sobotta Atlas der Anatomie, 25. Auflage
© Elsevier GmbH, 2022.
All rights reserved.
ISBN 978-3-437-44140-0

This translation of Sobotta Atlas der Anatomie, 25th edition by Friedrich Paulsen and Jens Waschke was undertaken by Elsevier GmbH.

Elsevier GmbH, Bernhard-Wicki-Str. 5, 80636 Munich, Germany
We are grateful for any feedback and suggestions sent to:
kundendienst@elsevier.com

ISBN 978-0-7020-6766-2

Notice

Practitioners and researchers must always rely on their own experience and knowledge in evaluating and using any information, methods, compounds or experiments described herein. Because of rapid advances in the medical sciences, in particular, independent verification of diagnoses and drug dosages should be made. To the fullest extent of the law, no responsibility is assumed by Elsevier, authors, editors or contributors for any injury and/or damage to persons or property as a matter of products liability, negligence or otherwise, or from any use or operation of any methods, products, instructions, or ideas contained in the material herein.

Bibliographical information published by the Deutsche Nationalbibliothek
The Deutsche Nationalbibliothek lists this publication in the Deutsche Nationalbibliografie: detailed bibliographic data are available on the internet at https://www.dnb.de

23 24 25 26 27   5 4 3 2 1

For copyright details for illustrations, see the credits for respective images.

Content strategist: Sonja Frankl
Project management: Dr. Andrea Beilmann, Sibylle Hartl
Editing and translating: Marieke O'Connor, Oxford, U.K.
Media rights management: Sophia Höver, Munich, Germany
Production management: Dr. Andrea Beilmann, Sibylle Hartl
Design: Nicola Kerber, Olching, Germany
Typesetting: abavo GmbH, Buchloe, Germany
Printing and binding: Drukarnia Dimograf Sp. z o. o., Bielsko-Biała, Poland
Cover design: Stefan Hilden, hilden_design, Munich; SpieszDesign, Neu-Ulm, Germany

This atlas was founded by Johannes Sobotta †, former Professor of Anatomy and Director of the Anatomical Institute of the University in Bonn, Germany.

German editions:
1st Edition: 1904–1907 J. F. Lehmanns Verlag, Munich, Germany
2nd–11th Edition: 1913–1944 J. F. Lehmanns Verlag, Munich, Germany
12th Edition: 1948 and following editions Urban & Schwarzenberg, Munich, Germany
13th Edition: 1953, ed. H. Becher
14th Edition: 1956, ed. H. Becher
15th Edition: 1957, ed. H. Becher
16th Edition: 1967, ed. H. Becher
17th Edition: 1972, eds. H. Ferner and J. Staubesand
18th Edition: 1982, eds. H. Ferner and J. Staubesand
19th Edition: 1988, ed. J. Staubesand
20th Edition: 1993, eds. R. Putz and R. Pabst, Urban & Schwarzenberg, Munich, Germany
21st Edition: 2000, eds. R. Putz and R. Pabst, Urban & Fischer, Munich, Germany
22nd Edition: 2006, eds. R. Putz and R. Pabst, Urban & Fischer, Munich, Germany
23rd Edition: 2010, eds. F. Paulsen and J. Waschke, Urban & Fischer, Elsevier, Munich, Germany
24th Edition: 2017, eds. F. Paulsen and J. Waschke, Elsevier, Munich, Germany
25th Edition: 2022, eds. F. Paulsen and J. Waschke, Elsevier, Munich, Germany

Foreign Editions:
Arabic
Chinese
Croatian
Czech
English (nomenclature in English or Latin)
French
Greek
Hungarian
Indonesian
Italian
Japanese
Korean
Polish
Portuguese
Russian
Spanish
Turkish
Ukrainian

Updated information is available on the internet at **www.elsevier.de**

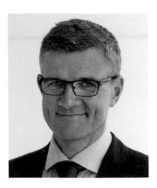

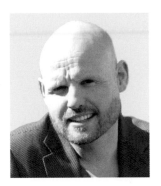

Prof. Dr. Friedrich Paulsen
Dissecting courses for students

In his teaching, Friedrich Paulsen puts great emphasis on students actually being able to dissect the cadavers of body donors. *'The hands-on experience in dissection is extremely important not only for the three-dimensional understanding of anatomy and as the basis for virtually every medical profession, but for many students also clearly addresses the issue of death and dying for the first time. The members of the dissection team not only study anatomy but also learn to deal with a particular situation. Medical students will never again come into such close contact with their classmates and teachers.'*
Friedrich Paulsen was born in Kiel in 1965. After completing his school education in Brunswick he first trained as a nurse. He then studied human medicine at the Christian-Albrecht University of Kiel (CAU). After acting as an AiP (Doctor in Practice) at the university clinic for Oral and Maxillofacial Surgery, and after acting as a doctor's assistant at the University ENT Clinic, he took on the position of assistant at the Anatomical Institute of the CAU in 1998, during an *'Ärzteschwemme',* obtaining a qualification in the subject of anatomy under Prof Dr Bernhard Tillmann, MD. In 2003 he was appointed to the posts of C3-Professor for Anatomy at the Ludwig-Maximilians-University in Munich and the Martin Luther University, Halle-Wittenberg. In Halle he founded a further Education Centre for Clinical Anatomy. Further posts followed at the ordinariat at the Universities of Saarland, Tübingen and Vienna, as well as at the Friedrich Alexander University (FAU), Erlangen-Nuremberg, where he has been the Professor for Anatomy and the Institute Director since 2010. From 2016 to 2018 he was Vice President for Education and from 2018 until 2022 Vice President for the People, and thereby a part of the FAU university leadership. Since 2006 he has been the publisher of the magazine 'Annals of Anatomy' and since 2014 he has belonged to the Commission of Experts of the IMPP (Institute for medical and pharmaceutical examination issues). Friedrich Paulsen is honorary member of the Anatomical Society (Great Britain and Ireland) as well as of the Societatea Anatomistilor (Rumania). Since 2006 he has been the secretary of the Anatomical Society, from 2009 to 2019 he was the Secretary-General of the International Federation of Associations of Anatomy (IFAA), the international governing body of the anatomists and since 2021 he has been the president of the European Federation of Experimental Morphology (EFEM), the governing body of European anatomists. In addition, he is the Visiting Professor at the Department of Topographic Anatomy and Operative Surgery of the Sechenov University (Moscow/Russia) and was Visiting Professor at the Wroclaw Medical University (Wroclaw/Poland) and the Khon-Kaen University (Khon-Kaen/Thailand). He has received numerous scientific awards, including the Dr. Gerhard Mann SICCA research award from the professional organisation of ophthalmologists in Germany (Berufsverband der Augenärzte Deutschland), the Golden Lion from the German Ophthalmosurgeons, the Commemorative Medal from the Comenius University Bratislava as well as numerous awards for outstanding teaching.
His areas of focus in research concerns the surface of the eye, the protein and peptides in tears and the lacrimal system, as well as the causes of dry eyes.

Prof. Dr. med. Friedrich Paulsen

Prof. Dr. Jens Waschke
More clinical relevance in teaching

For Jens Waschke, one of the most important challenges of modern anatomy is to target the actual demands of clinical training and practice. *'The clinical aspects in the atlas direct the students within the first semester towards anatomy and show them how important the subject is for clinical practice in the future. The biggest challenge for modern anatomy is to focus on the relevant educational objectives. In our books we want to consolidate the important anatomical details, leaving out the unnecessary clinical knowledge aimed at specialists. At the start of their training, students are unable to differentiate between basic and specialist knowledge, and we need to avoid our young colleagues being overloaded instead of concentrating on the basics.'*
Jens Waschke (born 1974 in Bayreuth) studied medicine at the University of Würzburg and graduated in 2000 in Anatomy. After his AiP in Anatomy and Internal Medicine, he became qualified in 2007 in Anatomy and Cell Biology. Between 2003 and 2004 he completed a nine-month research placement in Physiology at the University of California in Davis, USA. From 2008 he held the newly founded Chair III at the University of Würzburg, before being appointed to the Ludwig-Maximilians-University in Munich, where he has been the head of Chair I at the Institute of Anatomy. He has turned down further appointments to Vienna (MUW) and Hanover (MHH).
Since 2012 he has been the head of the software company quo WADIS-Anatomie with Dr. Andreas Dietz. In 2018, Jens Waschke was chosen to be the president of the Anatomical Society and is a member of its board until 2022. In addition, he is a honorary founding member of the Anatomical Society of Ethiopia and member of the Commission of Experts of the IMPP.
In 2019, Jens Waschke published the book *Humans – Simply Genius!,* to make anatomy more easily understandable to the wider public. In 2021 he published his first anatomical crime novel *One Leg.* In his research as a cell biologist, Jens Waschke examines the mechanisms controlling the adherence between cells and the binding function of the outer and inner barriers of the human body. His main focus of interest is the mechanisms leading to the malfunctioning of cell adherence which variously cause the blister-forming skin disease pemphigus, arrhythmogenic cardiomyopathy or CROHN's disease. His goal is to understand cell adherence better and to discover new forms of treatment.

Prof. Dr. med. Jens Waschke

Translators

Prof. Dr. Thomas Klonisch

Professor Thomas Klonisch studied human medicine at the Ruhr-University Bochum and the Justus-Liebig-University (JLU) Giessen. He completed his doctoral thesis at the Institute of Biochemistry at the Faculty of Medicine of the JLU Giessen before joining the Institute of Medical Microbiology, University of Mainz (1989–1991). As an Alexander von Humboldt Fellow he joined the University of Guelph, Ontario, Canada, from 1991–1992 and, in 1993–1994, continued his research at the Ontario Veterinary College, Guelph, Ontario. From 1994–1996, he joined the immunoprotein engineering group at the Department of Immunology, University College London, UK, as a senior research fellow. From 1996–2004 he was a scientific associate at the Department of Anatomy and Cell Biology, Martin Luther University of Halle-Wittenberg, where he received his accreditation as anatomist (1999), completed his habilitation (2000), and held continuous national research funding. In 2004, he was appointed Full Professor and Head at the Department of Human Anatomy and Cell Science (HACS) at the College of Medicine, Faculty of Health Science, University of Manitoba, Winnipeg, Canada, where he was the Department Head until 2019. He remains a Professor at HACS and is currently the director of the Histology Services and Ultrastructural Imaging Platform.

His research areas include mechanisms employed by cancer stem/progenitor cells to enhance tissue invasiveness and survival strategies in response to anticancer treatments. A particular focus is the role of endocrine factors, such as the relaxin-like ligand-receptor system, in promoting carcinogenesis.

Prof. Dr. Sabine Hombach-Klonisch

Teaching clinically relevant anatomy and clinical case-based anatomy learning are the main teaching focuses of Sabine Hombach-Klonisch at the Rady Faculty of Health Sciences of the University of Manitoba. Since her appointment in 2004, Professor Hombach has been nominated annually for teaching awards by the Manitoba Medical Student Association (MMSA) and received the MMSA award for teaching in the small group setting in 2020 and 2021.

Sabine Hombach graduated from Medical School at the Justus-Liebig-University Giessen in 1991 and successfully completed her doctoral thesis in 1994. Following a career break to attend to her two children she re-engaged as a sessional lecturer at the Department of Anatomy and Cell Biology of the Martin-Luther-University Halle-Wittenberg in 1997 and received a post-doctoral fellowship from the province of Saxony-Anhalt 1998–2000. Thereafter, she joined the Department of Anatomy and Cell Biology as a scientific associate. Professor Hombach received her accreditation as anatomist in 2003 from the German Society of Anatomists and from the Medical Association of Saxony-Anhalt, and completed her habilitation at the Medical Faculty of the Martin-Luther-University Halle-Wittenberg in 2004. In 2004, Professor Hombach was appointed to the Department of Human Anatomy and Cell Science, Faculty of Medicine of the University of Manitoba. Appointed as department head in January 2020, she strongly promotes postgraduate clinical anatomy training for residents.

Her main research interests are in the field of breast and brain cancer. Her focus is to identify the molecular mechanisms that regulate metastasis and cell survival under treatment stress. She employs unique cell and animal models and human primary cells to study the influence of the tumour microenvironment on brain metastatic growth.

Preface of the 25th German edition

In the foreword to the first edition of his atlas, Johannes Sobotta wrote in May 1904: 'Many years of experience in anatomical dissection prompted the author to create a pictorial representation of the peripheral nervous system and blood vessels in the way that the student has got used to seeing the relevant parts on a dissection, i.e. showing vessels and nerves in the same area in conjunction to each other. In addition, the atlas alternately contains text and tables. The images form the core of the atlas, with additional ancillary and schematic illustrations, and the figure legends give a short and succinct clarification for quick orientation when using the book in the dissection lab.'

As with fashion, students' reading and study habits change regularly. The multimedia presence and availability of information as well as stimuli are surely the main reasons for these habits to be changing more quickly than ever before. These developments and thereby also the changing requirements students demand from the atlases and textbooks they wish to use, as well as the digital availability of the contents, need to be taken into consideration by the authors, editors and publishers. Interviews and systematic surveys with students are useful in guaging their expectations. Until now, the textbook market has also been an indicator for change: detailed textbooks claiming complete integrity are brushed aside for textbooks and lecture notes targeted at the didactic needs of the students at particular universities as well as the study content of human medicine, dentistry and biomedical sciences and the corresponding examinations involved. Equally, the illustrations in atlases such as the Sobotta, which have fascinated many generations of doctors and health professionals from all over the world with their exact and naturalistic depictions of real anatomical specimens, are sometimes regarded by students as too complicated and detailed. This realisation requires some consideration as to how to adapt the strengths of the atlas – which has developed over 25 editions into a reference work of accuracy and quality – to modern didactic concepts without comprimising its unique characteristics and originality.

Looking at it didactically, we have retained the concept of the three volumes, as used by Sobotta in his first edition: General Anatomy and Musculoskeletal System (1), Internal Organs (2) and Head, Neck and Neuroanatomy (3). We have also adopted although slightly modified the approach mentioned in the preface of the first edition of combining the figures in the atlas with explanatory text, a trend which has regained popularity. Hereby each image is accompanied by a short explanation which gives an introduction to the image and explains why the particular dissection and area were chosen. The individual chapters were systematically divided according to current study habits and various images were supplemented or replaced. Most of these new images are conceptualised in such a way that the studying of the relevant pathways supplying blood and innervation is made easier pedagogically. In addition, we have reviewed many existing figures, shortened the descriptions and have highlighted the important terms, to make the anatomical content more accessible. Numerous clinical cases are referred to, most now including illustrations, and turn the sometimes lifeless subject of anatomy into a clinical and lively one. This helps the beginner to visualize a possible future career and gives them a taste of what's to come. Introductions to the individual chapters gives a succinct overview of the contents and the most important themes, as well as presenting a relevant case in everyday clinical practice. Each chapter ends with a number of typical questions as they may be given in an oral or written anatomy exam. As with the 24th edition, every chapter contains a short introduction to the embryology of the relevant theme. Included for the first time are the lifesize poster of the skeleton and musculature of a woman and a man, as well as the instructional poster.

Two points should be taken into account:
1. The atlas in the 25th edition does not replace any accompanying textbook.
2. No matter how good the didactical concept, it cannot replace the study process, but it can at least try to make it more vivid. To study anatomy is not difficult but it is very time-consuming. Time well worth spending, as both the doctor and the patient will eventually benefit. The goal of the 25th edition of the Sobotta Atlas is not only to ease the study process but also to make it an exciting and interesting time, so that one turns to it eagerly when studying, as well as in the course of one's professional career.

Erlangen and Munich in the summer of 2022,
exactly 118 years after publication of the first German edition.

Friedrich Paulsen and Jens Waschke

Any errors?

 https://else4.de/978-0-7020-6766-2

We demand a lot from our contents. Despite every precaution it is still possible that an error can slip through or that the factual contents needs updating. For all relevant errors, a correction will be provided. With this QR code, quick access is possible.

We are grateful for each and every suggestion which could help us to improve this publication. Please send your proposals, praise and criticism to the following email address: kundendienst@elsevier.com

Acknowledgements of the 25th German edition

It has again been very exciting to work on the 25th edition of the Sobotta Atlas, with which we feel increasingly closely connected.

Now more than ever, a comprehensive atlas such as the Sobotta demands a dedicated team run by a well-organised publishing company. The entire process for this 25th edition has been coordinated by the content strategist Sonja Frankl, to whom we are very grateful. Additionally, not much would have been possible without the longstanding and all-encompassing experience of Dr Andrea Beilmann, who was entrusted with many of the previous editions and who forms the foundation of the Sobotta team. We thank her warmly for all her help and support. We fondly remember the monthly telephone conferences in which Dr Beilman and Sonja Frankl were on hand to lend support with the design, bringing together their distinct and diverse working styles in a quite remarkable fashion. Along with Dr Beilmann, Sibylle Hartl coordinated the project and was responsible for the production as a whole. We thank her wholeheartedly. Without the determination and vigilance of Kathrin Nühse, this edition would not have been possible in its present form. We are further enormously grateful to Martin Kortenhaus (editing), the team at the abavo GmbH (formal image processing and setting), and Nicola Kerber (layout development), who were involved with the editorial side and in making the outcome a success.

In particular, we are grateful to our illustrators, Dr Katja Dalkowski, Anne-Kathrin Hermanns, Martin Hoffmann, Sonja Klebe and Jörg Mair, who helped us to revise many existing images as well as creating numerous new ones.

For their help in creating the clinical images, we sincerely thank: PD Dr Frank Berger, MD, Institute for Clinical Radiology at the Ludwig-Maximilians-University, Munich; Prof Dr Christopher Bohr, MD, Clinic and Polyclinic for Ear, Nose and Throat, University Hospital, Regensburg – previously UK-Erlangen/FAU; Dr Eva Louise Brahmann, MD, Clinic for Ophthalmology at the Heinrich Heine University, Düsseldorf; Prof Dr Andreas Dietz, MD, Director of the Clinic and Polyclinic for Ear, Nose and Throat, University of Leipzig; Prof Dr Arndt Dörfler, MD, Institute for Radiology, Neuroradiology, Friedrich Alexander University, Erlangen-Nuremberg; Prof Dr Gerd Geerling, MD, Clinic for Ophthalmology at the Heinrich-Heine University of Düsseldorf; Dr Berit Jordan, MD, University Clinic and Polyclinic for Neurology, Martin Luther University of Halle-Wittenberg; Prof Dr Marco Kesting, MD, Dentistry, Oral Maxillofacial Clinic, Friedrich Alexander University, Erlangen-Nuremberg; PD Dr Axel Kleespies, MD; Surgical Clinic, Ludwig-Maximilians-University, Munich; Prof Dr Norbert Kleinsasser, MD, University Clinic for Ear, Nose and Throat, Julius Maximilian University, Würzburg; PD Dr Hannes Kutta, MD, ENT Practice, Hamburg-Altona/Ottensen; Dr Christian Markus, MD, Clinic for Anaesthesiology, Julius Maximilian University, Würzburg; MTA Hong Nguyen and PD Doctor of Science Martin Schicht, Institute for Functional and Clinical Anatomy, Friedrich Alexander University at Erlangen-Nuremberg; Jörg Pekarsky, Institute for Anatomy, Functional and Clinical Anatomy, Friedrich Alexander University, Erlangen-Nuremberg; Dr Dietrich Stövesand, MD, Clinic for Diagnostic Radiology, Martin Luther University of Halle-Wittenberg; Prof Dr Jens Werner, MD, Surgical Clinic, Ludwig-Maximilians-University, Munich; Dr Tobias Wicklein, MD Dentristry, Erlangen, and Prof Dr Stephan Zierz, MD, Director of University Clinic and Polyclinic for Neurology, Martin Luther University of Halle-Wittenberg.

Finally we thank our families, who have had to share us with the Sobotta Atlas in the context of the 25th edition, as well as being on hand with advice when needed and strong support.

Erlangen and Munich, summer of 2022

Friedrich Paulsen and Jens Waschke

Adresses of the editors in chief

Prof. Dr. Friedrich Paulsen
Institute of Anatomy, Department of Functional and Clinical Anatomy
Friedrich Alexander University Erlangen-Nuremberg
Universitätsstraße 19
91054 Erlangen
Germany

Prof. Dr. Jens Waschke
Institute of Anatomy and Cell Biology, Department I
Ludwig-Maximilians-University (LMU) Munich
Pettenkoferstraße 11
80336 Munich
Germany

Adresses of the translators

Prof. Dr. Thomas Klonisch
Dept. of Human Anatomy and Cell Science
Max Rady College of Medicine, Rady Faculty of Health Sciences
University of Manitoba
130–745 Bannatyne Avenue
Winnipeg, Manitoba, R3E 0J9, Canada

Prof. Dr. Sabine Hombach-Klonisch
Dept. of Human Anatomy and Cell Science
Max Rady College of Medicine, Rady Faculty of Health Sciences
University of Manitoba
130–745 Bannatyne Avenue
Winnipeg, Manitoba, R3E 0J9, Canada

True-to-life representation is the top priority

Sabine Hildebrandt*, Friedrich Paulsen, Jens Waschke

'To practise as a doctor without profound anatomical knowledge is unthinkable. For the diagnosing, treatment and prognosis of illnesses, a detailed knowledge of the structure, positional relationships and the neurovascular pathways which supply the regions and organs of the body is central.'

Anatomical knowledge is gained through cognitive, tactile and especially visual learning processes, and can only be fully acquired when working with the human body itself. Images, graphics and three-dimensional programmes depicting the essential elements help to develop a three-dimensional perception of the relationships in the human body, and help the student to memorise and name structures.

The visual principle of learning did not always apply in anatomical teaching. The writings of the great anatomists of antiquity, such as the school of **Hippocrates of Kos** (460–370 BC) and **Galen of Pergamon** (131–200), did not include any illustrations of human anatomy, because a life-like representation of the human form in books was technically impossible; nor did these authors perform dissections on humans.[1,2,3,4] Even the reformer of anatomy, **Mondino di Luzzi** (1270–1326), had to do without illustrations. He introduced the dissection of human bodies for anatomical education in Bologna and wrote the first modern anatomy 'book' in 1316. This 77-page collection of folios became the standard reference for medical training for the next few centuries.[1,4] Images from another contemporary medical compendium were included for visual instruction; however, their lack of detail and overt inaccuracies did not add much of practical value to the volume.

The Renaissance brought an increased awareness of nature and the relevance of trueness to life in art, and in this it was **Leonardo da Vinci** (1452–1519) who emphasised the visual representation of anatomy. His depictions of human anatomy were based on his own dissections.[5] Unfortunately, he never completed his planned anatomical volume, but did leave behind his anatomical sketches. It was thus in 1543 that **Andreas Vesalius'** (1514–1564) '*De humani corporis fabrica libri septem*' became the first book to depict human anatomy entirely based on the dissection of bodies. The numerous illustrations were high-quality woodcut prints but were not coloured.[6,7] Image quality evolved over the next few centuries and reached another peak with the work of anatomist **Jean Marc Bourgery** (1797–1849) and his draftsman **Nicolas Henri Jakob** (1782–1871). Bougery and Jakob jointly created an eight-volume anatomy atlas over a period of more than 20 years. However, this work as well as the one created by Vesalius, were published in folio format and thus so expensive and unwieldy that they were – and still are – highly valued by wealthy doctors and art connoisseurs, but unsuitable for students and their foundational anatomy education. In the English-speaking world this changed in 1858, when **Henry Gray** (1827–1861) published the textbook 'Anatomy, Descriptive and Surgical'. It contained non-coloured illustrations based on dissections of the human body, and was quickly established as an affordable and popular alternative for students.[8]

Around 1900, **August Rauber** (1841–1917), along with **Friedrich Wilhelm Kopsch** (1868–1955), **Carl Heitzmann** (1836–1896), as well as **Carl Toldt** (1840–1920), **Werner Spalteholz** (1861–1940) and several other authors, created volumes on anatomy for various publishers. These atlases, sometimes in combination with a textbook, claimed to present human anatomy in full. The anatomist **Johannes Sobotta** (1869–1945), who worked in Würzburg, complained that the books were too detailed and therefore unsuitable for foundational medical education. In addition, he believed the prices for these volumes were unjustifiably high for the quality of the images. Sobotta therefore endeavored to '*produce an atlas with lifelike images and suitable for use by medical students in the dissecting room*'.[9] The publishers and editors of the Sobotta Atlas have followed this basic principle ever since.

The first edition of the Sobotta Atlas was published in 1904 by J.F. Lehmanns under the title 'Atlas of the descriptive anatomy of humans in 3 volumes' and contained 904 mostly coloured illustrations. The majority of these were created by the illustrator **Karl Hajek** (1878–1935), who thus had a large share in the quality and success of the Sobotta Atlas. The atlas seems to have had a ground-breaking effect after its publication in that it brought the further development of anatomical textbooks a big step forward.

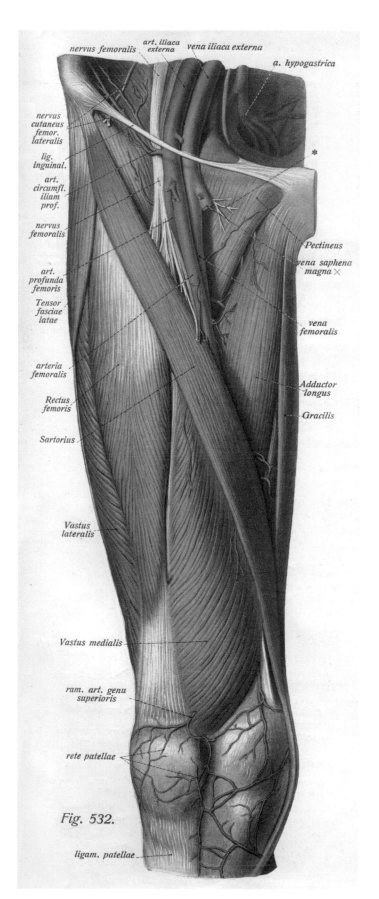

Fig. 1 Illustration of the ventral femoral musculature based on a dissection (1st edition of the Sobotta Atlas). [S700]

At the time of the first edition of the Sobotta Atlas, there were other atlases featuring muscles that were coloured, and neurovascular bundles highlighted in colour. However, it was only the Sobotta atlas which gave a complete and true-to-life colouring of the images of a situs or extremity, and this was only possible through a high-quality printing technique. This is illustrated by → Fig. 1 from the first edition with the example of the dissection of an anterior thigh. Even more than 100 years later, these images still look fresh and life-like and are therefore timeless. Many illustrations were added over the following editions, and the existing illustrations were continuously revised and adapted to match contemporary learning habits and aesthetic perceptions.

Unfortunately, we cannot mention all the illustrators over the course of 25 editions who have made the Sobotta Atlas what it is today; there are simply too many. Individual artists will therefore be singled out as being representative for all. From 1925, **Erich Lepier** (1898–1974) worked as illustrator for Urban & Schwarzenberg; first for various clinicians and then for the anatomist Eduard Pernkopf. After the Second World War, when Urban & Schwarzenberg had taken over publication of the Sobotta Atlas from J.F. Lehmanns, Lepier produced numerous illustrations for this atlas. Late in life he was awarded the title of professor because of his outstanding work.

From the 20th edition in 1993, **Sonja Klebe** contributed to the atlas and her outstanding creations need to be highlighted. The editors still work with her in a productive collaborative team, as can be seen in → Fig. 2, with an image of the topography of the head.

For later editions, images from other works by the Elsevier publishing company have also been included in the Sobotta Atlas. Since the turn of the millennium, most anatomical images from many of the publishing houses have been created digitally. Technical advances make it possible to create anatomical images in an inverse way to before. Previously, as in the Sobotta Atlas, new images were drawn exclusively using real human specimens. Schematic representations for simplification were derived by deduction.

Today, simple line drawings and schematics are first drawn up by computer programmes, to then incorporate the textures of various tissues by induction. Ultimately this produces the impression of a real representation of an anatomical specimen. The results are remarkably vivid despite being artificial. It is an attractive option for organisational as well as economic reasons. Today – in contrast to the times leading up to the postwar period – hardly any anatomical institute still employs its own illustrators, who, along with the anatomists and the dissected specimen, would create images of the quality required for the Sobotta Atlas. In addition, there are hardly any anatomists whose work time can be dedicated to producing anatomical specimens of the highest quality. Anatomists today are not only university professors and textbook

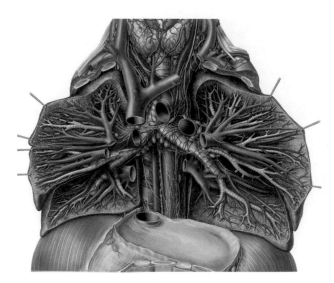

Fig. 3 Illustration of a dissection of the lungs from the Pernkopf Atlas (25th edition of the Sobotta Atlas, → Fig. 5.113). [S700-L238]/ [Q300]

authors, but scientists who conduct research and depend on performance-oriented financial resources. Due to these developments, it is next to impossible for today's anatomists to collaborate with illustrators over several months in the creation of a single optimal illustration. As a result, this manner of image creation has been almost entirely abandoned, and there are practically no representations that exceed or even compete with the images in older atlases. This is also the reason for the Sobotta Atlas to continue including images from atlases such as the Pernkopf Atlas as a model for new editions. The quality of some of the Pernkopf images is still unsurpassed, as → Fig. 3 shows, with a dissection of the lungs as an example – the editors know of no other comparable illustration of the lung structure and its associated neurovasculature that represents all vascular details, including the lymphatics, correctly.

This decision to reproduce an illustration from the Pernkopf Atlas can only be justified on the basis of a conscious examination[10] of the egregious ethical transgressions of anatomy during National Socialism (Nazi Germany), in memory of the victims of the Nazi regime whose bodies are depicted here. Since this applies to all anatomical representations in atlases that already existed and were further developed during this period, we discuss this historical background in more detail here.[11]

Anatomical work in teaching and research, as well as in the production of new teaching materials, including atlases, was and is dependent on an adequate supply of dead human bodies. Traditional legal anatomical body procurement in Germany and worldwide was based on the bodies of so-called 'unclaimed' people, i.e. those who died in public institutions and whose relatives did not claim them for a burial. It was only in the second half of the 20th century that this changed fundamentally – in Germany as in other countries – with the advent of effective body donation programmes.[12,13] Before that, the sources of anatomical body procurement primarily included psychiatric institutions, prisons, people who committed suicide and – historically the first legally regulated source – bodies of the executed. Anatomy laws were repeatedly adapted by the respective governments, including Nazi Germany.[14,15] With rare exceptions, a constant theme in the history of anatomy has been the lack of bodies for teaching and research. This changed significantly under National Socialism. In the first years after 1933 there were still the usual missives by anatomists to the authorities, complaining about the scant body supply. Very soon, however, their inquiries became specific, and they asked for access to execution sites and the bodies of the executed, or asked for the bodies of prisoners of war to be delivered to their institutes. Thus, anatomists were not only passive recipients of the bodies of Nazi victims, but actively requested them for teaching, and above all for research.[16]

In the 'Third Reich', the bodies from psychiatric hospitals included those of people murdered as part of the 'euthanasia' killing programme, as documented for various anatomical institutes.[17,18] From 1933 on there

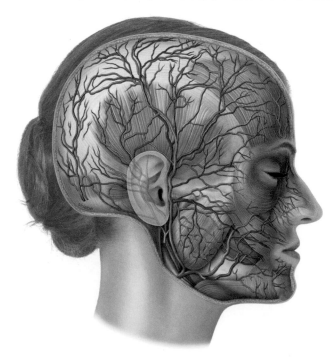

Fig. 2 Illustration by Sonja Klebe of the vascular pathways of the head (25th edition of the Sobotta Atlas, → Fig. 8.83). [S700-L238]

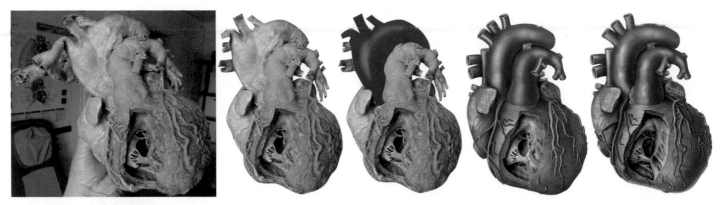

Fig. 4 Step-by-step development of one of Sonja Klebe's drawings of the topography of the heart, based on a plastinate and photos. [L238]

was also an increase in persecuted Jewish citizens among the suicides.[19] Due to the changes in Nazi legislation and the persecution of the so-called 'enemies of the German people', the number of political prisoners increased, not only in the normal penal system and in the Gestapo prisons, but above all in the constantly expanding network of concentration camps and decentralised camps for prisoners of war and forced labourers. The escalating violence and inhumane living conditions in these facilities resulted in high death rates, and the dead were delivered to many of the anatomical institutes. The number of executions after civilian and military trials also rose exponentially under the National Socialists, especially during the war years.[20] All anatomical institutes received the bodies of the executed, without exception, and regardless of the political convictions of the individual anatomists who worked with these bodies.

More than 80% of the anatomists who remained in Nazi Germany had joined the NSDAP, the Nazi party, but not all of them were such avid National Socialist ideologues as **Eduard Pernkopf** (1888–1955), the Viennese Dean of the Medical Faculty and Director of the Institute of Anatomy. He used the unrestricted access to the bodies of executed Nazi victims not primarily for scientific studies, as many of his colleagues did, but instead created the subsequent volumes of his 'Topographical Anatomy of Humans'. Together with his assistants and a group of medical illustrators, he had begun this work in the early 1930s. It is highly likely that the majority of the pictures in the atlas created during the war years show victims of the Nazi regime, because Pernkopf's institute received the bodies of more than 1,377 executed people from the Vienna prison system between 1938 and 1945, more than half of them convicted of treason.[21] Erich Lepier and his illustrator colleagues Karl Endtresser (1903–1978) and Franz Batke (1903–1983) left clear signs of their political sympathies with the Nazi regime in their signatures on images that were created during the war. Lepier often integrated a swastika in his signature, and Endtresser and Batke SS runes. These peculiarities of the atlas initially remained without comment, and the work enjoyed great popularity with anatomists, surgeons and medical illustrators alike, due to the true-to-nature details, a colour palette intensified by a new printing process, and Pernkopf's so-called 'stratigraphic' method of representation, in which a body region is presented in dissection steps from the surface to the deep layers in a sequence of dissections. After the war, Lepier copied a number of Pernkopf originals for the Sobotta Atlas to replace illustrations by Karl Hajek. Interestingly, very detailed illustrations of the body cavities and their organs which also depicted the neurovascular system were not copied. Leaving out these drawings across many editions of the Sobotta Atlas can be explained by the fact that, for many years, the relevance of neurovascular structures to the diagnostics and treatment of malignant tumours were not fully explored. As this very important function of the lymph vessels is now well-known, the current publishers regard further appropriation of the high-quality Pernkopf images as well-justified.

Soon after the publication of the first American edition of the Pernkopf Atlas in 1963/64, questions arose about the political background of the work. The rumours were only followed up on in the 1980s with investigations by American authors, before a public debate on the ethics of the use of the Pernkopf Atlas ensued in the mid-1990s.[22] Recommendations ranged from complete removal of the atlas from libraries to its historically informed use.[23] Urban and Schwarzenberg ended the publication of the work, but this did not stop its use, especially by surgeons.[24,25] When results of the systematic study of anatomy in Nazi Germany became known to a wider audience, a new inquiry emerged about the ethical use of the Pernkopf images in special surgical situations in 2016.[26] This question found an answer, based on Jewish medical ethics, in the *Responsum Vienna Protocol* by Rabbi Joseph Polak.[27,28,29] A responsum is a traditional scholarly and legal answer to a question put to a rabbi. Rabbi Polak concludes that most authorities would certainly allow the use of the Pernkopf images if they help save human life (according to the principle of *piku'ach nefesh*). However, this use is tied to the absolute condition that it is made known to one and all what these images are. Only in this way will the dead be granted at least some of the dignity to which they are entitled.

Following the argument of the *Vienna Protocol* and the condition that the victims of National Socialism whose bodies are shown in the images of the Pernkopf Atlas are remembered explicitly, the editors see it as justifiable to include new re-drawn copies of Pernkopf images in this new edition of the Sobotta Atlas: **to save future patients through the best possible anatomical visual instruction, in memory of the victims.**

In the 25th edition, the number of images has now grown to 2,500. It remains the highest priority to continue creating images with the various illustrators and graphic artists that are in no aspect inferior to dissected specimens. → Fig. 4 shows the example of a plastinated heart from a body donor, which the illustrator Sonja Klebe used, together with photographs from different perspectives, to create a new image. The spatial depth allows for three-dimensional understanding of the anatomy. It is the result of the artist's exploration process, in which she was able to observe, 'grasp' and understand the specimen.

The editors would like to thank all the illustrators and artists involved, as well as the Elsevier publishing team, without whom the atlas would not have been possible in this form.

Boston, Erlangen and Munich, 2022

Sabine Hildebrandt*, Friedrich Paulsen and Jens Waschke

Literature

1   Persaud TVN. Early history of human anatomy. Springfield: Charles C Thomas, 1984.

2   Persaud TVN. A history of human anatomy: the post-Vesalian era. Springfield: Charles C Thomas, 1997: 298, 309.

3   Rauber A, Kopsch F. Anatomie des Menschen. 7. Aufl. Leipzig: Thieme, 1906.

4   Roberts KB, Tomlinson JDW. The fabric of the body. Oxford: Oxford University Press, 1992.

5   Clayton M, Philo R. Leonardo da Vinci Anatomist. London: Royal Collection Trust, 2017.

6   Garrison DH, Hast MH. The fabric of the human body (kommentierte Übersetzung des Werks von Andreas Vesalius). Basel: Karger, 2014.

7   Vollmuth R. Das anatomische Zeitalter. München: Verlag Neuer Merkur, 2004.

8   Hayes B. The Anatomist: A True story of Gray's Anatomy. Ballantine, 2007. ISBN 978-0-345-45689-2

9   Sobotta, J. Atlas der Anatomie des Menschen. 1. Aufl. München: J. F. Lehmanns-Verlag, 1904–1907.

10 Arbeitskreis »Menschliche Präparate in Sammlungen« (2003): Empfehlungen zum Umgang mit Präparaten aus menschlichem Gewebe in Sammlungen, Museen und öffentlichen Räumen, in: Deutsches Ärzteblatt 2003; 100: A1960–A1965. As well as other points, it explains: 'If it is shown that the deceased has died because of their genealogy, idealogy or political persuasion due to state-controlled and-managed acts of violence or due to the well-founded probability of this having been the case, this is seen as a grave injury to their personal dignity. If such a context of wrongdoing is established, the specimens from the collections in question will be removed and interred in a dignified manner or will cease to be used, in a comparably dignified manner.' Distinct priority is especially given to specimens from the Nazi era, 'dealing with these specimens in a specialised way – after extensive research of the source – indiscriminately removing all dissections from collections between 1933 and 1945.' For specimens with an uncertain source and date of origin, the following is recommended: 'If after a first assessment, the specimen is of unknown origin and appears to be from the 20th century, it should then be separated and be subjected to a thorough examination. If no unambiguous allocation can be made, these specimens need to be categorically interred, unless there are certain cases in which contradictory overall aspects can be presented, documented and established.'

11 A full presentation of the history of anatomy in Nazi Germany is here: Hildebrandt S. The Anatomy of Murder: Ethical Transgressions and Anatomical Science in the Third Reich. New York: Berghahn Books, 2016.

12 Garment A, Lederer S, Rogers N, et al. Let the Dead Teach the Living: The Rise of Body Bequeathal in 20th-century America. Academic Medicine 2007; 82, 1000–1005.

13 Habicht JL, Kiessling C, Winkelmann A. Bodies for anatomy education in medical schools: An overview of the sources of cadavers worldwide. Acad Med 2018; 93: 1293–1300.

14 Stukenbrock K. Der zerstückte Coerper: Zur Sozialgeschichte der anatomischen Sektionen in der frühen Neuzeit (1650–1800). Stuttgart: Franz Steiner Verlag, 2001.

15 Hildebrandt S. Capital Punishment and Anatomy: History and Ethics of an Ongoing Association. Clinical Anatomy 2008; 21: 5–14.

16 Noack T, Heyll U. Der Streit der Fakultäten. Die medizinische Verwertung der Leichen Hingerichteter im Nationalsozialismus. In: Vögele J, Fangerau H, Noack T (Hrsg.). Geschichte der Medizin – Geschichte in der Medizin. Hamburg: Literatur Verlag, 2006: 133–142.

17 Overview in: Hildebrandt S. The Anatomy of Murder: Ethical Transgressions and Anatomical Science in the Third Reich. New York: Berghahn Books, 2016.

18 Czech H, Brenner E. Nazi victims on the dissection table – the anatomical institute in Innsbruck. Ann Anat 2019; 226: 84–95.

19 Goeschel C. Suicide in Nazi Germany. Oxford: Oxford University Press, 2009.

20 Numbers in Hildebrandt 2016 , see footnote 17.

21 Angetter DC. Anatomical Science at University of Vienna 1938–45. The Lancet 2000; 355: 1445–57.

22 Weissmann G. Springtime for Pernkopf. Reprinted 1987. In: Weissmann G (ed.). They All Laughed at Christopher Columbus. New York: Times Books; Williams, 1988: 48–69.

23 Hildebrandt S. How the Pernkopf Controversy Facilitated a Historical and Ethical Analysis of the Anatomical Sciences in Austria and Germany: A Recommendation for the Continued Use of the Pernkopf Atlas. Clinical Anatomy 2006; 19: 91–100.

24 Yee A, Coombs DM, Hildebrandt S, et al. Nerve surgeons' assessment of the role of Eduard Pernkopf 's Atlas of Topographic and Applied Human Anatomy in surgical practice. Neurosurgery 2019; 84: 491–498.

25 Yee A, Li J, Lilly J, et al. Oral and maxillofacial surgeons' assessment of the role of Pernkopf's atlas in surgical practice. Ann Anat 2021; 234: 1–10.

26 Complete documentation pertaining to this enquiry and the history of the perception of the Pernkopf Atlas, as well as the 'Vienna Protocol' in: Vol. 45 No. 1 (2021): Journal of Biocommunication Special Issue on Legacies of Medicine in the Holocaust and the Pernkopf Atlas, https://journals.uic.edu/ojs/index.php/jbc/article/view/10829 (last assessed: 27. November 2021).

27 Polak J. A. Vienna Protocol for when Jewish or possibly-Jewish human remains were discovered. Wiener Klinische Wochenschrift 2018; 130: S239–S243.

28 Vienna Protocol 2017. How to deal with Holocaust era human remains: recommendations arising from a special symposium. 'Vienna Protocol' for when Jewish or Possibly-Jewish Human Remains are Discovered. Im Internet: https://journals.uic.edu/ojs/index.php/jbc/article/view/10829/9795 (last assessed: 21. October 2021).

29 Hildebrandt S, Polak J, Grodin MA, et al. The history of the Vienna Protocol. In: Hildebrandt S, Offer M, Grodin MA (eds.). Recognizing the past in the present: medicine before, during and after the Holocaust. New York: Berghahn Books, 2021: 354–372.

*   Sabine Hildebrandt, MD;
    Associate Scientific Researcher, Assistant Professor of Pediatrics, Harvard Medical School; Boston, U.S.A.

1. List of abbreviations

Singular:

			Plural:					
A.	=	Arteria	Aa.	=	Arteriae	♀	=	female
Lig.	=	Ligamentum	Ligg.	=	Ligamenta	♂	=	male
M.	=	Musculus	Mm.	=	Musculi			
N.	=	Nervus	Nn.	=	Nervi			
Proc.	=	Processus	Procc.	=	Processus			
R.	=	Ramus	Rr.	=	Rami			
V.	=	Vena	Vv.	=	Venae			
Var.	=	Variation						

Percentages:

In the light of the large variation in individual body measurements, the percentages indicating size should only be taken as approximate values.

2. General terms of direction and position

The following terms indicate the position of organs and parts of the body in relation to each other, irrespective of the position of the body (e.g. supine or upright) or direction and position of the limbs. These terms are relevant not only for human anatomy but also for clinical medicine and comparative anatomy.

General terms

anterior – posterior = in front – behind (e.g. Arteriae tibiales anterior et posterior)
ventralis – dorsalis = towards the belly – towards the back
superior – inferior = above – below (e.g. Conchae nasales superior et inferior)
cranialis – caudalis = towards the head – towards the tail
dexter – sinister = right – left (e.g. Arteriae iliacae communes dextra et sinistra)
internus – externus = internal – external
superficialis – profundus = superficial – deep (e.g. Musculi flexores digitorum superficialis et profundus)
medius, intermedius = located between two other structures (e.g. the Concha nasalis media is located between the Conchae nasales superior and inferior)
medianus = located in the midline (Fissura mediana anterior of the spinal cord). The median plane is a sagittal plane which divides the body into right and left halves.
medialis – lateralis = located near to the midline – located away from the midline of the body (e.g. Fossae inguinales medialis et lateralis)
frontalis = located in a frontal plane, but also towards the front (e.g. Processus frontalis of the maxilla)

longitudinalis = parallel to the longitudinal axis (e.g. Musculus longitudinalis superior of the tongue)
sagittalis = located in a sagittal plane
transversalis = located in a transverse plane
transversus = transverse direction (e.g. Processus transversus of a thoracic vertebra)

Terms of direction and position for the limbs

proximalis – distalis = located towards or away from the attached end of a limb or the origin of a structure (e.g. Articulationes radioulnares proximalis et distalis)

for the upper limb:
radialis – ulnaris = on the radial side – on the ulnar side (e.g. Arteriae radialis et ulnaris)

for the hand:
palmaris – dorsalis = towards the palm of the hand – towards the back of the hand (e.g. Aponeurosis palmaris, Musculus interosseus dorsalis)

for the lower limb:
tibialis – fibularis = on the tibial side – on the fibular side (e.g. Arteria tibialis anterior)

for the foot:
plantaris – dorsalis = towards the sole of the foot – towards the back of the foot (e.g. Arteriae plantares lateralis et medialis, Arteria dorsalis pedis)

3. Use of brackets

[ ]: Latin terms in square brackets refer to alternative terms as given in the Terminologia Anatomica (1998), e.g. Ren [Nephros]. To keep the legends short, only those alternative terms have been added that differ in the root of the word and are necessary to understand clinical terms, e.g. nephrology. They are primarily used in figures in which the particular organ or structure plays a central role.

( ): Round brackets are used in different ways:
– for terms also listed in round brackets in the Terminologia Anatomica, e.g. (M. psoas minor)
– for terms not included in the official nomenclature but which the editors consider important and clinically relevant, e.g. (Crista zygomaticoalveolaris)
– to indicate the origin of a given structure, e.g. R. spinalis (A. vertebralis).

4. Colour chart

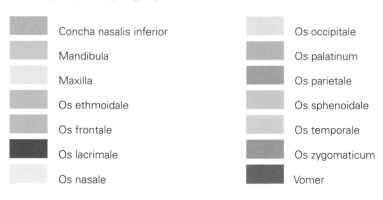

Concha nasalis inferior	Os occipitale	In the newborn the following cranial bones are indicated by only one colour:
Mandibula	Os palatinum	
Maxilla	Os parietale	Os nasale, Os temporale, Mandibula
Os ethmoidale	Os sphenoidale	Maxilla, Os incisivum
Os frontale	Os temporale	Os occipitale, Os palatinum
Os lacrimale	Os zygomaticum	
Os nasale	Vomer	

Picture credits

The reference for all image sources in this work appears at the end of each figure legend in square brackets.
Explanation of the special characters:
[…]/[…] = after submission of
[.../...] = collaboration between author and illustrator
[…~…] = modified by author and/or illustrator
[…-…] = work combined with illustrator

All unlabelled graphics and illustrations © Elsevier GmbH, Munich. We are very grateful to all clinical colleagues named below who have made available ultrasound, computed tomographic and magnetic resonance images as well as endoscopic images and colour photos of operation sites and patients.

B500   Benninghoff-Archiv: Benninghoff A, Drenckhahn D. Anatomie, div. Bd. und Aufl. Elsevier/Urban & Fischer

B501   Benninghoff. Drenckhahn D, Waschke J. Taschenbuch Anatomie, div. Aufl. Elsevier/Urban & Fischer

C155   Földi M, Kubik S. Lehrbuch der Lymphologie. 3. A. Gustav Fischer, 1993

C185   Voss H, Herrlinger R. Taschenbuch der Anatomie. Gustav Fischer, 1963

E102-005   Silbernagl S. Taschenatlas der Physiologie. 3. A. Thieme, 2009

E107   Blechschmidt E. Die vorgeburtlichen Entwicklungsstadien des Menschen. S. Karger AG, 1961

E262-1   Rauber A, Kopsch F. Anatomie des Menschen. Band I. Thieme, 1987

E282   Kanski, J. Clinical Ophthalmology: A Systematic Approach. 5th ed. Butterworth-Heinemann, 2003

E288   Forbes C, Jackson W. Color Atlas and Text of Clinical Medicine. 3rd A. Elsevier/Mosby, 2003

E329   Pretorius ES, Solomon JA. Radiology Secrets Plus. 3rd ed. Elsevier/Mosby, 2011

E336   LaFleur Brooks, M.: Exploring Medical Language. 7th ed. Elsevier/Mosby, 2008

E339-001   Asensio JA, Trunkey DD. Current Therapy of Trauma and Surgical Critical Care. 1st ed. Elsevier/Mosby, 2008

E347-09   Moore KL, Persaud TVN, Torchia MG. The Developing Human. 9th ed. Elsevier/Saunders, 2013

E347-11   Moore KL, Persaud TVN, Torchia MG. The Developing Human. 11th ed. Elsevier/Saunders, 2020

E377   Eisenberg RL, Johnson N. Comprehensive Radiographic Pathology, Skeletal System. Elsevier/Mosby, 2012

E380   Eiff MP, Hatch RL. Fracture Management for Primary Care. 3rd ed. Elsevier/Saunders, 2012

E393   Adam A, Dixon AK. Grainger & Allison's Diagnostic Radiology. 5th ed. Elsevier/Churchill Livingstone, 2008

E402   Drake R, Vogl AW, Mitchell A. Gray's Anatomy for Students. 1st ed. Elsevier, 2005

E402-004   Drake R, Vogl AW, Mitchell A. Gray's Anatomy for Students. 4th ed. Elsevier, 2020

E404   Herring JA. Tachdjian's Pediatric Orthopaedics. 4th ed. Elsevier/Saunders, 2008.

E458   Kelley LL, Petersen C. Sectional Anatomy for Imaging Professionals. 2nd ed. Elsevier, 2007

E460   Drake R, et al. Gray's_Atlas of Anatomy. 1st ed. Elsevier, 2008

E475   Baren JM, et al. Pediatric Emergency Medicine. 1st ed. Elsevier/Saunders, 2008

E513-002   Herring W. Learning Radiology- Recognizing the Basics. 2nd ed. Elsevier/Saunders, 2012

E530   Long B, Rollins J, Smith B. Merrill's Atlas of Radiographic Positioning and Procedures. 11th ed. Elsevier/Mosby, 2007

E563   Evans R. Illustrated Orthopedic Physical Assessment. 3rd ed. Elsevier/Mosby, 2008

E602   Adams JG, et al. Emergency Medicine. Expert Consult. Elsevier/Saunders, 2008

E625   Myers E, Snyderman C. Operative Otolaryngology: Head and Neck Surgery. 3rd ed. Elsevier/Saunders, 2008

E633-002   Tillmann BN. Atlas der Anatomie. 2. A. Springer, 2010

E633-003   Tillmann BN. Atlas der Anatomie. 3. A. Springer, 2017

E684   Herrick AL, et al. Orthopaedics and Rheumatology in Focus. 1st ed. Elsevier/Churchill Livingstone, 2006

E708   Marx J, Hockberger RS, Walls RM. Rosen's Emergency Medicine 7th revised ed. Elsevier/Mosby, 2009

E748   Seidel H, et al. Mosby's Guide to Physical Examination. 7th ed. Elsevier/Mosby, 2011

E761   Fuller G, Manford MR. Neurology. An Illustrated Colour Text. 3rd ed. Elsevier/Churchill Livingstone, 2010

E813   Green M, Swiontkowski M. Skeletal Trauma in Children. 4th ed. Elsevier/Saunders, 2009

E821   Pauwels F. Gesammelte Abhandlungen zur funktionellen Anatomie des Bewegungsapparates. Springer, 1965

E838   Mitchell B, Sharma R. Embryology. An Illustrated Colour Text. 1st ed. Elsevier/Churchill Livingstone, 2005

E867   Winn HR. Youmans Neurological Surgery. 6th ed. Elsevier/Saunders, 2011

E908-003   Corne J, Pointon K. Chest X-ray Made Easy. 3rd ed. Elsevier/Churchill Livingstone, 2010

E943   Kanski J. Clinical Ophthalmology. A Systemic Approach. 6th ed. Butterworth-Heinemann, 2007

E984   Klinke R, Silbernagl S. Lehrbuch Physiologie. 5. A. Thieme; 2005

E993   Auerbach P, Cushing T, Harris NS. Auerbach's Wilderness Medicine. 7th ed. Elsevier, 2016

E1043   Radlanski RJ, Wesker KH. Das Gesicht. Bildatlas klinische Anatomie. 2. A. KVM, 2012

F201-035   Abdul-Khaliq H, Berger F. Angeborene Herzfehler: Die Diagnose wird häufig zu spät gestellt. Dtsch Arztebl 2011;108:31-2

F264-004   Hwang S. Imaging of Lymphoma of the Musculoskeletal System. Radiologic Clinics of North America 2008;46/2:75-93

F276-005   Frost A, Robinson C. The painful shoulder. Surgery 2006;24/11:363-7

F276-006   Marsh H. Brain tumors. Surgery. 2007; 25/12:526-9

F276-007   Hobbs C, Watkinson J. Thyroidectomy. Surgery 2007;25/11:474-8

F698-002   Meltzer CC, et al. Serotonin in Aging, Late-Life Depression, and Alzheimer's Disease: The Emerging Role of Functional Imaging. Neuropsychopharmacology 1998;18:407-30

F702-006   Stelzner F, Lierse W. Der angiomuskuläre Dehnverschluss der terminalen Speiseröhre. Langenbecks Arch. klin. Chir. 1968;321:35–64

F885   Senger M, Stoffels HJ, Angelov DN. Topography, syntopy and morphology of the human otic ganglion: A cadaver study. Ann Anat 2014;196: 327-35

F1062-001   Bajada S, Mofidi A, Holt M, Davies AP. Functional relevance of patellofemoral thickness before and after unicompartmental patellofemoral replacement. The Knee. 2012;19/3:155-228

F1067-001   Lee MW, McPhee RW, Stringer MD. An evidence-based approach to human dermatomes. Clin Anat 2008;21(5):363-73

F1082-001   Weed LH. Forces concerned in the absorption of cerebrospinal fluid. Am J Physiol1935;114/1:40-5

G056   Hochberg MC, et al. Rheumatology. 5th ed. Elsevier/Mosby, 2011

G123   DeLee JC, Drez D, Miller MD. DeLee & Drez's Orthopaedic Sports Medicine. 2nd ed. Elsevier/Saunders, 2003

G159   Forbes A. et al. Atlas of Clinical Gastroenterology. 3rd ed. Elsevier/Mosby, 2004

G198   Mettler F. Essentials of Radiology. 2nd ed. Elsevier/Saunders, 2005

G210   Standring S. Gray's Anatomy. 42nd ed. Elsevier, 2020

G211 Ellenbogen R, Abdulrauf S, Sekhar L. Principles of Neuro-logical Surgery. 3rd ed. Elsevier/Saunders, 2012

G217 Waldman S. Physical Diagnosis of Pain. 2nd ed. Elsevier/Saunders, 2009

G305 Hardy M, et al.: Musculoskeletal Trauma. A guide to assessment and diagnosis. 1st ed. Elsevier/Churchill Livingstone, 2011

G322 Larsen WJ. Human embryology. 1st ed. Elsevier/Churchill Livingstone, 1993

G343 Netter FH. Atlas of Human Anatomy. 5th ed. Elsevier/Saunders, 2010

G435 Perkin GD, et al. Atlas of Clinical Neurology. 3rd ed. Elsevier/Saunders, 2011

G463 DeLee JC, Drez D, Miller MD. DeLee & Drez's Orthopaedic Sports Medicine. Principles and Practices. 3rd ed. Elsevier/Saunders, 2010

G465 Tang JB, et al. Tendon Surgery of the Hand. 1st ed. Elsevier/Saunders, 2012

G548 Swartz MH. Textbook of Physical Diagnosis. 7th ed. Elsevier, 2014

G568 Applegate E. J. The Sectional Anatomy Learning System-Concepts. 3rd ed. Elsevier/Saunders, 2009

G570 Wein AJ, et al. Campbell-Walsh Urology. 10th ed. Elsevier/Saunders, 2012

G617 Folkerth RD, Lidov H. Neuropathology. Elsevier, 2012

G645 Douglas G, Nicol F, Robertson C. Macleod's Clinical Examination. 13th ed. Elsevier/Churchill Livingstone, 2013

G704 Hagen-Ansert SL. Textbook of Diagnostic Sonography. 7th ed. Elsevier/Mosby, 2012

G716 Pagorek S, et al. Physical Rehabilitation of the Injured Athlete. 4th ed. Elsevier/Saunders, 2011

G717 Milla S, Bixby S. The Teaching Files- Pediatrics. 1st ed. Elsevier/Saunders, 2010

G718 Soto J, Lucey B. Emergency Radiology- The Requisites. 1st ed. Elsevier/Mosby, 2009

G719 Thompson SR, Zlotolow A.: Handbook of Splinting and Casting (Mobile Medicine). 1st ed. Elsevier/Mosby, 2012

G720 Slutsky DJ. Principles and Practice of Wrist Surgery. 1st ed. Elsevier/Saunders, 2010

G721 Canale ST, Beaty J. Campbell's Operative Orthopaedics (Vol.1). 11th ed. Elsevier/Mosby, 2008

G723 Rosenfeld JV. Practical Management of Head and Neck Injury. 1st ed. Elsevier/Churchill Livingstone, 2012

G724 Broder J. Diagnostic Imaging for the Emergency Physician. 1st ed. Elsevier/Saunders, 2011

G725 Waldmann S, Campbell R. Imaging of Pain. 1st ed. Elsevier/Saunders, 2011

G728 Sahrmann S. Movement System Impairment Syndromes of the Extremities, Cervical and Thoracic Spines. 1st ed. Elsevier/Mosby, 2010

G729 Browner BD, Fuller RP. Musculoskeletal Emergencies. 1st ed. Elsevier/Saunders, 2013

G744 Weir J, et al. Imaging Atlas of Human Anatomy. 4th ed. Elsevier/Mosby, 2011

G749 Le Roux P, Winn H, Newell D. Management of cerebral aneurysms. Elsevier/Saunders, 2004

G1060-001 Schünke M, Schulte E, Schumacher U. Prometheus. All-gemeine Anatomie und Bewegungsapparat. Band 1. 5. A. Thieme, 2018

G1060-002 Schünke M, Schulte E, Schumacher U. Prometheus. Innere Organe. Band 2. 5. A. Thieme, 2018

G1060-003 Schünke M, Schulte E, Schumacher U. Prometheus. Kopf, Hals, Neuroanatomie. Band 3. 5. A. Thieme, 2018

G1061 Debrunner HU. Orthopädisches Diagnostikum. 4. A. Thieme, 1982

G1062 Liniger H, Molineus G. Der Unfallmann. J.A. Barth, 1974

G1063 Vossschulte KF, et al. Lehrbuch der Chirurgie. Thieme, 1982

G1064 Schmidt H-M, Lanz U. Chirurgische Anatomie der Hand. Hippokrates, 1992

G1065 Tubiana R. The Hand, Vol. 1. Saunders, 1981

G1066 Gegenbaur C, Göpfert E. Lehrbuch der Anatomie des Menschen, Band III/1: Das Blutgefäßsystem. W. Engel-mann, 1913

G1067 Baumgartl E. Das Kniegelenk. Springer, 1964

G1068 Tondler J. Lehrbuch der systematischen Anatomie, 3. Band. Das Gefäßsystem. F.C.W. Vogel, 1926

G1069 Loeweneck H, Feifel G. Bauch. In: Praktische Anatomie (begründet von von Lanz T, Wachsmuth W). Springer, 2004

G1070 Debrunner HU, Jacob AC. Biomechanik des Fußes. 2. A. Ferdinand Enke, 1998

G1071 Carpenter MB. Core Text of Neuroanatomy. 2nd ed. Williams & Wilkins, 1978

G1072 Schultze O, Lubosch W. Atlas und kurzgefasstes Lehrbuch der topographischen und angewandten Anatomie. 4. A. Lehmanns, 1935

G1073 Kubik S. Visceral lymphatic system. In: Viamonte Jr M, Rüttmann A (eds.). Atlas of Lymphography. Thieme, 1980

G1076 Schiebler TH, Korf H-W. Anatomie. 10. A. Steinkopff bei Springer, 2007

G1077 Zilles K, Rehkämper G. Funktionelle Neuroanatomie. 3. A. Springer, 1998

G1078 Stelzner F. Die anorectalen Fisteln. 3. A. Springer, 1981

G1079 Bourgery JM, Jacob NH. Atlas of Human Anatomy and Surgery. TASCHEN, 2007

G1080 Tillmann B. Farbatlas der Anatomie: Zahnmedizin – Humanmedizin. Thieme, 1997

G1081 Purves D, et al. NeuroScience. 3rd ed. Sinauer Associates Inc, 2004

G1082 von Hagens G, Whalley A, Maschke R, Kriz W. Schnitt-anatomie des menschlichen Gehirns. Steinkopff, 1990

G1083 Braus H, Elze C. Anatomie des Menschen, Band 3. Periphere Leitungsbahnen II, Centrales Nervensystem, Sinnesorgane. Springer, 1960

G1084 Martini FH, Timmons MJ, Tallitsch RB. Anatomie. 1. A. Pearson, 2017

G1085 Brodmann K. Vergleichende Lokalisationslehre der Groß-hirnrinde in ihren Prinzipien, dargestellt aufgrund des Zellenbaues. J.A. Barth, 1909

G1086 Rohen JW. Anatomie für Zahnmediziner. Schattauer, 1994

G1087 Spoendlin H. Strukturelle Organisation des Innenohres. In: Oto-Rhino-Laryngologie in Klinik und Praxis. Band 1. (Hrsg. Helms J, Herberhold C, Kastenbauer E). Thieme, 1994: 32-74

G1088 Nieuwenhuys R, Voogd J, van Huijzen C. Das Zentral-nervensystem des Menschen. Ein Atlas mit Begleittext. 2. A. Springer, 1991

G1089 Berkovitz KB, et al. Oral Anatomy, Histology and Embryology. 5th ed. Elsevier/Mosby, 2017

G1091 Kandel ER, Koester JD, Mack SH, Siegelbaum SA. Principles of Neuroscience. 6th ed. McGraw Hill, 2021

G1192 O'Dowd G, Bell S, Wright S. Wheater's Pathology: A Text, Atlas and Review of Histopathology. 6th ed. Elsevier, 2019

H043-001 Mutoh K, Hidaka Y, Hirose Y, Kimura M. Possible induction of systemic lupus erythematosus by zonisamide. Pediatr Neurol 2001; 25(4):340-3

H061-001 Dodds SD, et al. Radiofrequency probe treatment for subfailure ligament injury: a biomechanical study of rabbit ACL. Clin Biomech 2004; 19(2):175-83

H062-001 Sener RN. Diffusion MRI: apparent diffusion coefficient (ADC) values in the normal brain and a classification of brain disorders based on ADC values. Comput Med Imaging Graph 2001; 25(4):299-326

H063-001 Heller AC, Kuether T, Barnwell SL, Nesbit G, Wayson KA. Spontaneous brachial plexus hemorrhage-case report. Surg Neurol 2000; 53(4):356-9

H064-001 Philipson M, Wallwork N. Traumatic dislocation of the sternoclavicular joint. Orthopaedics and Trauma 2012; 26(6):380-4

H081 Yang B, et al. A Case of Recurrent In-Stent Restenosis with Abundant Proteoglycan Component. Korean Circulation 2003; 33(9):827-31

H084-001 Custodio C, et al. Neuromuscular Complications of Cancer and Cancer Treatments. Physical Med Rehabilitation Clin North America 2008; 19(1):27-45

H102-002 Armour JA, et al. Gross and microscopic anatomy of the human intrinsic cardiac nervous system. Anat Rec 1997; 247:289–98

H230-001 Boyden EA. The anatomy of the choledochoduodenal junction in man. Surg Gynec Obstet 1957; 104:641–52

H233-001 Perfetti R, Merkel P. Glucagon-like peptide-1: a major regulator of pancreatic b-cell function. Eur J Endocrinol 2000; 143:717–25.

H234-001 Braak H. Architectonics as seen by lipofuscin stains. In: Peters A, Jones EG (eds.): Cerebral Cortex. Cellular Components of the Cerebral Cortex. Cellular Components of the Cerebral Cortex, Vol I. Plenum Press, 1984:59–104

J787 Colourbox.com

J803 Biederbick & Rumpf, Adelsdorf, Germany

K383 Cornelia Krieger, Hamburg, Germany

L106 Henriette Rintelen, Velbert, Germany

L126 Dr. med. Katja Dalkowski, Buckenhof, Germany

L127 Jörg Mair, München, Germany

L131 Stefan Dangl, München, Germany

L132 Michael Christof, Würzburg, Germany

L141 Stefan Elsberger, Planegg, Germany

L157 Susanne Adler, Lübeck, Germany

L190 Gerda Raichle, Ulm, Germany

L231 Stefan Dangl, München, Germany

L238 Sonja Klebe, Löhne, Germany

L240 Horst Ruß, München, Germany

L266 Stephan Winkler, München, Germany

L271 Matthias Korff, München, Germany

L275 Martin Hoffmann, Neu-Ulm, Germany

L280 Johannes Habla, München, Germany

L281 Luitgard Kellner, München, Germany

L284 Marie Davidis, München, Germany

L285 Anne-Katrin Hermanns, „Ankats Art", Maastricht, Netherlands

L303 Dr. med. Andreas Dietz, Konstanz, Germany

L316 Roswitha Vogtmann, Würzburg, Germany

L317 H.-C. Thiele, Gießen, Germany

L318 Tamas Sebesteny, Bern, Suisse

L319 Marita Peter, Hannover, Germany

M282 Prof. Dr.med. Detlev Drenckhahn, Würzburg, Germany

M492 Prof. Dr. med. Peter Kugler, Würzburg, Germany

M580 Prof. Dr. med. W. Kriz, Heidelberg, Germany

M1091 Prof. Dr. Reinhard Pabst, Hannover, Germany

O534 Prof. Dr. Arnd Dörfler, Erlangen, Germany

O548 Prof. Dr. med Andreas Franke, Kardiologie, Klinikum Region Hannover, Germany

O1107 Dr. Helmuth Ferner- Privatklinik Döbling, Wien, Austria

O1108 Prof. Hans-Rainer Duncker, Gießen, Germany

O1109 August Vierling (1872–1938), Heidelberg, Germany

P310 Prof. Dr. med. Friedrich Paulsen, Erlangen, Germany

P498 Prof. Dr. med. Philippe Pereira, SLK-Kliniken, Klinik für Radiologie, Heilbronn, Germany

Q300 Pernkopf-Archiv: Pernkopf E. Atlas der topgraphischen und angewandten Anatomie des Menschen, div. Bd. und Aufl. Elsevier/Urban & Fischer

R110-20 Rüther W, Lohmann C. Orthopädie und Unfallchirurgie. 20. A. Elsevier, 2014

R170-5 Welsch U, Kummer W, Deller T. Histologie – Das Lehrbuch: Zytologie, Histologie und mikroskopische Anatomie. 5. A. Elsevier/Urban & Fischer, 2018

R234 Bruch H-P, Trentz O. Berchtold Chirurgie. 6. A. Elsevier/Urban & Fischer, 2008

R235 Böcker W, Denk H, Heitz P, Moch H. Pathologie. 4. A. Elsevier/Urban & Fischer, 2008

R236 Classen M, Diehl V, Kochsiek K. Innere Medizin. 6. A. Elsevier/Urban & Fischer, 2009

R242 Franzen A. Kurzlehrbuch Hals-Nasen-Ohren-Heilkunde 3. A. Elsevier/Urban & Fischer, 2007

R247 Deller T, Sebesteny T. Fotoatlas Neuroanatomie. 1. A. Elsevier/Urban & Fischer, 2007

R252 Welsch U. Atlas Histologie. 7. A. Elsevier/Urban & Fischer, 2005

R254 Garzorz N. Basics Neuroanatomie. 1. A. Elsevier/Urban & Fischer, 2009

R261 Sitzer M, Steinmetz H. Neurologie. 1. A. Elsevier/Urban & Fischer, 2011

R306 Illing St, Classen M. Klinikleitfaden Pädiatrie.8. A. Elsevier/Urban & Fischer, 2009

R314 Böckers T, Paulsen F, Waschke J. Sobotta Lehrbuch Anatomie. 2. A. Elsevier/Urban & Fischer, 2019

R316-007 Wicke L. Atlas der Röntgenanatomie. 7. A. Elsevier/Urban & Fischer, 2005

R317 Trepel M. Neuroanatomie. 5. A. Elsevier/Urban& Fischer, 2011

R331 Fleckenstein P, Tranum-Jensen J. Röntgenanatomie. 1. A. Elsevier/Urban & Fischer, 2004

R333 Scharf H-P, Rüter A. Orthopädie und Unfallchirurgie. 2. A. Elsevier/Urban & Fischer, 2018

R349 Raschke MJ, Stange R. Alterstraumatologie – Prophylaxe, Therapie und Rehabilitation 1. A. Elsevier/Urban & Fischer, 2009,

R388 Weinschenk S. Handbuch Neuraltherapie. Diagnostik und Therapie mit Lokalanästhetika. 1. A. Elsevier/Urban & Fischer, 2010

R389 Gröne B. Schlucken und Schluckstörungen: Eine Einführung. 1. A. Elsevier/Urban & Fischer, 2009

R419 Menche N. Biologie- Anatomie- Physiologie. 9. A. Elsevier/Urban & Fischer, 2020

R449 Hansen JT. Netter's Clinical Anatomy. 4th ed. Elsevier/Urban & Fischer, 2018

R476 Kienzle-Müller B, Wilke-Kaltenbach G. Babies in Bewegung. 4. A. Elsevier, 2020

S002-5 Lippert H. Lehrbuch Anatomie. 5. A. Elsevier/Urban & Fischer, 2000

S002-7 Lippert H. Lehrbuch Anatomie. 7. A. Elsevier/Urban & Fischer, 2006

S008-4 Kauffmann GW, Sauer R, Weber WA. Radiologie. 4. A. Elsevier/Urban & Fischer, 2008

S100 Classen M, et al. Differentialdiagnose Innere Medizin 1. A. Urban & Schwarzenberg, 1998

S124 Breitner B. Chirurgische Operationslehre, Band III, Chirurgie des Abdomens. 2. A. Urban & Schwarzenberg, 1996

S130-6 Speckmann E-J, Hescheler J, Köhling R. Physiologie. 6. A. Elsevier/Urban & Fischer, 2013

S133 Wheater PR, Burkitt HG, Daniels VG. Funktionelle Histologie. 2. A. Urban & Schwarzenberg, 1987.

S700 Sobotta-Archiv: Sobotta. Atlas der Anatomie des Menschen, div. Aufl. Elsevier/Urban & Fischer

S701 Sobotta-Archiv: Hombach-Klonisch S, Klonisch T, Peeler J. Sobotta. Clinical Atlas of Human Anatomy. 1st ed. Elsevier/Urban & Fischer, 2019

S702 Sobotta-Archiv: Böckers T, Paulsen F, Waschke J. Sobotta. Lehrbuch Anatomie, div. Aufl. Elsevier/Urban & Fischer

T127 Prof. Dr. Dr. Peter Scriba, München, Germany

T419 Jörg Pekarsky, Institut für Anatomie LST II, Universität Erlangen-Nürnberg, Germany

T534 Prof. Dr. med. Matthias Sitzer, Klinik für Neurologie, Klinikum Herford, Germany

T663 Prof. Dr. Kurt Fleischhauer, Hamburg, Germany

T719 Prof. Dr. Norbert Kleinsasser, HNO-Klinik, Universitätsklinikum Würzburg, Germany

T720 PD Dr. med. Hannes Kutta, Universitätsklinikum Hamburg-Eppendorf, Germany

T786 Dr. Stephanie Lescher, Institut für Neuroradiologie, Klinikum der Goethe-Universität, Frankfurt, Prof. Joachim Berkefeld, Institut für Neuroradiologie, Klinikum der Goethe-Universität, Frankfurt, Germany

T832 PD Dr. Frank Berger, Institut für Klinische Radiologie der LMU, München, Germany

T863 C. Markus, Uniklinik Würzburg, Germany

T867 Prof. Dr. Gerd Geerling, Universitätsklinikum Düsseldorf, Germany

T872 Prof. Dr. med. Micheal Uder, Universitätsklinikum Erlangen, Germany

T882 Prof. Dr. med Christopher Bohr, Universitätsklinikum Regensburg, Germany

T884 Tobias Wicklein, Erlangen, Germany

T887 Prof. Dr. med Stephan Zierz, Dr. Jordan, Uniklinik Halle, Germany

Table of content

Organs of the thoracic cavity

Organs of the abdominal cavity

Retroperitoneal space and pelvic cavity

Organs of the thoracic cavity

5

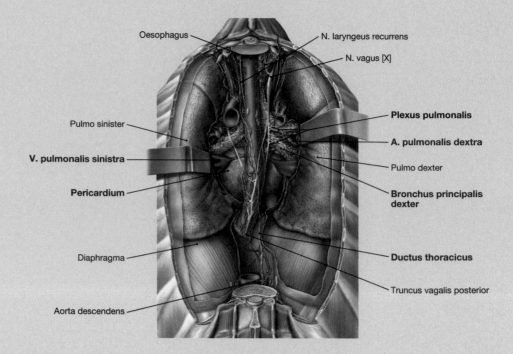

Oesophagus

N. laryngeus recurrens

N. vagus [X]

Pulmo sinister

Plexus pulmonalis

A. pulmonalis dextra

V. pulmonalis sinistra

Pulmo dexter

Pericardium

Bronchus principalis dexter

Diaphragma

Ductus thoracicus

Truncus vagalis posterior

Aorta descendens

Overview

In a dissection course, the opening of the **thoracic cavity** is one of the key processes which is met by teachers and students with a mixture of awe, suspense and interest. Exposing the heart and lungs as well as being allowed to grasp (literally and metaphorically) these vital organs of the body with one's own hands is considered a great privilege in these lessons.

The thoracic cavity (Cavitas thoracis) is enclosed by the thoracic cage (Cavea thoracis), consisting of ribs, thoracic spine and sternum. It is separated **below** by the **diaphragm; above** there is **no clear** boundary separating the neck. If the anterior thoracic wall, which is made up of important **muscles to aid breathing,** is removed, we can see the division of the Cavitas thoracis into **two pleural cavities** (Cavitates pleu-

rales) containing the lungs, and the connective tissue space of the **mediastinum** lying in-between becomes visible.

Directly behind the sternum, the **thymus** is embedded in the mediastinum. The **superior vena cava (V. cava superior)** is shifted to the right. The curved **main artery (aorta)** dominates the upper mediastinum. Among the major vessels are the **trachea,** which divides into the right and left main bronchi (Bronchi principales), and, dorsally of the trachea, the **oesophagus.** In its pericardial sac (pericardium) within the inferior mediastinum, facing the diaphragm, the **heart (Cor)** which rests broadly on the diaphragm, dominates. The **lungs (Pulmones)** are located in both pleural cavities.

Main topics

After working through this chapter, you should be able to:

Thoracic cavity
- describe the composition of the thoracic cavity with the mediastinum and pleural cavities, including their neurovascular pathways on a dissection;
- describe the position and function of the thymus;

Heart
- explain the development of the heart, including fetal circulation with any possible fundamental malformations;
- illustrate the position, orientation and projection of the heart, clearly showing the margins, on a dissection and an X-ray;
- describe the inner and outer structures of the heart chambers, as well as the wall layers, the pericardial sac and the cardiac skeleton on a dissection;
- explain the structure, function and projection as well as the auscultation type of the various heart valves with their malfunctions on a dissection;
- show the conduction system with accurate localisation of the sinoatrial and AV nodes on a dissection and understand the autonomic innervation of the heart;
- indicate the Aa. coronariae with all the important branches on a dissection and describe their importance in the development, di-

agnosis and treatment of coronary heart disease (CHD); with the veins, only the main features will be necessary;

Trachea and lungs
- describe the structure of the lower respiratory tract and its development and describe the sections of the trachea;
- indicate the projection of the lungs and their division into lobes and segments on a dissection, and also indicate the systematics of the bronchial tree;
- describe the Vasa publica and privata of the lungs including origin, pathway and function, as well as the lymph vessel systems and the autonomic innervation;

Oesophagus
- indicate the sections and constrictions of the oesophagus with their positional relationships on a dissection;
- describe the closing mechanisms of the proximal and distal oesophagus and their clinical significance;
- explain the neurovascular pathways of the different sections of the oesophagus, including the relationship of the veins to the portal venous system.

Clinical relevance

In order not to lose touch with prospective everyday clinical life with so many anatomical details, the following describes a typical case that shows why the content of this chapter is so important.

Pulmonary embolism

Case study
A 22-year-old student is admitted to the emergency department in the morning. She reports having woken up in the morning with shortness of breath and coughing the day after she had returned from a flight to the USA. When getting up she noticed that her left lower leg was significantly thicker.

Result of examination
Cardiac (120/min) and respiratory rates (35/min) are significantly raised. The patient is conscious, awake and fully oriented. She has severe pain in the region of her left leg and is complaining of shortness of breath and chest pain. The lower left leg is reddened and shows expanded veins; the affected area has extended to the ankle and thigh.

Diagnostic procedure
The blood gas analysis shows a lowering of oxygen content in the blood. Due to a suspected pulmonary embolism, it is primarily coagulation values and D-dimers, formed by coagulated blood clots (thrombi), which are determined in blood sampling. The CT angiography of the Cavitas thoracis shows that several branches of the pulmonary arteries are displaced. The ultrasound examination of the heart (echocardiography) indicates stress on the right ventricle. A colour-coded duplex ultrasound confirms that the deep veins in the area of the femoral vein on the left-hand side of the leg are displaced by a blood clot (thrombus).

Diagnosis
A pulmonary embolism from deep vein thrombosis (→ Fig. a). The clot from the V. femoralis seems to have detached in part and blocked the pulmonary arteries as an embolism. Before the exclusion of a clotting disorder, the transatlantic flight, the taking of oral contraceptives ('the pill'), as well as smoking, are already present as risk factors.

Treatment
Via venous access, a breakdown (thrombolysis) of the blood clots is initiated with a plasminogen activator. In addition, the patient is supplied with oxygen via a nasogastric tube. The thrombolysis is successful and the patient is largely symptom-free after a week.

Dissection lab
To understand this clinical case, we need to look at two body regions: the veins of the leg and the organs of the Cavitas thoracis. Veins are generally a little neglected in anatomy lessons and are usually just considered to be the supporting structures of the arteries, in the way their pathways through the body and their designations correspond. In some regions there are, however, deviations from this rule or certain clinical references that require an explanation. At the extremities there is a **superficial (epifascial)** venous system which flows independently of the arteries, and a **deep venous system (subfascial)** in which two veins usually accompany the corresponding artery distally (in the forearm/lower leg) and proximally merge further on. However, superficial veins are connected to the deep venous system via **perforating veins,** which feature semilunar valves and allow blood flow only in the direction of the deep veins. Thus, the majority (approximately 75 %) of venous blood flows through this deep venous system back to the heart.

Blood clots in the veins are potentially life-threatening, as they can be dislodged into the blood stream. As embolisms they then move through the **inferior vena cava (V. cava inferior)** into the right atrium of the heart (Atrium dextrum) and through the **right ventricle (Ventriculus dexter)** into the **pulmonary arteries (Aa. pulmonales),** which channel deoxygenated blood into the lungs.

 On the right-hand side the main bronchus is located above the artery, with the veins right at the front underneath. The black nodes on the surface of a removed lung are the hilum lymph nodes of the lung.

If one removes the parenchyma of the lung from the hilum onwards, one can see that the pulmonary arteries follow the branching of the bronchial tree, while the **pulmonary veins** (Vv. pulmonales) proceed independently. The yellow colour of the pulmonary arteries is characteristic because they, like all arteries proximal to the heart, are of the elastic type due to the many elastic fibres in their muscle layer. If, in the case of a pulmonary embolism, a considerable part of the vessel diameter is blocked, then a drastic diminution of the gas exchange surface results in acute laboured breathing. The life-threatening sign, however, is the rise in pressure in the pulmonary circulation, a condition the right ventricle can neither immediately nor permanently adapt to, and this can lead to right-sided heart failure (Cor pulmonale) and death. Therefore, when preparing the heart in the dissecting laboratory, one should always pay attention to the wall thickness of the right ventricle, which is normally 3–5 mm thick, approx. one third of the thickness of the left wall. A thicker wall diameter can be a sign of chronic damage to the right side of the heart.

 The first time one holds a heart in one's hands is a special feeling! In order to orientate oneself, one must always hold the heart in the same position in which it lies in the mediastinum. Then the right ventricle is at the front!

Back in the clinic
The treatment was changed to a six-month oral administration of Marcumar® for anticoagulation. Molecular biological investigation reveals a mutation of clotting factor V and thus an inherited genetic predisposition for the occurrence of thrombosis. The patient was therefore advised against 'the pill' and smoking. For long trips and in the case of a planned pregnancy, a subcutaneous injection of low molecular weight heparin and the wearing of compression hosiery were recommended to the patient.

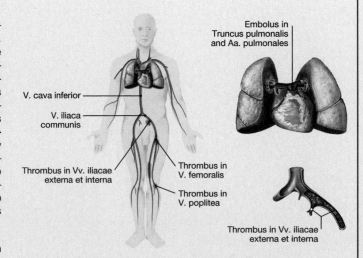

Embolus in
Truncus pulmonalis
and Aa. pulmonales

V. cava inferior

V. iliaca communis

Thrombus in Vv. iliacae externa et interna

Thrombus in V. femoralis

Thrombus in V. poplitea

Thrombus in Vv. iliacae externa et interna

Fig. a Deep vein thrombosis with the complication of a pulmonary embolism. [S702-L266]

Surface anatomy

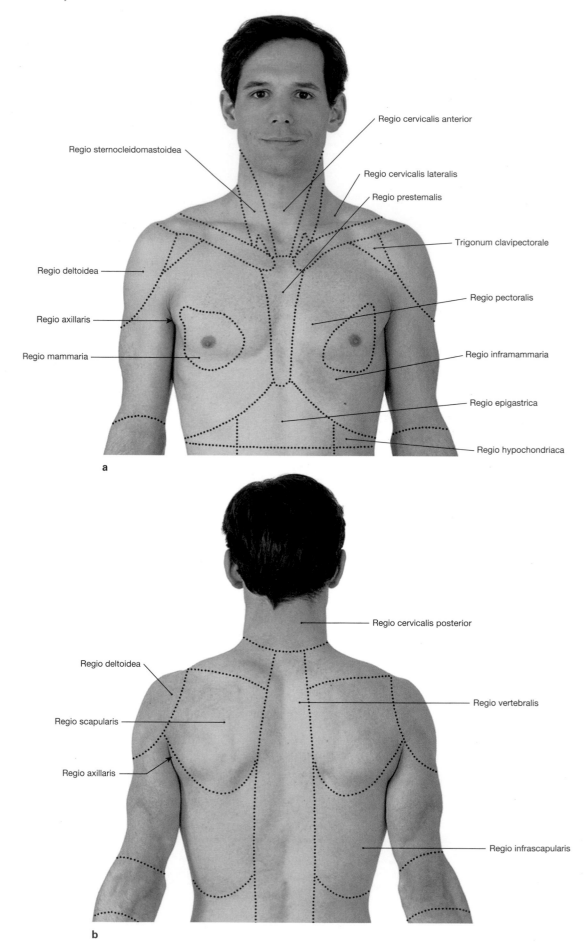

Regio cervicalis anterior

Regio sternocleidomastoidea

Regio cervicalis lateralis

Regio prestemalis

Trigonum clavipectorale

Regio deltoidea

Regio pectoralis

Regio axillaris

Regio mammaria

Regio inframammaria

Regio epigastrica

Regio hypochondriaca

a

Regio cervicalis posterior

Regio deltoidea

Regio vertebralis

Regio scapularis

Regio axillaris

Regio infrascapularis

b

Fig. 5.1a and b   Regions of the thorax. [S701-J803]
a Ventral view.
b Dorsal view.

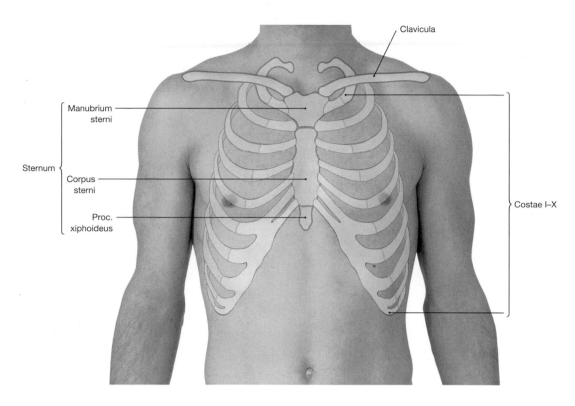

Clavicula

Manubrium
sterni

Sternum

Corpus
sterni

Proc.
xiphoideus

Costae I–X

Fig.5.2 Projection of the skeletal thoracic elements, Cavea thoracis, onto the ventral thoracic wall; ventral view. [S701-J803/L126]

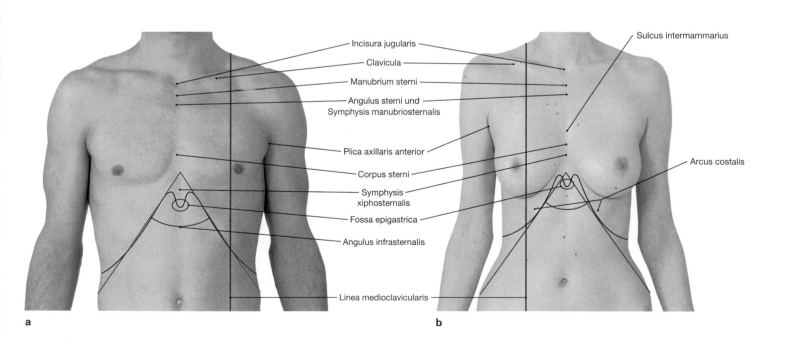

Incisura jugularis

Clavicula

Manubrium sterni

Angulus sterni und
Symphysis manubriosternalis

Plica axillaris anterior

Corpus sterni

Symphysis
xiphosternalis

Fossa epigastrica

Angulus infrasternalis

Linea medioclavicularis

Sulcus intermammarius

Arcus costalis

a

b

Fig.5.3a and b Surface landmarks of the ventral thoracic wall;
ventral view. [S701-J803]

a Male thorax.
b Female thorax.

Organs of the thoracic cavity

Pleural cavities and mediastinum

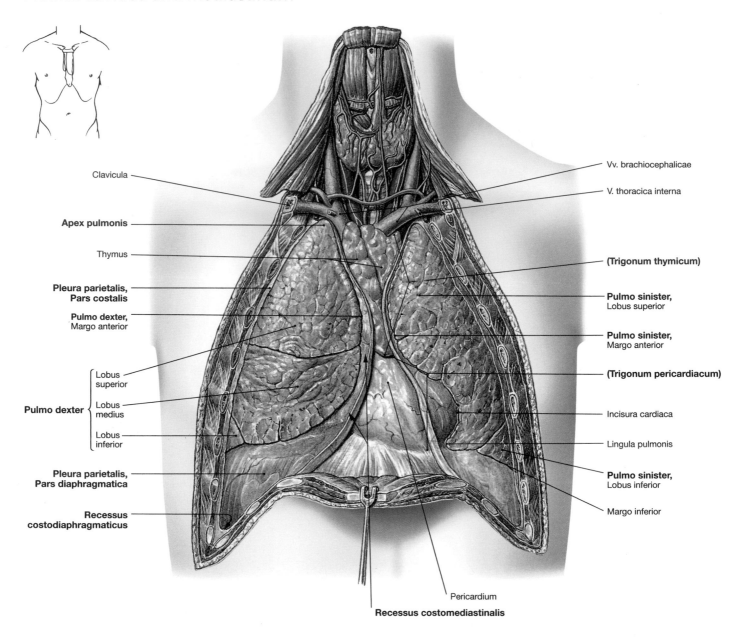

Clavicula

Apex pulmonis

Thymus

Pleura parietalis, Pars costalis

Pulmo dexter, Margo anterior

Lobus superior

Pulmo dexter — Lobus medius

Lobus inferior

Pleura parietalis, Pars diaphragmatica

Recessus costodiaphragmaticus

Vv. brachiocephalicae

V. thoracica interna

(Trigonum thymicum)

Pulmo sinister, Lobus superior

Pulmo sinister, Margo anterior

(Trigonum pericardiacum)

Incisura cardiaca

Lingula pulmonis

Pulmo sinister, Lobus inferior

Margo inferior

Pericardium

Recessus costomediastinalis

Fig. 5.4 Mediastinum and pleural cavities, Cavitates pleurales of an adolescent boy; ventral view; after removal of the thoracic wall. [S700]

After opening the **thoracic cavity,** the **Cavea thoracis,** the two pleural cavities, in which both lungs lie, become visible. The pleural cavities are separated in the middle by a connective tissue space, which is called the **mediastinum.** The mediastinum contains the heart, which is embedded in the **pericardium,** as well as the **thymus** and a number of **neurovascular pathways,** which connect the Cavitas thoracis with the neck via the upper thoracic aperture and with the abdomen via the diaphragm.

The pleural cavity (Cavitas pleuralis) is covered by the **parietal pleura (Pleura parietalis).** The parietal pleura is divided into the Pars mediastinalis, Pars costalis and Pars diaphragmatica. The **visceral pleura (Pleura visceralis)** covers the outer surface of the lungs. Both pleural mem-

branes form a capillary space that contains 5 ml in total of serous fluid, which helps the lung adhere to the wall of the torso.

Above, the pleural cavities protrude on both sides with the **cervical pleura (Cupula pleurae)** over the upper thoracic aperture by 2.5 to 5 cm. The medial pleural boundaries leave free between them the thymic trigone above and the pericardial trigone below. The pleural cavities have four paired **pleural recesses (Recessus pleurales),** in which the lung expands during deeper inspiration:

- **Recessus costodiaphragmaticus:** lateral, in the midaxillary line up to 5 cm deep
- **Recessus costomediastinalis:** on both sides ventral between the mediastinum and thoracic wall
- **Recessus phrenicomediastinalis:** caudal between the diaphragm and mediastinum
- **Recessus vertebromediastinalis:** dorsal, adjacent to the spine (→ Fig. 5.139b).

Clinical remarks

An increase in fluid in the Cavitas pleuralis **(pleural effusion)** may occur with pneumonia through inflammation of the pleura (pleurisy), through vascular congestion in the case of (left-sided) heart failure, or with tumours of the lung and the pleura. Chylous pleural effusions may also occur, in which lymphs burst from the Ductus thoracicus

into the Cavitas pleuralis. Pleural effusions cause dullness in percussion. Aspiration of pleural effusions is made from the costodiaphragmatic recess for diagnostic reasons and to improve respiratory excursion.

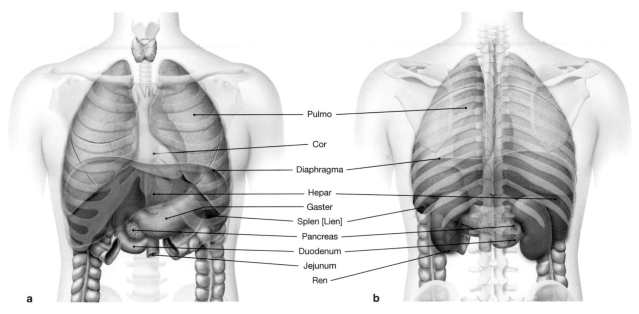

Pulmo
Cor
Diaphragma
Hepar
Gaster
Splen [Lien]
Pancreas
Duodenum
Jejunum
Ren

a

b

Fig. 5.5a and b   Thoracic cavity, Cavitas thoracis, and organs of the upper abdomen; schematic diagram. [S700-L275]
a Ventral view.
b Dorsal view.
Lying in the Cavitas thoracis is the **heart, Cor,** in its pericardium in the **mediastinum,** in between the two **pleural cavities, Cavitates pleurales,** which house the right and left **lungs, Pulmo dexter and Pulmo**

sinister. Since the diaphragmatic domes are relatively high (right, during expiration in the fourth intercostal space [ICS]; left, one half to a full ICS deeper), in addition to the organs of the Cavitas thoracis, the ribs also protect the **organs of the upper abdomen** (right, liver and gallbladder; left, stomach and spleen; dorsally on both sides, kidneys and adrenal glands). These organs are thereby relatively well protected from mechanical impact.

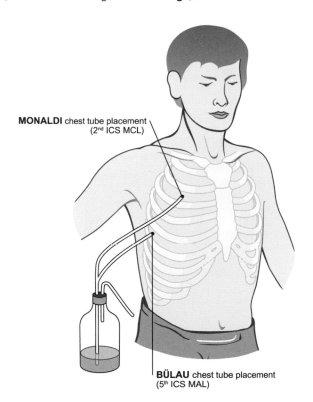

MONALDI chest tube placement
(2nd ICS MCL)

BÜLAU chest tube placement
(5th ICS MAL)

Fig. 5.6   Chest tube; ventral view from the right; schematic diagram. [S702-L126]
With a chest tube, there are two approaches: with the **MONALDI method,** the puncture is made in the second intercostal space (ICS) in the midclavicular line (MCL); with the **BÜLAU method,** it is made in the fifth ICS in the midaxillary line (MAL).

Clinical remarks

If lung excursion is impaired by an accumulation of blood in the pleural cavity (haemothorax) or by air congestion in the pleural cavity (tension pneumothorax), or if the lung collapses in the case of a pneumothorax, a **chest tube** is applied in order to siphon off the blood and re-inflate the lung. For this there are two access routes, whereby the risk of damage to the surrounding organs is kept as low as possible:
MONALDI drainage: in the second ICS in the MCL. There should be no further medial insertion in order to avoid damage to the parasternal flowing thoracic artery and vein. The axillary neurovascular pathways and the intercostobrachial nerves lie laterally against them.

BÜLAU drainage: in the fifth ICS in the MAL. The liver, which is located below the right diaphragmatic dome, must not be punctured here. In maximum expiration, the latter may extend up into the fourth ICS.
In preclinical emergency care, both access routes are sensible; however, in a hospital situation, the MONALDI method is chosen in the case of a pneumothorax.

Mediastinum

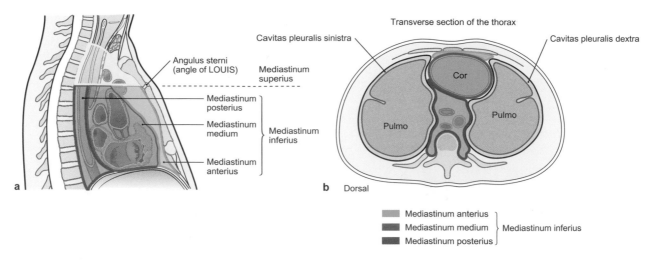

Transverse section of the thorax

Cavitas pleuralis sinistra
Cavitas pleuralis dextra

Cor

Pulmo
Pulmo

a

b Dorsal

Angulus sterni (angle of LOUIS)
Mediastinum superius

Mediastinum posterius
Mediastinum medium
Mediastinum anterius
Mediastinum inferius

- Mediastinum anterius
- Mediastinum medium ⎫ Mediastinum inferius
- Mediastinum posterius ⎭

Fig. 5.7a and b Structure of the mediastinum; schematic diagram.
a Sagittal section with view from the right. [S700-L126]
b Cross-section with view from below. [S701-L126]
The connective tissue space that separates the two pleural cavities is referred to as the **mediastinum.** The mediastinum is divided into the Mediastinum inferius, where the heart is, and the Mediastinum superi-

us. The lower mediastinum is further divided into the Mediastinum anterius in front of the heart, the Mediastinum medium with the pericardium, and the Mediastinum posterius behind the pericardium.
Clinical remark: The Angulus sterni (angle of LOUIS) is a palpable landmark for the separation of the upper mediastinum from the inferior.

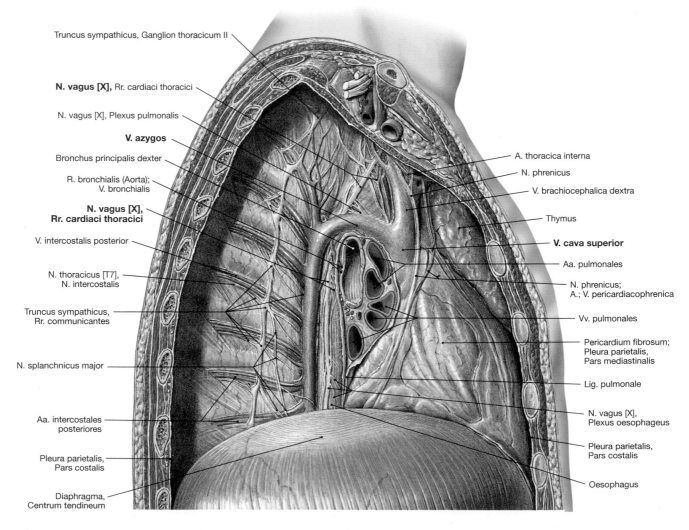

Truncus sympathicus, Ganglion thoracicum II

N. vagus [X], Rr. cardiaci thoracici

N. vagus [X], Plexus pulmonalis

V. azygos

Bronchus principalis dexter

R. bronchialis (Aorta); V. bronchialis

N. vagus [X], Rr. cardiaci thoracici

V. intercostalis posterior

N. thoracicus [T7], N. intercostalis

Truncus sympathicus, Rr. communicantes

N. splanchnicus major

Aa. intercostales posteriores

Pleura parietalis, Pars costalis

Diaphragma, Centrum tendineum

A. thoracica interna
N. phrenicus
V. brachiocephalica dextra
Thymus
V. cava superior
Aa. pulmonales
N. phrenicus; A.; V. pericardiacophrenica
Vv. pulmonales
Pericardium fibrosum; Pleura parietalis, Pars mediastinalis
Lig. pulmonale
N. vagus [X], Plexus oesophageus
Pleura parietalis, Pars costalis
Oesophagus

Fig. 5.8 Mediastinum and pleural cavity, Cavitas pleuralis, of an adolescent boy; view from the right side; after removal of the lateral thoracic wall and the right lung. [S700]
In the view from the right, what is particularly prominent in the posterior mediastinum is the **V. azygos,** which ascends alongside the spine, crosses the root of the right lung and then, at the level of the fourth/fifth

thoracic vertebrae, flows dorsally into the V. cava superior. The other structures run in a similar way to the left pleural cavity (→ Fig. 5.9). The **N. vagus [X]** runs behind the right main bronchus (Bronchus principalis dexter) to the oesophagus, while the **N. phrenicus** in front of the V. cava superior reaches the pericardium.

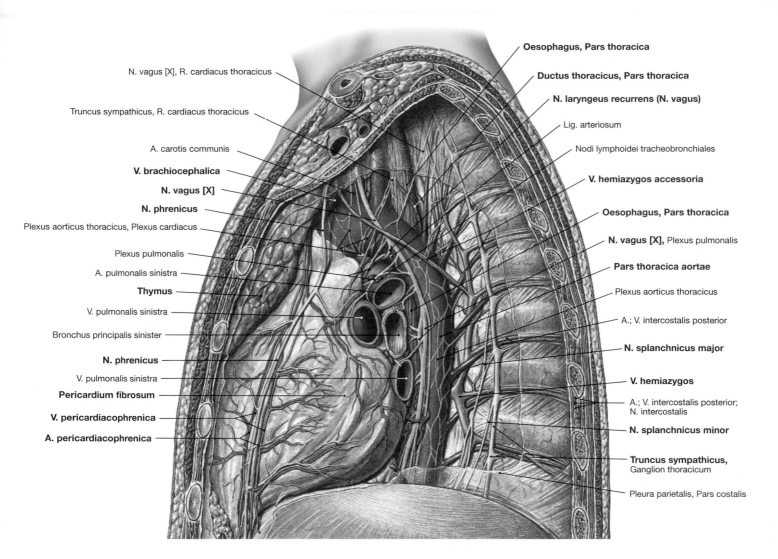

N. vagus [X], R. cardiacus thoracicus

Truncus sympathicus, R. cardiacus thoracicus

A. carotis communis

V. brachiocephalica

N. vagus [X]

N. phrenicus

Plexus aorticus thoracicus, Plexus cardiacus

Plexus pulmonalis

A. pulmonalis sinistra

Thymus

V. pulmonalis sinistra

Bronchus principalis sinister

N. phrenicus

V. pulmonalis sinistra

Pericardium fibrosum

V. pericardiacophrenica

A. pericardiacophrenica

Oesophagus, Pars thoracica

Ductus thoracicus, Pars thoracica

N. laryngeus recurrens (N. vagus)

Lig. arteriosum

Nodi lymphoidei tracheobronchiales

V. hemiazygos accessoria

Oesophagus, Pars thoracica

N. vagus [X], Plexus pulmonalis

Pars thoracica aortae

Plexus aorticus thoracicus

A.; V. intercostalis posterior

N. splanchnicus major

V. hemiazygos

A.; V. intercostalis posterior; N. intercostalis

N. splanchnicus minor

Truncus sympathicus, Ganglion thoracicum

Pleura parietalis, Pars costalis

Fig. 5.9 Mediastinum and pleural cavity, Cavitas pleuralis, of an adolescent boy; view from the left; after removal of the lateral thoracic wall and the left lung. [S700]
In the view from the left, the posterior mediastinum is dominated by the **aorta (Pars thoracica),** which descends to the left in front of the spine. Laterally, on the vertebral body, lies the **V. hemiazygos,** which flows between the 10th and seventh thoracic vertebrae into the V. azygos. It usually communicates with the **V. hemiazygos accessoria** which receives the blood of the upper Vv. intercostales. Even further laterally, on

the rib heads, are the ganglia of the **Truncus sympathicus** of the **sympathetic nervous system** from which the **Nn. splanchnici major and minor** proceed. The **N. vagus [X]** runs behind the root of the lung to the oesophagus, after it has given rise to the **N. laryngeus recurrens,** which loops around the Arcus aortae on the left-hand side. In the middle mediastinum is the pericardium and on this lies the **N. phrenicus,** which is accompanied by the **Vasa pericardiacophrenica.** In the upper mediastinum, the thymus covers the large vessels ventrally.

Structures of the mediastinum	
Structures of the Mediastinum superius	**Structures of the Mediastinum inferius**
<ul><li>Thymus</li><li>Trachea</li><li>Oesophagus</li><li>Arcus aortae</li><li>Vv. brachiocephalicae and V. cava superior</li><li>Lymphatic pathways: lymphatic trunks (Ductus thoracicus, Trunci bronchomediastinales) and mediastinal lymph nodes</li><li>Autonomic nervous system (Truncus sympathicus, N. vagus [X] with the N. laryngeus recurrens)</li><li>N. phrenicus</li></ul>	<ul><li>**Mediastinum anterius:** retrosternal lymphatic drainage of the mammary gland, the anterior mediastinal lymph nodes</li><li>**Mediastinum medium:** pericardium with vessels near the heart (Aorta ascendens, Truncus pulmonalis, V. cava superior) N. phrenicus with the Vasa pericardiacophrenica, medial mediastinal lymph nodes</li><li>**Mediastinum posterius:** Aorta descendens, Oesophagus with Plexus oesophageus of the N. vagus, N. vagus (Truncus vagalis anterior and posterior), Ductus thoracicus, Truncus sympathicus with Nn. splanchnici, V. azygos and V. hemiazygos, as well as intercostal neurovascular pathways, posterior mediastinal lymph nodes</li></ul>

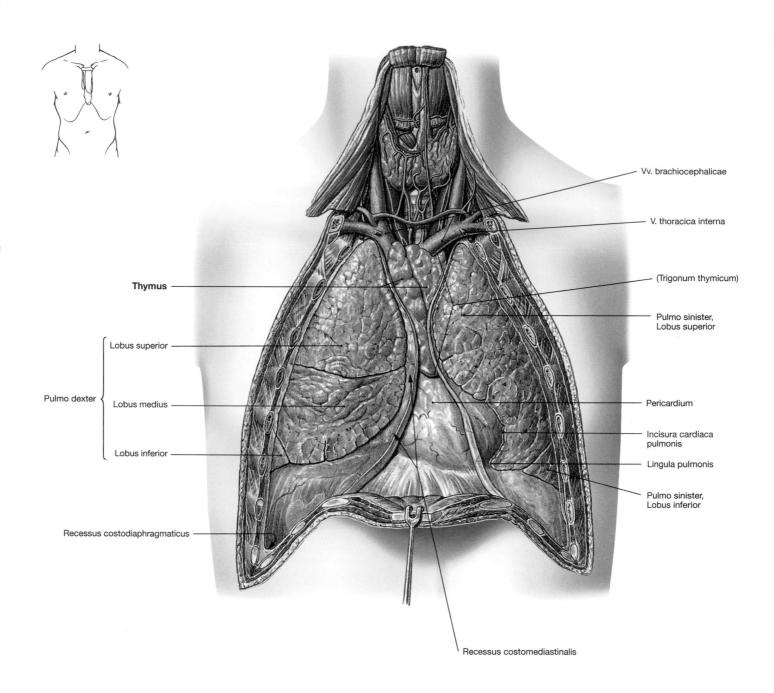

Vv. brachiocephalicae

V. thoracica interna

(Trigonum thymicum)

Pulmo sinister,
Lobus superior

Thymus

Lobus superior

Pulmo dexter

Lobus medius

Pericardium

Incisura cardiaca
pulmonis

Lobus inferior

Lingula pulmonis

Pulmo sinister,
Lobus inferior

Recessus costodiaphragmaticus

Recessus costomediastinalis

Fig. 5.10   Upper mediastinum with thymus of an adolescent boy; ventral view; after removal of the ventral thoracic wall. [S700]
The **thymus** lies in the upper mediastinum in the Trigonum thymicum between the medial walls of the pleural cavities. The thymus weighs 20 g in the adult and changes its tissue composition during its life cycle. Since its total volume remains almost the same in the process (5 cm x 3 cm x 1 cm), it is much larger relatively speaking in a newborn than in an adult (→ Fig. 5.12). The thymus is still relatively large in a young adult. After puberty, adaptive thymus tissue is increasingly replaced by fat

tissue so that the thymus as an organ is often difficult to identify in older people. In older people, it is almost completely replaced by fatty tissue. For this reason, it is often only the thymus carcass that is found in dissections, identified macroscopically solely on the basis of small arterial branches from the A. thoracica interna/A. thyroidea inferior and venous connections to the Vv. brachiocephalicae, mostly at the upper margin of the thymus. Nevertheless, adaptive thymus tissue always remains extant to allow for an immune response.

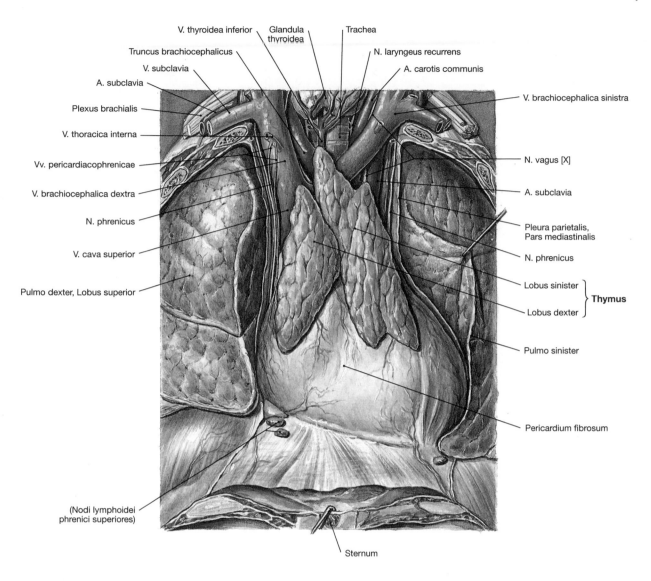

Fig. 5.11 **Thymus of an adolescent boy;** ventral view. [S700]
The thymus is a **primary lymphatic organ.** It serves for the proliferation and selection of T-lymphocytes which then leave the thymus in order to settle in the secondary lymphatic organs, dealing with specifically cellular immune responses.

The thymus develops from the entoderm of the third pharyngeal pouch and the ectoderm of the third pharyngeal groove. Macroscopically it consists of two lobes (Lobi dexter and sinister), which overlie the large vessels in the front section of the upper mediastinum. Microscopically these lobes are divided into lobules.

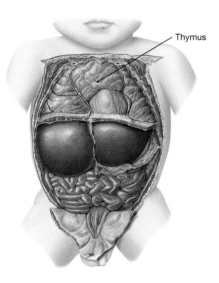

Fig. 5.12 **Position of the thymus of a newborn;** ventral view; after removal of the ventral abdominal wall. [S700]

N. phrenicus

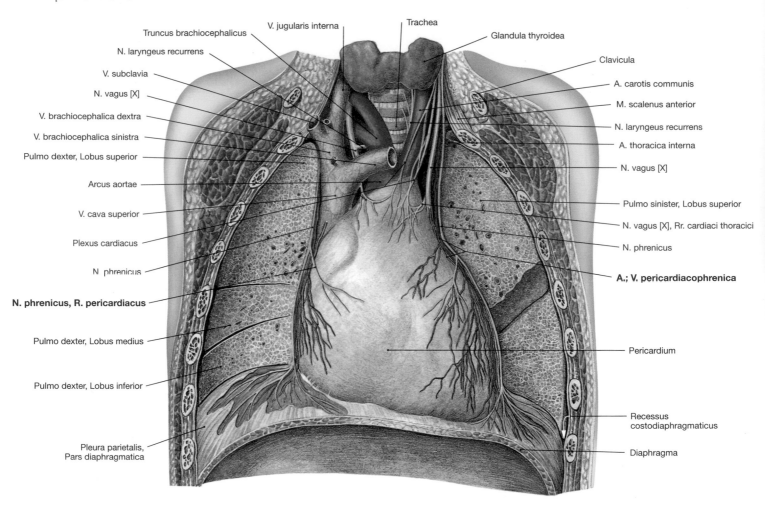

Truncus brachiocephalicus
N. laryngeus recurrens
V. subclavia
N. vagus [X]
V. brachiocephalica dextra
V. brachiocephalica sinistra
Pulmo dexter, Lobus superior
Arcus aortae
V. cava superior
Plexus cardiacus
N. phrenicus
N. phrenicus, R. pericardiacus
Pulmo dexter, Lobus medius
Pulmo dexter, Lobus inferior
Pleura parietalis, Pars diaphragmatica

V. jugularis interna
Trachea
Glandula thyroidea
Clavicula
A. carotis communis
M. scalenus anterior
N. laryngeus recurrens
A. thoracica interna
N. vagus [X]
Pulmo sinister, Lobus superior
N. vagus [X], Rr. cardiaci thoracici
N. phrenicus
A.; V. pericardiacophrenica
Pericardium
Recessus costodiaphragmaticus
Diaphragma

Fig. 5.13 Middle mediastinum; ventral view; after removal of the ventral thoracic wall, lungs dissected in the frontal plane. [S700]

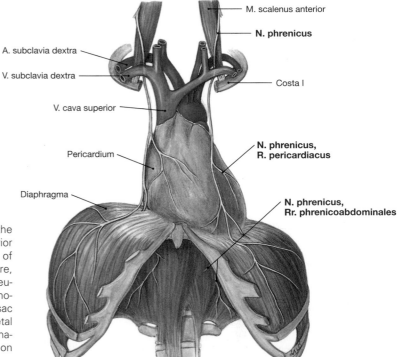

M. scalenus anterior
N. phrenicus
A. subclavia dextra
V. subclavia dextra
Costa I
V. cava superior
N. phrenicus, R. pericardiacus
Pericardium
Diaphragma
N. phrenicus, Rr. phrenicoabdominales

Fig. 5.14 Pathway of the N. phrenicus. [S700]
The **N. phrenicus** originates from segments C3 to C5 (mainly C4) of the cervical plexus, runs caudally at the neck on the M. scalenus anterior (key muscle!) and then in the lower **middle mediastinum** in front of the root of the lung it reaches the pericardial sac **(pericardium),** where, accompanying the Vasa pericardiacophrenica, and covered by the Pleura mediastinalis, it descends to the diaphragm which it innervates motorically. In addition, it provides sensory branches to the pericardial sac (R. pericardiacus), for the Pleura diaphragmatica as well as the parietal peritoneum on the underside of the diaphragm (Rr. phrenicoabdominales). The Rr. phrenicoabdominales innervate the visceral peritoneum on the liver and gallbladder.

Clinical remarks

The evolutionary pathway of the N. phrenicus has clinical significance in **paraplegia.** Caudal spinal cord lesions from C4 do not lead to any breathing dysfunction, while an injury to the C4 segment can lead to suffocation.

The innervation of **liver and gallbladder** via the phrenicoabdominal branches can lead to **referred pain in the right shoulder** (in the case of liver aspiration, a gallbladder inflammation). Splenic ruptures can cause a similar radiating pain in the left shoulder.

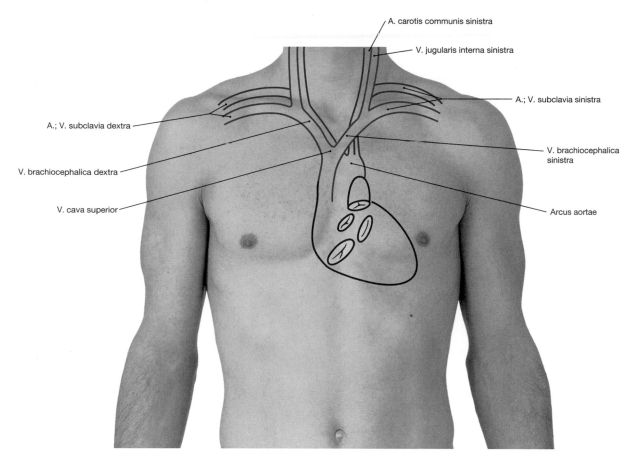

A. carotis communis sinistra

V. jugularis interna sinistra

A.; V. subclavia sinistra

A.; V. subclavia dextra

V. brachiocephalica sinistra

V. brachiocephalica dextra

V. cava superior

Arcus aortae

Fig. 5.15   Projection of the large vessels of the upper mediastinum onto the ventral thorax wall; ventral view. [S701-J803/L126]

The V. brachiocephalica sinistra crosses the upper mediastinum behind the Manubrium sterni and joins the V. brachiocephalica dextra behind the first sternocostal joint to form the **V. cava superior.**

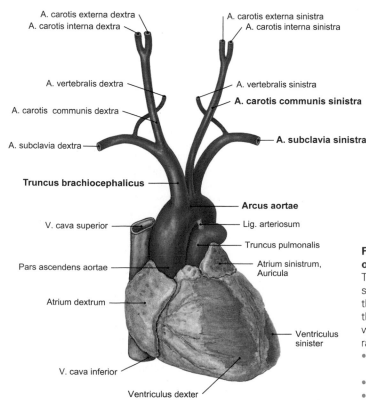

A. carotis externa dextra
A. carotis interna dextra

A. carotis externa sinistra
A. carotis interna sinistra

A. vertebralis dextra

A. vertebralis sinistra
A. carotis communis sinistra

A. carotis communis dextra

A. subclavia dextra

A. subclavia sinistra

Truncus brachiocephalicus

Arcus aortae

V. cava superior

Lig. arteriosum

Truncus pulmonalis

Pars ascendens aortae

Atrium sinistrum, Auricula

Atrium dextrum

Ventriculus sinister

V. cava inferior

Ventriculus dexter

Fig. 5.16   Aorta ascendens and Arcus aortae with outflow tracts of the large arteries; ventral view. [S700]

The **ascending aorta (Pars ascendens aortae** or **Aorta ascendens)** is still in the pericardium and thus in the lower mediastinum. It moves in the upper mediastinum into the **Arcus aortae,** which is connected to the Truncus pulmonalis via the Lig. arteriosum, and then continues within the descending side (Pars descendens aortae) of the Aorta thoracica (→ Fig. 5.18). The Arcus aortae provides the following branches:
* Truncus brachiocephalicus (right), which branches into the A. subclavia dextra and the A. carotis communis dextra
* A. carotis communis sinistra
* A. subclavia sinistra.

Arcus aortae with outflow tracts

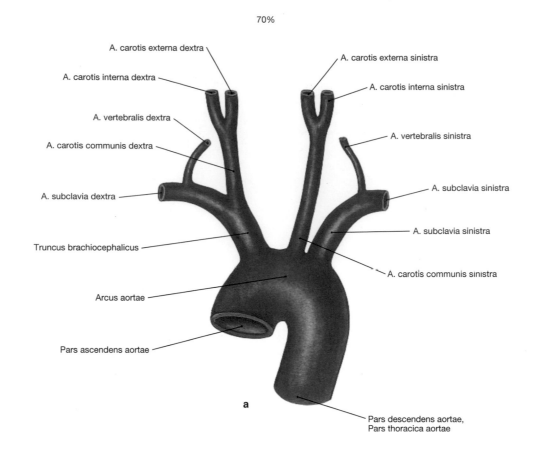

70%

A. carotis externa dextra

A. carotis interna dextra

A. vertebralis dextra

A. carotis communis dextra

A. subclavia dextra

Truncus brachiocephalicus

Arcus aortae

Pars ascendens aortae

A. carotis externa sinistra

A. carotis interna sinistra

A. vertebralis sinistra

A. subclavia sinistra

A. subclavia sinistra

A. carotis communis sinistra

Pars descendens aortae,
Pars thoracica aortae

a

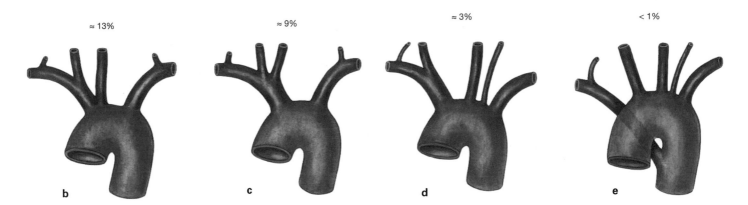

≈ 13%

≈ 9%

≈ 3%

< 1%

b   c   d   e

Fig. 5.17a–e   Outflow tract variants of the large vessels from the Arcus aortae. [S700]
a 'Textbook case'.
b Common origin of Truncus brachiocephalicus and A. carotis communis sinistra.
c Common branch for Truncus brachiocephalicus and A. carotis communis sinistra.
d Independent outflow tract of the A. vertebralis sinistra from the Arcus aortae.

e Outflow tract of the A. subclavia dextra as the last branch out of the Arcus aortae. This unusual artery mostly runs behind the oesophagus to the right and may cause problems with swallowing (dysphagia) **(Arteria lusoria).**
The occurrence of a stand-alone **Arcus aortae** running to the thyroid gland, which originates from the Truncus brachiocephalicus or from the Arcus aortae as a second branch, is relatively rare.

Clinical remarks

During **surgical procedures involving the aortic arch,** the cardiothoracic surgeon needs to consider the pathway of the thoracic nerves. Lesions of the **left N. laryngeus recurrens** may cause hoarseness of the voice and shortness of breath when exercising. Lesions of the **left N. phrenicus** may compromise respiratory function. The N. phrenicus runs **laterally** to the A. carotis communis sinistra and crosses the A. subclavis sinistra **ventrally** while remaining

dorsal of the V. subclavia sinistra. It then crosses the Arcus aortae and the pulmonary vessels at the hilum of the lung **ventrally** (→ Fig. 5.81). The N. vagus sinister descends **dorsally** of the V. brachiocephalica sinistra, **laterally** of the A. carotis communis sinistra and **medially** of the A. subclavia sinistra, and crosses the aortic arch ventrally before branching off the N. laryngeus recurrens. The N. vagus then runs **dorsally** and descends behind the hilum of the lung.

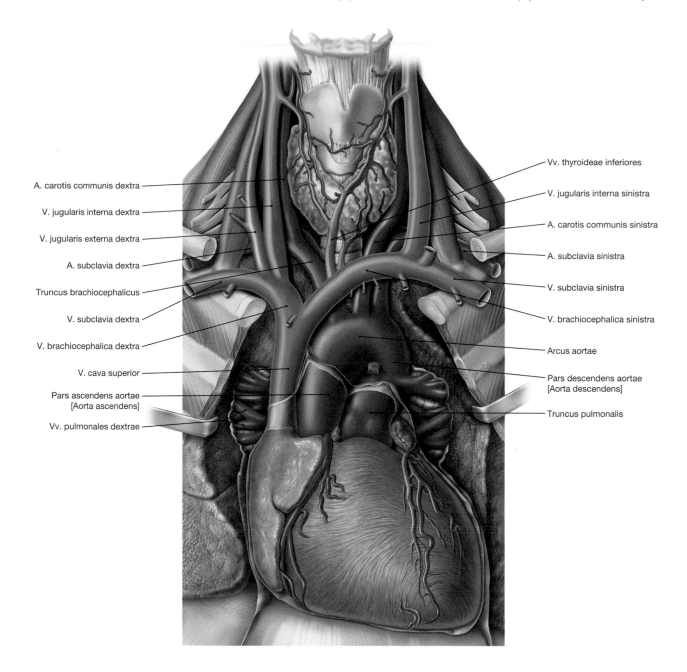

A. carotis communis dextra

V. jugularis interna dextra

V. jugularis externa dextra

A. subclavia dextra

Truncus brachiocephalicus

V. subclavia dextra

V. brachiocephalica dextra

V. cava superior

Pars ascendens aortae [Aorta ascendens]

Vv. pulmonales dextrae

Vv. thyroideae inferiores

V. jugularis interna sinistra

A. carotis communis sinistra

A. subclavia sinistra

V. subclavia sinistra

V. brachiocephalica sinistra

Arcus aortae

Pars descendens aortae [Aorta descendens]

Truncus pulmonalis

Fig. 5.18 Blood vessels of the upper mediastinum and the upper thoracic aperture, Apertura thoracis superior; ventral view. [S701-L238]

The A. subclavia passes through the **scalene gap** together with the brachial plexus. The scalene gap is bordered by the M. scalenus anterior, the M. scalenus medius and below by the muscular attachment of the first rib.

Clinical remarks

The scalene gap can be narrowed by an additional cervical rib at the seventh cervical vertebra. In this case, the Proc. transversus is elongated and comprises a rudimentary rib. Alternatively, an additional M. scalenus minimus may narrow the gap. Narrowing of the scalene gap causes the **thoracic-outlet syndrome,** a compression of the Plexus brachialis and the A. subclavia with elevation of the arm which may lead to a pulse deficit and numbness of the arm. [E402]

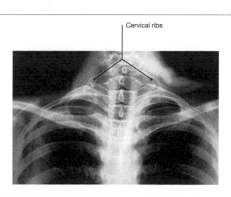

Cervical ribs

Organs of the thoracic cavity

Arcus aortae with outflow tracts

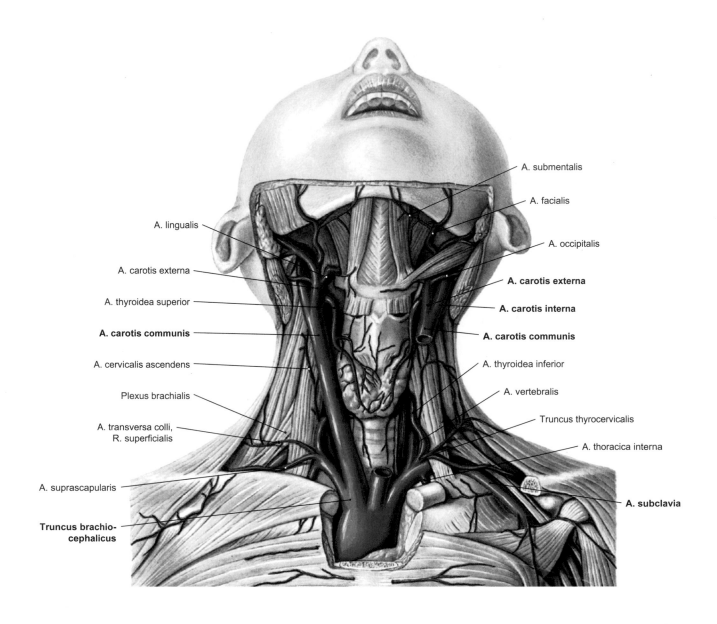

A. submentalis

A. facialis

A. occipitalis

A. lingualis

A. carotis externa

A. carotis externa

A. carotis interna

A. thyroidea superior

A. carotis communis

A. carotis communis

A. thyroidea inferior

A. cervicalis ascendens

A. vertebralis

Plexus brachialis

Truncus thyrocervicalis

A. transversa colli,
R. superficialis

A. thoracica interna

A. suprascapularis

A. subclavia

**Truncus brachio-
cephalicus**

Fig. 5.19   Arcus aortae with outflow tracts of the large arteries; ventral view; after removal of the Manubrium sterni. [G1068]
In the upper mediastinum, the **Arcus aortae** firstly provides the Truncus brachiocephalicus on the right, dividing into the A. subclavia dextra and the A. carotis communis dextra. The A. carotis communis sinistra and the A. subclavia sinistra then follow as outflow tracts.
A distinction is made between a **Pars thoracica** of the aorta (Pars thoracica aortae or Aorta thoracica) and a **Pars abdominalis** (Pars abdominalis aortae or Aorta abdominalis).

The **Aorta thoracica** is divided into the:
* **ascending aorta** (Pars ascendens aortae or Aorta ascendens) with the Aa. coronariae
* **aortic arch** (Arcus aortae): see illustration
* **descending aorta** (Pars descendens aortae or Aorta descendens) with parietal branches to supply the thoracic wall and visceral branches for the thoracic organs.

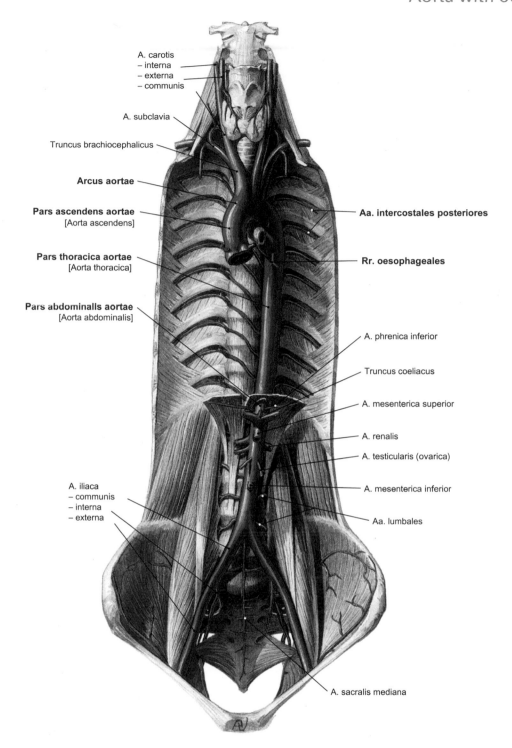

A. carotis
– interna
– externa
– communis

A. subclavia

Truncus brachiocephalicus

Arcus aortae

Pars ascendens aortae
[Aorta ascendens]

Pars thoracica aortae
[Aorta thoracica]

Pars abdominalis aortae
[Aorta abdominalis]

A. iliaca
– communis
– interna
– externa

Aa. intercostales posteriores

Rr. oesophageales

A. phrenica inferior

Truncus coeliacus

A. mesenterica superior

A. renalis

A. testicularis (ovarica)

A. mesenterica inferior

Aa. lumbales

A. sacralis mediana

Fig. 5.20 Sections of the aorta with outflow tracts of the large arteries; ventral view after removal of the ventral thoracic wall, all organs and all other neurovascular pathways of the thoracic, abdominal and pelvic cavities. [G1066-O1109]

Parietal branches of the Aorta thoracica:
* **Posterior Aa. intercostales:** nine pairs (the first two Aa. intercostales emerge from the Truncus costocervicalis of the A. subclavia)
* **A. subcostalis** (under the 12th rib)
* **A. phrenica superior:** to the upper side of the diaphragm.

Visceral branches of the Aorta thoracica:
* **Rr. bronchiales:** Vasa privata of the lung
* **Rr. oesophageales:** 3–6 branches on the oesophagus
* **Rr. mediastinales:** small branches to supply the mediastinum and the pericardium.

The aorta emerges at the level of the 12th thoracic vertebra through the aortic hiatus of the diaphragm, which is formed by the two lumbar arms of the diaphragm, and which continues within the **abdominal aorta.** This also has parietal and visceral branches, whereby the abdominal parietal branches continue the branch system in the Pars thoracica, and it then divides at the level of the fourth lumbar vertebra into its terminal branches.

Parietal branches of the abdominal aorta:
* **A. phrenica inferior:** on the underside of the diaphragm
* **Aa. lumbales** (four pairs; the last pair originates from the A. sacralis mediana).

Visceral branches of the abdominal aorta:
* **Truncus coeliacus:** first unpaired branch at the level of the 12th thoracic vertebra directly beneath the aortic hiatus
* **Aa. suprarenales mediae:** small branches to the adrenal glands
* **A. mesenterica superior:** unpaired vessel at the level of the first lumbar vertebra
* **Aa. renales:** the Aa. renales originate at the level of the second lumbar vertebra
* **Aa. testiculares/ovaricae:** descending vessels to supply the testes in men and the ovaries in women
* **A. mesenterica inferior:** unpaired vessel at the level of the third lumbar vertebra.

The two **iliac arteries (Aa. iliacae communes)** and the unpaired **A. sacralis mediana** at the front of the sacrum are **terminal branches** of the abdominal aorta.

Veins of the posterior mediastinum

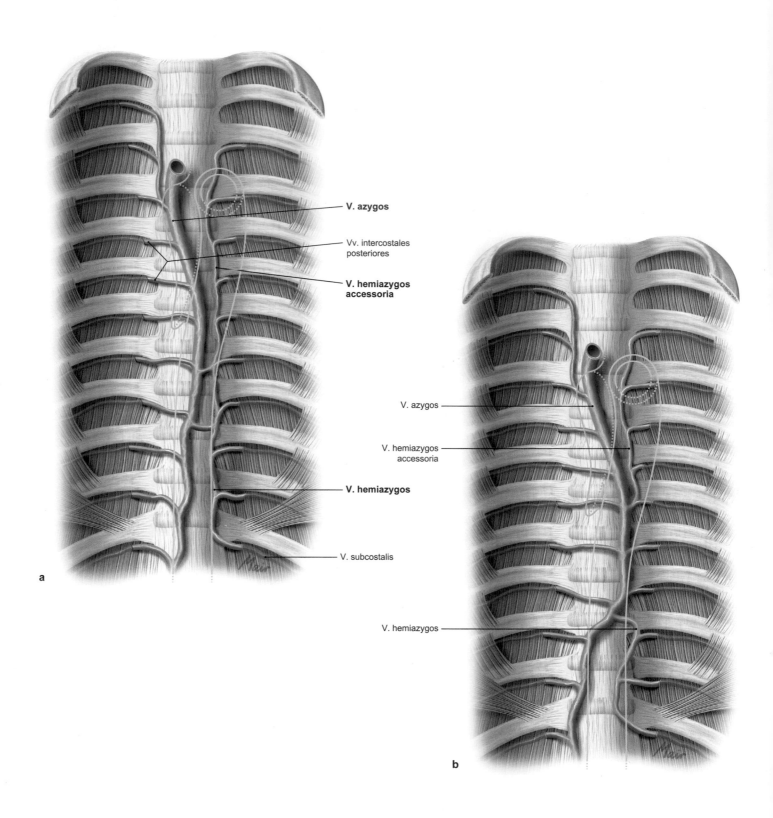

V. azygos

Vv. intercostales
posteriores

**V. hemiazygos
accessoria**

V. azygos

V. hemiazygos
accessoria

V. hemiazygos

V. hemiazygos

V. subcostalis

a

b

Fig. 5.21a and b   Azygos venous system; ventral view; after removal of all organs and all other neurovascular pathways of the thoracic cavity. [S700-L127]/[G210]

a The **V. cava superior** forms to the right of the spine behind the first sternocostal joint through the merging of the two Vv. brachiocephalicae (→ Fig. 5.22). Before discharging into the right atrium of the heart at the level of the fourth and fifth thoracic vertebrae, it receives the V. azygos, which crosses the main bronchus on the right beforehand. The V. azygos, together with the corresponding V. hemiazygos, forms the **azygos system.** The system with its parietal and visceral tributaries corresponds to the branches of the Aorta descendens.

Parietal branches of the V. azygos:
- Vv. intercostales posteriores: from the posterior thoracic wall
- V. subcostalis: below the lowest pair of ribs
- Vv. phrenicae superiores: from the top side of the diaphragm.

Visceral branches of the V. azygos:
- venous blood from the mediastinum with all its organs (Vv. mediastinales, Vv. oesophageales, Vv. bronchiales, Vv. pericardiacae).

b The V. azygos runs along the lower half of the mediastinum, often to the ventral side of the spine, or even to its right, so that a **V. hemiazygos** is not always formed in this section. If present, it enters between the 10th and seventh thoracic vertebrae into the V. azygos, whereby its pathway continues up through the **V. hemiazygos accessoria.**

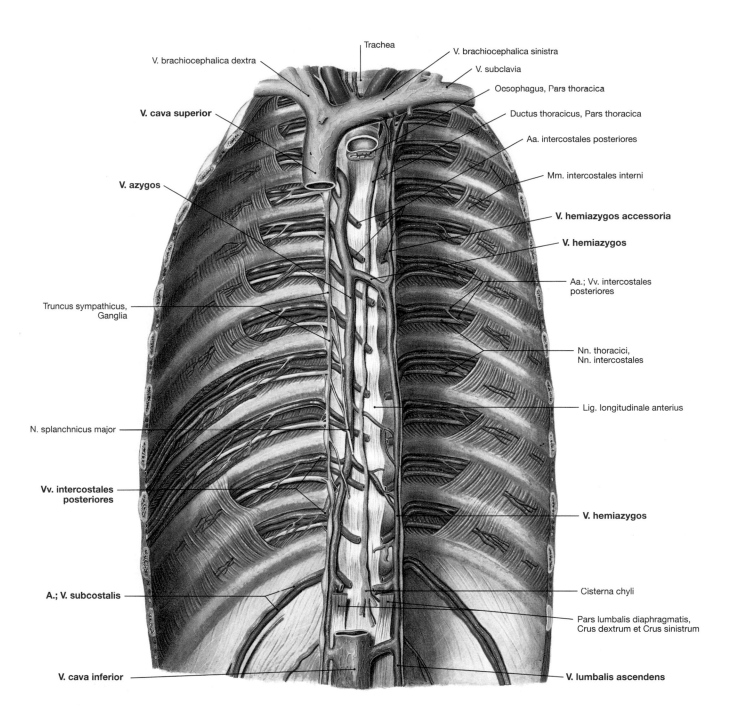

Trachea

V. brachiocephalica dextra

V. brachiocephalica sinistra

V. subclavia

V. cava superior

Oesophagus, Pars thoracica

Ductus thoracicus, Pars thoracica

Aa. intercostales posteriores

V. azygos

Mm. intercostales interni

V. hemiazygos accessoria

V. hemiazygos

Aa.; Vv. intercostales posteriores

Truncus sympathicus, Ganglia

Nn. thoracici, Nn. intercostales

Lig. longitudinale anterius

N. splanchnicus major

Vv. intercostales posteriores

V. hemiazygos

A.; V. subcostalis

Cisterna chyli

Pars lumbalis diaphragmatis, Crus dextrum et Crus sinistrum

V. cava inferior

V. lumbalis ascendens

Fig. 5.22 Veins of the azygos system; ventral view of the posterior thoracic wall; after removal of the diaphragm. [S700]
The azygos system connects Vv. cavae superior and inferior to each other, and its tributaries correspond to the branches of the Aorta thoracica. It is on the **right side** of the spine that the **V. azygos** ascends and it flows dorsally at the level of the fourth/fifth thoracic vertebrae into the V. cava superior. Correspondingly **on the left** to it is the **V. hemiazygos**, which drains between the 10th and seventh thoracic vertebrae into the V. azygos. The blood is received by a **V. hemiazygos accessoria** from the upper Vv. intercostales. Below the diaphragm, the pathway of the left and right azygos veins are respectively continued by a V. lumbalis ascendens, linking up in the V. cava inferior. In this way, the azygos system is involved in a collateral circulation system between the two

Vv. cavae. These **cavocaval anastomoses** include the following **tributaries:**
- **V. epigastrica superior** (connection to V. thoracica interna) and **V. epigastrica inferior** (connection to V. iliaca externa)
- **V. thoracoepigastrica** (connection to axillary vein) and **V. epigastrica superficialis** (connection to femoral vein)
- **Vv. azygos/hemiazygos** (confluence into V. cava superior) and **Vv. lumbales** (confluence into V. cava inferior)
- **Plexus venosus vertebralis** with confluence via Vv. intercostales/ Vv. lumbales into the azygos system, into the V. iliaca interna or directly into the V. cava inferior.

Organs of the thoracic cavity

Arteries of the posterior mediastinum

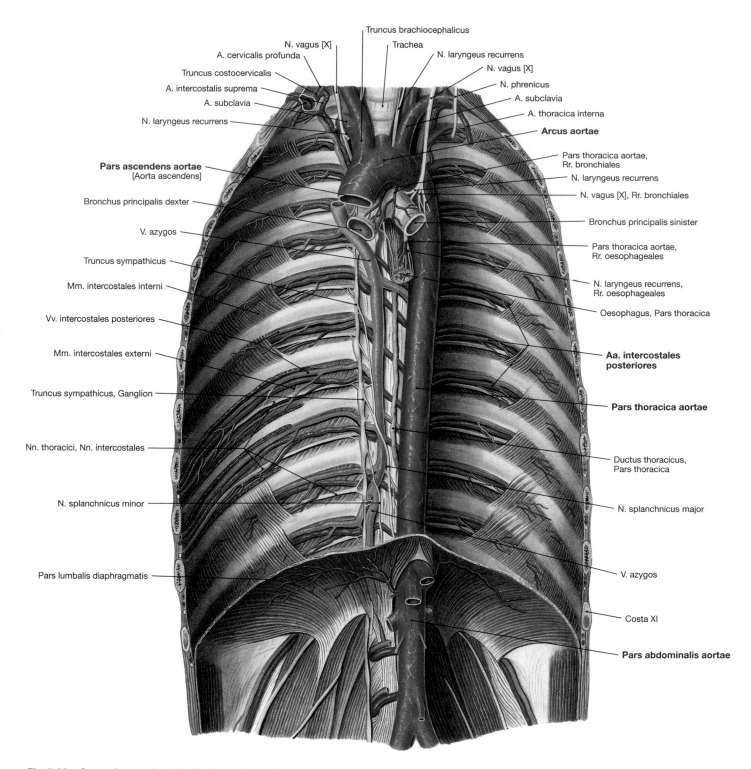

Truncus brachiocephalicus
N. vagus [X]
Trachea
A. cervicalis profunda
N. laryngeus recurrens
Truncus costocervicalis
N. vagus [X]
A. intercostalis suprema
N. phrenicus
A. subclavia
A. subclavia
N. laryngeus recurrens
A. thoracica interna
Arcus aortae
Pars thoracica aortae, Rr. bronchiales
Pars ascendens aortae [Aorta ascendens]
N. laryngeus recurrens
N. vagus [X], Rr. bronchiales
Bronchus principalis dexter
Bronchus principalis sinister
V. azygos
Pars thoracica aortae, Rr. oesophageales
Truncus sympathicus
N. laryngeus recurrens, Rr. oesophageales
Mm. intercostales interni
Oesophagus, Pars thoracica
Vv. intercostales posteriores
Mm. intercostales externi
Aa. intercostales posteriores
Truncus sympathicus, Ganglion
Pars thoracica aortae
Nn. thoracici, Nn. intercostales
Ductus thoracicus, Pars thoracica
N. splanchnicus minor
N. splanchnicus major
V. azygos
Pars lumbalis diaphragmatis
Costa XI
Pars abdominalis aortae

Fig. 5.23 **Aorta descendens in the thoracic section;** ventral view of the posterior thoracic wall. [S700]

The Pars descendens of the aorta descends into the posterior mediastinum **(Pars thoracica aortae)** and then crosses the diaphragm **(Pars abdominalis aortae).**

Branches of the Pars thoracica aortae [Aorta thoracica]	
Branches	**Individual arteries**
Parietal branches on the thoracic wall	• Aa. intercostales posteriores: nine pairs (the first two are branches of the costocervical trunk of the A. subclavia) • A. subcostalis: the last pair under rib 12 • A. phrenica superior: on the upper side of the diaphragm.
Visceral branches on the chest viscera	• Rr. bronchiales: Vasa privata of the lung (on the right side mostly from the A. intercostalis posterior dextra III) • Rr. oesophageales: 3–6 branches on the oesophagus • Rr. mediastinales: small branches on the mediastinum and pericardium.

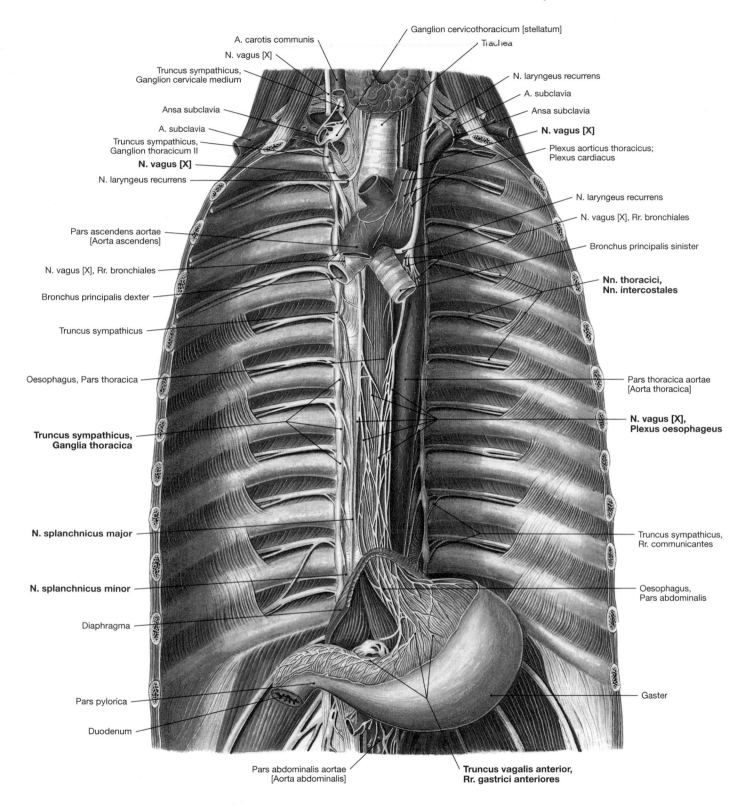

Fig. 5.24 Nerves of the posterior mediastinum; ventral view of the posterior thoracic wall; after removal of the diaphragm. [S700]

In the posterior mediastinum are, firstly, the intercostal nerves (Nn. intercostales) of the **somatic nervous system** and, secondly, sections of the sympathetic nervous system (Truncus sympathicus) and the parasympathetic nervous system (Nn. vagi) as part of the **autonomic nervous system.** The **Truncus sympathicus** forms a paravertebral chain of 12 thoracic ganglia in the posterior mediastinum, which are connected by the Rr. interganglionares. The preganglionic neurons of the sympathetic nervous system are located in the lateral horns (C8–L3) of the spinal cord and exit the spinal canal along with the spinal nerves. The white Rr. communicantes guide the fibres to the ganglia of the Truncus

sympathicus, in which the perikarya of the postganglionic neurons are located. Their axons return via the grey Rr. communicantes to the spinal nerves and their branches. Some preganglionic neurons are not switched in the Truncus sympathicus, but instead run along the Nn. splanchnici major and minor to the nerve plexuses on the Aorta abdominalis, where the switch happens. The preganglionic neurons of the **Nn. vagi** adduct behind the root of the lung to the oesophagus and form the Plexus oesophageus. Two trunks, the Trunci vagales anterior and posterior, are formed here and proceed with the oesophagus through the diaphragm to reach the autonomic nerve plexuses of the abdominal aorta. Here, however, there is no interconnection, as the postganglionic neurons are usually found in the vicinity of the respective organs.

Lymph vessels and lymph nodes of the mediastinum

Organs of the thoracic cavity

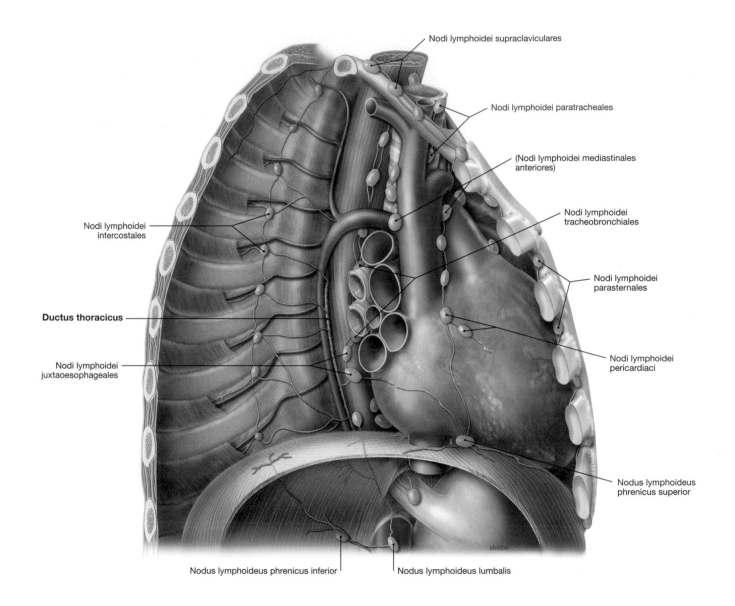

Nodi lymphoidei supraclaviculares

Nodi lymphoidei paratracheales

(Nodi lymphoidei mediastinales anteriores)

Nodi lymphoidei tracheobronchiales

Nodi lymphoidei parasternales

Nodi lymphoidei intercostales

Ductus thoracicus

Nodi lymphoidei juxtaoesophageales

Nodi lymphoidei pericardiaci

Nodus lymphoideus phrenicus superior

Nodus lymphoideus phrenicus inferior

Nodus lymphoideus lumbalis

Fig. 5.25   Lymph vessels and lymph nodes of the mediastinum; view from the right ventrolateral side after removal of the lateral thoracic wall. [S700-L238]/[C155]

There are various groups of lymph nodes in the mediastinum which are categorised into parietal lymph nodes (drainage of the thoracic walls) and visceral lymph nodes (drainage of the chest viscera). From there, the lymph flows into the major lymphatic trunks.

Parietal lymph nodes:

- **Nodi lymphoidei parasternales:** on both sides of the sternum. They receive lymph from the anterior thoracic wall, the mammary gland and the diaphragm. The lymph passes from them into the Truncus subclavius.

- **Nodi lymphoidei intercostales:** between the rib heads. They filter lymph of the posterior thoracic wall. The efferent lymph vessels drain directly into the Ductus thoracicus.

Visceral lymph nodes with connection to the Trunci bronchomediastinales:

- **Nodi lymphoidei mediastinales anteriores:** on both sides of the large vessels, tributaries from lungs and pleura, diaphragm (Nodi lymphoidei phrenici superiores), heart and pericardium (Nodi lymphoidei pericardiaci), and thymus.

- **Nodi lymphoidei mediastinales posteriores:** on bronchi and trachea (Nodi lymphoidei tracheobronchiales and paratracheales) and oesophagus (Nodi lymphoidei juxtaoesophageales).

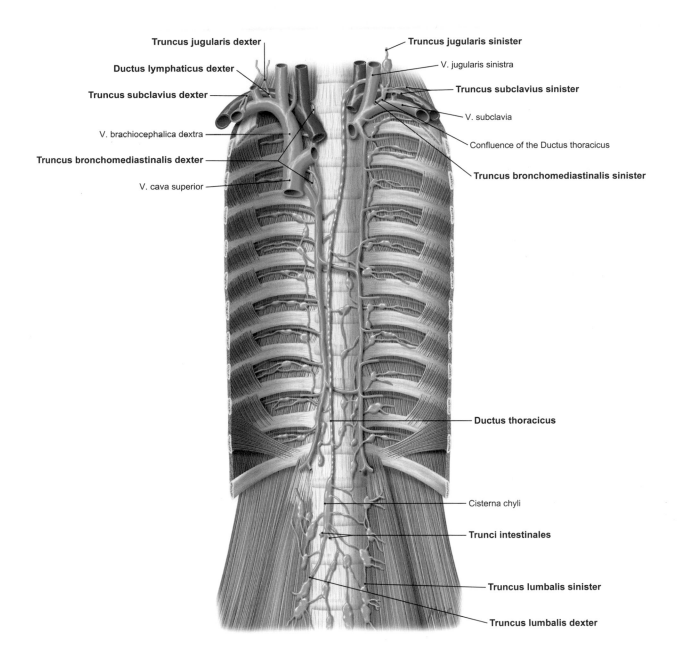

Truncus jugularis dexter

Ductus lymphaticus dexter

Truncus subclavius dexter

V. brachiocephalica dextra

Truncus bronchomediastinalis dexter

V. cava superior

Truncus jugularis sinister

V. jugularis sinistra

Truncus subclavius sinister

V. subclavia

Confluence of the Ductus thoracicus

Truncus bronchomediastinalis sinister

Ductus thoracicus

Cisterna chyli

Trunci intestinales

Truncus lumbalis sinister

Truncus lumbalis dexter

Fig. 5.26 Lymphatic trunks of the thorax, Cavitas thoracis; ventral view of the posterior thorax wall with the diaphragm removed. [S700-L127]/[G210]

The **Ductus thoracicus** originates just inferior to the diaphragm at the junction of the **Trunci intestinales** and the **Trunci lumbales**. This junction is frequently extended to the **Cisterna chyli** and normally positioned at the level of the second lumbar vertebra. The Ductus thoracicus passes through the diaphragm anterior to the 12th thoracic vertebra and ascends in the posterior mediastinum to the aorta, then posterior to the oesophagus to the level of the fourth thoracic vertebra where it crosses over the left pleural dome (3–4 cm above the clavicle) to join dorsally in the area of the left venous angle (between the V. subclavia and V. jugularis interna). Shortly before the confluence, it receives the **Truncus bronchomediastinalis sinister,** which runs autonomously in the mediastinum, as do the **Truncus subclavius sinister** (from the arm) and the **Truncus jugularis sinister** (from the neck). The equivalent collecting system on the right side is the short (mostly 1 cm) **Ductus lymphaticus dexter** that joins the right jugular-subclavian venous angle.

Clinical remarks

In cases of injury to the Ductus thoracicus during thoracic surgery involving the aortic arch or the oesophagus, or with oesophageal cancer or lymphoma in the posterior mediastinum, lymph leaks from the abdominal area into the pleural cavities, causing a **chylothorax.** The lymph from the Ductus thoracicus has a milky appearance as it contains the lipids resorbed from the intestinal tract. Since 1–2 liters of lymph pass through the Ductus thoracicus daily, the milky effusions from a chylothorax usually have to be drained frequently. In addition, patients require total parenteral nutrition until the leak in the Ductus thoracicus is healed, and cannot receive any oral nutrition.

Posterior mediastinum

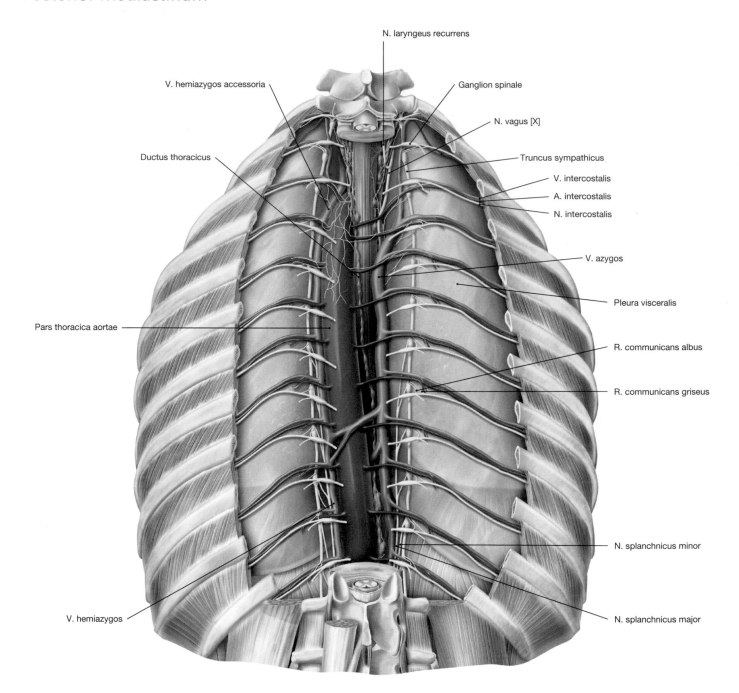

N. laryngeus recurrens

V. hemiazygos accessoria

Ganglion spinale

N. vagus [X]

Ductus thoracicus

Truncus sympathicus

V. intercostalis

A. intercostalis

N. intercostalis

V. azygos

Pleura visceralis

Pars thoracica aortae

R. communicans albus

R. communicans griseus

N. splanchnicus minor

V. hemiazygos

N. splanchnicus major

Fig. 5.27 Posterior mediastinum, Mediastinum posterius; dorsal view; after removal of the posterior thoracic wall including the spine. [S700-L275]/[Q300]
This view illustrates the topography of the neurovascular pathways in the posterior mediastinum. Because this depiction is generally not used in dissection courses, it is particularly useful for understanding positional relationships. The intercostal vascular, lymphatic and nervous systems (from cranial to caudal: **V.** intercostalis, **A.** intercostalis, **N.** intercostalis; **VAN**), which are situated on the lower rim of the respective ribs, run dorsally of the Pleura costalis to the lateral side. The Aa. intercostales originate segmentally from the **Aorta descendens,** which runs to the left of the median plane. To the right of the spine, displaced

to the lumbar and cervical area, ascends the **V. azygos,** which receives the Vv. intercostales. Corresponding to it on the left-hand side is the **V. hemiazygos,** which features here, at the level of the eighth and ninth ribs, anastomoses with the V. azygos, and cranially the **V. hemiazygos accessoria.** The Nn. intercostales correspond to the Rr. anteriores of the spinal nerves. From the spinal nerves, the Rr. communicantes branch out to connect to the **Truncus sympathicus** of the autonomic nervous system. The main lymph vessel of the human body, the **Ductus thoracicus,** ascends ventrally to the spine between the aorta and V. azygos. In the upper mediastinum, the oesophagus lies directly next to the spine.

Clinical remarks

A **surgical interruption (sympathicotomy)** or **resection (sympathectomy)** of the thoracic sympathetic trunk is performed in rare cases when other therapies have failed, to reduce excessive sweating (hyperhidrosis) of the face, neck or arm or when excessive vasoconstriction in RAYNAUD syndrome causes pain in the fingers when

cold. This is possible because the **sudomotor neurons,** which run via the sympathetic trunk to the sweat glands, arise from the T2–T7 segments to join the **vasoconstrictive fibres.** Visceral-afferent fibres also run along the sympathetic trunk.

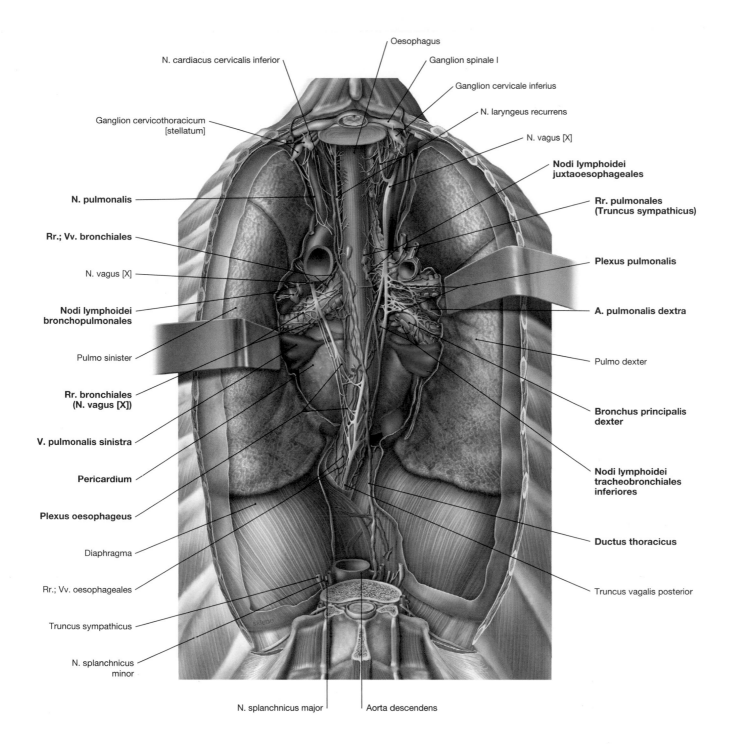

Oesophagus

N. cardiacus cervicalis inferior

Ganglion spinale I

Ganglion cervicale inferius

Ganglion cervicothoracicum [stellatum]

N. laryngeus recurrens

N. vagus [X]

N. pulmonalis

Nodi lymphoidei juxtaoesophageales

Rr.; Vv. bronchiales

Rr. pulmonales (Truncus sympathicus)

N. vagus [X]

Plexus pulmonalis

Nodi lymphoidei bronchopulmonales

A. pulmonalis dextra

Pulmo sinister

Pulmo dexter

Rr. bronchiales (N. vagus [X])

Bronchus principalis dexter

V. pulmonalis sinistra

Pericardium

Nodi lymphoidei tracheobronchiales inferiores

Plexus oesophageus

Diaphragma

Ductus thoracicus

Rr.; Vv. oesophageales

Truncus sympathicus

Truncus vagalis posterior

N. splanchnicus minor

N. splanchnicus major

Aorta descendens

Fig. 5.28 Posterior mediastinum, Mediastinum posterius; dorsal view; after removal of the posterior thoracic wall including the spine. The Pleura costalis is opened, and the lungs are secured on both sides to lateral. In addition, the Aorta descendens and the azygos system as well as the Truncus sympathicus have been displaced on their passage through the diaphragm. [S700-L238]/[Q300]

The **Ductus thoracicus** ascends ventrally of the spine. It is formed from the lumbar and intestinal trunks under the diaphragm and emerges to the right dorsal of the aorta via the Hiatus aorticus. The entire Pars thoracica of the **oesophagus** and, ventrally, of the **pericardium** and the **root of the lung (Radix pulmonis)** are visible here. The oesophagus emerges through the oesophageal hiatus in the lumbar part of the diaphragm. It is accompanied by an autonomic nerve plexus **(Plexus oesophageus),** the parasympathetic parts of which become condensed above the oesophageal hiatus to the **vagal trunks.** The Truncus vagalis posterior visible here emerges during development, predominantly from the fibres of the N. vagus on the right, due to stomach rotation. The autonomic **Plexus pulmonalis** is formed particularly strongly dorsally and accompanies the main bronchi to the hilum of the lung. It receives its parasympathetic fibres from the Nn. vagi and its sympathetic neurons from the Truncus sympathicus (not shown here).

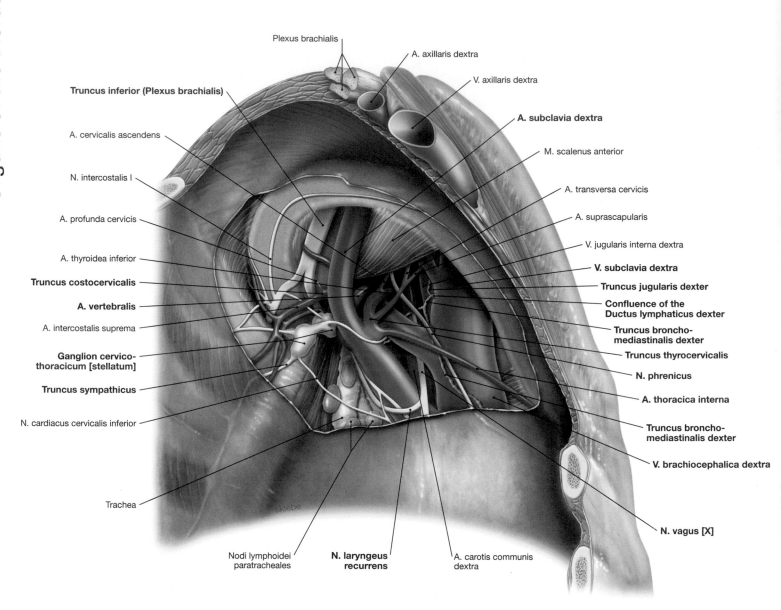

Plexus brachialis

A. axillaris dextra

V. axillaris dextra

A. subclavia dextra

Truncus inferior (Plexus brachialis)

A. cervicalis ascendens

M. scalenus anterior

N. intercostalis I

A. transversa cervicis

A. profunda cervicis

A. suprascapularis

V. jugularis interna dextra

A. thyroidea inferior

V. subclavia dextra

Truncus costocervicalis

Truncus jugularis dexter

A. vertebralis

Confluence of the Ductus lymphaticus dexter

A. intercostalis suprema

Truncus broncho-mediastinalis dexter

Ganglion cervico-thoracicum [stellatum]

Truncus thyrocervicalis

Truncus sympathicus

N. phrenicus

N. cardiacus cervicalis inferior

A. thoracica interna

Truncus broncho-mediastinalis dexter

V. brachiocephalica dextra

Trachea

N. vagus [X]

Nodi lymphoidei paratracheales

N. laryngeus recurrens

A. carotis communis dextra

Fig. 5.29 **Neurovascular pathways of the upper thoracic aperture, right side;** caudal view; after removal of the pleural dome. [S700-L238]/[Q300]

The pleural dome is bridged in front of the M. scalenus anterior by the V. subclavia and behind the muscle **(scalene gap)** by the A. subclavia and Plexus brachialis. Originating from the A. subclavia are the **A. thoracica interna,** which descends to the lateral surface of the sternum, the **A. vertebralis,** as well as the **Truncus thyrocervicalis** with its branches. Emerging dorsally of the M. scalenus anterior is the **Truncus costocervicalis,** which divides into the A. profunda cervicis and the A.

intercostalis suprema. The **N. phrenicus** lies ventrally on the V. brachiocephalica. Further dorsally the **N. vagus** releases the **N. laryngeus** recurrens, which winds around the A. subclavia on the right side, before it ascends again to the neck. Behind the A. subclavia lies the **Truncus sympathicus** with its **Ganglion cervicothoracicum** (stellate ganglion). Most difficult to identify is the short **Ductus lymphaticus dexter,** which drains into the right venous angle (between the V. subclavia and the V. jugularis interna) after merging with the Truncus bronchomediastinalis and the Truncus subclavius.

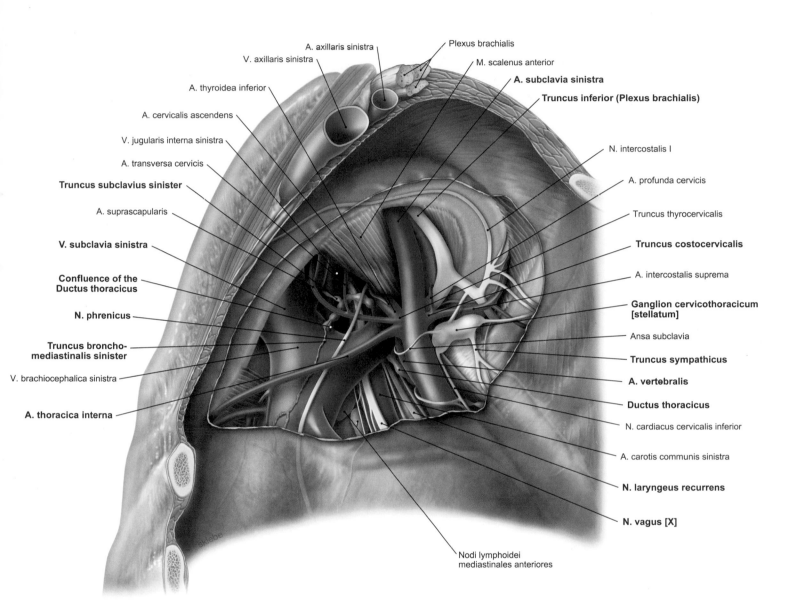

A. axillaris sinistra
Plexus brachialis
V. axillaris sinistra
M. scalenus anterior
A. thyroidea inferior
A. subclavia sinistra
A. cervicalis ascendens
Truncus inferior (Plexus brachialis)
V. jugularis interna sinistra
A. transversa cervicis
N. intercostalis I
Truncus subclavius sinister
A. profunda cervicis
A. suprascapularis
Truncus thyrocervicalis
V. subclavia sinistra
Truncus costocervicalis
Confluence of the
Ductus thoracicus
A. intercostalis suprema
N. phrenicus
Ganglion cervicothoracicum
[stellatum]
Truncus broncho-
mediastinalis sinister
Ansa subclavia
V. brachiocephalica sinistra
Truncus sympathicus
A. vertebralis
A. thoracica interna
Ductus thoracicus
N. cardiacus cervicalis inferior
A. carotis communis sinistra
N. laryngeus recurrens
N. vagus [X]
Nodi lymphoidei
mediastinales anteriores

Fig. 5.30 Neurovascular pathways of the upper thoracic aperture, left side; caudal view; after removal of the pleural dome. [S700-L238]/ [Q300]
Only those structures that vary in their pathway from the neurovascular pathways of the right side will be described here (→ Fig. 5.29). On the left side of the body, the **N. vagus [X]** descends further caudally before releasing its **N. laryngeus recurrens,** which then winds around the Arcus aortae (not in view) before it ascends again to the neck. Particular

attention should be paid to the pathway of the **Ductus thoracicus,** as it is often injured during dissection in this area. The **Ductus thoracicus** ascends in the posterior mediastinum and runs to the left pleural dome, before draining dorsally into the left venous angle (between the V. subclavia and the V. jugularis interna). Before reaching its outflow tract it receives the Truncus bronchomediastinalis, the Truncus subclavius and the Truncus jugularis (not shown).

Organisation of the cardiovascular system

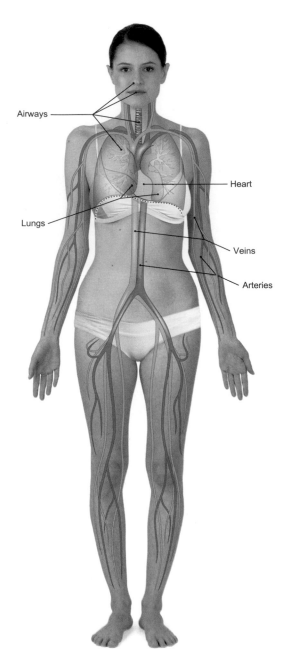

Airways

Heart

Lungs

Veins

Arteries

Fig. 5.31 The cardiorespiratory system; blue: deoxygenated blood, red: oxygenated blood. [S701-J803/L126]

The heart and blood vessels **(cardiovascular system)** together with the lungs and airways **(respiratory system)** form a functional unit that is referred to as the **cardiorespiratory system.**

The heart functions as a pump that is connected to all body parts and organs via the blood vessels. Oxygen enrichment occurs in the lungs to supply the peripheral organs and in turn, the metabolism product CO_2 is transported from the periphery back to the lungs.

In this way, blood is pumped from the heart into **arteries** and returned via **veins** to the heart. The definition of arteries and veins is exclusively determined by the direction of the blood flow towards and away from the heart, respectively.

Arteries and veins are referred to as vessels of **macrocirculation** since they are visible to the naked eye. Within the periphery of the body and the organs, the vessels of **microcirculation** connect the arteries and veins. Here blood pressure is reduced in the **arterioles** so that oxygen and gas exchange can take place in the **capillaries.** The **venules** collect the blood from the capillaries and join the veins.

Clinical remarks

The occlusion of an artery by a blood clot (embolus) or through atherosclerosis causes a **reduction in blood flow (ischaemia)** to dependent organs **(infarction)** or body parts. The occlusion of veins through localised formation of blood clots **(thrombosis)** causes accumulation of blood in dependent body parts and increased venous pressure resulting in **oedema.** If venous thrombotic material dislodges from the vessel wall it travels as an **embolus** and may obstruct pulmonary blood vessels (pulmonary embolism) causing heart failure.

Pathologies of microvascular vessels may have similar consequences. Arteriosclerosis can cause high systemic blood pressure (arterial **hypertension**). Thrombosis or changes in the corpuscular or plasma composition of blood can cause leakage of fluid into the interstitium **(oedema).** A swelling caused by **inflammation** results from extravasation of fluid from venules.

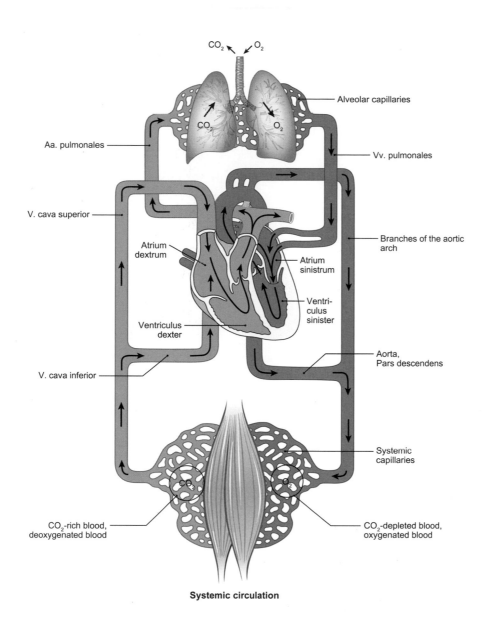

CO_2 O_2

Alveolar capillaries

CO_2 O_2

Aa. pulmonales

Vv. pulmonales

V. cava superior

Branches of the aortic arch

Atrium dextrum

Atrium sinistrum

Ventri-culus sinister

Ventriculus dexter

V. cava inferior

Aorta, Pars descendens

Systemic capillaries

CO_2 O_2

CO_2-rich blood, deoxygenated blood

CO_2-depleted blood, oxygenated blood

Systemic circulation

Fig. 5.32 **Organisation of the cardiovascular system;** blue: deoxygenated blood, red: oxygenated blood. [S701-L126]

A distinction is made between a **systemic circulation** and a **pulmonary circulation,** which are connected in a series. The heart is the parent organ of the cardiovascular system and drives the circulation as a suction and pressure pump. Accordingly, the heart is divided into two halves, which each consist of an atrium and a ventricle (ventriculus).

In this way, blood is pumped from the heart into **arteries** and returned via **veins** back to the heart. This definition of arteries and veins is independent of the oxygenation of the blood.

In the systemic circulation, oxygenated blood from the left ventricle (Ventriculus sinister) is directed via the main artery (aorta) and downstream arteries to the body periphery where the oxygen is used and carbon dioxide absorbed. The deoxygenated venous blood is returned to the heart via the veins, which join to form the superior and inferior Venae cavae (Vv. cavae superior and inferior) prior to entering the right

atrium (Atrium dextrum). Blood is then pumped from the right ventricle (Ventriculus dexter) through the Truncus pulmonalis and the pulmonary arteries into the pulmonary circulation, where renewed oxygen absorption into the blood and CO_2 exhalation take place. The pulmonary veins transport the oxygenated blood back into the left atrium (Atrium sinistrum) and the blood circulation is completed.

As the heart circulates blood in the body, its functions are identical to those of blood.

The **most important functions** of the cardiovascular system are:
- oxygen and nutrient supply of the organism (transport of gases and nutrients)
- thermal regulation (heat transfer in blood)
- immune defence function (transport of immune cells and antibodies)
- hormonal control (transport of hormones)
- haemostasis (transport of blood platelets and coagulation factors).

Structure of the heart

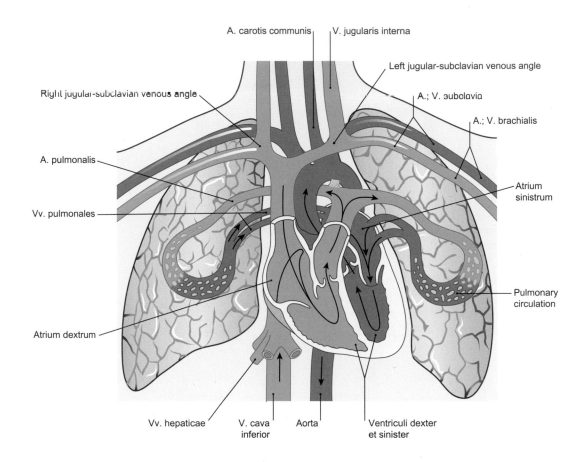

A. carotis communis

V. jugularis interna

Left jugular-subclavian venous angle

Right jugular-subclavian venous angle

A.; V. subclavia

A.; V. brachialis

A. pulmonalis

Atrium sinistrum

Vv. pulmonales

Atrium dextrum

Pulmonary circulation

Vv. hepaticae

V. cava inferior

Aorta

Ventriculi dexter et sinister

Fig. 5.33   Structure of the heart; blue: deoxygenated blood, red: oxygenated blood. [S702-L126]/[B500~M282]
The heart is divided into a **left and right side** by the cardiac septum. The two halves of the heart are each subdivided by valves (atrioventricular valves) into a right and left **atrium** and a right and left **ventricle.**

Thus, the septum also has two distinct parts:
- **Septum interatriale** between the atria
- **Septum interventriculare** between the ventricles. It consists of a narrow cranial membranous part (Pars membranacea), whereas the largest part consists of cardiac muscle (Pars muscularis).

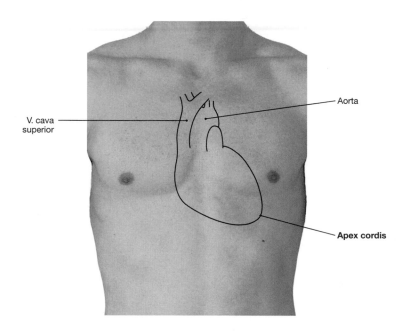

Fig. 5.34 Projection of the heart contour onto the ventral thoracic wall. The heart is displaced to the left side and thus does not lie in the centre of the thoracic cavity. [S700-J803/L126]
The right border of the heart projects from the third to sixth costal cartilage in a line which is 2 cm lateral to the right sternal border. **The**

left border of the heart projects onto a connecting line between the lower rim of the third rib (2–3 cm parasternal) and the midclavicular line on the left.

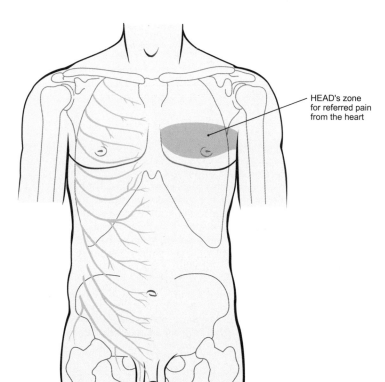

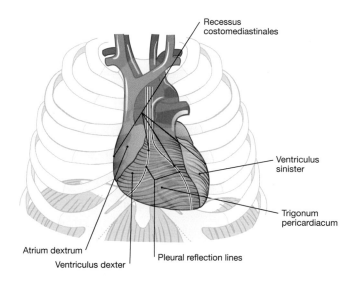

Fig. 5.36 Projection of the heart onto the thorax; schematic drawing. [S700-L126]/[B500~M282/L132]

Fig. 5.35 Zone of referred pain (HEAD's zone) of the heart.
[S700-L126]/[G1071]
Afferent nerve pathways from the heart, through which stimuli are transmitted to the central nervous system, merge in the respective spinal cord segments with nerve fibres that originate from corresponding skin areas (dermatomes). For the heart, these are the **dermatomes T3 and T4.** This organ-related skin area, where referred pain is localised, is referred to as the **HEAD's zone** of the heart.

Clinical remarks

Diseases of the heart, such as perfusion deficits in **angina pectoris** or a **heart attack** or myocardial infarction, sometimes cause pain and hypersensitivity to touch in the HEAD's zone of the heart, which corresponds to dermatomes T3 and T4 (= referred pain).

Heart

Projection of the heart

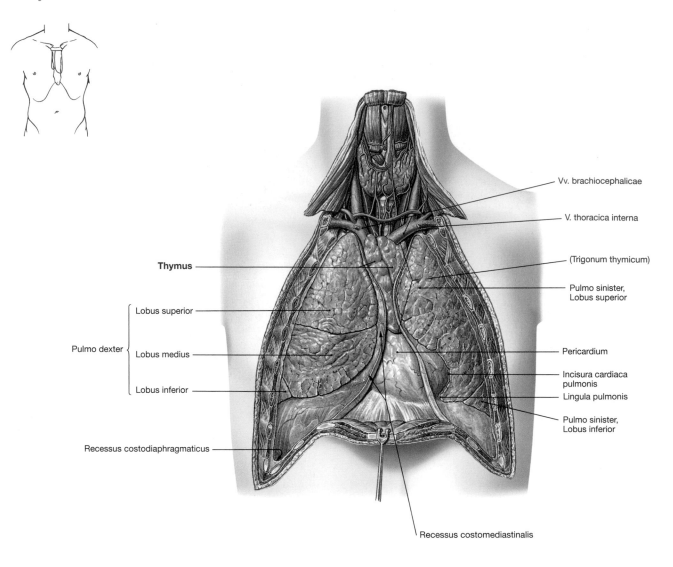

Thymus

Pulmo dexter — Lobus superior
— Lobus medius
— Lobus inferior

Recessus costodiaphragmaticus

Vv. brachiocephalicae

V. thoracica interna

(Trigonum thymicum)

Pulmo sinister,
Lobus superior

Pericardium

Incisura cardiaca
pulmonis

Lingula pulmonis

Pulmo sinister,
Lobus inferior

Recessus costomediastinalis

Fig. 5.37 Projection of the heart onto the thorax; mediastinum and Cavitates pleurales after removal of the thoracic wall; ventral view. [S700]

The heart is a cone-shaped, four-chambered, muscular hollow organ. Its size corresponds to the fist of each respective person; the weight is on average 250–300 g. The heart has **four sides:** the ventrally oriented **Facies sternocostalis** corresponds predominantly to the right ventricle. The caudally pointing **Facies diaphragmatica** is composed of parts from both ventricles. The **Facies pulmonalis** is formed to the right by the right atrium and to the left predominantly by the left ventricle. The result of this is that the right ventricle is not involved in the formation of

either the right or the left border of the heart. The posterior side of the heart has no official anatomical description. This part is taken up by the left atrium. Since the atria were viewed for a long time as part of the upstream veins, naming the posterior side was apparently neglected. The largest part of the Facies sternocostalis is covered on both sides by lung and pleura. These areas correspond to the **Recessus costomediastinales** of the Cavitas pleuralis. Underneath the fourth rib, the pleural edges move apart from each other and confine between them the **Trigonum pericardiacum,** in which the pericardium lies directly against the ventral thoracic wall.

Clinical remarks

From a **heart weight of 500 g (critical heart weight),** blood flow to the heart muscle is no longer sufficient so that perfusion deficiency (ischaemia) and death of cardiac tissue can ensue (heart attack). Enlargements of up to 1,100 g are known as **Cor bovinum** (bovine heart). Tapping of the heart **(percussion)** can give an initial indication of the **size** of the heart. The projection of the heart contours, which are covered by the pleura of the costomediastinal recess, reflect the area of **relative cardiac dullness,** since the air-filled lung makes the percussion sound less muffled. When this area extends to the left over the midclavicular line, it is an indication of left ventricular hyper-

trophy. The area where the heart is closely adjacent to the anterior thoracic wall is referred to as Trigonum pericardiacum and is the area of **absolute cardiac dullness,** since the percussion sound is muffled to the maximum (→ Fig. 5.36). This area has no diagnostic relevance, but can be used in case of emergency for injection into the right ventricle **(intracardiac injection),** without leading to an injury of the pleura, risking a pneumothorax. Intracardiac injections are performed in the fourth or fifth intercostal space, approximately 2 cm left parasternally. However, this measure is relatively risky and has therefore largely been abandoned.

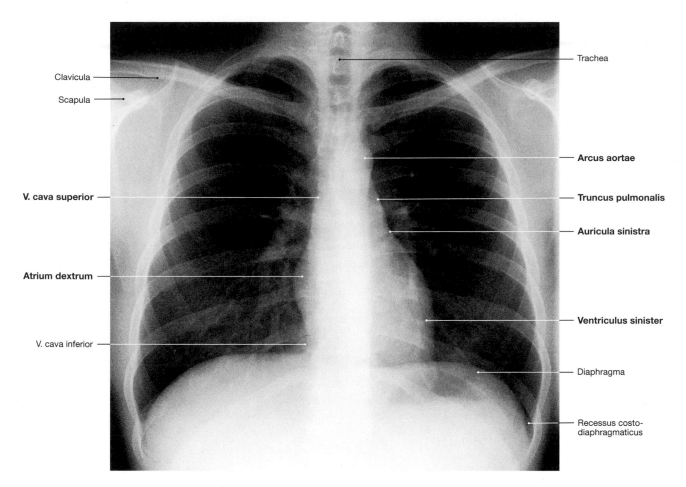

Fig. 5.38   Thoracic cage, Cavea thoracis, with thoracic viscera; X-ray in posteroanterior (PA) projection. [S700-T893]

The X-ray can be used to estimate the size of the heart. In addition to the overall size, knowledge of the structures contributing to the heart contours is of importance (→ Fig. 5.39).

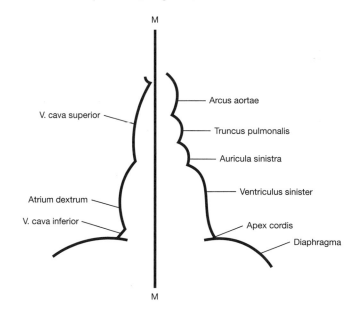

Fig. 5.39   Diagram of heart contours on an X-ray. [S700]
The **right border of the heart** is formed from top to bottom by the:
● upper caval vein (V. cava superior)
● right atrium (Atrium dextrum).
The **left border of the heart** is confined from top to bottom by the:
● aortic arch (Arcus aortae)
● Truncus pulmonalis
● left auricle (Auricula sinistra)
● left ventricle (Ventriculus sinister).
The right ventricle, therefore, does not form a border on any side!
M = median plane of the body

Clinical remarks

A chest radiograph provides information on the size of the heart. The transverse heart diameter is interindividually different. However, if it is larger than half the diameter of the thorax, an enlargement of the heart is present which may be caused by **hypertrophy** of the musculature or by **dilation** of the wall. In most cases, an enlargement on the left side (left pulmonary surface) is present, which points to an involvement of the left ventricle. This can be caused by **high blood pressure** (hypertension) in the systemic circulation, by **stenosis**, by

insufficiency of the **aortic valve,** or by **insufficiency** of the **mitral valve.** However, enlargements of the right ventricle, e.g. in pulmonary hypertension, in chronic obstructive pulmonary disease (asthma) or with occlusion of the pulmonary arteries (pulmonary embolism), are not visible on an X-ray in a sagittal projection, because the right ventricle is not border-forming. In this case, lateral or tomographic images such as computed tomography (CT) or magnetic resonance imaging (MRI) are required.

Development

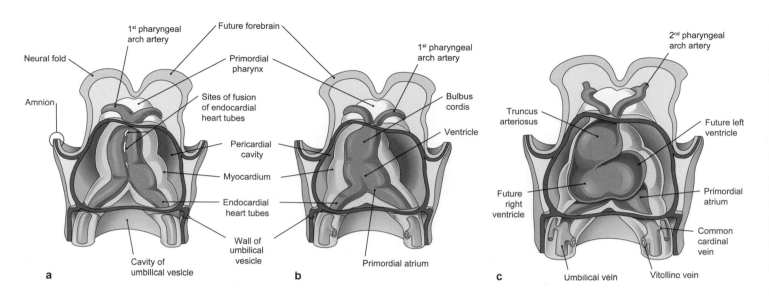

Fig. 5.40a–c   Stages of heart development in the third to fifth week. [E347-11]

In the **third week,** the initially horseshoe-shaped **endocardial tube** forms from a vessel plexus in the mesoderm of the cardiogenic zone. Gaps around the endocardial tube lead to the formation of the pericardial cavity which unites with the abdominal cavity. The inner layer of the pericardial cavity condenses into the myocardium. The epicardium develops from cells which migrate from the Septum transversum and the liver primordium. The sides of the endocardial tube fuse into a **tubular heart,** which from the end of the third week contracts rhythmically. The tubular heart is divided into what is first a paired atrium with the Sinus venosus as an inflow segment, with a ventricle and a Conus arteriosus as an outflow segment. Through varied lengthening of the individual parts and through redistribution, the tubular heart is transformed into the S-shaped **heart loop** in the **fourth to fifth week.** The connection between the atrium and ventricle is restricted to the unpaired atrioventricular canal which firstly flows into the left part of the ventricle, but later is diverted into the midline and divided by endocardial cushions into a right and a left atrioventricular opening. The endocardial cushions form the atrioventricular valves.

Week 10

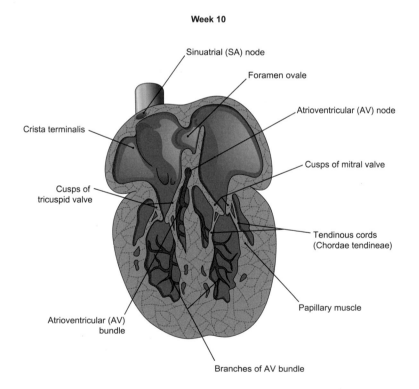

Fig. 5.41   Stages of heart development in the fifth to tenth week. [E347-11]

In the fifth to seventh week a **Septum interventriculare** (Pars muscularis) develops, which partially separates the two ventricles. They communicate with each other, however, until the end of the seventh week, when both ventricles are finally separated by the unification of the Pars membranacea of the septum. The Conus arteriosus of the outflow tract is divided spirally and, together with the adjacent Saccus aorticus, forms the **Truncus pulmonalis** and the **aorta.**

Pharyngeal arch arteries originate from the Saccus aorticus. Of the six pharyngeal arch arteries, however, only the third, fourth and sixth develop and form part of the arteries near the heart. The A. carotis communis emerges from the third pharyngeal arch artery; from the fourth pharyngeal arch artery parts of the A. subclavia emerge to the right and the aortic arch emerges to the left. The pulmonary arteries and the Ductus arteriosus develop from the sixth pharyngeal arch artery.

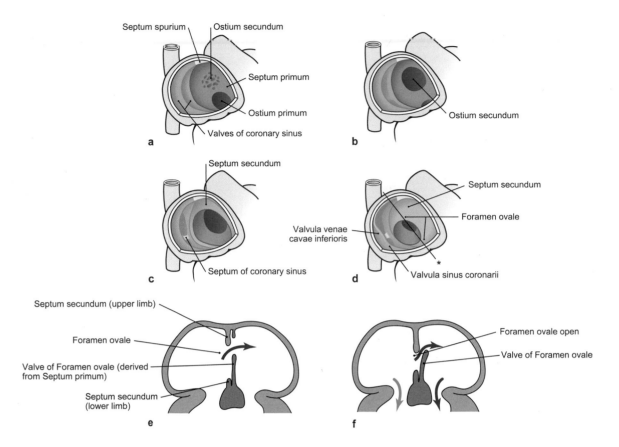

Fig. 5.42a–f Steps of atrial septation in the fifth (a, b), sixth (c, e), as well as the seventh and eighth week (d, f); view from the opened right atrium (**a–d**) and in the atrial septum (**e** and **f**). a–d [S702-L126]/[G1072], e,f [E347-11]

a Atrial septation occurs in the fifth to seventh week and begins with the formation of the **Septum primum,** which grows from dorsal upwards and leaves the **Ostium primum** free below.

b Within the upper part of the Septum primum, the **Ostium secundum** is created through programmed cell death (apoptosis).

c, e The **Septum secundum** develops to the right of the Septum primum. Both septa lie adjacent to each other and close off the Foramen ovale together.

d, f The Septum primum forms the **Valvula foraminis ovalis** which facilitates the directional blood flow from the right into the left atrium (→ Fig. 5.44). After birth, the Valvula foraminis ovalis closes the Foramen ovale due to the increased blood pressure in the left atrium (→ Fig. 5.46).

* sectional plane e, f

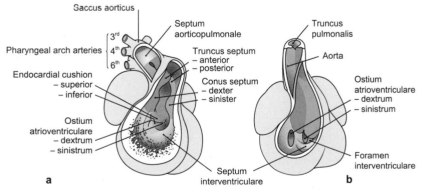

Fig. 5.43a and b Septation of the outflow tract; ventral view each time after exposure of the ventricular outflow tract. [S702-L126]/[G1072]

In the fifth to seventh week the outflow tract is also subdivided. In the process, the individual parts (Conus cordis, Truncus arteriosus, Saccus aorticus), which are already visible in the tubular heart (→ Fig. 5.40), are separated by bulbar ridges. Since these ridges are aligned perpendicularly to each other, the result is a twisted **Septum aorticopulmonale.** This divides the outflow tract into the Aorta ascendens and Truncus pulmonalis.

Clinical remarks

If the spiral-like subdivision of the outflow tract fails to appear, the Aorta ascendens and Truncus pulmonalis run directly next to each other. Thereby the aorta originates erroneously from the right ventricle and the Truncus pulmonalis from the left ventricle (**= transposition of the large vessels**). This malformation leads to the systemic and pulmonary circulations being completely separated from each other with no oxygenated blood entering the systemic circulation to reach the organs. In these cases, the ventricular and atrial septum do not close, which means that ventricular defects are present at birth. It is impossible to survive without these openings! These heart defects, comprising 5 % of all heart defects, are relatively rare.

Prenatal circulation

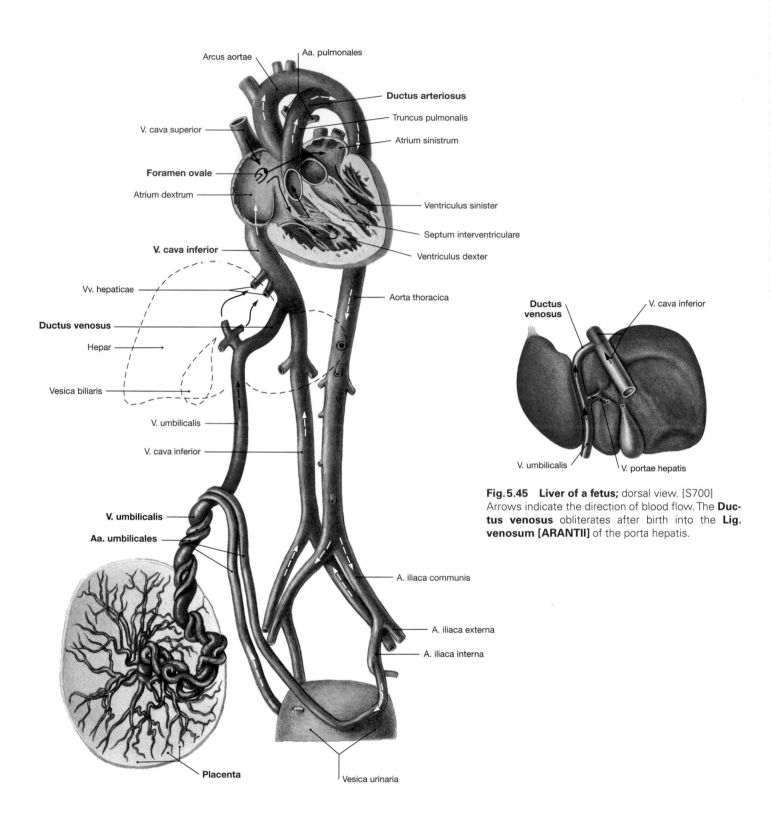

Arcus aortae

Aa. pulmonales

Ductus arteriosus

V. cava superior

Truncus pulmonalis

Atrium sinistrum

Foramen ovale

Atrium dextrum

Ventriculus sinister

Septum interventriculare

Ventriculus dexter

V. cava inferior

Vv. hepaticae

Aorta thoracica

Ductus venosus

Hepar

Vesica biliaris

V. umbilicalis

V. cava inferior

V. umbilicalis

Aa. umbilicales

A. iliaca communis

A. iliaca externa

A. iliaca interna

Placenta

Vesica urinaria

Ductus venosus

V. cava inferior

V. umbilicalis

V. portae hepatis

Fig. 5.45 Liver of a fetus; dorsal view. [S700]
Arrows indicate the direction of blood flow. The **Ductus venosus** obliterates after birth into the **Lig. venosum [ARANTII]** of the porta hepatis.

Fig. 5.44 Prenatal circulation (fetal circulation); schematic illustration. [S700]
In this illustration, the oxygen content of the blood is represented by colours: oxygenated (red), deoxygenated (blue), mixed blood (purple). Arrows indicate the direction of the blood flow.
Fetal circulation differs from postnatal circulation, by the umbilical vessels, the Ductus venosus, the Ductus arteriosus, the Foramen ovale, etc. (→ Fig. 5.46).
The deoxygenated blood of the fetus reaches the placenta via the **Aa. umbilicales,** which are provided by the Aa. iliacae internae. From there

it is brought back to the fetus after oxygenation via the V. umbilicalis and circumvents the liver via the **Ductus venosus (ARANTII)** since flow resistance in the liver is relatively high. Through a valve at the confluence of the V. cava inferior (Valvula venae cavae inferioris), the blood is channelled predominantly through the **Foramen ovale** into the left atrium. The oxygenated blood is thus taken on the shortest route to the organs. The blood of the V. cava superior enters the right ventricle and is channelled from there via the **Ductus arteriosus (BOTALLI)** as a bypass vessel from the Truncus pulmonalis into the aorta and thereby circumvents the non-functional pulmonary circulation.

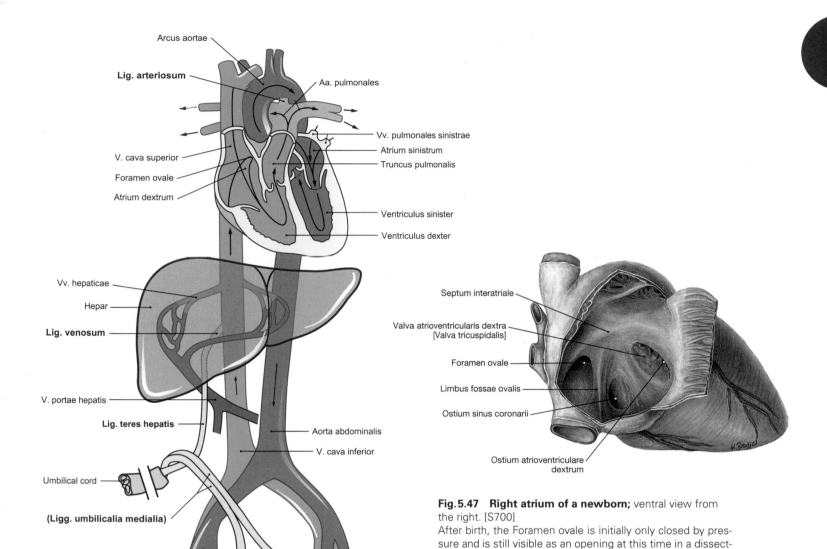

Arcus aortae

Lig. arteriosum

Aa. pulmonales

Vv. pulmonales sinistrae

Atrium sinistrum

Truncus pulmonalis

V. cava superior

Foramen ovale

Atrium dextrum

Ventriculus sinister

Ventriculus dexter

Vv. hepaticae

Hepar

Lig. venosum

V. portae hepatis

Lig. teres hepatis

Aorta abdominalis

V. cava inferior

Umbilical cord

(Ligg. umbilicalia medialia)

Septum interatriale

Valva atrioventricularis dextra
[Valva tricuspidalis]

Foramen ovale

Limbus fossae ovalis

Ostium sinus coronarii

Ostium atrioventriculare
dextrum

Fig. 5.47   Right atrium of a newborn; ventral view from
the right. [S700]
After birth, the Foramen ovale is initially only closed by pressure and is still visible as an opening at this time in a dissected heart.

Fig. 5.46   Postnatal circulation, schematic illustration. [S700-L126]/
[G1060-002]
At birth, the placental circulation is interrupted. Breathing inflates the
lungs and pulmonary circulation is opened, so that pressure in the left
atrium increases. With the change from fetal to postnatal circulation,
the following changes happen:
The valve-like connection of the Foramen ovale between the right and
left atria is passively closed by the increased pressure in the left atrium.
Later, the Valvula foraminis ovalis fuses with the Septum secundum. Of
the Foramen ovale, the **Fossa ovalis** remains.

The Ductus arteriosus closes within a few days and becomes the **Lig.
arteriosum** (→ Fig. 5.55).
The Ductus venosus obliterates after birth into the **Lig. venosum** of the
porta hepatis.
The umbilical vein obliterates into the **Lig. teres hepatis** between the
liver and the abdominal wall.
The distal part of the umbilical arteries becomes the right and left **Lig.
umbilicale mediale,** each forming the foundation of the Plica umbilicalis medialis on the inner surface of the abdominal wall.

Clinical remarks

Patent Ductus arteriosus: as prostaglandin E₂ has a dilating effect
on the ductus, an inhibitor of prostaglandin synthesis may cause a
closure of the patent ductus and possibly help to avoid an operation.
However, since these active substances are also used as anti-inflam-
matory agents and analgesics, they may also cause a premature closure of the fetal Ductus arteriosus in a pregnant woman.

Patent Foramen ovale: An opening in the Foramen ovale remains
present in approximately 20 % of adults. This is usually not relevant
from a functional point of view, but can lead to thrombi in the form of
emboli from the leg veins entering the systemic circulation and causing organ infarctions and ischaemic strokes in the brain.

Heart defects

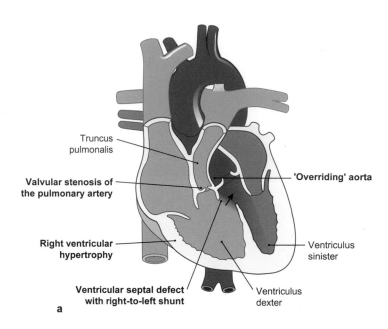

Truncus pulmonalis

Valvular stenosis of the pulmonary artery

'Overriding' aorta

Right ventricular hypertrophy

Ventriculus sinister

Ventricular septal defect with right-to-left shunt

Ventriculus dexter

a

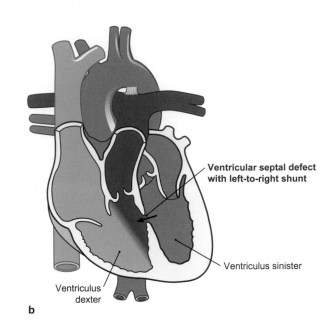

Ventricular septal defect with left-to-right shunt

Ventriculus sinister

Ventriculus dexter

b

Fig. 5.48a and b   Heart defect: Tetralogy of FALLOT and ventricular septal defect, schematic diagram; ventral view. [S702-L126]/[F201-035]

When the relatively complicated septation processes during heart development do not take place, children with heart defects are born. Understanding of the development is necessary for diagnostics and treatment, which is mostly operative.

a Tetralogy of FALLOT. If the outflow tract is not divided symmetrically, tetralogy of FALLOT ensues. This is the most common malformation

(9 % of all heart defects) with **right-to-left shunting,** where blood from the right ventricle flows out into the systemic circulation.

b Ventricular septal defect. The ventricular septal defect is the most common malformation of the heart overall (25 % of all heart defects). Here, the Septum interventriculare does not close completely, mostly in the area of the Pars membranacea, so that blood from the left ventricle is pumped into the pulmonary circulation described as **left-to-right shunting**.

Clinical remarks

Congenital heart defects occur in 0.75 % of all newborn babies and thus are the most common developmental disorders. Fortunately, however, not all heart defects **(vitia)** require treatment, as they are often not functionally relevant. To understand the genesis and clinical symptoms of major heart defects in paediatric and adolescent medicine, one must first become familiar with the fundamental development of the heart. Due to their medical importance and exam relevance in various subjects, the most important congenital heart defects are discussed briefly here. According to their pathophysiology, the most common heart defects can be divided into three groups:

* The most common group comprises defects with **left-to-right shunting** (ventricular septal defect 25 %, atrial septal defect 12 %, patent Ductus arteriosus 12 %) which present with increased pressure in the systemic circulation and blood flow from left to right into the pulmonary circulation. Pulmonary hypertension leads to right heart failure if the defect is not surgically corrected.

* Defects with **right-to-left shunting** (tetralogy of **FALLOT** 9 %, transposition of the large vessels 5 %) are, in contrast, characterised by a bluish colouring of the skin (cyanosis), because deoxygenated blood from the pulmonary circulation enters the systemic circulation.

* The third group comprises **defects with obstruction** (pulmonary valve stenosis, aortic valve stenosis, coarctation of the aorta, 6 % each) presenting with hypertrophy of the respective ventricle.

Tetralogy of FALLOT is a combination of a ventricular septal defect, pulmonary valve stenosis, right ventricular hypertrophy and an overriding aorta. Because of asymmetric septation of the Conus arteriosus, the pulmonary valve is too narrow and the aorta too wide and displaced over the septum ('overriding'). Resulting from the narrow pulmonary valve, a right ventricular hypertrophy ensues, which is responsible for the right-to-left shunting through the ventricular septal defect and thus the cyanosis.

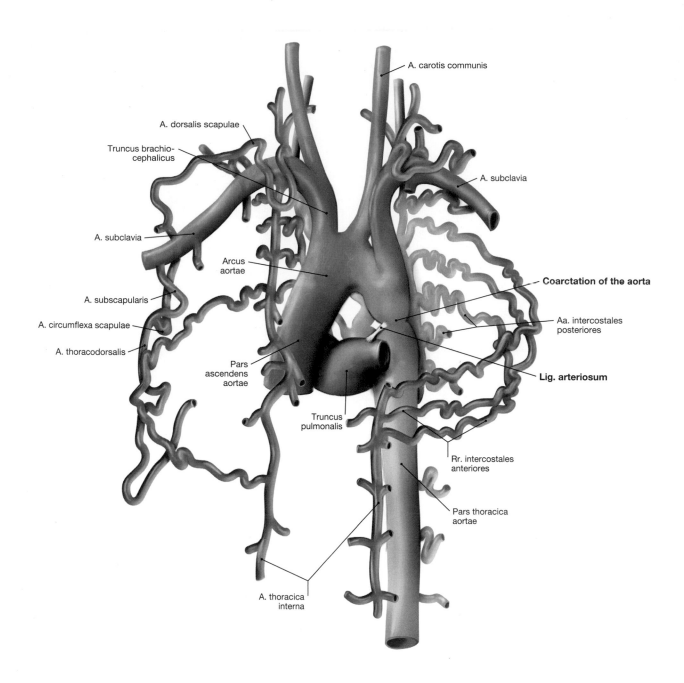

A. carotis communis

A. dorsalis scapulae

Truncus brachio-
cephalicus

A. subclavia

A. subclavia

Arcus
aortae

Coarctation of the aorta

A. subscapularis

Aa. intercostales
posteriores

A. circumflexa scapulae

A. thoracodorsalis

Lig. arteriosum

Pars
ascendens
aortae

Truncus
pulmonalis

Rr. intercostales
anteriores

Pars thoracica
aortae

A. thoracica
interna

Fig. 5.49 Coarctation of the aorta, semi-schematic diagram; ventral view. [S702-L266]
After birth, the Ductus arteriosus closes due to increased oxygen content in the blood. When the occlusion of the Ductus arteriosus en-croaches upon the surrounding parts of the Arcus aortae, a coarctation of the aorta ensues.

Clinical remarks

In a **coarctation of the aorta,** hypertrophy of the left heart with hypertension in the upper half of the body ensues. In contrast, pressure in the lower half of the body is very low. What stands out diagnostically is a systolic cardiac murmur between the shoulder blades as well as radiographically visible rib defects because of bypass circulations of the Aa. intercostales to the A. thoracica interna. The stenosis must be corrected via an operation or by dilation, otherwise heart failure and strokes can occur even at a young age. Since prostaglandins in the blood keep the Ductus arteriosus open through atony of the muscle, an inhibitor of prostaglandin synthesis may facilitate a closure after birth. Since these inhibitors are included in some medication for inflammation and pain relief, they can cause premature occlusion of the Ductus arteriosus in pregnant women with damage to the fetus.

Heart position

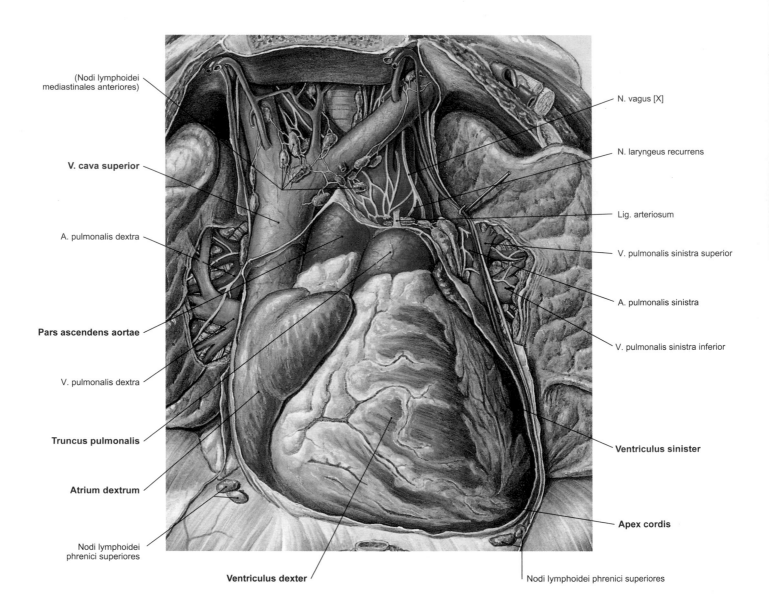

(Nodi lymphoidei mediastinales anteriores)

V. cava superior

A. pulmonalis dextra

Pars ascendens aortae

V. pulmonalis dextra

Truncus pulmonalis

Atrium dextrum

Nodi lymphoidei phrenici superiores

Ventriculus dexter

N. vagus [X]

N. laryngeus recurrens

Lig. arteriosum

V. pulmonalis sinistra superior

A. pulmonalis sinistra

V. pulmonalis sinistra inferior

Ventriculus sinister

Apex cordis

Nodi lymphoidei phrenici superiores

Fig. 5.50 Position of the heart, Cor, in the thorax, Situs cordis; ventral view; after opening of the pericardium. [S700]
The heart lies in the pericardial cavity (Cavitas pericardiaca) in the lower middle mediastinum. The heart has a broad base which is aligned upwards and to the right and which corresponds to the valve level at the source of the large vessels. The apex of the heart (Apex cordis) points downwards to the left and to the front. Base and apex are connected by the **longitudinal axis** (12 cm) which runs obliquely across the thorax from the right dorsally above to the left ventrally below and thus forms an **angle** of approximately 45° with all **three spatial planes.** The heart has four surfaces (→ Fig. 5.37). The anterior surface of the heart **(Facies sternocostalis)** is formed predominantly by the right ventricle. The inferior surface lies adjacent to the diaphragm **(Facies diaphragmatica)** and consists of parts of the right and left ventricles. Clinically, the inferior surface is a corresponding 'posterior wall' in ECG diagnostics, if, for example, it is a matter of posterior myocardial infarction. The **Facies pulmonalis** is encased by the right atrium on the right side and by the left ventricle on the left side.

Clinical remarks

For the physical exam of **trauma patients,** the abdominal anatomy is assessed by ultrasound (**FAST-sonography,** Focused Assessment with Sonography for Trauma) to identify internal bleeding. The ultrasound probe is positioned on the abdominal wall to scan longitudinal and cross-sections of the following four regions:
- Directed cranially below the costal arch to assess the **pericardium** for a potential pericardial tamponade

- Right side of the body to view the right **Recessus subphrenicus** and **Recessus subhepaticus** (Recessus hepatorenalis or MORISON's pouch), posterior and superior to the liver
- Left side of the body to view the left **Recessus subphrenicus** (Recessus splenorenalis or KOLLER's pouch) between the spleen and the kidney
- Above the pubic symphysis to view the **Excavatio rectouterina** (pouch of DOUGLAS) in women and the **Excavatio rectovesicalis** (PROUST's space) in men. (→ Fig. 6.19).

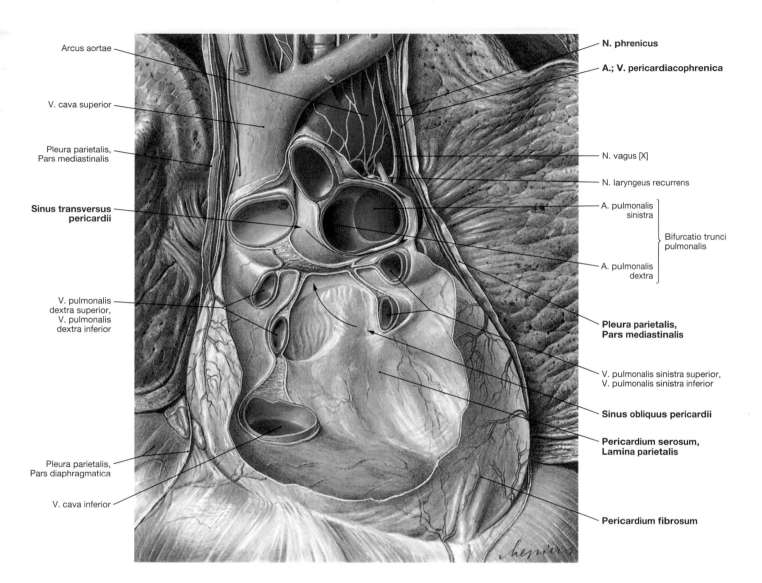

Arcus aortae

V. cava superior

Pleura parietalis,
Pars mediastinalis

**Sinus transversus
pericardii**

V. pulmonalis
dextra superior,
V. pulmonalis
dextra inferior

Pleura parietalis,
Pars diaphragmatica

V. cava inferior

N. phrenicus

A.; V. pericardiacophrenica

N. vagus [X]

N. laryngeus recurrens

A. pulmonalis
sinistra

Bifurcatio trunci
pulmonalis

A. pulmonalis
dextra

**Pleura parietalis,
Pars mediastinalis**

V. pulmonalis sinistra superior,
V. pulmonalis sinistra inferior

Sinus obliquus pericardii

**Pericardium serosum,
Lamina parietalis**

Pericardium fibrosum

Fig. 5.51 Pericardium; ventral view; after removal of the posterior wall of the pericardium and the heart. [S700]
The pericardium surrounds the heart, stabilises its position and enables the heart to contract without friction. The pericardium consists on the outside of a **Pericardium fibrosum** of dense connective tissue, on the inside of which and adjacent to lies a serosa as the **Pericardium serosum.** This part of the Pericardium serosum constitutes the Lamina parietalis, which, ventrally at the outflow of the large vessels, folds back onto the upper surface of the heart as the visceral layer (= **epicardium**). On the posterior side of the atria, the pericardial folds fold back onto the epicardium and form a vertical fold between the Vv. cavae inferior and superior and a horizontal fold between the upper pulmonary veins of the right and left sides. This creates two recesses on the posterior side of the pericardium (Sinus pericardii, see arrows):
- **Sinus transversus pericardii:** above the horizontal fold between the V. cava superior or aorta and Truncus pulmonalis
- **Sinus obliquus pericardii:** below the horizontal fold and between the pulmonary veins on both sides.

Structure and function

The **Pericardium fibrosum** is connected to:
- the Centrum tendineum of the diaphragm
- the posterior aspect of the sternum (Ligg. sternopericardiaca) and
- the tracheal bifurcation (Membrana bronchopericardiaca).

Adjacent to the Pericardium fibrosum is the **Pleura parietalis, Pars mediastinalis.** The N. phrenicus and the Vasa pericardiacophrenica runs between these two layers.
The epicardium is the visceral layer of the Pericardium serosum.

Pericardium

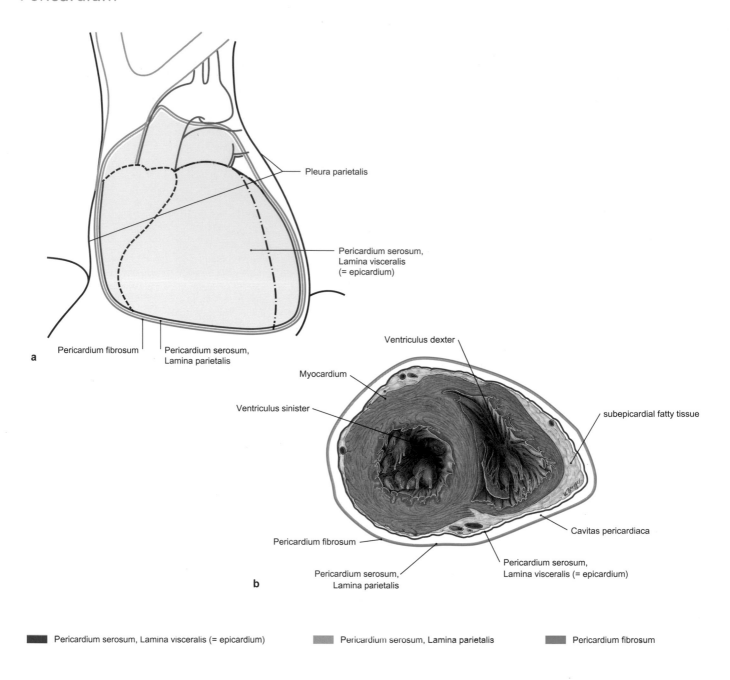

Pleura parietalis

Pericardium serosum,
Lamina visceralis
(= epicardium)

a Pericardium fibrosum · Pericardium serosum,
Lamina parietalis

Ventriculus dexter

Myocardium

Ventriculus sinister

subepicardial fatty tissue

Cavitas pericardiaca

Pericardium fibrosum

Pericardium serosum,
Lamina parietalis

Pericardium serosum,
Lamina visceralis (= epicardium)

b

Pericardium serosum, Lamina visceralis (= epicardium)   Pericardium serosum, Lamina parietalis   Pericardium fibrosum

Fig. 5.52a and b Layers of the pericardium; schematic illustration.
[S701-L231]
a Ventral view.
b Cross-section through the heart with caudal view.
The **Pericardium fibrosum** is the outer layer and consists of collagen-rich connective tissue. The inner Tunica serosa comprises simple epithelial cells (mesothelium) forming the **Pericardium serosum.** The

parietal layer (Lamina parietalis) of the serous pericardium is directly adjacent to the fibrous pericardium. At the proximal region of the large vessels of the heart, the parietal serous pericardium transitions onto the visceral layer (Lamina visceralis), covering the entire surface of the heart, the **epicardium.** Thus, the proximal parts of the Aorta ascendens, the Truncus pulmonalis and the V. cava superior are located within the pericardial sac at the level of the middle mediastinum.

┌ Clinical remarks

The pericardial cavity usually contains 15–35 ml of serous fluid. The pericardium, including the heart, has a total volume of 700–1,100 ml. With heart failure or inflammation of the pericardium **(pericarditis),** fluid can accumulate **(pericardial effusion)** and even affect cardiac output.
In the case of rupture of the heart wall after a heart attack or through an injury (knife stab), **cardiac tamponade** can ensue. Blood within the pericardial sac inhibits cardiac function which generally has a fatal result. [H043-001]

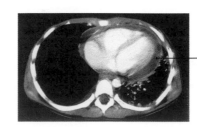

Pericardial effusion
(fluid in the pericardial sac)

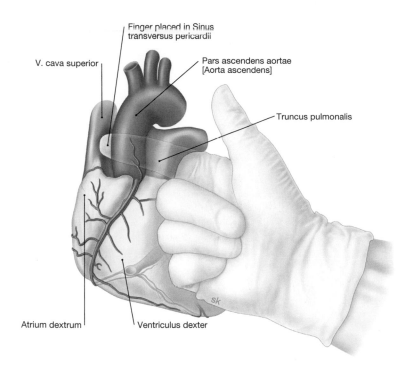

Fig. 5.53 **Sinus transversus pericardii;** schematic drawing, ventral view. [S701-L238]
The pericardial reflection onto the visceral layer (= epicardium) of the serous pericardium at the posterior aspects of the atria forms a vertical axis between Vv. cavae inferior and superior, and a horizontal axis between the superior pulmonary veins of the right and left side (→ Fig. 5.51). The Sinus transversus pericardii is positioned above the horizontal reflection line. When placing a finger in this sinus, the arteries (Aorta ascendens and Truncus pulmonalis) are positioned anterior and the V. cava superior is positioned posterior to the finger.

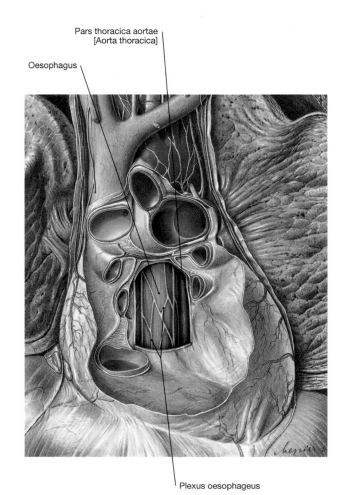

Fig. 5.54 **Sinus obliquus pericardii;** Ventral view after removal of the heart and fenestration of the posterior pericardium. [S700]
The **Sinus obliquus pericardii** is a pericardial space beneath the horizontal axis of the posterior pericardial reflection line and expands to the reflection line between the superior and inferior vena cava (V. cava superior and inferior) and is positioned between the pulmonary veins of both sides. The oesophagus and the vagus nerves (Plexus oesophageus) are located posterior to the Sinus obliquus pericardii.

Clinical remarks

The Sinus transversus pericardii and the Sinus obliquus pericardii are clinically important landmarks when connecting a **heart-lung machine** for open cardiac surgery or when an accessory **bundle for electrical conduction** needs to be **interrupted** to treat arrhythmias.

The proximity of the oesophagus to the left atrium of the heart (Atrium sinistrum) makes it possible to use ultrasound to show the heart valves emerging from the oesophagus **(transoesophageal echocardiography).**

Organs of the thoracic cavity

5

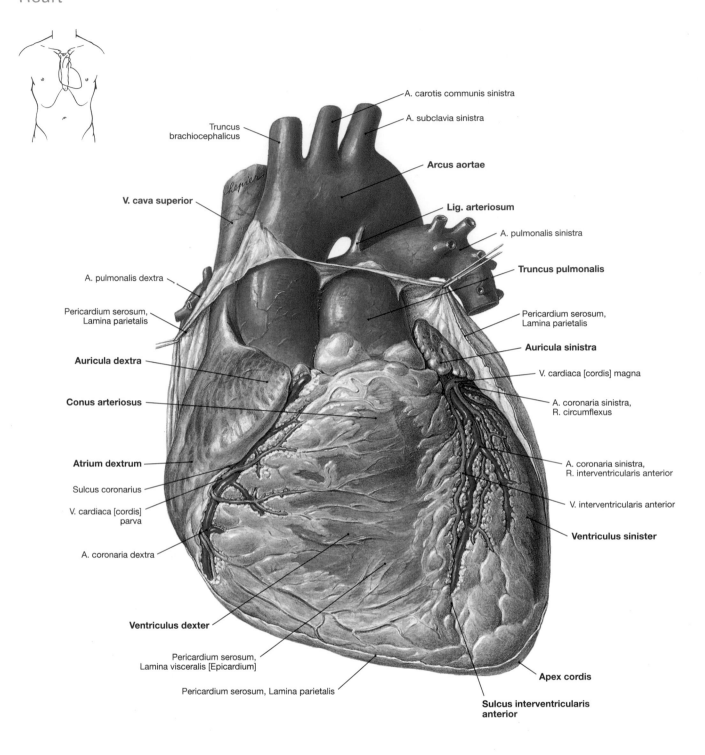

A. carotis communis sinistra

A. subclavia sinistra

Truncus brachiocephalicus

Arcus aortae

V. cava superior

Lig. arteriosum

A. pulmonalis sinistra

A. pulmonalis dextra

Truncus pulmonalis

Pericardium serosum, Lamina parietalis

Pericardium serosum, Lamina parietalis

Auricula dextra

Auricula sinistra

V. cardiaca [cordis] magna

Conus arteriosus

A. coronaria sinistra, R. circumflexus

Atrium dextrum

A. coronaria sinistra, R. interventricularis anterior

Sulcus coronarius

V. cardiaca [cordis] parva

V. interventricularis anterior

A. coronaria dextra

Ventriculus sinister

Ventriculus dexter

Pericardium serosum, Lamina visceralis [Epicardium]

Apex cordis

Pericardium serosum, Lamina parietalis

Sulcus interventricularis anterior

Fig. 5.55 Heart, Cor; ventral view. [S700]

The heart weighs 250–300 g and is approximately the size of the fist of each respective person. The apex of the heart (Apex cordis) faces downwards and to the left. The base corresponds to the position of the **Sulcus coronarius,** in which, among others, the A. coronaria dextra flows. The heart consists of a ventricular chamber (ventricle) and an atrial chamber (atrium) on the right and left side, respectively. On the anterior side (Facies sternocostalis), the **Sulcus interventricularis anterior** reveals the position of the cardiac septum (Septum interventriculare) and guides the R. interventricularis anterior of the A. coronaria sinistra. The boundary of the ventricle in the **Sulcus interventricularis**

posterior (→ Fig. 5.56) is on the inferior side (Facies diaphragmatica). Prior to its transition into the Truncus pulmonalis, the right ventricle expands to the Conus arteriosus. In contrast, the point of origin of the aorta from the left ventricle is not visible from outside due to the spiralling pathway of the aorta behind the Truncus pulmonalis. Therefore, the aorta originates to the right of the Truncus pulmonalis. The latter is connected to the Arcus aortae via the Lig. arteriosum, a developmental remnant of the Ductus arteriosus of the fetal circulation (→ Fig. 5.46). Both atria have a blind pouch, referred to as the right and left auricles (Auriculae dextra and sinistra). The Vv. cavae superior and inferior enter the right atrium, and the four pulmonary veins enter the left atrium.

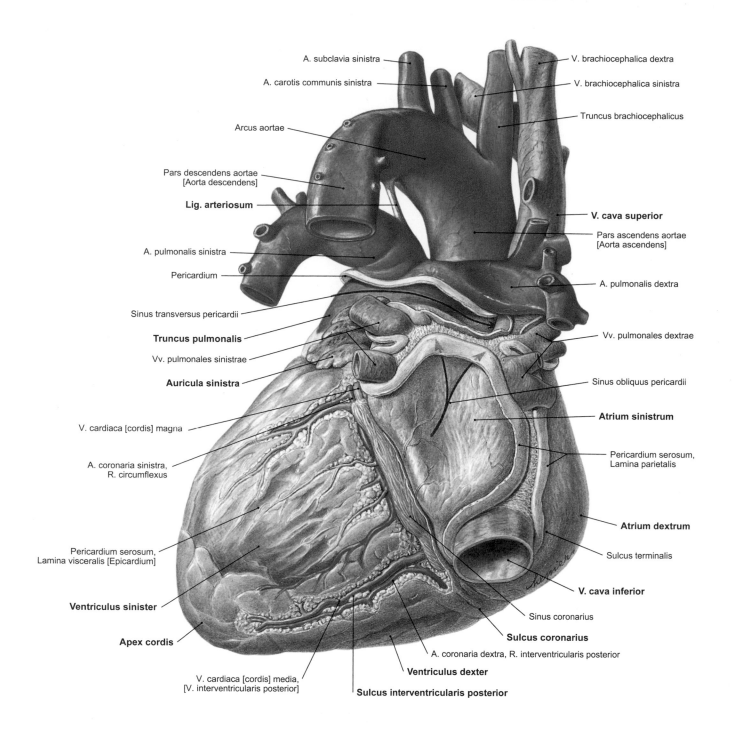

A. subclavia sinistra

A. carotis communis sinistra

Arcus aortae

Pars descendens aortae
[Aorta descendens]

Lig. arteriosum

A. pulmonalis sinistra

Pericardium

Sinus transversus pericardii

Truncus pulmonalis

Vv. pulmonales sinistrae

Auricula sinistra

V. cardiaca [cordis] magna

A. coronaria sinistra,
R. circumflexus

Pericardium serosum,
Lamina visceralis [Epicardium]

Ventriculus sinister

Apex cordis

V. cardiaca [cordis] media,
[V. interventricularis posterior]

V. brachiocephalica dextra

V. brachiocephalica sinistra

Truncus brachiocephalicus

V. cava superior

Pars ascendens aortae
[Aorta ascendens]

A. pulmonalis dextra

Vv. pulmonales dextrae

Sinus obliquus pericardii

Atrium sinistrum

Pericardium serosum,
Lamina parietalis

Atrium dextrum

Sulcus terminalis

V. cava inferior

Sinus coronarius

Sulcus coronarius

A. coronaria dextra, R. interventricularis posterior

Ventriculus dexter

Sulcus interventricularis posterior

Fig. 5.56 Heart, Cor; dorsal view (explanation → Fig. 5.55). [S700]

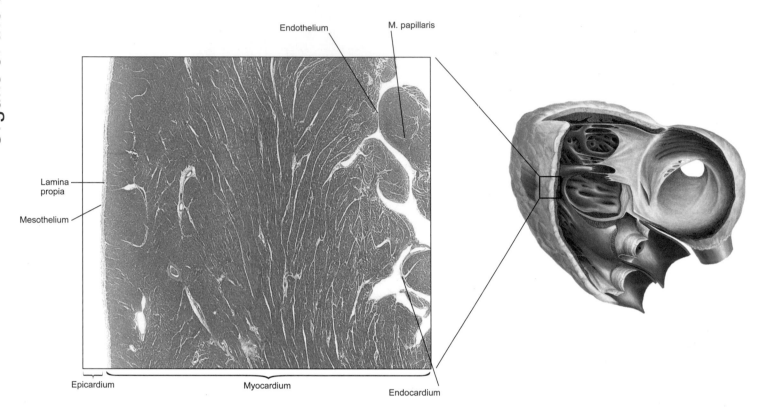

Fig. 5.57   Structure of the heart wall; section from the right atrium. [S700]/[G1192]

The wall of the heart is composed of three layers:

- **Endocardium:** inner surface consisting of endothelium and connective tissue

- **Myocardium:** cardiac muscle consisting of cardiomyocytes
- **Epicardium:** serosa and subserosa on the outer surface correspond to the visceral layer of the Pericardium serosum. In people, the subserosa contains a lot of fatty tissue, in which the blood vessels and nerves of the heart are embedded.

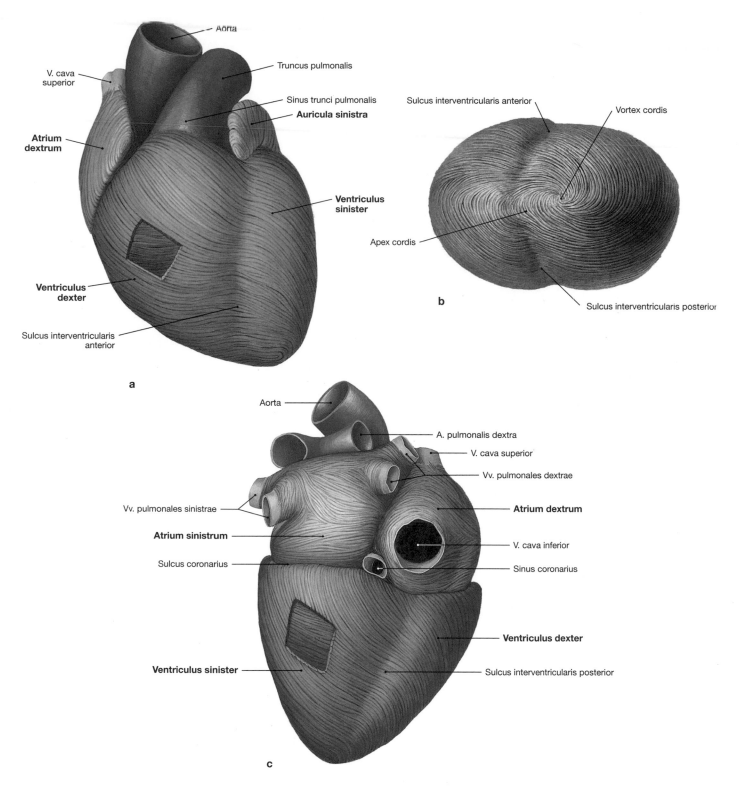

Fig. 5.58a–c Cardiac musculature, myocardium. [S700]
a Ventral view.
b View from the apex of the heart.
c Dorsal caudal view.
The heart muscle fibres are made up of individual cardiomyocytes and run spirally around the heart. In the wall of the atria and the right ventri-

cle they form two layers; in the case of the left ventricle even three layers. The myocardium and thereby also the entire heart wall is much thicker in the area of the left ventricle because the left ventricle has to pump blood into the systemic circulation at a higher pressure than the right ventricle. Wall thickness on the right is 3–5 mm, but 8–12 mm on the left.

Clinical remarks

Hypertrophy presents when the wall thickness of the **left ventricle is over 15 mm,** which may be caused by arterial hypertension or an aortic valve stenosis. With the **right ventricle,** hypertrophy is already present at **more than 5 mm.** In addition to pulmonary valve stenosis,

another cause that should be considered is pulmonary hypertension caused by chronic obstructive pulmonary diseases such as asthma or by a pulmonary embolism.

Organs of the thoracic cavity

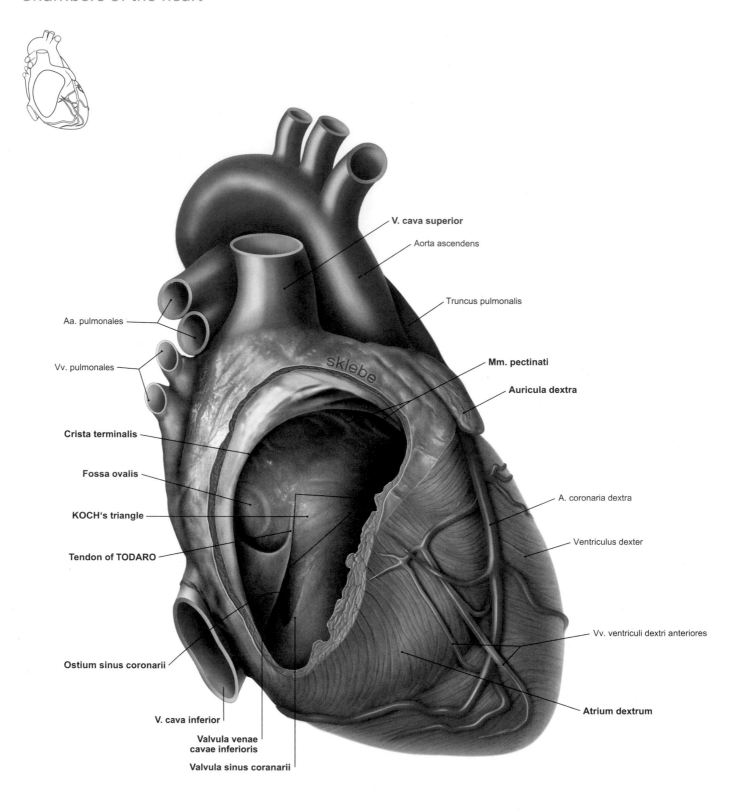

- V. cava superior
- Aorta ascendens
- Truncus pulmonalis
- Aa. pulmonales
- Vv. pulmonales
- sklebe
- **Mm. pectinati**
- **Auricula dextra**
- **Crista terminalis**
- **Fossa ovalis**
- **KOCH's triangle**
- **Tendon of TODARO**
- A. coronaria dextra
- Ventriculus dexter
- Vv. ventriculi dextri anteriores
- **Ostium sinus coronarii**
- **V. cava inferior**
- **Valvula venae cavae inferioris**
- **Valvula sinus coranarii**
- **Atrium dextrum**

Fig. 5.59 Right atrium, Atrium dextrum; view from the right side after fenestration of the right atrium. [S700-L238]

The right atrium **(Atrium dextrum)** is the most complex chamber of the heart featuring several specific structures. The superior and inferior venae cavae **(V. cava superior** and **V. cava inferior)** as well as the coronary sinus **(Sinus coronarius)** enter the right atrium. The inferior vena cava and the coronary sinus both have a valve which confines the opening **(Valvula venae cavae inferioris** and **Valvula sinus coronarii).** The valve of the inferior vena cava continues as the **TODARO's tendon** (Tendo valvulae venae cavae inferioris) and inserts into the cardiac skel-

eton beneath the endocardium. The TODARO's tendon and the valve of the coronary sinus together with the septal cusp of the atrioventricular valve form the boundary of the **KOCH's triangle,** a landmark for the position of the AV-node of the cardiac conduction system. Opposite to the opening of the inferior vena cava is the **Fossa ovalis,** a relict of the fetal circulation. Unusually, this illustration clearly visualises the **Crista terminalis,** a crest-like protrusion separating the smooth-walled part of the atrium between the two venae cavae from the muscular part featuring the **Mm. pectinati.** Anteriorly, the atrium extends to connect to the right auricle **(Auricula dextra).**

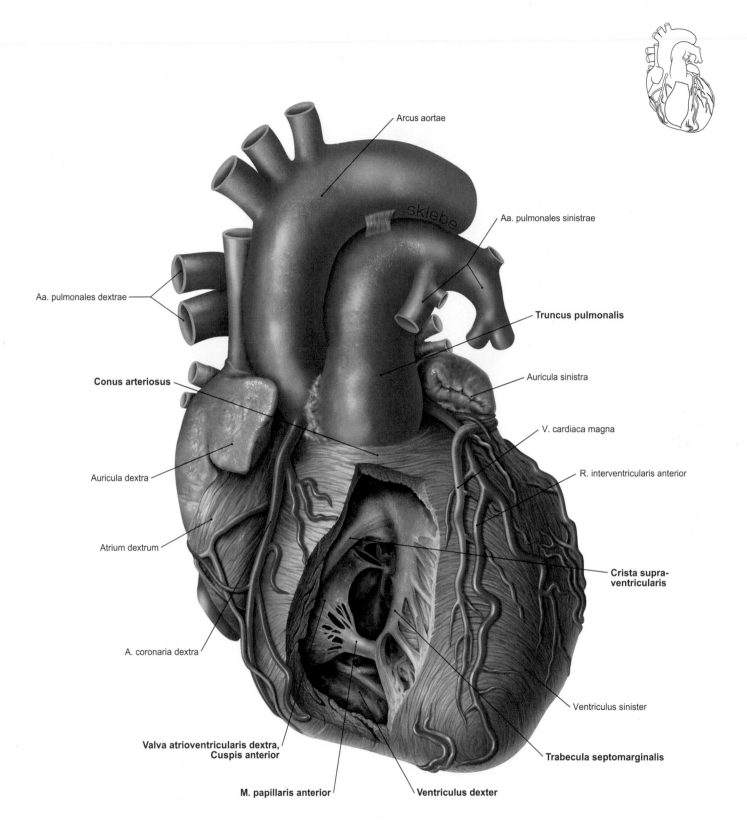

Arcus aortae

Aa. pulmonales sinistrae

Truncus pulmonalis

Auricula sinistra

V. cardiaca magna

R. interventricularis anterior

Crista supra-
ventricularis

Ventriculus sinister

Trabecula septomarginalis

Ventriculus dexter

Aa. pulmonales dextrae

Conus arteriosus

Auricula dextra

Atrium dextrum

A. coronaria dextra

Valva atrioventricularis dextra,
Cuspis anterior

M. papillaris anterior

Fig. 5.60 Right ventricle, Ventriculus dexter; ventral view after fenestration of the right chamber. [S700-L238]
The opening in the anterior wall of the **right ventricle (Ventriculus dexter)** reveals the inner structures in place. The **right atrioventricular valve (Valva atrioventricularis)** connects to the right atrium. Blood entering the right ventricle from the right atrium (inflow tract) is directed around the **Crista supraventricularis** through the wide **Conus arteriosus** into the Truncus pulmonalis (outflow tract).

The prominent **Trabecula septomarginalis** connects the interventricular septum to the anterior papillary muscle **(M. papillaris anterior).** It contains fibres of the conducting system (LEONARDO DA VINCI's moderator band).

Chambers of the heart

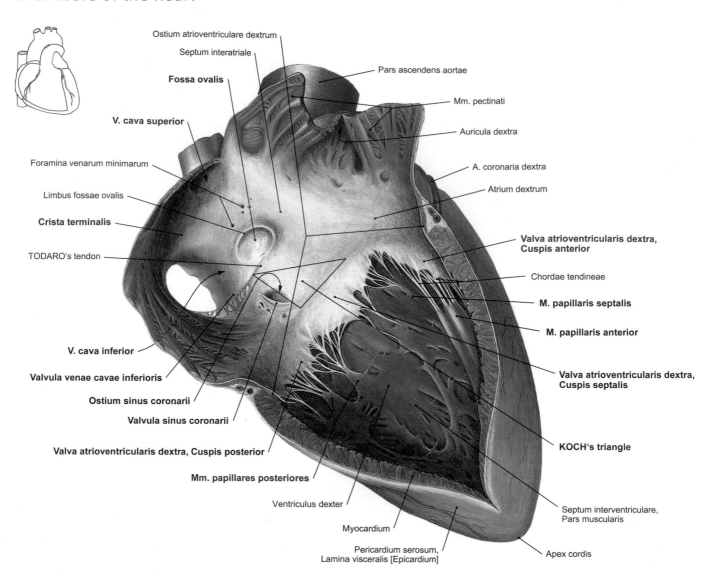

Fig. 5.61 **Right atrium, Atrium dextrum, and right ventricle, Ventriculus dexter;** ventral view. [S700]

The right atrium consists of a part with a smooth inner surface, the atrial sinus (Sinus venarum cavarum), and the rough inner surface of a muscular part, which consists of pectinate muscles (Mm. pectinati). Between the two parts lies the **Crista terminalis,** which serves as an important landmark because the sinus node of the electrical stimulation and conduction system is located on the outside (subepicardial) between the opening of the V. cava superior and the right auricle (Auricula dextra; → Fig. 5.67). The interatrial septum (Septum interatriale) shows a remnant of the Foramen ovale, the **Fossa ovalis,** the edge of which is raised to the Limbus fossae ovalis. The opening of the **Sinus coronarius** (Ostium sinus coronarii), which depicts the largest cardiac vein, is flanked by a valve (Valvula sinus coronarii) similar to the opening of the V. cava inferior (Valvula venae cavae inferioris); both of them, however, do not close the lumen. Even small cardiac veins discharge directly into the right atrium (Foramina venarum minimarum). The TODARO's tendon (Tendo valvulae venae cavae inferioris) is an extension of the Valvula venae cavae inferioris. It also serves as a significant landmark because together with the opening of the coronary sinus and the tricuspid valve (Valva atrioventricularis dextra), it delineates the **KOCH's triangle,** in which the AV node is located (→ Fig. 5.74 to → Fig. 5.76). In the right ventricle, the three cusps are attached via tendinous cords (Chordae tendineae) to three **papillary muscles** (Mm. papillares anterior, posterior and septalis). Of the Septum interventriculare only the muscular part is visible here. Fibres (not visible here) of the electrical conduction system (LEONARDO DA VINCI's moderator band) reach from here to the anterior papillary muscle. This connection is referred to as the **Trabecula septomarginalis** (→ Fig. 5.76).

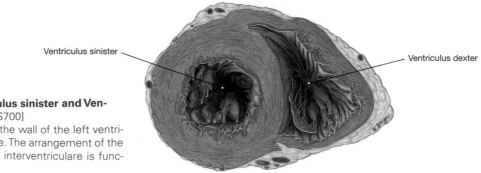

Fig. 5.62 **Left and right ventricles, Ventriculus sinister and Ventriculus dexter;** cross-section, cranial view. [S700]

With the substantially stronger muscle layer, the wall of the left ventricle is thicker than the wall of the right ventricle. The arrangement of the heart muscle cells indicates that the Septum interventriculare is functionally a part of the left ventricle.

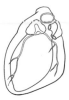

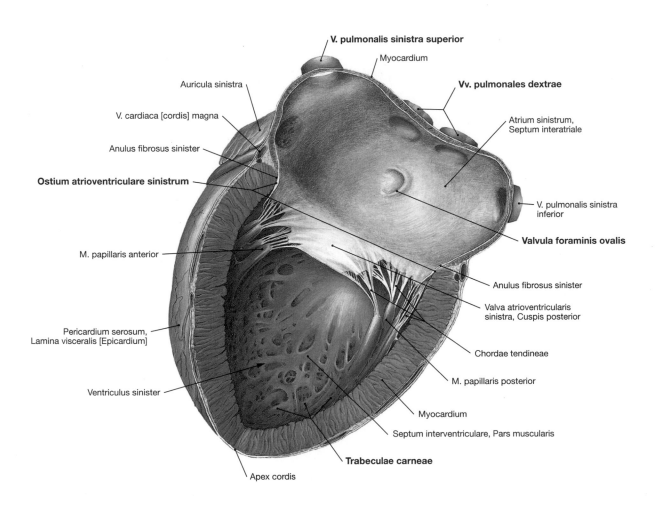

V. pulmonalis sinistra superior

Myocardium

Auricula sinistra

V. cardiaca [cordis] magna

Anulus fibrosus sinister

Ostium atrioventriculare sinistrum

M. papillaris anterior

Pericardium serosum,
Lamina visceralis [Epicardium]

Ventriculus sinister

Apex cordis

Vv. pulmonales dextrae

Atrium sinistrum,
Septum interatriale

V. pulmonalis sinistra
inferior

Valvula foraminis ovalis

Anulus fibrosus sinister

Valva atrioventricularis
sinistra, Cuspis posterior

Chordae tendineae

M. papillaris posterior

Myocardium

Septum interventriculare, Pars muscularis

Trabeculae carneae

Fig. 5.63   Left atrium, Atrium sinistrum, and left ventricle, Ventriculus sinister; lateral view. [S700]
The left atrium contains the left auricle (Auricula sinistra). Four pulmonary veins (Vv. pulmonales) enter the atrium. The Valvula foraminis ovalis obtrudes as a crescent-shaped mucosal fold at the septal wall. It is a

remnant of the Septum primum during the heart development (→ Fig. 5.42). The Ostium atrioventriculare sinistrum contains the Valva mitralis and connects to the left ventricle. The wall of the ventricle is not smooth but roughened by muscle trabeculae (Trabeculae carneae).

Chambers of the heart

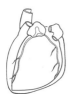

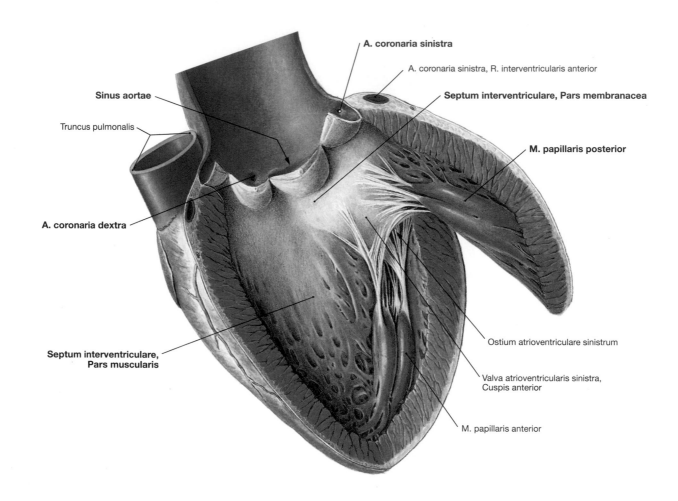

A. coronaria sinistra

A. coronaria sinistra, R. interventricularis anterior

Sinus aortae

Septum interventriculare, Pars membranacea

Truncus pulmonalis

M. papillaris posterior

A. coronaria dextra

Septum interventriculare, Pars muscularis

Ostium atrioventriculare sinistrum

Valva atrioventricularis sinistra, Cuspis anterior

M. papillaris anterior

Fig. 5.64   Left ventricle, Ventriculus sinister; lateral view. [S700] Beneath the left atrioventricular valve lies the roughly 1 cm² large area of the **membranous part (Pars membranacea)** of the ventricular septum. In contrast, the largest part of the ventricular septum consists of the muscular part (Pars muscularis). Behind the semilunar valves of the aortic valve are the **Sinus aortae (VALSALVIA),** in which the right and left **coronary arteries** (Aa. coronariae dextra and sinistra) originate.

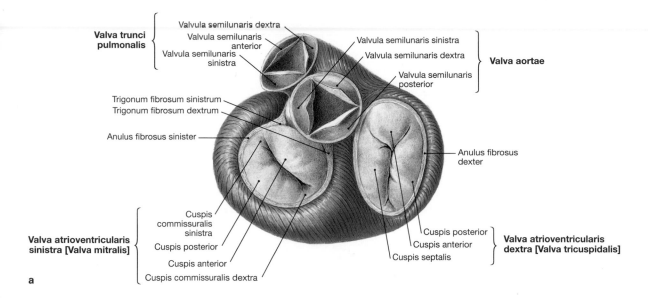

Valva trunci pulmonalis
Valvula semilunaris dextra
Valvula semilunaris anterior
Valvula semilunaris sinistra

Valvula semilunaris sinistra
Valvula semilunaris dextra
Valvula semilunaris posterior
Valva aortae

Trigonum fibrosum sinistrum
Trigonum fibrosum dextrum

Anulus fibrosus sinister

Anulus fibrosus dexter

Cuspis commissuralis sinistra
Cuspis posterior
Cuspis anterior
Cuspis commissuralis dextra

Valva atrioventricularis sinistra [Valva mitralis]

Cuspis posterior
Cuspis anterior
Cuspis septalis

Valva atrioventricularis dextra [Valva tricuspidalis]

a

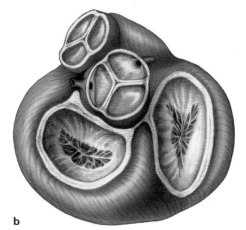

b

Fig. 5.65a and b   Heart valves, Valvae cordis; cranial view, after removal of the atria, aorta and Truncus pulmonalis.
a View with open semilunar valves during systole. [S700]
b View with open atrioventricular valves during diastole. [S701-L285]
The heart has two **cuspidal valves** (Valvae cuspidales), each of them between the atria and the ventricles. The right atrioventricular valve (Valva atrioventricularis dextra) consists of three cusps **(tricuspid valve).** The left atrioventricular valve (Valva atrioventricularis sinistra) is formed from two cusps **(mitral valve).** Both atrioventricular valves comprise a thinner peripheral (atrial) zone and a thicker central coaptation zone that facilitates the tight closure of the valves. The cuspidal valves are anchored to the papillary muscles via tendinous cords (Chordae tendineae), which prevent prolapse of the valves. Between the ventricles and large vessels there is the **aortic valve** (Valva aortae**)** on the left and the **pulmonary valve** (Valva trunci pulmonalis) on the right side, both of which are formed by three semilunar cusps (Valvulae semilunares). In the ejection phase of the **systole,** when blood is ejected from the ventricles into the large vessels, the **semilunar valves are open** and the cuspidal valves closed. In the filling phase of the **diastole,** the **cuspidal valves are open** in order to take blood from the atria into the ventricles. The semilunar valves are closed.

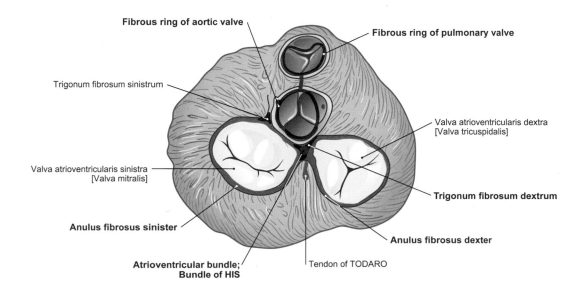

Fibrous ring of aortic valve

Fibrous ring of pulmonary valve

Trigonum fibrosum sinistrum

Valva atrioventricularis dextra [Valva tricuspidalis]

Valva atrioventricularis sinistra [Valva mitralis]

Trigonum fibrosum dextrum

Anulus fibrosus sinister

Anulus fibrosus dexter

Atrioventricular bundle; Bundle of HIS

Tendon of TODARO

Fig. 5.66   Cardiac skeleton; cranial view, schematic diagram. [S700-L126]/[(B500~M282/L240]
The cardiac valves are anchored to the cardiac skeleton. This consists of connective tissue that forms a ring (Anuli fibrosi dexter and sinister) each time around the atrioventricular valves (Valvae atrioventriculares) as well as a fibrous ring around the semilunar valves. Between the Anuli fibrosi lies the Trigonum fibrosum dextrum through which the bundle

of HIS of the cardiac conduction system passes from the right atrium into the Septum interventriculare. In addition to the **stabilisation of the heart valves** the cardiac skeleton also serves as an **electrical insulation of the atria and ventricles,** because all the muscle cells of the heart are attached to the cardiac skeleton and thus do not encroach on the ventricles from the atria. Thus, the stimulus is transmitted to the ventricles only via the bundle of HIS.

Heart valves

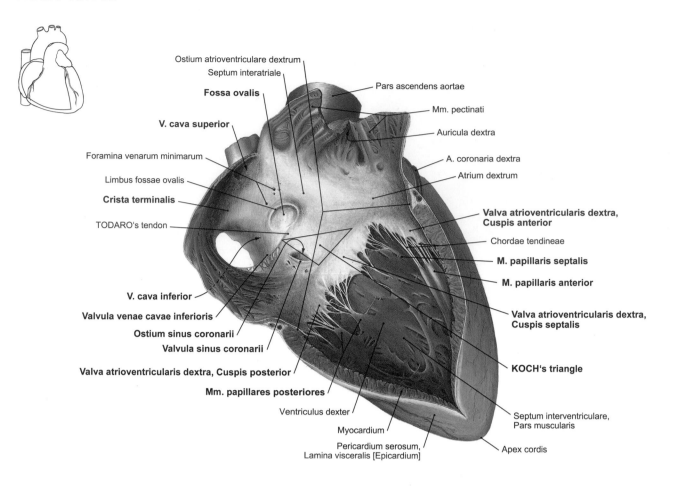

Ostium atrioventriculare dextrum
Septum interatriale
Fossa ovalis
V. cava superior
Foramina venarum minimarum
Limbus fossae ovalis
Crista terminalis
TODARO's tendon
V. cava inferior
Valvula venae cavae inferioris
Ostium sinus coronarii
Valvula sinus coronarii
Valva atrioventricularis dextra, Cuspis posterior
Mm. papillares posteriores
Ventriculus dexter
Myocardium
Pericardium serosum, Lamina visceralis [Epicardium]

Pars ascendens aortae
Mm. pectinati
Auricula dextra
A. coronaria dextra
Atrium dextrum
Valva atrioventricularis dextra, Cuspis anterior
Chordae tendineae
M. papillaris septalis
M. papillaris anterior
Valva atrioventricularis dextra, Cuspis septalis
KOCH's triangle
Septum interventriculare, Pars muscularis
Apex cordis

Fig. 5.67 Right atrioventricular valve, Valva atrioventricularis dextra; ventral view. [S700]
The right atrium and the right ventricle are separated by the tricuspid valve (Valva atrioventricularis dextra). This consists of **three cusps (Cuspis anterior, posterior, septalis)** which are attached via tendinous cords (Chordae tendineae) to three **papillary muscles** (Mm. papillares anterior, posterior and septal). Through active contraction of the papillary muscles during ventricle contraction, the cusps can be prevented from prolapsing back into the atrium.

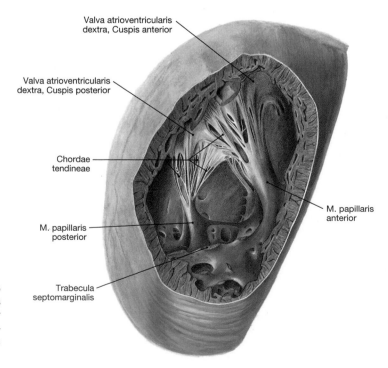

Valva atrioventricularis dextra, Cuspis anterior
Valva atrioventricularis dextra, Cuspis posterior
Chordae tendineae
M. papillaris posterior
Trabecula septomarginalis
M. papillaris anterior

Fig. 5.68 Papillary muscles of the right atrioventricular valve, Valva atrioventricularis dextra; dorsal view. [S700]
The right ventricle is opened from the septum onwards, showing two of the three **papillary muscles** (Mm. papillares). The **tendinous cords** (Chordae tendineae) connect the M. papillaris anterior with the anterior cusp (Cuspis anterior) of the tricuspid valve (Valva atrioventricularis dextra) and the posterior papillary muscle with the posterior cusp (Cuspis posterior).

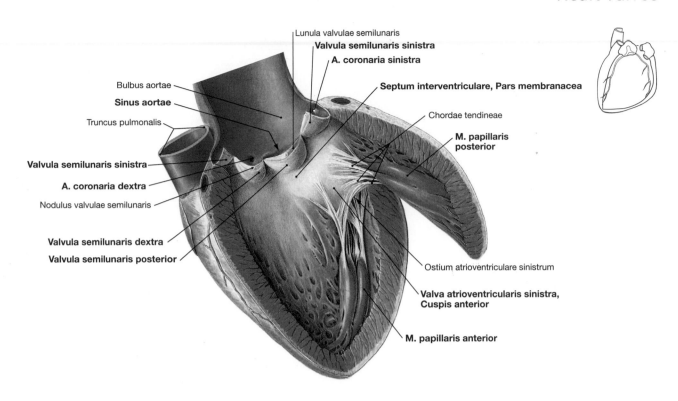

Lunula valvulae semilunaris
Valvula semilunaris sinistra
A. coronaria sinistra
Septum interventriculare, Pars membranacea

Bulbus aortae
Sinus aortae
Truncus pulmonalis

Chordae tendineae
M. papillaris posterior

Valvula semilunaris sinistra
A. coronaria dextra
Nodulus valvulae semilunaris

Valvula semilunaris dextra
Valvula semilunaris posterior

Ostium atrioventriculare sinistrum
Valva atrioventricularis sinistra, Cuspis anterior

M. papillaris anterior

Fig. 5.69   Left atrioventricular valve, Valva atrioventricularis sinistra, and aortic valve, Valva aortae; lateral view. [S700]
The mitral valve (Valva atrioventricularis sinistra) is only composed of **two cusps (Cuspis anterior and posterior)** which are further subdivided anterolaterally and posteromedially into smaller parts (Cuspides commissurales). Correspondingly there are only two **papillary muscles** (Mm. papillares anterior and posterior). Blood is ejected via the **aortic valve (Valva aortae),** which consists of three semilunar valves (Valvulae semilunares dextra, sinistra and posterior), into the expanded part of the aorta (Bulbus aortae).

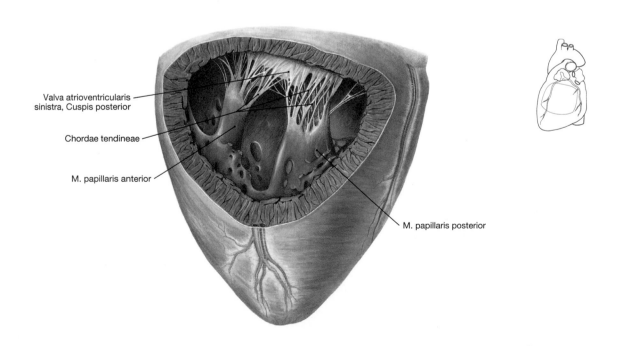

Valva atrioventricularis sinistra, Cuspis posterior

Chordae tendineae

M. papillaris anterior

M. papillaris posterior

Fig. 5.70   Papillary muscles of the left atrioventricular valve, Valva atrioventricularis sinistra; ventral cranial view. [S700]
The left ventricle is opened in such a way that the two **papillary muscles** of the mitral valve can be identified. The **tendinous cords (Chordae tendineae)** connect the M. papillaris anterior with the anterior cusp (Cuspis anterior) of the Valva atrioventricularis sinistra, and the M. papillaris posterior with the posterior cusp (Cuspis posterior).

Heart

Projection of the heart valves

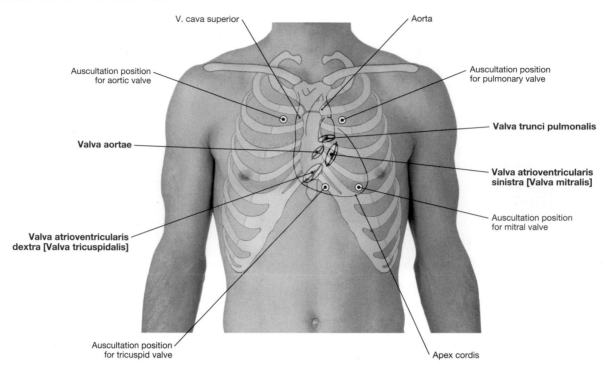

V. cava superior

Aorta

Auscultation position
for aortic valve

Auscultation position
for pulmonary valve

Valva trunci pulmonalis

Valva aortae

**Valva atrioventricularis
sinistra [Valva mitralis]**

Auscultation position
for mitral valve

**Valva atrioventricularis
dextra [Valva tricuspidalis]**

Auscultation position
for tricuspid valve

Apex cordis

Fig. 5.71 Projection of the heart valves and auscultation sites on the anterior thoracic wall. [S701-J803/L126]
The **projection of the four heart valves** forms a cross, slightly shifted to the left from the median plane. The projection of the valves is of mi-nor practical importance as heart sounds and also heart murmurs, which may arise in the region of the valves, are transmitted with the blood stream to points of auscultation (circles).

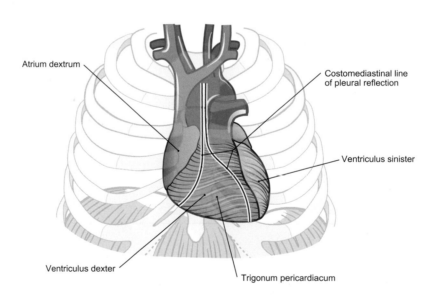

Atrium dextrum

Costomediastinal line
of pleural reflection

Ventriculus sinister

Ventriculus dexter

Trigonum pericardiacum

Fig. 5.72 Projection of the heart onto the rib cage; ventral view.
[S701-L126]/[B500-L240~M282]

The right atrium points to the right, while the right ventricle is positioned anteriorly and thereby directly behind the sternum. The left atrium and the left ventricle are located on the left side of the body.

Projection and points of auscultation of the cardiac valves		
Heart valves	**Projection points**	**Auscultation sites**
Pulmonary valve	Left (!) sternal border, third costal cartilage	Second ICS left parasternal
Aortic valve	Left sternal border, third ICS	Second ICS right parasternal
Mitral valve	Fourth to fifth costal cartilages on the left	Fifth ICS left in the midclavicular line
Tricuspid valve	Behind the sternum, fifth costal cartilage	Fifth ICS right parasternal

ICS = intercostal space

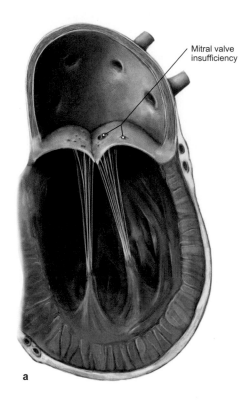

Mitral valve
insufficiency

a

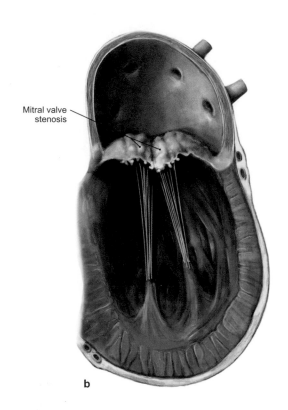

Mitral valve
stenosis

b

Fig. 5.73 Pathological change of the heart valves using the example of the mitral valve. [S702-L266]
a Mitral insufficiency.
b Mitral stenosis.
Besides congenital stenoses of the heart valves, which are regarded as heart defects (vitia), other defects or deformations of the heart valves, which accompany an **insufficiency or stenosis of the valves,** can en-

sue, caused for example by **inflammatory processes** or **degenerative changes.**
Malfunctioning heart valves can be replaced by **artificial valves or porcine heart valves** if the heart function is compromised. Valves can be introduced surgically in transthoracic open heart surgery or via a catheter (TAVI, transcatheter aortioc valve implantation). Mitral and aortic valves are increasingly repaired in the case of cardiac failure.

Clinical remarks

When listening to the heart with a stethoscope **(auscultation)**, one hears the **heart sounds** at various points, resulting from cardiac output:
- The **first heart sound** is created at the beginning of the systole by the ventricular contraction and snapping shut of the cuspidal valves.
- The **second heart sound** is generated at the beginning of the diastole by the closure of the semilunar valves.

Heart murmurs, however, are not present in healthy people and are caused by malfunction of the valves. Both narrowing (stenosis) as well as insufficient closure (failure) of the valves may cause murmurs. The timing of the murmur and its localisation give information on the malfunction of the respective valves.

The murmurs are loudest at the respective auscultation points of the valves. If during the **systole** (i. e. between the first and second heart sounds), a murmur occurs above a **cuspidal valve,** this means there is a **failure** because the valve should be closed at this stage. If a murmur can be heard in the **diastole** above the cuspidal valve, this suggests a **stenosis** since the valve should be open in the filling phase. With the **semilunar valves** it is exactly **the opposite.** Stenoses can be either congenital or acquired (rheumatic diseases, bacterial endocarditis). Failures are usually acquired and can also be caused by heart attacks if the papillary muscles, which anchor the cuspidal valves, are damaged.

Electrical stimulation and conduction system of the heart

Organs of the thoracic cavity

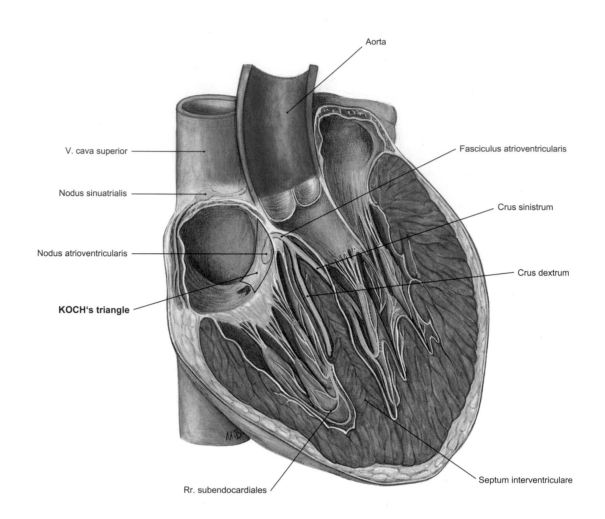

Aorta

V. cava superior

Nodus sinuatrialis

Nodus atrioventricularis

KOCH's triangle

Fasciculus atrioventricularis

Crus sinistrum

Crus dextrum

Septum interventriculare

Rr. subendocardiales

Fig. 5.74 Electrical stimulation and conduction system along the cardiac axis of a sectioned heart. [S700]

The heart has an electrical stimulation and conduction system that is built from modified heart muscle cells (no nerve fibres!). It is divided into four parts:

• **Sinus nodes** (Nodus sinuatrialis, KEITH-FLACK nodes)
• **AV nodes** (Nodus atrioventricularis, ASCHOFF-TAWARA nodes)
• **Atrioventricular bundle** (Fasciculus atrioventricularis, bundle of HIS)
• **Bundle branches** (Crura dextrum and sinistrum, TAWARA branches).

The electrical stimulation is initiated independently within the sinus node by spontaneous depolarisation of the muscle cells and has a frequency of approximately 70/min. The **Nodus sinuatrialis (sinus node)** is approximately 3 × 10 mm large and is located in the wall of the right atrium subepicardially within a groove (Sulcus terminalis cordis) between the confluence of the V. cava superior and the right auricle, which corresponds to the Crista terminalis on the inner surface. Sometimes the node is covered by subepicardial fat so that it is visible to the naked eye. The sinus node has its own artery (R. nodi sinuatrialis), which usually originates from the A. coronaria dextra. From the Nodus sinuatrialis, stimulation is conducted via the myocardium of the atrium to the **AV node,** which slightly delays the stimulation in order to allow adequate filling of the ventricle.

The AV node is approx. 5 × 3 mm large and is located at the tip of KOCH's triangle, embedded into the myocardium of the atrioventricular septum. The KOCH's triangle is confined by the TODARO's tendon, the opening of the Sinus coronarius and the septal cusp of the tricuspid valve (→ Fig. 5.67). The AV node also has its own arterial supply (R. nodi atrioventricularis), which usually originates from the dominant coronary artery (in most cases the A. coronaria dextra) near the outflow of the R. interventricularis posterior.

From the AV node, the electrical signal is conveyed by the **bundle of HIS** (approx. 4 × 20 mm), which passes through the right fibrous trigone, into the ventricular septum.

In the membranous part of the septum, the bundle of HIS divides into the **bundle branches.** The left TAWARA branch divides into an anterior, a septal and a posterior fascicle to the respective parts of the myocardium, including to the papillary muscles as well as to the apex of the heart. The right bundle branch descends subendocardially within the septum to the apex of the heart and reaches the anterior papillary muscle via the Trabecula septomarginalis (→ Fig. 5.76).

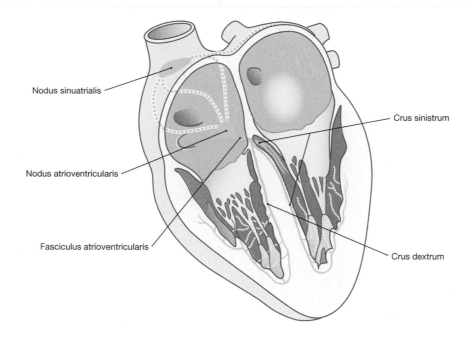

Nodus sinuatrialis

Nodus atrioventricularis

Fasciculus atrioventricularis

Crus sinistrum

Crus dextrum

Fig. 5.75 Electrical stimulation and conduction system of the heart; schematic diagram. [S700-L126]

The dotted lines in the area of the atria indicate that the area of stimulation here does not occur through specialised myocardial tissue, but through the normal working myocardium.

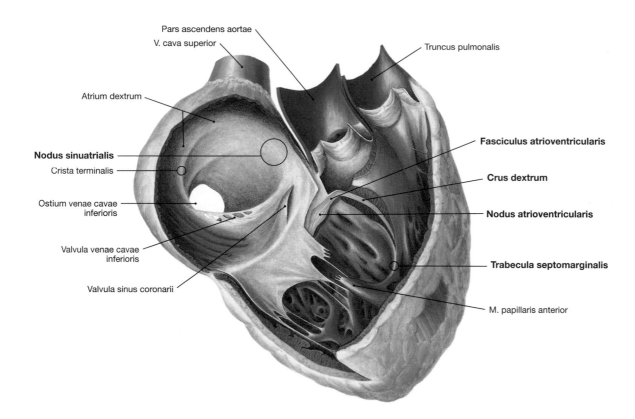

Pars ascendens aortae

V. cava superior

Truncus pulmonalis

Atrium dextrum

Nodus sinuatrialis

Crista terminalis

Ostium venae cavae inferioris

Valvula venae cavae inferioris

Valvula sinus coronarii

Fasciculus atrioventricularis

Crus dextrum

Nodus atrioventricularis

Trabecula septomarginalis

M. papillaris anterior

Fig. 5.76 Electrical stimulation and conduction system of the heart. [S700]

The electrical stimulation and conduction system is divided into **four parts** (→ Fig. 5.74).

In the illustration it is clearly visible how a part of the right bundle branch (Crus dextrum) reaches the right anterior papillary muscle via the **Trabecula septomarginalis**.

Electrical stimulation and conduction system of the heart

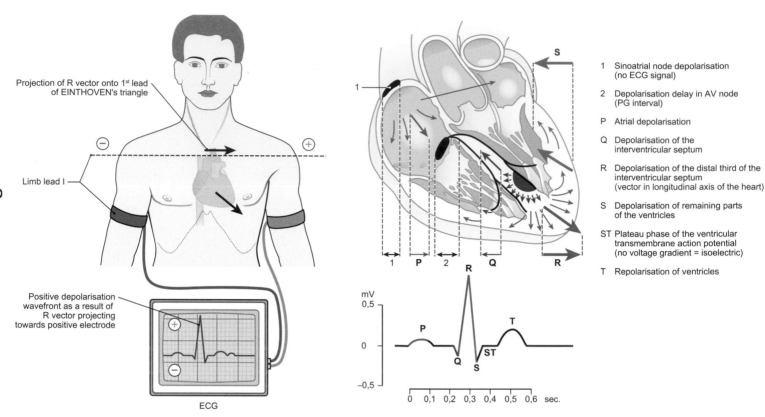

Projection of R vector onto 1st lead of EINTHOVEN's triangle

Limb lead I

Positive depolarisation wavefront as a result of R vector projecting towards positive electrode

ECG

1　Sinoatrial node depolarisation (no ECG signal)

2　Depolarisation delay in AV node (PG interval)

P　Atrial depolarisation

Q　Depolarisation of the interventricular septum

R　Depolarisation of the distal third of the interventricular septum (vector in longitudinal axis of the heart)

S　Depolarisation of remaining parts of the ventricles

ST　Plateau phase of the ventricular transmembrane action potential (no voltage gradient = isoelectric)

T　Repolarisation of ventricles

Fig. 5.77　Anatomical fundamentals of an electrocardiogram (ECG). [S700-L126]/[B500~M282/L132]

The electrical stimulation or excitation spreads from the sinus node and, after conduction delay in the AV node, is transmitted by the bundle of HIS to the Septum interventriculare. The bundle branches divide and finally stimulate the ventricle muscles. This excitation propagation can be diverted by electrodes to the surface of the body. If the excitation travels towards the electrodes on the surface of the body, a positive upsurge ensues. Sinus node stimulation is not discernible due to the small volume of the node. The **P wave** corresponds to the stimulation of the atria. The stimulation delay in the AV node occurs during the PQ segment, in which the entire atrial myocardium is stimulated and thus no change in potential is discernible. The **Q wave** results from a temporary downward excitation propagation in the interventricular septum. The ascending branch of the **R wave** is caused by excitation propagation to the apex of the heart, the descending branch and the **S wave** due to propagation away from the apex of the heart. During the ST segment, the entire ventricular myocardium is stimulated. Since repolarisation occurs in reverse order, the **T wave** shows a positive upsurge on the ECG again. Because typically at least three limb leads are taken up, one can determine the electrical axis and thereby the normal axis from the deflection with the largest R wave. The electrical cardiac axis is, however, not identical to the anatomical cardiac axis, because the muscle mass of the two ventricles and the electrical excitability of the tissue also have an influence.

Clinical remarks

An ECG can establish heart rhythm disorders, where the heart beats too quickly **(tachycardia, > 100/min),** too slowly **(bradycardia, < 60/min)** or simply irregularly **(arrhythmia).** In addition, however, circulatory disorders in coronary heart disease (e. g. heart attack) and other diseases, such as inflammation of the myocardium, also influence excitation propagation. The ECG is of particular importance for the identification of a myocardial infarction.

If atrial fibres bypass the AV node and directly link to the bundle of HIS or the ventricular myocardium (bundle of KENT), cardiac arrhythmias can also ensue **(WOLFF-PARKINSON-WHITE syndrome).** If these arrhythmias produce unpleasant symptoms and do not respond to medication, then the accessory pathways must by cut off by cardiac catheters.

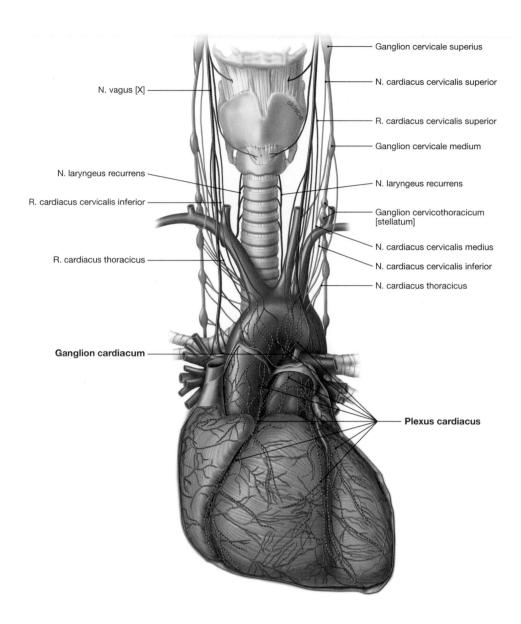

N. vagus [X]

N. laryngeus recurrens

R. cardiacus cervicalis inferior

R. cardiacus thoracicus

Ganglion cardiacum

Ganglion cervicale superius

N. cardiacus cervicalis superior

R. cardiacus cervicalis superior

Ganglion cervicale medium

N. laryngeus recurrens

Ganglion cervicothoracicum [stellatum]

N. cardiacus cervicalis medius

N. cardiacus cervicalis inferior

N. cardiacus thoracicus

Plexus cardiacus

Fig. 5.78 Innervation of the heart: Plexus cardiacus with sympathetic (green) and parasympathetic (purple) nerve fibres; schematic diagram. [S700-L238]

The function of the electrical conduction system and the working myocardium can be adapted by autonomic innervation to the capacity needs of the whole body. This part of the autonomic nervous system is the **Plexus cardiacus,** which contains both sympathetic and parasympathetic nerve fibres. The **sympathetic fibres** are postganglionic nerve fibres, the cell bodies (perikarya) of which are localised within the neck ganglia of the Truncus sympathicus, and reach the Plexus cardiacus via three nerves (the Nn. cardiaci cervicales superior, medius and inferior). The **sympathetic nervous system** increases the heart rate (positive chronotropic effect), conduction speed (positive dromotropic effect), and the excitability (positive bathmotropic effect) of the cardiomyo-

cytes. In addition, the contractile force (positive inotropic effect) is increased, atony is accelerated (positive lusitropic effect), and cell cohesion is enhanced (positive adhesiotropic effect). The **parasympathetic nervous system** has negative chronotropic, dromotropic and bathmotropic effects as well as negative inotropic effects on the atria. Although parasympathetics were previously described as exclusively acting on the atria, clear evidence now exists that parasympathetic fibres reach the myocardium of all four chambers of the heart. The **parasympathetic nerve fibres** are preganglionic nerve fibres from the N. vagus [X] and reach the Rr. cardiaci cervicales superior and inferior or the Rr. cardiaci thoracici of the Plexus cardiacus, where they are converted from up to 500 mostly microscopic ganglia (Ganglia cardiaca) into postganglionic neurons.

Clinical remarks

An increased sympathetic tone, e. g. caused by stress, is accompanied by an increased heart rate **(tachycardia)** and rise in blood pressure **(hypertension)**. Damage of the parasympathetic nerve fibres can also lead to tachycardia. The escalation of cardiac output increas-

es the oxygen requirements of the cardiomyocytes and, with narrowing of the coronary vessels (coronary heart disease), can lead to angina pectoris and myocardial infarction.

Innervation of the heart

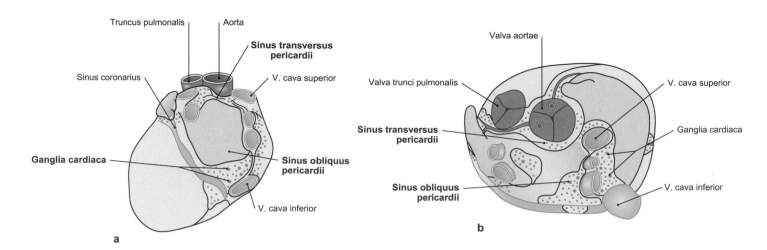

Fig. 5.79a and b   Plexus cardiacus with ganglia; schematic diagram. [(B500~M282/L132)/H102-002]
a Dorsal view.
b Cranial view.
The synapsing of the **parasympathetic nerve fibres** of the **Plexus cardiacus** is carried out in distinct ganglia **(Ganglia cardiaca).** As with other organs, with these ganglia often embedded in the walls, the parasympathetic Ganglia cardiaca are usually microscopically small and therefore not visible to the naked eye in a dissection. The ganglia contain the cell bodies (perikarya) of the postganglionic parasympathetic

neurons and lie in large numbers predominantly on the large vessels as well as embedded in the epicardium on the surface of the heart. The up to 500 small ganglia thus allow a **superficial, anterior group** located on the ascending aorta to be identified. The **deep, posterior group** extends into the Sinus transversus pericardii and thereby between the arterial vessels (Aorta ascendens and Truncus pulmonalis) and the venous vessels (V. cava superior and Vv. pulmonales). This posterior group spreads caudally to the dorsal layer of the pericardium into the Sinus obliquus pericardii.

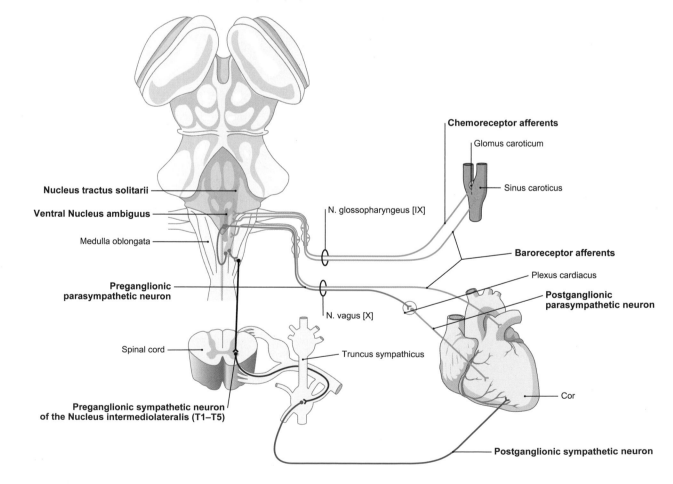

Fig. 5.80   Regulation of the autonomic innervation of the heart; schematic drawing. [S701-L127]
Chemoreceptors of the Glomus caroticum and baroreceptors in the vessel wall of the Sinus caroticus and the large vessels of the heart transmit information about the oxygen and carbondioxide concentration of the blood and the arterial blood pressure via the N. glossopharyn-

geus [IX] and N. vagus [X] to the **Nucleus tractus solitarii** in the brainstem. From the **ventral part of the Nucleus ambiguus,** the N. vagus [X] passes through the Plexus cardiacus to reduce cardiac output. Activation of the sympathetic nervous system increases cardiac output. Preganglionic sympathetic neurons are located in the lateral horn of the spinal cord segments T1–T5.

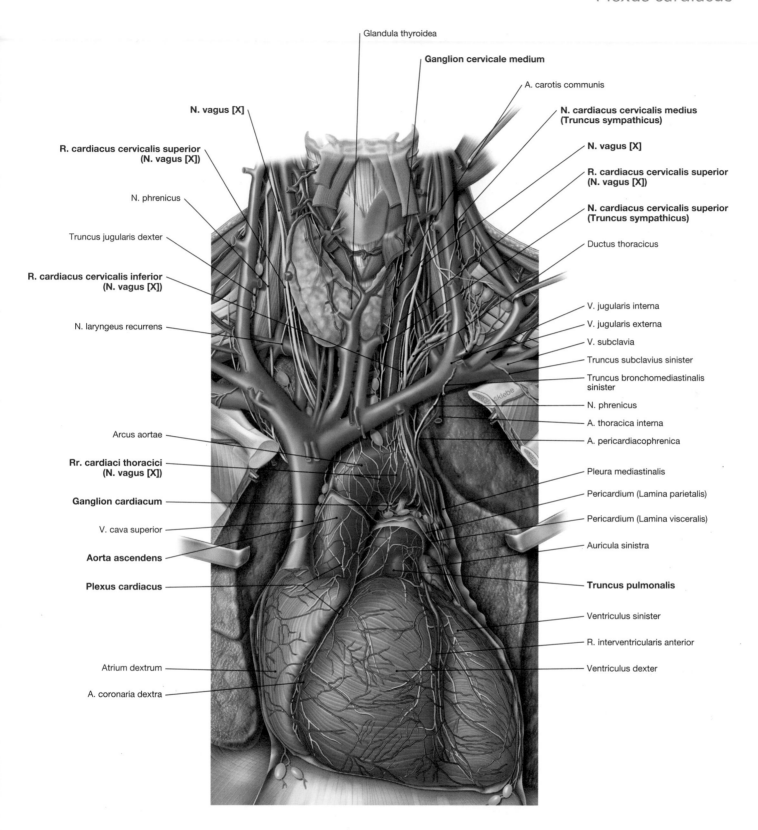

Glandula thyroidea

Ganglion cervicale medium

A. carotis communis

N. vagus [X]

**N. cardiacus cervicalis medius
(Truncus sympathicus)**

**R. cardiacus cervicalis superior
(N. vagus [X])**

N. vagus [X]

N. phrenicus

**R. cardiacus cervicalis superior
(N. vagus [X])**

Truncus jugularis dexter

**N. cardiacus cervicalis superior
(Truncus sympathicus)**

Ductus thoracicus

**R. cardiacus cervicalis inferior
(N. vagus [X])**

N. laryngeus recurrens

V. jugularis interna

V. jugularis externa

V. subclavia

Truncus subclavius sinister

Truncus bronchomediastinalis
sinister

N. phrenicus

Arcus aortae

A. thoracica interna

A. pericardiacophrenica

**Rr. cardiaci thoracici
(N. vagus [X])**

Pleura mediastinalis

Pericardium (Lamina parietalis)

Ganglion cardiacum

Pericardium (Lamina visceralis)

V. cava superior

Auricula sinistra

Aorta ascendens

Plexus cardiacus

Truncus pulmonalis

Ventriculus sinister

R. interventricularis anterior

Atrium dextrum

Ventriculus dexter

A. coronaria dextra

Fig. 5.81 Plexus cardiacus in situ; ventral view; the anterior thoracic wall is removed, the mediastinum and pericardium have been opened to reveal the heart. [S700-L238]/[Q300]

The illustration shows the Mediastinum superius as well as the lower middle mediastinum (Mediastinum medium). The **Plexus cardiacus** in the centre is in its natural position (in situ) and shows the pathways of the autonomic neurons. The postganglionic **sympathetic neurons** run as the **Nn. cardiaci cervicales superior, medius and inferior** from the Truncus sympathicus to the Plexus cardiacus. The superficial, anterior part of the plexus spreads anterior to the Aorta ascendens and the Trun-

cus pulmonalis. The neurons then follow the branches of the cardiac vessels and spread from there onto the surface of the heart. The **parasympathetic neurons,** on the other hand, are preganglionic nerve fibres from the N. vagus [X] and its N. laryngeus recurrens. They reach the Plexus cardiacus as **Rr. cardiaci cervicales superior and inferior** or as **Rr. cardiaci thoracici,** where they are converted from up to 500 mostly microscopic **ganglia (Ganglia cardiaca)** into postganglionic neurons. A larger ganglion is noticeable to the right of the Lig. pulmonale between the Truncus pulmonalis and the Arcus aortae.

Organs of the thoracic cavity

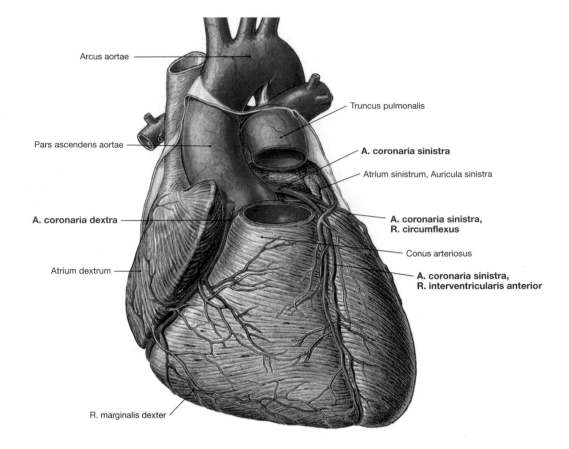

Arcus aortae

Truncus pulmonalis

Pars ascendens aortae

A. coronaria sinistra

Atrium sinistrum, Auricula sinistra

A. coronaria dextra

A. coronaria sinistra,
R. circumflexus

Conus arteriosus

Atrium dextrum

A. coronaria sinistra,
R. interventricularis anterior

R. marginalis dexter

Fig. 5.82   Coronary arteries, Aa. coronariae; ventral view. [S700]
The **right coronary artery** (A. coronaria dextra) originates in the right coronary sinus of the aorta, flows within the Sulcus coronarius to the lower border (Margo dexter), and changes over to the Facies diaphragmatica, where the **R. interventricularis posterior** usually originates as a terminal branch.
The **left coronary artery** (A. coronaria sinistra) emerges from the left coronary sinus of the aorta and divides after 1 cm into the **R. interven-**

tricularis anterior, which stretches to the apex of the heart, and into the **R. circumflexus,** which flows within the Sulcus coronarius around the left ventricle border onto the posterior surface.
Usually, the coronary artery that provides the R. interventricularis posterior is referred to as 'dominant'. Thereby, in balanced (→ Fig. 5.86, → Fig. 5.89, → Fig. 5.90a) and right-dominant coronary circulation (→ Fig. 5.88, → Fig. 5.90c), together in 75 % of cases (→ Fig. 5.90), the A. coronaria dextra is therefore dominant.

Branches of the coronary arteries	
Coronary arteries	**Branches**
Right coronary artery (A. coronaria dextra)	• R. coni arteriosi • R. nodi sinuatrialis (two-thirds of cases): to the **sinus node** (Nodus sinuatrialis) • R. marginalis dexter • R. posterolateralis dexter • R. nodi atrioventricularis: to the **AV node** (in dominance) • The R. interventricularis posterior (in dominance) and the Rr. interventriculares septales supply the **bundle of HIS**
Left coronary artery (A. coronaria sinistra)	**R. interventricularis anterior:** • R. coni arteriosi • R. lateralis (clin.: R. diagonalis) • Rr. interventriculares septales **R. circumflexus:** • R. nodi sinuatrialis (one-third of cases): to the **sinus node** (Nodus sinuatrialis) • R. marginalis sinister • R. posterior ventriculi sinistri

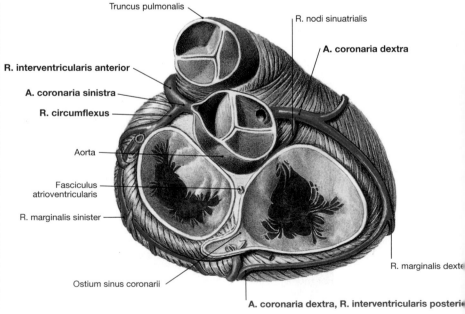

Truncus pulmonalis

R. nodi sinuatrialis

A. coronaria dextra

R. interventricularis anterior

A. coronaria sinistra

R. circumflexus

Aorta

Fasciculus atrioventricularis

R. marginalis sinister

R. marginalis dexter

Ostium sinus coronarii

A. coronaria dextra, R. interventricularis posterior

Fig. 5.83   Coronary arteries, Aa. coronariae; cranial view. [S700]

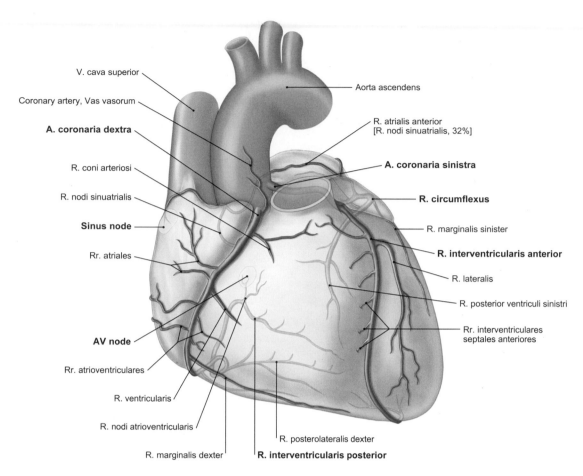

Fig. 5.84 **Branches of the coronary arteries, Aa. coronariae.**
[S700-L238]/[B500~M282/L132)/O1107]
The **right coronary artery (A. coronaria dextra)** descends within the Sulcus coronarius almost completely perpendicularly. Here, branching off to the right as the first branch is the **R. nodi sinuatrialis,** which runs, initially covered, from the right auricle to the sinus node. In addition, further branches on the Facies sternocostalis supply the right atrium and ventricle. Before the A. coronaria dextra switches over to the Facies diaphragmatica, the **R. marginalis dexter** emerges. On the caudal surface of the heart, the A. coronaria dextra usually (balanced circulation) flows into the **R. interventricularis posterior.** The **R. nodi**

atrioventricularis starts where the R. interventricularis posterior turns off almost perpendicularly into the Sulcus interventricularis posterior.
In contrast to the A. coronaria dextra, the **A. coronaria sinistra** soon divides into its two main branches: the **R. interventricularis anterior** continues its pathway caudally on the Facies sternocostalis and provides the **R. lateralis** in the direction of the apex of the heart. The **R. circumflexus,** together with the **left marginal artery,** supplies the left pulmonary surface, before it turns onto the Facies diaphragmatica. There, the R. circumflexus forms the **posterior left ventricular branch** as a terminal branch.

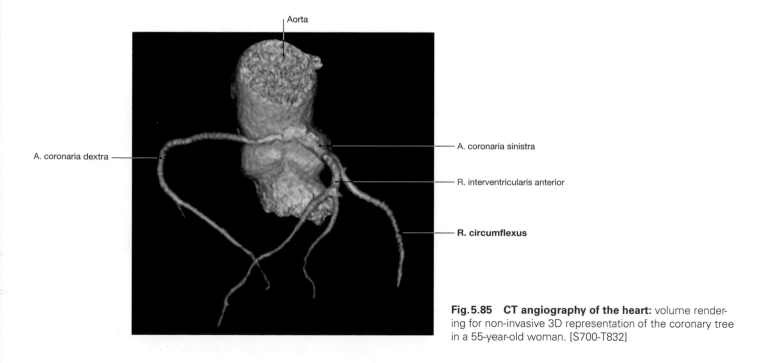

Fig. 5.85 **CT angiography of the heart:** volume rendering for non-invasive 3D representation of the coronary tree in a 55-year-old woman. [S700-T832]

Circulation of the coronary arteries

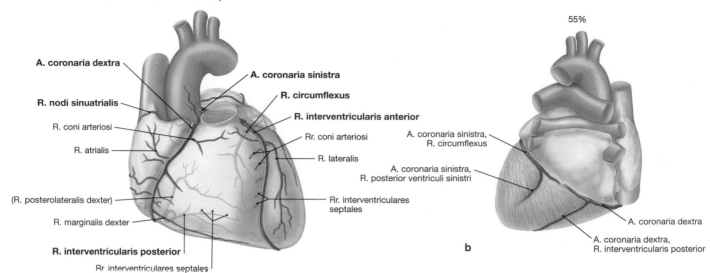

Fig. 5.86a and b   Balanced circulation of the Aa. coronariae.
[S700-L238]
a Ventral view.
b Dorsal view.

The coronary circulation determines the severity and the clinical presentation of a myocardial infarction. Generally (in 55 % of cases), the R. interventricularis posterior originates from the A. coronaria dextra but does not overlap onto the posterior aspect of the left ventricle. This is referred to as **balanced (codominant) circulation.**

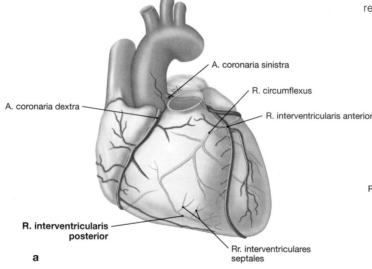

Fig. 5.87a and b   Left-dominant circulation of the Aa. coronariae.
[S700-L238]
a Ventral view.

b Dorsal view.
In 11–20 % of cases, the R. interventricularis posterior originates from the left coronary artery, which is referred to as **left-dominant circulation (left coronary dominance).**

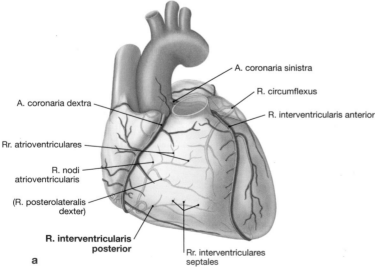

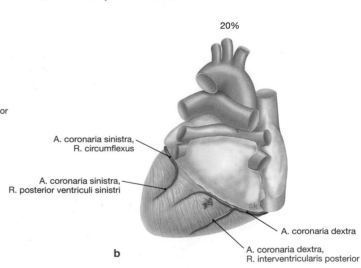

Fig. 5.88a and b   Right-dominant circulation of the Aa. coronariae. [S700-L238]
a Ventral view.
b Dorsal view.

In 14–25 % of cases, the A. coronaria dextra provides not only the R. interventricularis posterior, but also supplies parts of the posterior aspect of the left ventricle. In this case it is referred to as **right-dominant circulation (right coronary dominance).**

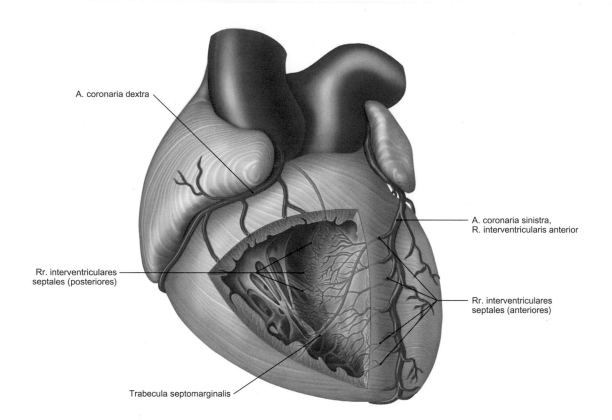

A. coronaria dextra

A. coronaria sinistra,
R. interventricularis anterior

Rr. interventriculares
septales (posteriores)

Rr. interventriculares
septales (anteriores)

Trabecula septomarginalis

Fig. 5.89 Arterial supply of the Septum interventriculare, balanced circulation; ventral view. [S700-L238]/[B500-O1107~M282/L132]

The anterior **two thirds of the interventricular septum,** including the moderator band and the right anterior papillary muscle, are supplied by the septal branches of the **R. interventricularis anterior.** Only the **posterior third** receives blood from the septal branches of the R. interventricularis posterior, which emerges from the A. coronaria dextra in balanced and right-dominant circulation. Therefore, as well as differentiating between the types of circulation, there is another classification according to the 'dominance' of a coronary artery, which is mainly used as a clinical term. Here, the differentiation depends on which coronary artery provides the R. interventricularis posterior and is thus involved in

the supply of the posterior part of the Septum interventriculare and of the part of the left ventricle which connects to the Facies diaphragmatica ('posterior wall' of clinicians). In over 80 % of the cases in balanced and right-dominant circulation the dominant artery is the A. coronaria dextra. Only in up to 20 % of cases is the A. coronaria sinistra dominant. The **dominant artery** also supplies the **AV node** and the **bundle of HIS.** The branch to the AV node usually penetrates into the heart wall, where the R. interventricularis posterior from the Sulcus coronarius branches off into the Sulcus interventricularis posterior. The bundle of HIS is fed by the proximal septal branches of the R. interventricularis posterior. Thus, in the majority of cases (as a rule), the sinus node, as the primary cardiac pacemaker, as well as the AV node and the bundle of HIS are supplied by the A. coronaria dextra.

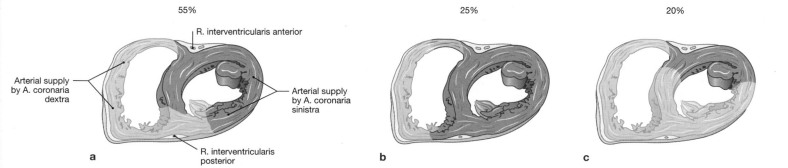

55%   25%   20%

R. interventricularis anterior

Arterial supply
by A. coronaria
dextra

Arterial supply
by A. coronaria
sinistra

R. interventricularis
posterior

a   b   c

Fig. 5.90a–c Area of the heart supplied by the A. coronaria dextra (light red) and the A. coronaria sinistra (dark red) in cross-sections; caudal view. [S700-L126]/[B500~M282/L132]/[E1120]

a Balanced circulation: The A. coronaria sinistra supplies approx. the two anterior thirds of the septum from the R. interventricularis anterior via the Rr. interventriculares septales. Corresponding branches from the R. interventricularis posterior of the A. coronaria dextra reach the posterior third of the Septum interventriculare.

b Left-dominant circulation: The A. coronaria sinistra supplies the entire septum and also the AV node.

c Right-dominant circulation: Two thirds of the septum and large areas of the posterior aspect of the left ventricle are supplied with blood by the A. coronaria dextra.

This distribution pattern has implications for the severity of a heart attack when there is an occlusion of one of the Aa. coronariae.

Coronary heart disease

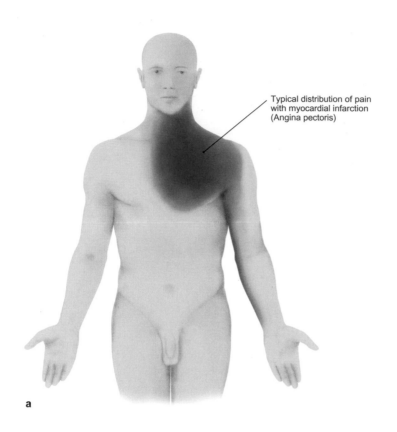

Typical distribution of pain
with myocardial infarction
(Angina pectoris)

a

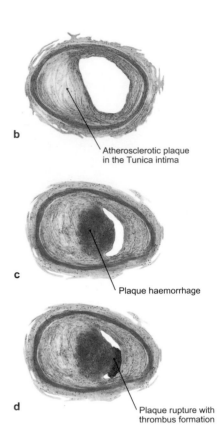

b

Atherosclerotic plaque
in the Tunica intima

c

Plaque haemorrhage

d

Plaque rupture with
thrombus formation

Fig. 5.91a–d   Coronary heart disease. [S702-L266]

a Clinical presentation: In coronary heart disease (CHD) when there is sudden underperfusion (ischaemia) of the myocardium (acute coronary syndrome), tightness of the chest is often felt and is known as **angina pectoris (a).** This presentation allows no distinction as to whether a minor perfusion of the myocardium still occurs or whether in the case of a complete blockage muscle cell destruction (necrosis) is imminent. If the myocardium is dying, then a **heart attack (myocardial infarction)** is present which may lead to sudden cardiac death. In accordance with the area of the referred pain (HEAD's zone), pain is mainly perceived in the left-hand chest region and radiates into the left arm and the left half of the neck. It should however be noted that pain radiation to the right side, or no pain at all, is also possible, since the risk factors which result in CHD often also damage the afferent nerve fibres, e. g. diabetes mellitus. It is therefore impossible to exclude a heart attack without thorough diagnostics!

b–d Arteriosclerosis as the cause of CHD: In most cases, CHD is caused by **atherosclerosis** of the Aa. coronariae and their branches. Accompanying risk factors are diabetes mellitus, high blood pressure

(hypertension), elevated cholesterol levels in the blood (hypercholesterolaemia) and smoking. In these cases, an inflammatory process originates in the Tunica intima of the Aa. coronariae, which is triggered by cholesterol-containing lipid deposits. This **chronic inflammatory process** forms atherosclerotic plaques **(b)** which narrow the vessel lumen and into which haemorrhages can occur **(c).** Due to flow conditions, the outflow tracts of the Aa. coronariae from the ascending aorta or those of the branches of the Aa. coronariae are often particularly affected by the plaque formation. If these plaques rupture, the protective layer of endothelial cells is lost, so that blood clots (thrombi) form **(d)** which can completely displace the lumen. If the occlusion is complete and a recanalisation does not occur spontaneously, myocardial tissue disintegrates and **myocardial infarction results.** It is important to note that arteriosclerosis is often a **systemic disease** and affects the whole systemic circulation, in which blood pressure is high. Therefore, myocardial infarction patients have an increased risk of stroke, kidney or bowel infarction or peripheral artery disease (PAD), in which walking is painfully restricted due to inadequate blood flow.

Clinical remarks

For diagnosis and therapeutic approaches to coronary heart disease (CHD) it is essential to know the branches of the coronary arteries and the areas of the heart supplied by these branches (→ Fig. 5.86, → Fig. 5.87, → Fig. 5.88). The clinical terms for the coronary arterial branches deviate from the anatomical terms, and abbreviations of their English terms are used:

- The A. coronaria sinistra is identified as **LCA** (left coronary artery) and the A. coronaria dextra as **RCA** (right coronary artery).
- The R. interventricularis anterior is referred to as **LAD** (left anterior descending coronary artery) and the R. interventricularis posterior as **RPD** (right posterior descending coronary artery).
- The R. circumflexus is called **RCX.**

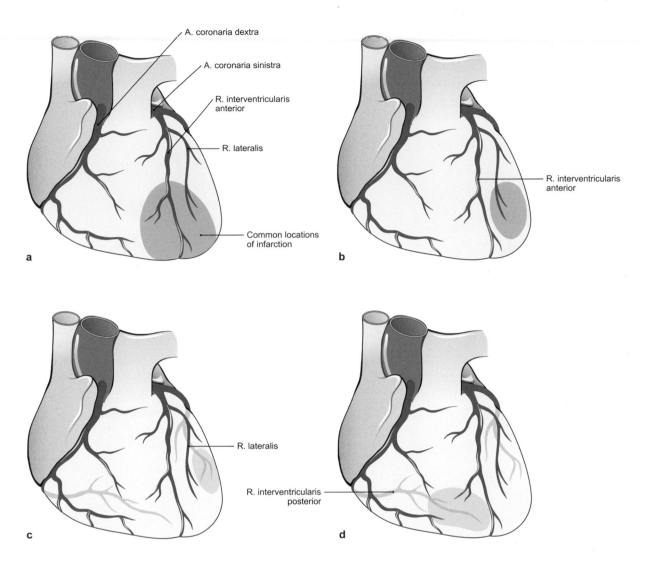

A. coronaria dextra

A. coronaria sinistra

R. interventricularis anterior

R. lateralis

Common locations of infarction

a

R. interventricularis anterior

b

R. lateralis

R. interventricularis posterior

c

d

Fig. 5.92a–d   Infarction pattern in occlusion of the coronary arteries. [S700-L126]/[G1060-002]
a With isolated occlusion of the R. interventricularis anterior it is a case of **anterior wall myocardial infarction.**
b In the case of distal occlusion of the R. lateralis the result is an **apical myocardial infarction.**

c An occlusion of the R. circumflexus results in an infarction in the region of the Facies diaphragmatica, referred to as **posterior wall myocardial infarction.**
d Importantly, the occlusion of the R. interventricularis posterior also leads to a **posterior wall myocardial infarction.**

Clinical remarks

As the Aa. coronariae are functional terminal arteries, an occlusion of individual branches leads to circumscribed infarction patterns. These can often already be determined in the various deflections of an ECG. The safest confirmation method is achieved by cardiac catheter examination, using an X-ray contrast agent. In **posterior wall myocardial infarction** the perfusion of the AV node is typically also impaired because its artery usually originates at the branching point of the R. interventricularis posterior (→ Fig. 5.84). This can result additionally in bradycardiac arrhythmias. Since the muscle wall of the right ventricle has a lower oxygen demand than that of the left ventricle, due to pressure conditions, a proximal occlusion of the right coronary artery (A. coronaria dextra) commonly also results in an isolated posterior wall myocardial infarction. In this case, the bradycardia can be very pronounced due to insufficient perfusion of the sinus node. [H081]

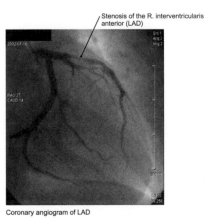

Stenosis of the R. interventricularis anterior (LAD)

Coronary angiogram of LAD

Heart

Circulation of the coronary arteries

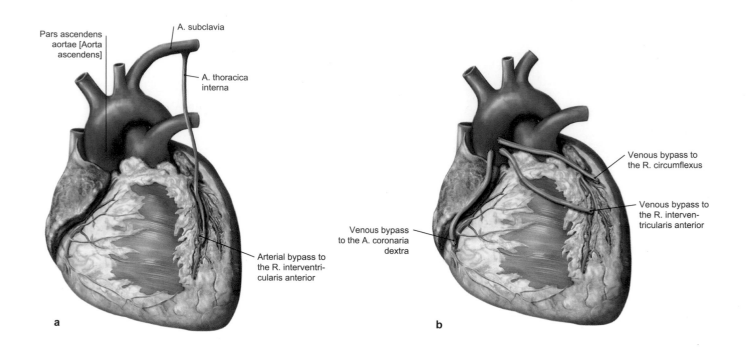

Fig. 5.93a and b Bypass options with coronary artery occlusions.
[S702-L266]
a Arterial bypass.
b Venous bypass.
A pronounced coronary artery occlusion necessitates bypass surgery, especially if more than one of the major branches are affected (RCA, RCX and LAD).
The **arterial bypass** utilises the proximal **A. thoracica interna** to connect to the coronary artery distal of the occlusion. The benefit here is that the anatomy of the proximal part is preserved. The arterial wall is adapted to the blood pressure and therefore an arterial bypass remains patent. As there are only two Aa. thoracicae internae, only two arterial bypass placements can be made.
With more than two stenoses, **venous bypass grafts are necessary.** Here the **V. saphena magna** from the leg is mostly used and is connected to the respective vessel branches from the aorta as this epifascial vein is long and easily accessible. Venous bypass graft occlusions occur more frequently.

Clinical remarks

The acute situation of a myocardial infarction requires the inhibition of platelet aggregation and potentially the lysis of a thrombus to restore blood flow. If pharmacological intervention is not possible in an acute situation, invasive measures are necessary. An occlusion of two of the three main coronary arteries (RCA, RCX, LAD) with compromised cardiac ejection requires bypass surgery. If cardiac ejection is only marginally affected with one or two occluded coronary arteries, bypass surgery may not be necessary if **coronary catheterisa-** **tion** allows for a **balloon dilation** or placement of a small mesh tube (**stent**).
There is clinical evidence that the dilation of an existing coronary stenosis does not improve the prognosis with CHD. This is in part due to the fact that atherosclerotic plaques can rupture at locations other than the ones with visible stenoses. Because these plaques have not been verifiable, however, depicting a cardiac catheterisation of the stenoses is not possible.

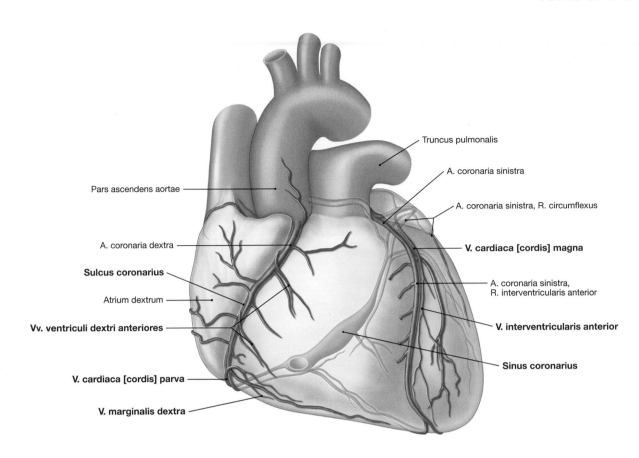

Fig. 5.94 **Cardiac veins, Vv. cordis**; ventral view. [S700-L238]
Venous blood from the heart flows via **three major systems.** Of the venous blood, 75 % is received by the **coronary sinus** and carried into the right atrium. The remaining 25 % of the venous blood reaches the atria and ventricles directly via the **transmural** and **endomural** systems.

Labels (Fig. 5.94):
Truncus pulmonalis
A. coronaria sinistra
A. coronaria sinistra, R. circumflexus
V. cardiaca [cordis] magna
A. coronaria sinistra, R. interventricularis anterior
V. interventricularis anterior
Sinus coronarius
Pars ascendens aortae
A. coronaria dextra
Sulcus coronarius
Atrium dextrum
Vv. ventriculi dextri anteriores
V. cardiaca [cordis] parva
V. marginalis dextra

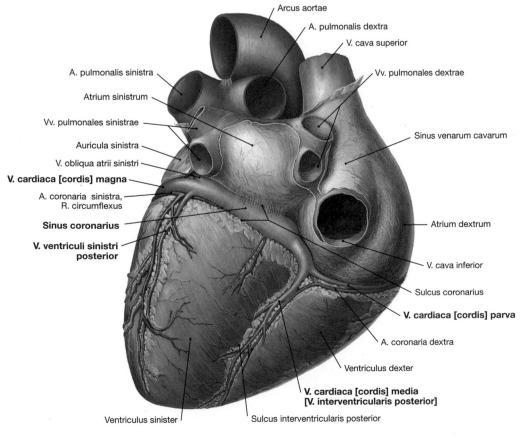

Fig. 5.95 **Cardiac veins, Vv. cordis**; dorso-caudal view. [S700]

Labels (Fig. 5.95):
Arcus aortae
A. pulmonalis dextra
V. cava superior
Vv. pulmonales dextrae
Sinus venarum cavarum
Atrium dextrum
V. cava inferior
Sulcus coronarius
V. cardiaca [cordis] parva
A. coronaria dextra
Ventriculus dexter
V. cardiaca [cordis] media [V. interventricularis posterior]
Sulcus interventricularis posterior
Ventriculus sinister
V. ventriculi sinistri posterior
Sinus coronarius
A. coronaria sinistra, R. circumflexus
V. cardiaca [cordis] magna
V. obliqua atrii sinistri
Auricula sinistra
Vv. pulmonales sinistrae
Atrium sinistrum
A. pulmonalis sinistra

Cardiac veins (Vv. cordis)	
System	**Veins**
Coronary sinus system	• V. cardiaca magna: corresponds to the supply area of the A. coronaria sinistra • V. interventricularis anterior • V. marginalis sinistra • Vv. ventriculi sinistri posteriores • V. cardiaca media: in the Sulcus inter-ventricularis posterior • V. cardiaca parva: in the right Sulcus coronarius, present in 50 % • V. obliqua atrii sinistri
Transmural system	• Vv. ventriculi dextri anteriores • Vv. atriales
Endomural system	Vv. cardiacae minimae (THEBESIAN veins)

Projection of the trachea and bronchi

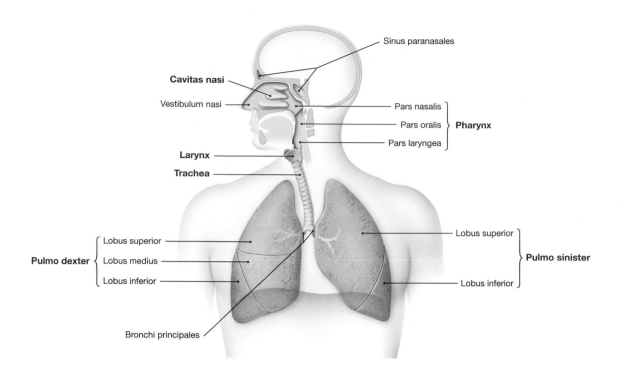

Fig. 5.96 Upper and lower respiratory tracts; schematic diagram. [S700-L275]
The respiratory system is divided into upper and lower respiratory tracts.
The **upper** respiratory tract includes:
* Nasal cavity (Cavitas nasi)
* Pharynx.

The **lower** respiratory tract comprises:
* Larynx
* Trachea
* Lungs (Pulmones).
The right lung (Pulmo dexter) has three lobes, the left lung (Pulmo sinister) has two.

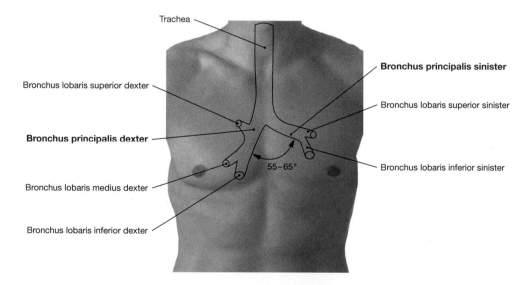

Fig. 5.97 Projection of the trachea and main bronchi onto the anterior thoracic wall. [S700]
The trachea is 10–13 cm long and during deep inspiration extends by up to 5 cm. Originating at the cricoid cartilage of the larynx, it projects onto the seventh cervical vertebra; its bifurcation, where it divides into the two main bronchi, projects onto the fourth to fifth thoracic vertebrae (second to third ribs). The angle between the main bronchi is 55° to 65°. The **right main bronchus (Bronchus principalis dexter)** is stronger, 1–2.5 cm long and is **almost vertically** positioned, while the left main bronchus (Bronchus principalis sinister) is almost twice as long and is positioned diagonally.

Clinical remarks

Because of the vertical position of the right main bronchus, when breathing in foreign bodies **(aspiration)**, the aspirated material usually enters the **right lung.** In the event of imminent suffocation this knowledge may provide a doctor with a crucial time advantage! The asymmetrical position of the main bronchi should also be taken into account for **intubations:** with this, a rubber tube (tubus) is inserted via the mouth into the lower respiratory tract in order to enable ventilation. If this tube is inserted too far, it usually inserts into the vertically positioned right main bronchus, so that only the right lung is ventilated. After intubation, one should therefore use sounding of the lung (auscultation) to ensure the tube has been correctly positioned in the trachea!

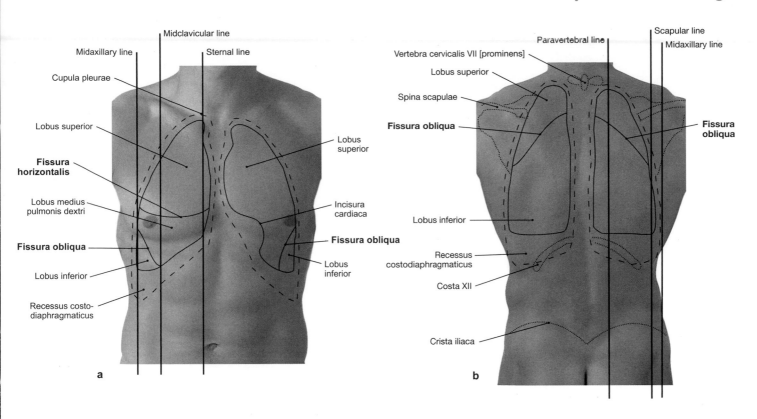

Fig. 5.98a and b   Projection of pulmonary and pleural margins.
[S700]
a Projection onto the anterior thoracic wall.
b Projection onto the back.
The **right lung** has three lobes which are demarcated by the **Fissura obliqua** and the **Fissura horizontalis.** The Fissura obliqua follows the fourth rib dorso-laterally and separates the upper and lower lobes. From the midaxillary line it then descends steeply and reaches the sixth rib in the midclavicular line. On the anterior surface of the lung, the Fissura obliqua therefore divides the middle and lower lobes from each other (→ Fig. 5.105). Anteriorly, the Fissura horizontalis continues along the fourth rib and separates the upper and middle lobes.

The **left lung** only has two lobes which are separated by the **Fissura obliqua.** Because the heart causes the mediastinum to extend to the left (Incisura cardiaca), the volume of the left lung is smaller and its position also differs in the sternal and midclavicular lines from the right lung (→ table below).
Each **pleural cavity** (Cavitas pleuralis) is covered by **parietal pleura** (Pleura parietalis). The Pleura parietalis is divided into the Pars mediastinalis, Pars costalis and Pars diaphragmatica (→ Fig. 5.4). The pleural cavities feature four pleural recesses (Recessus pleurales). The largest is the **Recessus costodiaphragmaticus** which expands laterally up to 5 cm within the midaxillary line.
Pulmonary margins = solid line, pleural margins = dotted line

Lungs and pleural margins		
Anatomical lines	**Right pulmonary margins**	**Left pulmonary margins**
Sternal line	Cutting at rib 6	Cutting at rib 4
Midclavicular line	Parallel to rib 6	Cutting at rib 6
Midaxillary line	Cutting at rib 8	Same as the right
Scapular line	Cutting at rib 10	Same as the right
Paravertebral line	Cutting at rib 11	Same as the right
Pleural boundaries: one rib deeper each time		

Clinical remarks

The margins of the lungs and the pleura play a role in physical examinations in order to determine the **size and respiratory expansion** of the lungs and the **localisation of pathological changes,** which can be indicative of a pulmonary inflammation (pneumonia) or an increased volume of fluid in the Cavitas pleuralis (pleural effusion). **Pleural effusions** are drained in the costodiaphragmatic recess.

Only the **Pleura parietalis** is nociceptively innervated and therefore **sensitive to pain.** If pneumonia or lung tumours are accompanied by chest pain, then one can assume involvement of the parietal pleura. If air penetrates the Cavitas pleuralis, the lung partially or completely collapses **(pneumothorax).** During percussion, one hears a loud (hypersonorous) percussion sound.

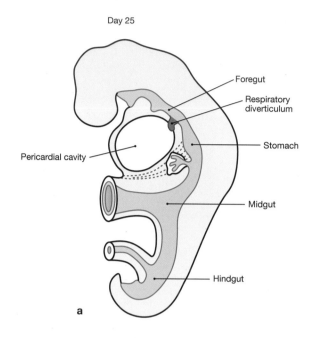

Lung

Development

Day 25

Foregut

Respiratory diverticulum

Stomach

Pericardial cavity

Midgut

Hindgut

a

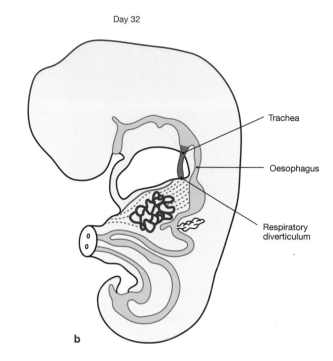

Day 32

Trachea

Oesophagus

Respiratory diverticulum

b

Fig. 5.99a and b   Development of the lower respiratory tract.
[S700-L126]/[B501-O1108/L317]
a Development on day 25.
b Development on day 32.
Epithelial tissues of the larynx, trachea and lungs develop from the fourth week from the entoderm of the foregut. Connective tissue, smooth muscles and blood vessels are derived from the surrounding mesoderm. Firstly, a **lung bud forms,** which extends to the **laryngotracheal groove,** and where at its lower end, the **bronchial buds** emerge as precursors of the main bronchi.

Clinical remarks

A disruption of the division of oesophagus and trachea can cause abnormal collateral connections **(tracheo-oesophageal fistulas),** often associated with a blind-ended oesophagus **(oesophageal atresia).**
From the **28th week, surfactant** is produced in the pulmonary alveoli, a secretion that reduces the surface tension of the alveoli. From the 35th week, the production is usually sufficient to enable **spontaneous breathing** if necessary. Insufficient surfactant production results in **respiratory distress syndrome** (RDS) which is the most common cause of death in premature babies. In the case of birth before the 30th week, up to 60 % of premature babies develop RDS. Because it is only at birth that the lungs are filled with air, a coroner can use a **flotation test** to establish whether the child was born dead (lung sinks) or alive (lung floats). However, this indication of a stillbirth is no longer recognised in forensic medicine.

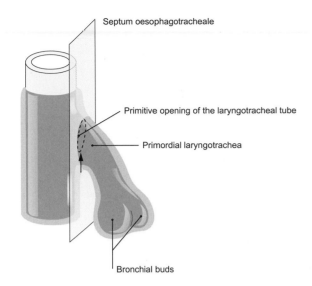

Septum oesophagotracheale

Primitive opening of the laryngotracheal tube

Primordial laryngotrachea

Bronchial buds

Fig. 5.100   Development of the Septum oesophagotracheale.
[E347-09]
During the fourth and fifth weeks, mesenchymal folds form on both sides; the folds join to the Septum oesophagotracheale and thereby separate the primordium of the lower respiratory tract from the oesophagus.

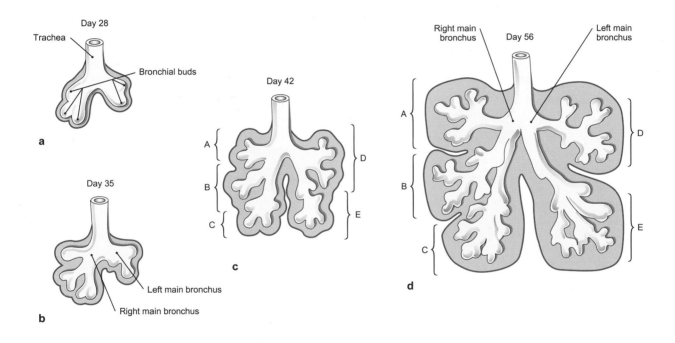

Day 28
Trachea
Bronchial buds
a

Day 35
Left main bronchus
Right main bronchus
b

Day 42
A
B
C
D
E
c

Right main bronchus   Day 56   Left main bronchus
A
B
C
D
E
d

A Right upper lobe   D Left upper lobe
B Right middle lobe   E Left lower lobe
C Right lower lobe

Fig. 5.101a–d   Stages of lung development. [E347-09]
a Development on day 28.
b Development on day 35.
c Development on day 42.
d Development on day 56.
A distinction is made between three phases of lung development, which partially overlap:

- **Pseudoglandular phase** (seventh–17th week): formation of the conducting part of the respiratory system
- **Canalicular phase** (13th–26th week): early development of the respiratory part (gas exchange) of the respiratory system
- **Alveolar phase** (23rd week–eighth year of life): formation of the alveoli. Lung development is therefore not completed at birth, but continues into childhood!

Clinical remarks

If the Septum oesophagotracheale does not form properly below the larynx to separate the lower respiratory tract from the oesophagus, **fistelation** between the trachea and the oesophagus may occur.

These frequently coexist with **atresia of the oesophagus,** causing infants to aspirate breast milk into the lungs and exhale milk through the nose and mouth.

Trachea and bronchi

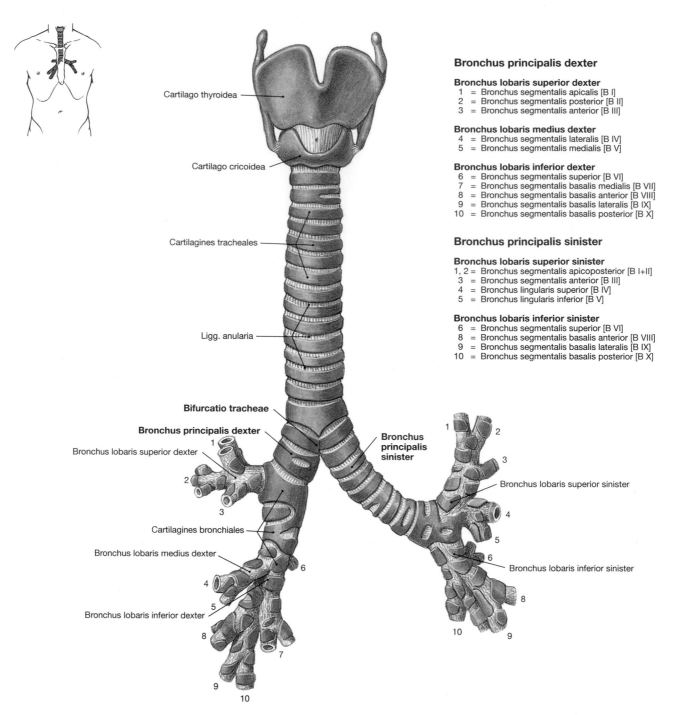

Cartilago thyroidea

Cartilago cricoidea

Cartilagines tracheales

Ligg. anularia

Bifurcatio tracheae

Bronchus principalis dexter

Bronchus lobaris superior dexter

Cartilagines bronchiales

Bronchus lobaris medius dexter

Bronchus lobaris inferior dexter

Bronchus principalis sinister

Bronchus lobaris superior sinister

Bronchus lobaris inferior sinister

Bronchus principalis dexter

Bronchus lobaris superior dexter
1 = Bronchus segmentalis apicalis [B I]
2 = Bronchus segmentalis posterior [B II]
3 = Bronchus segmentalis anterior [B III]

Bronchus lobaris medius dexter
4 = Bronchus segmentalis lateralis [B IV]
5 = Bronchus segmentalis medialis [B V]

Bronchus lobaris inferior dexter
6 = Bronchus segmentalis superior [B VI]
7 = Bronchus segmentalis basalis medialis [B VII]
8 = Bronchus segmentalis basalis anterior [B VIII]
9 = Bronchus segmentalis basalis lateralis [B IX]
10 = Bronchus segmentalis basalis posterior [B X]

Bronchus principalis sinister

Bronchus lobaris superior sinister
1, 2 = Bronchus segmentalis apicoposterior [B I+II]
3 = Bronchus segmentalis anterior [B III]
4 = Bronchus lingularis superior [B IV]
5 = Bronchus lingularis inferior [B V]

Bronchus lobaris inferior sinister
6 = Bronchus segmentalis superior [B VI]
8 = Bronchus segmentalis basalis anterior [B VIII]
9 = Bronchus segmentalis basalis lateralis [B IX]
10 = Bronchus segmentalis basalis posterior [B X]

Fig. 5.102 Lower respiratory tract with larynx, trachea and bronchi; ventral view. [S700]

The trachea is 10–13 cm long and extends from the cricoid cartilage of the larynx to its division (Bifurcatio tracheae) into the two main bronchi **(Bronchi principales).** It is divided into a neck part (Pars cervicalis) and a sternum part (Pars thoracica). Projection and topography are described in → Fig. 5.96. The main bronchi further divide into three right-sided and two left-sided lobar bronchi **(Bronchi lobares).** The segmental bronchi **(Bronchi segmentales)** emerge from the lobar bronchi. On the right-hand side, there are 10 lung segments and thus 10 segmental bronchi. In the left lung, however, segment 7 and the corresponding bronchus are missing. A more detailed systematic description of the bronchial tree is not illustrated here. The bronchi divide six to twelve times and then pass into the

bronchioles, which have a diameter of less than 1 mm and are therefore only clearly visible with a microscope. Bronchioles are easily distinguished from bronchi as they no longer contain cartilage and glands in their walls. Each bronchiole supplies a pulmonary lobule (Lobulus pulmonis) and further divides three to four times to become **terminal bronchioles.** These represent the last of the **conducting parts** of the respiratory system which has a volume of 150–170 ml. A terminal bronchiole supplies a pulmonary acinus **(Acinus pulmonis),** which generates ten further generations of respiratory bronchioles with Ductus and Sacculi alveolares. All parts of the acinus have alveoli and therefore belong to the **respiratory or gas exchange part** of the respiratory system.

Clinical remarks

The volume of the conducting parts of the respiratory system **(150–170 ml)** is equivalent to the **anatomical dead space** and has practical relevance for **resuscitation.** During ventilation, a volume greater than 170 ml needs to be exchanged, otherwise no oxygenated air

reaches the alveoli, but stale air is simply moved around within the respiratory tract. Therefore, it is better to ventilate slowly with more volume than quickly with too little volume.

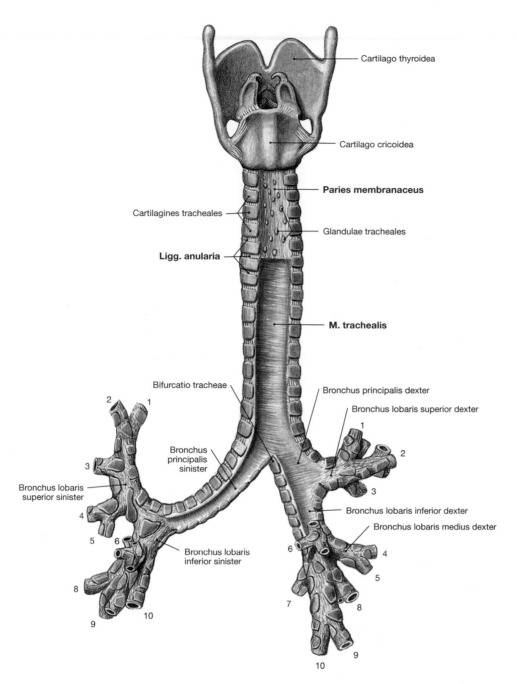

Fig. 5.103 Lower respiratory tract with larynx, trachea, and bronchi; dorsal view. [S700]
The systematic composition of the bronchial tree is described in → Fig. 5.102. The dorsal view clearly shows that the dorsal walls of the trachea and the main bronchi do not have any cartilage (Paries membranaceus) but consist predominantly of smooth muscles (M. trachealis). The individual links are connected by Ligg. anularia of elastic connective tissue, so that the trachea can extend during deep inhalation by up to 5 cm.

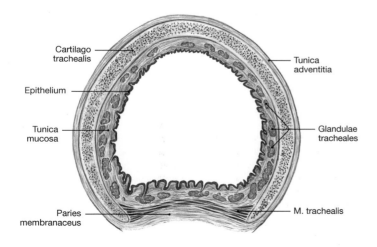

Fig. 5.104 Trachea; cross-section, microscopic view. [S700]
The wall of the trachea and main bronchi comprises a mucous membrane (Tunica mucosa), to which the Tunica fibromusculocartilaginea and the Tunica adventitia attach themselves on the outside. The Tunica fibromusculocartilaginea consists of 16 to 20 horseshoe-shaped tracheal cartilages of hyaline cartilage, which are open at the back where they are bridged posteriorly by smooth muscles (M. trachealis).

Clinical remarks

The posterior wall of the trachea is directly adjacent to the oesophagus (→ Fig. 5.135), allowing **proximal tumours of the oesophagus** to infiltrate the tracheal wall. This is associated with a poor prognosis as tracheal resections are not possible.

Organs of the thoracic cavity

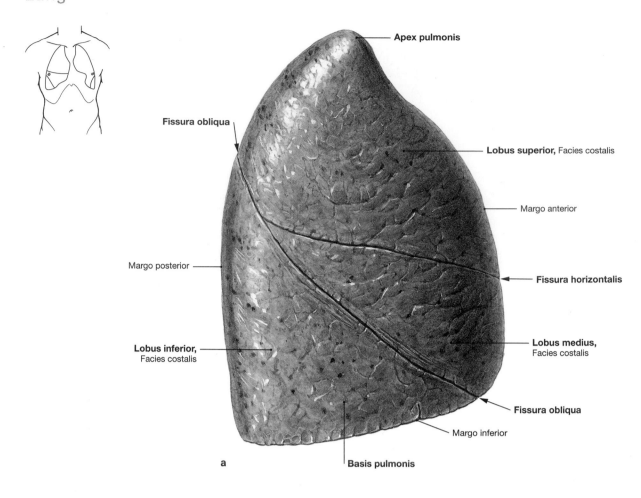

- Apex pulmonis
- Fissura obliqua
- Lobus superior, Facies costalis
- Margo anterior
- Margo posterior
- Fissura horizontalis
- Lobus inferior, Facies costalis
- Lobus medius, Facies costalis
- Fissura obliqua
- Margo inferior
- Basis pulmonis

a

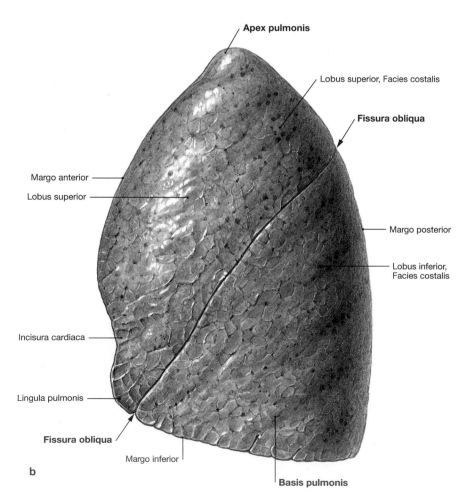

- Apex pulmonis
- Lobus superior, Facies costalis
- Fissura obliqua
- Margo anterior
- Lobus superior
- Margo posterior
- Lobus inferior, Facies costalis
- Incisura cardiaca
- Lingula pulmonis
- Fissura obliqua
- Margo inferior
- Basis pulmonis

b

Fig. 5.105a and b   Right and left lung; lateral view. [S700]

a Pulmo dexter; lateral view.
b Pulmo sinister; lateral view.

The **right lung** has **three lobes (Lobi superior, medius and inferior),** which are separated by the oblique fissure and the horizontal fissure. The **left lung,** however, consists of **two lobes (Lobi superior and inferior)** and has just a Fissura obliqua. Corresponding to the middle lobe is the Lingula pulmonis of the superior lobe; the lingula forms a tongue-shaped projection underneath the Incisura cardiaca. The fissures can however be incomplete, so that the lobes are not completely separated, which happens in the Fissura horizontalis in up to 50 % of cases. Or the Lingula pulmonis on the left side can be separated to create a third lobe.

The volume of the right lung encompasses 2–3 l, and even 5–8 l during maximum inspiration. Corresponding to this volume is a gas exchange surface area of 70–140 m². The volume of the left lung, due to the heart tilting slightly to the left, has a 10–20 % smaller volume.

Cranially the lungs form an **apex (Apex pulmonis)** and caudally a wide **base (Basis pulmonis).** The surface is covered by the Pleura visceralis and can be divided into three areas in accordance with the topographical relationships. The lateral **Facies costalis** passes below at the Margo inferior into the **Facies diaphragmatica** (→ Fig. 5.106), at the Margo anterior and at the blunt Margo posterior, into the **Facies mediastinalis** on the medial side.

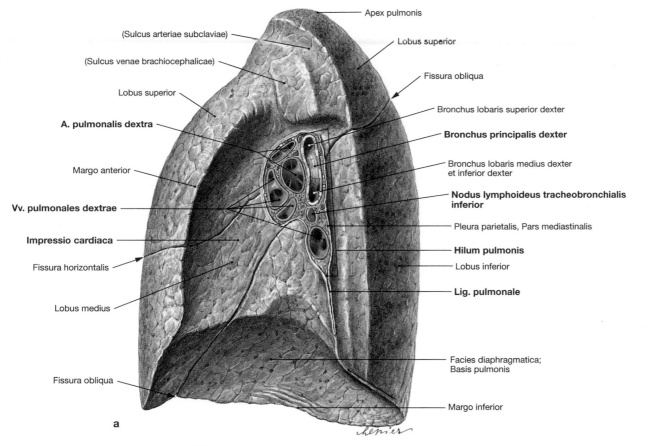

Apex pulmonis
(Sulcus arteriae subclaviae)
(Sulcus venae brachiocephalicae)
Lobus superior
A. pulmonalis dextra
Margo anterior
Vv. pulmonales dextrae
Impressio cardiaca
Fissura horizontalis
Lobus medius
Fissura obliqua

Lobus superior
Fissura obliqua
Bronchus lobaris superior dexter
Bronchus principalis dexter
Bronchus lobaris medius dexter et inferior dexter
Nodus lymphoideus tracheobronchialis inferior
Pleura parietalis, Pars mediastinalis
Hilum pulmonis
Lobus inferior
Lig. pulmonale
Facies diaphragmatica; Basis pulmonis
Margo inferior

a

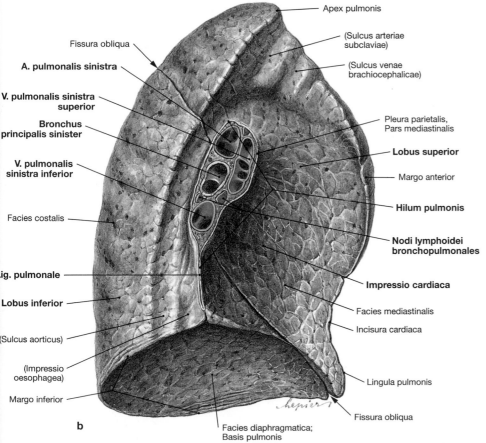

Fissura obliqua
A. pulmonalis sinistra
V. pulmonalis sinistra superior
Bronchus principalis sinister
V. pulmonalis sinistra inferior
Facies costalis
Lig. pulmonale
Lobus inferior
(Sulcus aorticus)
(Impressio oesophagea)
Margo inferior

Apex pulmonis
(Sulcus arteriae subclaviae)
(Sulcus venae brachiocephalicae)
Pleura parietalis, Pars mediastinalis
Lobus superior
Margo anterior
Hilum pulmonis
Nodi lymphoidei bronchopulmonales
Impressio cardiaca
Facies mediastinalis
Incisura cardiaca
Lingula pulmonis
Fissura obliqua

b

Facies diaphragmatica; Basis pulmonis

Fig. 5.106a and b Right and left lung; medial view. [S700]
a Pulmo dexter; medial view.
b Pulmo sinister; medial view.
The medial aspect reveals the **hilum of the lung (Hilum pulmonis),** where the main bronchi and the neurovascular pathways of the lung enter and exit, the so-called **root of the lung (Radix pulmonis).** At the hilum, the **visceral pleura (Pleura visceralis)** also passes from the lung surface onto the **parietal pleura (Pleura parietalis),** that lines the Cavitas pleuralis. This pleural fold extends inferiorly into the Lig. pulmonale. The arrangement of the main bronchi and the large vessels in the hilum of the lung is characteristic in both lungs. On the **right lung,** the **Bronchus principalis** lies furthest **above,** while on the left side it is located underneath the A. pulmonalis. The Vv. pulmonales are in front and below. During dissection of the root of the lung some tracheobronchial lymph nodes (Nodi lymphoidei tracheobronchiales) in the area of the hilum of the lung are usually also cut; these nodes are usually black due to coal dust deposits. The mediastinal surface (left more than right) is concave because of the heart (Impressio cardiaca). Both lungs exhibit depressions which are caused by adjacent blood vessels or, on the left side, by the oesophagus. These indentations are, like the margins of the lung, only visible in the fixed lung (fixation artefacts), but they clarify the positional relationships of the lungs.

Clinical remarks

Since the apex of the lung extends above the upper thoracic aperture by 2.5 to 5 cm, when applying a **central venous catheter** (CVC) via the V. subclavia there is the danger of injuring the lung and of 'lancing', as clinicians say, a **pneumothorax,** thus causing lung collapse by opening the pleural space. This risk also exists in principle with a CVC in the V. jugularis interna at the neck since the catheter is pointed in the direction of the sternoclavicular joint and thus towards the apex of the lung. However, the risk is much greater when applying a CVC in the V. subclavia since it lies directly in contact with the Cavitas pleuralis (→ Fig. 5.135) before it continues into the V. brachiocephalica.

Organs of the thoracic cavity

Bronchopulmonary segments

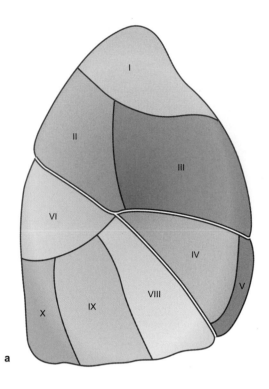

a

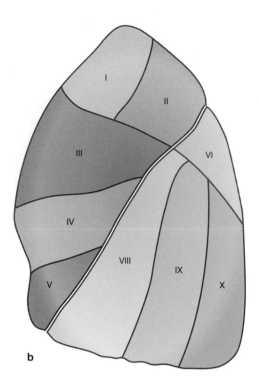

b

Pulmo dexter

Lobus superior

Segmentum apicale [S I]

Segmentum posterius [S II]

Segmentum anterius [S III]

Lobus medius

Segmentum laterale [S IV]

Segmentum mediale [S V]

Lobus inferior

Segmentum superius [S VI]

Segmentum basale mediale [cardiacum] [S VII]

Segmentum basale anterius [S VIII]

Segmentum basale laterale [S IX]

Segmentum basale posterius [S X]

Pulmo sinister

Lobus superior

Segmentum apicoposterius [S I + II]

Segmentum anterius [S III]

Segmentum lingulare superius [S IV]

Segmentum lingulare inferius [S V]

Lobus inferior

Segmentum superius [S VI]

Segmentum basale anterius [S VIII]

Segmentum basale laterale [S IX]

Segmentum basale posterius [S X]

Fig. 5.107a and b   Bronchopulmonary segments, Segmenta bronchopulmonalia; lateral view. [S700-L126]
a Right lung; lateral view.
b Left lung; lateral view.
The lung lobes subdivide into cone-shaped lung segments, which are separated incompletely from each other by connective tissue septa, so that the segment boundaries are not discernible on the surface of the lungs. The segments have corresponding **segmental bronchi** and segmental branches of the pulmonary arteries. The **right lung** has **ten seg-**ments: three in the superior, two in the middle and five in the inferior lobe. The **left lung** only has **nine segments,** because, due to the larger expansion of the mediastinum on the left-hand side, the segment VII (Segmentum basale mediale, → Fig. 5.108a) is missing or severely reduced in size and merged with segment VIII. Otherwise, the segmental subdivision is relatively similar, since the segments of the middle lobe on the right side correspond to two segments on the left in the Lingula pulmonis.

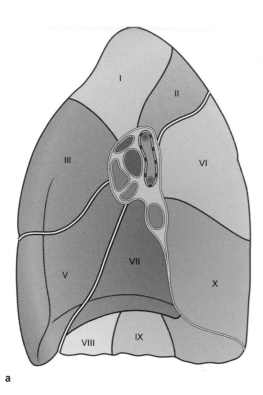

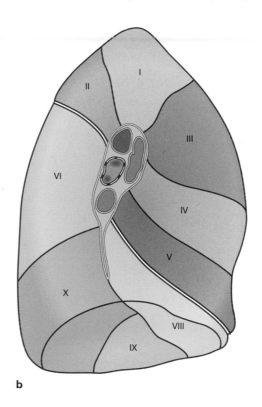

a

b

Fig. 5.108a and b   Bronchopulmonary segments, Segmenta bron-chopulmonalia; medial view. [S700-L126]
a Right lung; medial view.

b Left lung; medial view.
The right lung has 10 segments. In contrast, the left lung has only nine segments, as segment VII (Segmentum basale mediale) is missing.

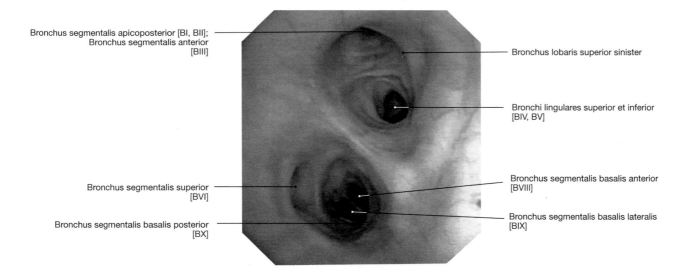

Bronchus segmentalis apicoposterior [BI, BII];
Bronchus segmentalis anterior
[BIII]

Bronchus lobaris superior sinister

Bronchi lingulares superior et inferior
[BIV, BV]

Bronchus segmentalis superior
[BVI]

Bronchus segmentalis basalis anterior
[BVIII]

Bronchus segmentalis basalis posterior
[BX]

Bronchus segmentalis basalis lateralis
[BIX]

Fig. 5.109   Bronchi; bronchoscopy with view of the segmental bronchi of the left lung. [S700]
As can be seen, the segmental bronchus VII is missing on the left side (→ Fig. 5.108b).

Clinical remarks

To aid orientation when performing a **bronchoscopy,** knowledge of the lung segments is important. A bronchoscopy is performed when diagnostic imaging reveals unclear mass lesions that need to be clarified through a biopsy, e.g. in order to exclude or diagnose a tumour. Another indication is a treatment-resistant pneumonia. Here the aim is to identify the pathogen.

Respiratory volume measurements are made pre-operatively to assess lung function and to what extent respiratory function will be restricted following resection of individual lung segments. Thus, knowledge of the number of segments of the affected lung helps to decide whether an operation would be sensible and would not significantly compromise the function of the remaining lung.

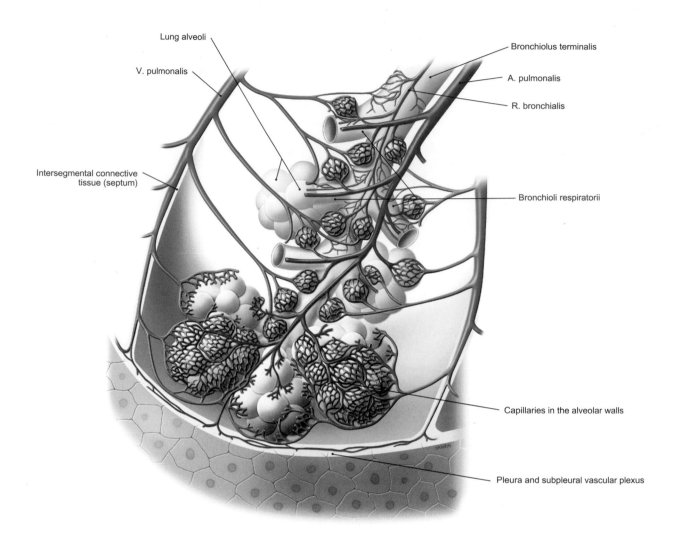

Lung alveoli

V. pulmonalis

Intersegmental connective tissue (septum)

Bronchiolus terminalis

A. pulmonalis

R. bronchialis

Bronchioli respiratorii

Capillaries in the alveolar walls

Pleura and subpleural vascular plexus

Fig. 5.110 Acinus of the lung, Acinus pulmonis, with blood supply. [S700-L238]

The lung has two blood vessel systems which communicate through their terminal branches in the walls of the alveoli (alveolar septa). The Aa. and Vv. pulmonales of the pulmonary circulation constitute the **Vasa publica** which take care of the gas exchange in the blood. The branches of the Aa. pulmonales run in the peribronchial and subpleural connective tissue and transport the deoxygenated blood from the right heart to the alveoli. In contrast, the Vv. pulmonales are located in the intersegmental connective tissue and transport the oxygenated blood to the left atrium.

The **Vasa privata** of the lung supply the lung tissue itself. The arterial Rr. bronchiales and the Vv. bronchiales run alongside the bronchi. The Vv. bronchiales discharge into the veins of the azygos system (→ Fig. 5.21, → Fig. 5.127).

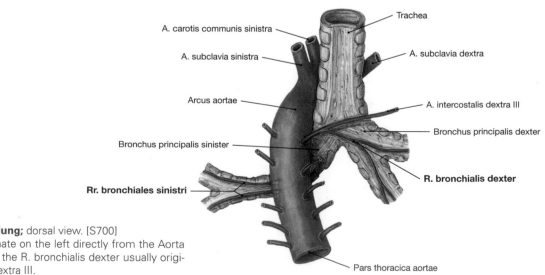

A. carotis communis sinistra

A. subclavia sinistra

Arcus aortae

Bronchus principalis sinister

Rr. bronchiales sinistri

Trachea

A. subclavia dextra

A. intercostalis dextra III

Bronchus principalis dexter

R. bronchialis dexter

Pars thoracica aortae

Fig. 5.111 Vasa privata of the lung; dorsal view. [S700]

The arterial Rr. bronchiales originate on the left directly from the Aorta thoracica; on the right, however, the R. bronchialis dexter usually originates from the A. intercostalis dextra III.

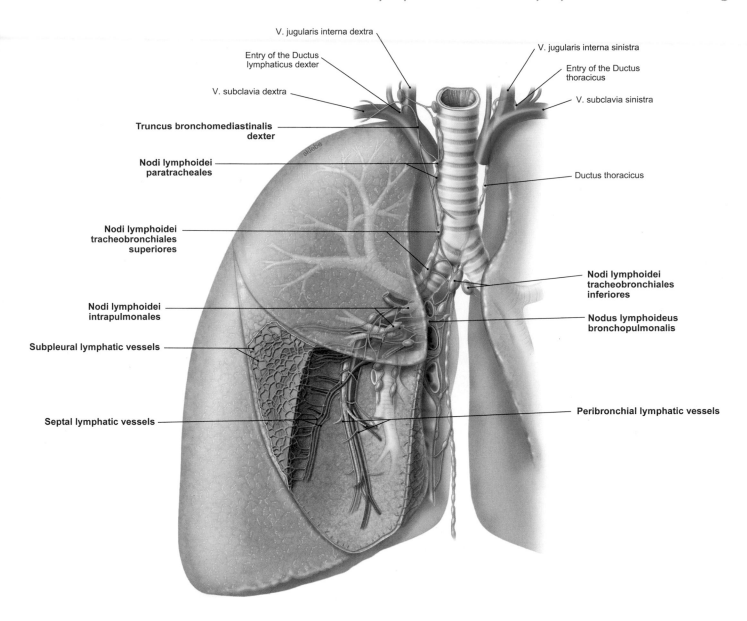

V. jugularis interna dextra

Entry of the Ductus
lymphaticus dexter

V. subclavia dextra

**Truncus bronchomediastinalis
dexter**

**Nodi lymphoidei
paratracheales**

**Nodi lymphoidei
tracheobronchiales
superiores**

**Nodi lymphoidei
intrapulmonales**

Subpleural lymphatic vessels

Septal lymphatic vessels

V. jugularis interna sinistra

Entry of the Ductus
thoracicus

V. subclavia sinistra

Ductus thoracicus

**Nodi lymphoidei
tracheobronchiales
inferiores**

**Nodus lymphoideus
bronchopulmonalis**

Peribronchial lymphatic vessels

**Fig. 5.112 Lymph vessels, Vasa lymphatica, and lymph nodes,
Nodi lymphoidei, of the lung;** ventral view; schematic drawing.
[S700-L238]/[B501-O1108/L137]

The lung has two lymph vessel systems which converge at the hilum.
The **peribronchial system** follows the bronchi and includes several
lymph nodes on its way. The first station is the **Nodi lymphoidei,** which
lie adjacent to the branching of the lobes into the segmental bronchi.
The second station is the **Nodi lymphoidei bronchopulmonales** at
the hilum of the lung. The subsequent **Nodi lymphoidei tracheobronchiales** are positioned at the root of the lung. A distinction is made between Nodi lymphoidei tracheobronchiales superiores and inferiores
above and below the tracheal bifurcation. These nodes also collect the

lymph from the heart. There is no distinct drainage pathway from the
right and left heart.
From the tracheobronchial nodes, the lymph flows into the **Nodi lymphoidei paratracheales** or into the **Trunci bronchomediastinales** of
both sides, so that there is no strict alignment to either side of the
lymphatic pathways.
In contrast, the first station for the **subpleural** and the **septal lymph
vessel systems** are the Nodi lymphoidei tracheobronchiales. The fine
lymphatic pathways form a polygonal network on the surface of the
lung, the mesh of which corresponds to the boundaries of the individual lung lobules. Due to carbon dust deposits (exhaust fumes and ciga-
rette smoke), these lymphatic pathways and thus the boundaries of the
lobules are clearly visible in a dissection.

Clinical remarks

Clinicians usually collectively call all tracheobronchial lymph nodes of
the lung **hilar lymph nodes.** This is deceptive as the Nodi lymphoidei intrapulmonales spread relatively widely into the lung parenchyma. Due to this linguistic inaccuracy, mass lesions in the parenchy-

ma may be prematurely considered to be independent disease
processes and not as enlargements of the lymph nodes, and unnecessary diagnostic steps for their clarification are initiated.

Neurovascular pathways of the lung in situ and innervation of the lung

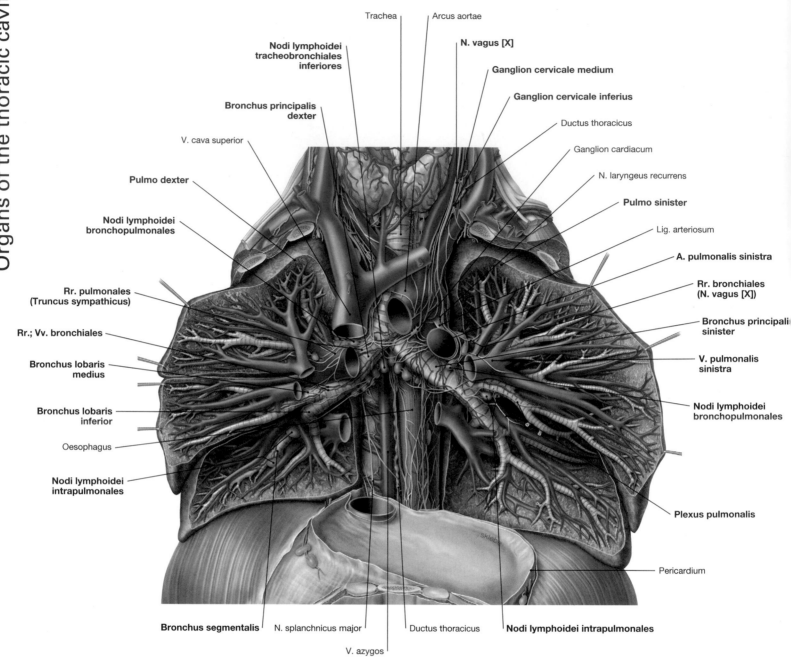

Trachea

Arcus aortae

N. vagus [X]

Nodi lymphoidei
tracheobronchiales
inferiores

Ganglion cervicale medium

Ganglion cervicale inferius

Bronchus principalis
dexter

Ductus thoracicus

V. cava superior

Ganglion cardiacum

Pulmo dexter

N. laryngeus recurrens

Pulmo sinister

Nodi lymphoidei
bronchopulmonales

Lig. arteriosum

A. pulmonalis sinistra

Rr. pulmonales
(Truncus sympathicus)

Rr. bronchiales
(N. vagus [X])

Rr.; Vv. bronchiales

Bronchus principalis
sinister

Bronchus lobaris
medius

V. pulmonalis
sinistra

Bronchus lobaris
inferior

Nodi lymphoidei
bronchopulmonales

Oesophagus

Nodi lymphoidei
intrapulmonales

Plexus pulmonalis

Pericardium

Bronchus segmentalis   N. splanchnicus major   Ductus thoracicus   Nodi lymphoidei intrapulmonales

V. azygos

Fig. 5.113 Bronchial tree of the lungs with neurovascular pathways; ventral view; after removal of the heart with pericardium. [S700-L238]/[Q300]

The **main bronchi (Bronchi principales)** commence at the hilum of the lungs. Together with the neurovascular pathways of the lungs these form the **root of the lung (Radix pulmonis)**. The main bronchi divide into the **lobar and segmental bronchi (Bronchi lobares and Bronchi segmentales)** accompanied by the branches of the **pulmonary arteries (Aa. pulmonales)**. In contrast, the **pulmonary veins (Vv. pulmonales)** are isolated within the subpleural and intersegmental connective tissue, which has been removed. These large vessels are merged as vasa publica, as they serve to oxygenate the blood and thus the supply of the whole body. They can be seen clearly in a dissection. The illustration also shows the finer neurovascular pathways that are usually not distinct in a dissection: the arterial **Rr. bronchiales** and the **Vv. bronchiales** constitute the vasa privata of the lung since they supply the lung tissue. They run directly along the bronchi. The lymphatic pathways of the peribronchial lymph vessel system are connected to the Nodi lym-

phoidei intrapulmonales, which are located as the first lymph node station at the branching of the lobes into the segmental bronchi. The second station of the **Nodi lymphoidei bronchopulmonales** is right inside the hilum.

The autonomic nerve fibres of the **Plexus pulmonalis** form a network on the main bronchi that includes both efferent as well as afferent nerve fibres. The sympathetic nerve fibres **(Rr. pulmonales)** are postganglionic and come from the lower ganglion of the sympathetic chain (Ganglion cervicale inferius), as well as the upper ganglia of the thoracic sympathetic chain. The parasympathetic nerve fibres **(Rr. bronchiales)** from the N. vagus [X] and N. laryngeus recurrens are still preganglionic. Their synaptic switch happens in the mostly microscopically small ganglia of the Plexus pulmonalis. The **Truncus sympathicus** effects an expansion of the bronchi **(bronchial dilation)** for better ventilation of the lung, while the **parasympathetic trunk** narrows the bronchi **(bronchial constriction)** and activates the secretion of mucous-forming glands. The N. vagus [X] also leads afferent nerve fibres from the lung to the brainstem in order to be able to convey stretch and pain stimuli.

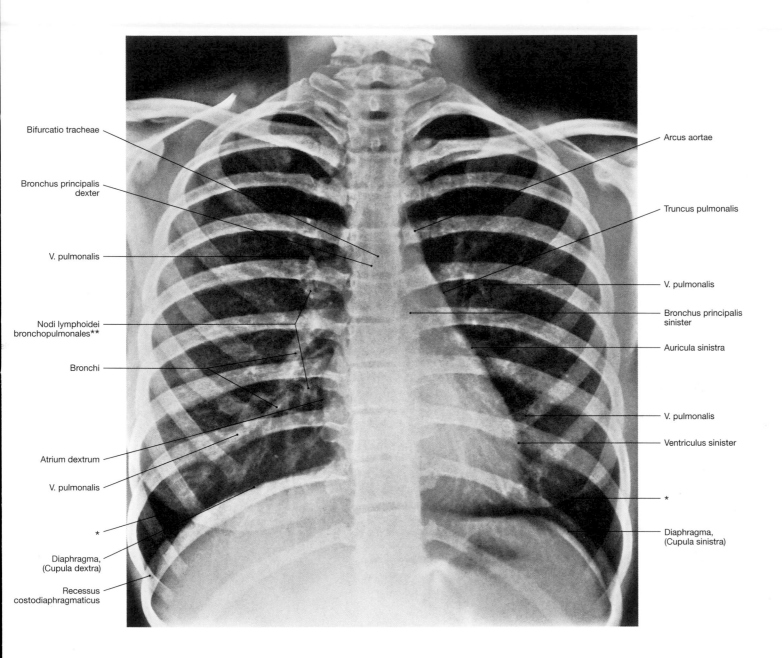

Bifurcatio tracheae

Bronchus principalis dexter

V. pulmonalis

Nodi lymphoidei bronchopulmonales**

Bronchi

Atrium dextrum

V. pulmonalis

*

Diaphragma, (Cupula dextra)

Recessus costodiaphragmaticus

Arcus aortae

Truncus pulmonalis

V. pulmonalis

Bronchus principalis sinister

Auricula sinistra

V. pulmonalis

Ventriculus sinister

*

Diaphragma, (Cupula sinistra)

Fig. 5.114   Thoracic cage, Cavea thoracis, with organs of the Cavitas thoracis; X-ray in posteroanterior (PA) projection. [R316-007] The bronchi are partially discernible on the pathway. On the right side, clusters of lymph nodes in the area of the hilum of the lung are also discernible.

*   mammary shadow (contour)
** clin.: hilar lymph nodes

Clinical remarks

X-ray images of the thorax are frequently taken if **pathological processes** of the lungs and the pleura are suspected, such as inflammations (pneumonia, pleurisy) or tumours (bronchial carcinoma). Changes in the parenchyma often stand out as 'shadows' because radiolu-

cency is usually lower than in intact lung tissue. In the case of a pleural effusion, the costodiaphragmatic recess is blunted with an upright body position, resulting in a horizontal fluid level.

Oesophagus

Projection of the oesophagus

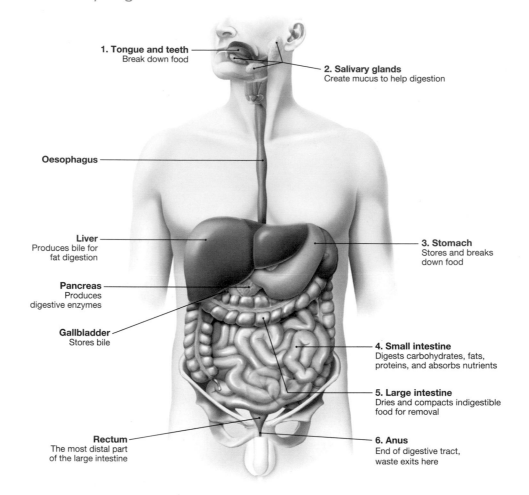

1. **Tongue and teeth**
Break down food

2. **Salivary glands**
Create mucus to help digestion

Oesophagus

Liver
Produces bile for
fat digestion

Pancreas
Produces
digestive enzymes

Gallbladder
Stores bile

3. **Stomach**
Stores and breaks
down food

4. **Small intestine**
Digests carbohydrates, fats,
proteins, and absorbs nutrients

5. **Large intestine**
Dries and compacts indigestible
food for removal

Rectum
The most distal part
of the large intestine

6. **Anus**
End of digestive tract,
waste exits here

Fig. 5.115 Overview of the digestive system. [S701-L275]
The digestive system extends from the oral cavity via the pharynx to the gastrointestinal tract and also comprises the accessory glands, such as oral and pancreatic glands, liver and gallbladder.
The **oesophagus** is a muscular tube, which connects the **pharynx** with the **stomach (Gaster)** and transports the swallowed food. The oesophagus is **25 cm long** and reaches from the cricoid cartilage which projects onto the sixth cervical vertebra to the stomach entrance (cardia) at the height of the 10th thoracic vertebra (below the Proc. xiphoideus of

the breastbone). The anatomical length of the oesophagus is relatively negligible for diagnostics. Here, the distance from the dental arch is given, since in an endoscopic examination of the upper gastrointestinal tract (gastroscopy) the length of the oral cavity and pharynx must be taken into account. The oesophagus develops from the foregut (→ Fig. 5.100), with the epithelium derived from the intestinal tube and the muscle and connective tissue of the oesophageal wall from the surrounding mesoderm.

Fig. 5.116 HEAD's zone of the oesophagus and the heart; schematic diagram of the sensory innervation of the ventral torso wall; ventral view. [S700-L126]/[G1071]
Afferent nervous pathways from the heart, through which stimuli are transmitted to the central nervous system, run in the respective spinal cord segments together with nerve fibres that originate from the dedicated skin areas (dermatomes). In the oesophagus, these are the dermatomes T4 and T5. This organ-dependent skin area where pain is perceived is referred to as the **HEAD's zone of the oesophagus.** Since the **HEAD's zone of the heart** is closely adjacent, pain in the area of the ventral thoracic wall is always initially regarded as angina pectoris until CHD is excluded.

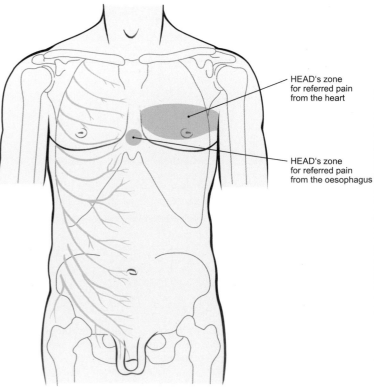

HEAD's zone
for referred pain
from the heart

HEAD's zone
for referred pain
from the oesophagus

Clinical remarks

The projection of the oesophagus makes it understandable why a mucosal inflammation caused by gastric juices **(reflux oesophagitis)** causes pain and retrosternal burning in a similar location as a heart attack. From these two organs, the afferent nerve fibres go into the same spinal cord segments as nerve fibres of the anterior thoracic wall, so that the brain cannot properly differentiate whether the pain stems from the body surface or from one of the internal organs.

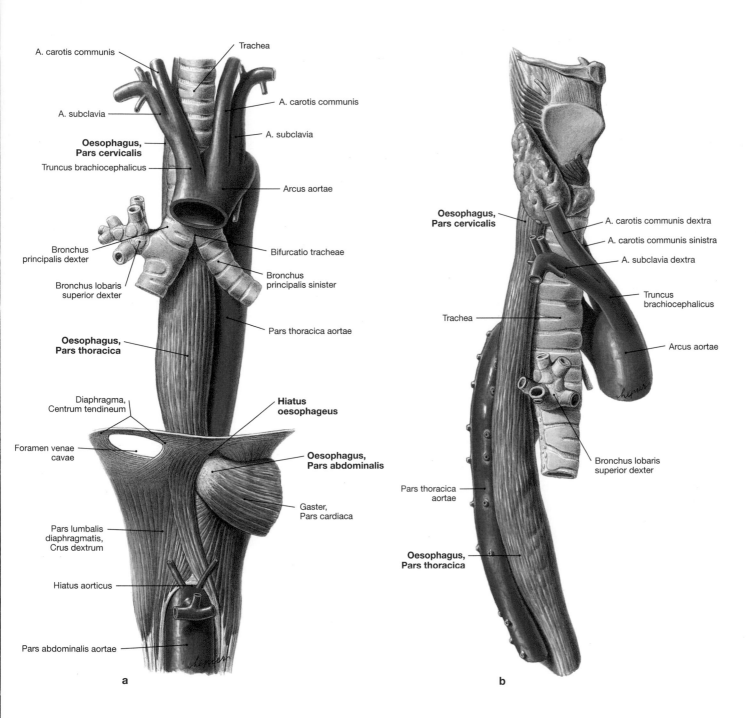

A. carotis communis

Trachea

A. subclavia

A. carotis communis

Oesophagus, Pars cervicalis

A. subclavia

Truncus brachiocephalicus

Arcus aortae

Bronchus principalis dexter

Bifurcatio tracheae

Bronchus lobaris superior dexter

Bronchus principalis sinister

Pars thoracica aortae

Oesophagus, Pars thoracica

Diaphragma, Centrum tendineum

Hiatus oesophageus

Foramen venae cavae

Oesophagus, Pars abdominalis

Gaster, Pars cardiaca

Pars lumbalis diaphragmatis, Crus dextrum

Hiatus aorticus

Pars abdominalis aortae

a

Oesophagus, Pars cervicalis

A. carotis communis dextra

A. carotis communis sinistra

A. subclavia dextra

Truncus brachiocephalicus

Trachea

Arcus aortae

Bronchus lobaris superior dexter

Pars thoracica aortae

Oesophagus, Pars thoracica

b

Fig. 5.117a and b   Oesophagus, trachea, and Pars thoracica of the aorta. [S700]
a Ventral view.
b View from the right.
The oesophagus is 25 cm long and is divided into three parts:
*   Pars cervicalis (5–8 cm)
*   Pars thoracica (16 cm)
*   Pars abdominalis (1–4 cm).

The **Pars cervicalis** is located in the spine. The **Pars thoracica** crosses the Arcus aortae, which is situated dorsally from the left, runs past the left main bronchus and moves increasingly away to the ventral side of the spine. In the dorsal view, it is clear that the Pars thoracica has direct contact to the pericardium and therefore enters into close proximity to the left atrium (→ Fig. 5.118). The short intraperitoneally located Pars abdominalis commences after passing through the oesophageal hiatus.

Structure of the oesophagus

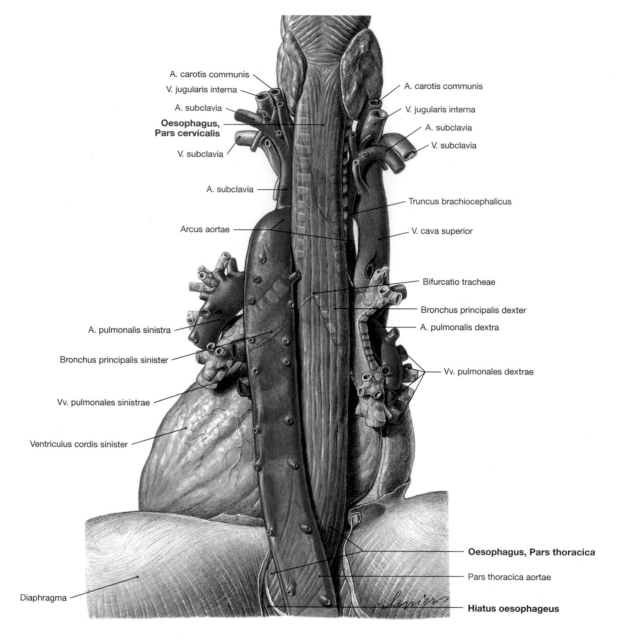

A. carotis communis
V. jugularis interna
A. subclavia
Oesophagus, Pars cervicalis
V. subclavia

A. subclavia

Arcus aortae

A. pulmonalis sinistra

Bronchus principalis sinister

Vv. pulmonales sinistrae

Ventriculus cordis sinister

Diaphragma

A. carotis communis
V. jugularis interna
A. subclavia
V. subclavia

Truncus brachiocephalicus

V. cava superior

Bifurcatio tracheae

Bronchus principalis dexter

A. pulmonalis dextra

Vv. pulmonales dextrae

Oesophagus, Pars thoracica

Pars thoracica aortae

Hiatus oesophageus

Fig. 5.118 Oesophagus, pericardium and Pars thoracica aortae; dorsal view. [S700]
The Pars thoracica of the oesophagus runs adjacent and to the right of the **Aorta descendens.** The neck part and the upper part of the Pars thoracica are situated directly on the dorsal side of the **trachea.** The caudal part of the Pars thoracica, which is situated below the tracheal bifurcation, dorsally abuts the left atrium **(Atrium sinistrum),** which is only separated by the pericardium. The tracheal bifurcation abuts the oesophagus at a distance of approximately 23 cm from the dental arch.

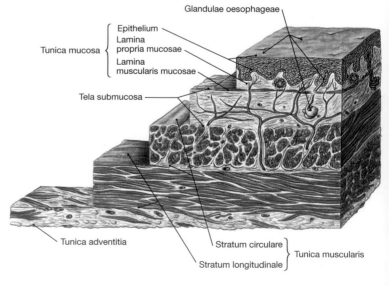

Glandulae oesophageae

Epithelium
Lamina propria mucosae

Tunica mucosa

Lamina muscularis mucosae

Tela submucosa

Tunica adventitia

Stratum circulare
Stratum longitudinale

Tunica muscularis

Fig. 5.119 Wall composition of the oesophagus; microscopic view. [S700]
Similar to the entire gut, the wall of the oesophagus consists of a luminal mucous membrane **(Tunica mucosa)** which is separated by a loose connective tissue layer **(Tela submucosa)** from the muscular layer **(Tunica muscularis).** The cervical and thoracic parts are covered by the **Tunica adventitia.** Only in the intraperitoneally located Pars abdominalis is the outer surface covered by visceral peritoneum, the Tunica serosa.

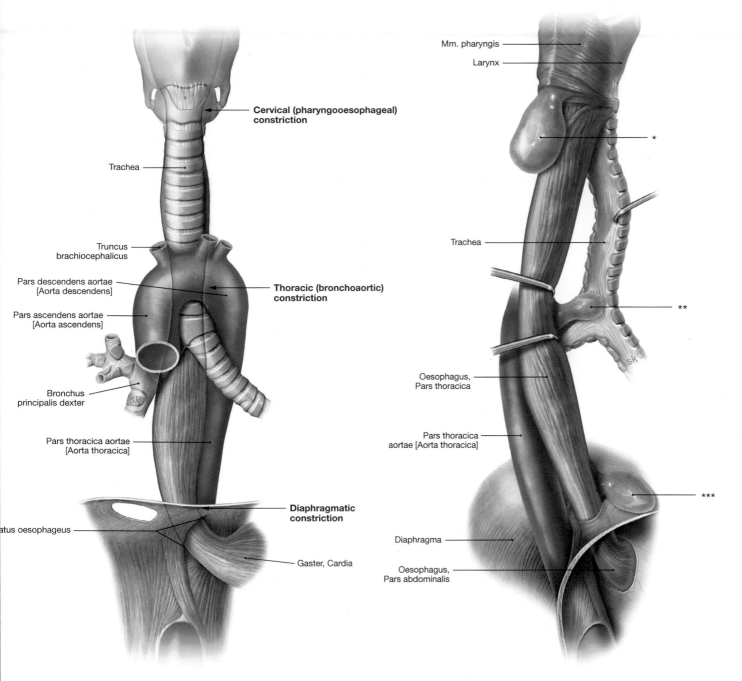

Fig. 5.120   Constrictions, Angustiae, of the oesophagus; ventral view. [S700-L238]

The oesophagus has three constrictions:
- Pharyngoesophageal constriction (Angustia cricoidea)
- Aortic constriction (Angustia aortica)
- Diaphragmatic constriction (Angustia diaphragmatica).

The **pharyngoesophageal constriction** is the narrowest point in the area of the upper oesophageal sphincter at the level of the sixth cervical vertebra. The **aortic constriction** is brought forth dorsally on the left by the accretion of the Arcus aortae (height of the fourth thoracic vertebra). The **diaphragmatic constriction** lies in the oesophageal hiatus of the diaphragm (height 10th thoracic vertebra). There is no real sphincter here, only an angiomuscular extension closure. The oesophagus is secured with elastic connective tissue (Lig. phrenicooesophageale) to the outside of the Hiatus oesophageus.

Fig. 5.121   Diverticula of the oesophagus; dorsal right view. [S700-L238]

*   clin.: ZENKER's diverticulum
**   clin.: traction diverticulum
*** clin.: epiphrenic diverticulum

Clinical remarks

Swallowed foreign bodies (e. g. fish bones) can get stuck at the constrictions. Diverticula of the entire oesophageal wall can occur at different points. **ZENKER's diverticula** (70 %) are the most common. These diverticula bulge through the KILLIAN's triangle of the hypopharynx (→ Fig. 5.123) and are falsely regarded as diverticula of the oesophagus. The cause is a weakening of the lower pharyngeal constrictor muscle. **Traction diverticula** (22 %) are phylogenetically caused by a defective separation of the oesophagus and trachea (→ Fig. 5.100). **Epiphrenic diverticula** (8 %) are believed to be caused by a fault of the lower oesophageal sphincter.

Closing mechanisms of the oesophagus – upper oesophageal sphincter

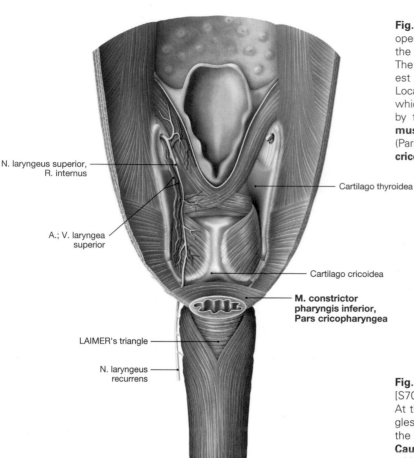

N. laryngeus superior, R. internus

A.; V. laryngea superior

LAIMER's triangle

N. laryngeus recurrens

Cartilago thyroidea

Cartilago cricoidea

M. constrictor pharyngis inferior, Pars cricopharyngea

Fig. 5.122 **Upper oesophageal sphincter;** dorsal view onto the opened pharynx, the mucous membrane of which was resected on the anterior side. [S700-L275]/[G1060-002]
The oesophagus starts at the cricoid cartilage constriction. This narrowest part of the oesophagus projects onto the sixth cervical vertebra. Located here is a true sphincter **(upper oesophageal sphincter)**, which is also morphologically distinguishable. It is formed on the **inside** by the transverse striated muscle fibres (Stratum circulare) of the **muscular layer of the oesophagus.** On the **outside,** muscle fibres (Pars transversa) of the **M. constrictor pharyngis inferior, the Pars cricopharyngea,** contribute to this sphincter.

Fig. 5.123 **KILLIAN's triangle and LAIMER's triangle;** dorsal view. [S700]
At the transition between the pharynx and oesophagus are two triangles with sparse muscular coverage. **Cranially** of the transverse part of the inferior pharyngeal constrictor muscle lies the **KILLIAN's triangle. Caudally** of the transverse fibres, the **LAIMER's triangle** as an area with sparce muscles can be distinguished.

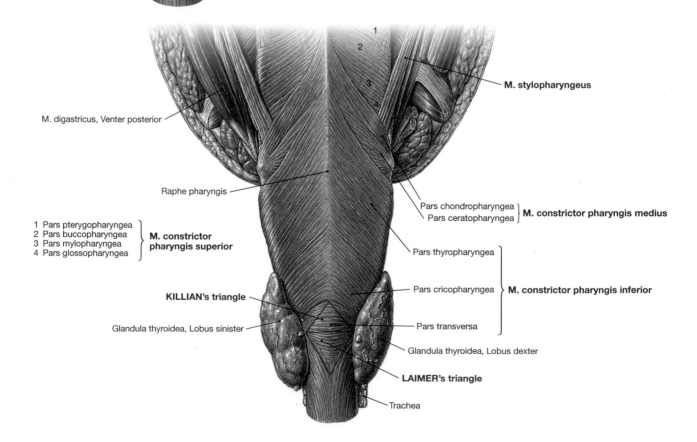

M. digastricus, Venter posterior

Raphe pharyngis

1 Pars pterygopharyngea
2 Pars buccopharyngea
3 Pars mylopharyngea
4 Pars glossopharyngea } **M. constrictor pharyngis superior**

KILLIAN's triangle

Glandula thyroidea, Lobus sinister

M. stylopharyngeus

Pars chondropharyngea
Pars ceratopharyngea } **M. constrictor pharyngis medius**

Pars thyropharyngea

Pars cricopharyngea } **M. constrictor pharyngis inferior**

Pars transversa

Glandula thyroidea, Lobus dexter

LAIMER's triangle

Trachea

Clinical remarks

If during swallowing, the transverse fibres of the inferior pharyngeal constrictor do not relax in time, thereby causing increased pressure above the sphincter, **ZENKER's diverticula** can emerge as protru-

sions (→ Fig. 5.121). They can lead to swallowing difficulties (dysphagia) as they compress the oesophagus from the outside.

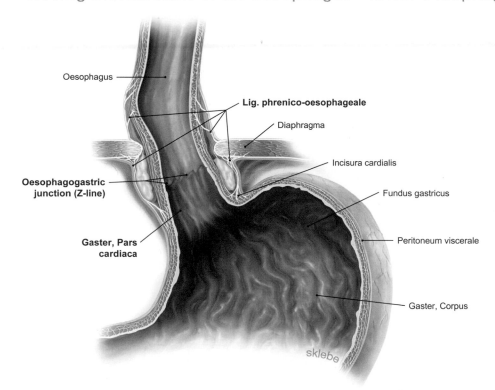

Fig. 5.124 Anchoring of the oesophagus in the oesophageal hiatus of the diaphragm; ventral view, after removal of the anterior wall of the oesophagus and stomach. [S700-L238]/[G343]

At its caudal aspect the oesophagus does not have a morphologically demarcated sphincter. There is, however, a functional closure which relies on different mechanisms. (→ Fig. 5.125).

- **Neuromuscular oesophageal sphincter:** The spiral muscle fibres of the Tunica muscularis (Stratum longitudinale) are twisted due to the longitudinal tension of the oesophagus. Together with venous cushions under the mucous membranes this results in a closure.
- **Mucosal fold in the angle of HIS:** Between the stomach entrance (cardia) and fundus of the stomach is a constriction (Incisura cardialis) with a sharp angle of 65°. In this angle of HIS a mucosal fold

which is raised by the notch (Incisura cardialis) emerges into the lumen of the stomach and prevents the reflux of stomach contents.
- **Lig. phrenico-oesophageale:** This fibrous anchoring of the oesophagus in the Hiatus oesophageus of the diaphragm stabilises its position and counteracts a reflux.
- **Pressure gradient between abdominal and thoracic cavities:** The higher pressure in the abdominal cavity supports the closure.

The mucosal transition between the oesophagus and stomach is macroscopically visible due to the epithelial change. Due to its jagged structure, it is called the **Z-line.** This line is mostly located in the area of the oesophagus (70 %) and thus proximal to the supposed border on the outside between the oesophagus and stomach.

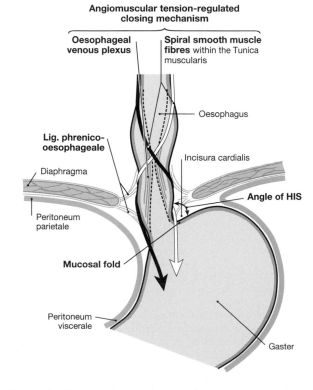

Fig. 5.125 Angiomuscular tension-regulated closure mechanism and angle of HIS at the terminal oesophagus; schematic illustration; ventral view. [S700-L126]/[B500~M282/T663]/[F702-006]

Clinical remarks

If the inferior closing mechanism fails, a reflux of the stomach contents and, in the longer term, an inflammation of the oesophageal mucosa **(oesophageal reflux)** ensue. A typical symptom is heartburn. As a result, the oesophageal mucosa may convert to the mucosa of the stomach so that the Z-line no longer presents regularly or has deflected proximally. This metaplasia is referred to as a **BARRETT's oesophagus.** It is associated with an increased risk for development of oesophageal cancer. These **adenocarcinomas of the oesophagus** are not very common, but represent one of the most rapidly growing tumour diseases in the Western world as the risk factors for reflux are associated with nutritional habits.

Because the Z-line can shift due to pathological processes, it cannot be used clinically as a demarcation between the oesophagus and stomach. However, an unambiguous boundary is important as the treatment of **oesophageal cancer** (removal of the oesophagus with stomach interposition or small intestine interposition) fundamentally differs from the treatment of gastric cancer (removal of the stomach, gastrectomy). Therefore, since 2010, the first mucosal fold of the stomach is used as the boundary between the stomach and oesophagus, and tumours positioned at the oesophagogastric junction are treated as oesophageal tumours.

Arteries of the oesophagus

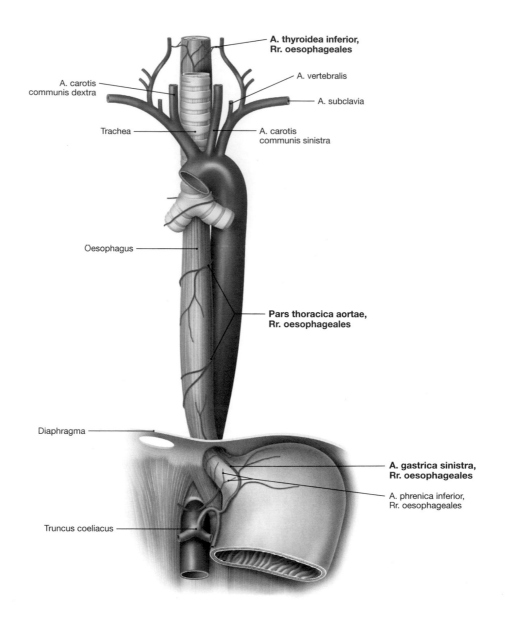

Fig. 5.126 Arteries of the oesophagus; ventral view. [S700-L275]
The individual parts of the oesophagus are supplied by surrounding arteries:

- **Pars cervicalis:** A. thyroidea inferior
- **Pars thoracica:** Rr. oesophageales of the Aorta thoracica
- **Pars abdominalis:** A. gastrica sinistra and A. phrenica inferior.

The arterial and venous supply of the trachea correspond to the blood vessels of the cervical and thoracic parts of the oesophagus.

Clinical remarks

In contrast to the other organs of the gastrointestinal tract, the oesophagus **lacks proprietary arteries**, but is supplied from adjacent blood vessels. This poses a challenge for surgery, and oesophageal surgery is categorised as high risk.

Surgeries for **oesophageal carcinoma** involve two body cavities in order to mobilise both the abdominal and the thoracic parts of the section to be removed, and to tie off relevant blood vessels and remove the lymph nodes. This method is used in surgeries for adeno-

carcinomas which are increasingly occurring in the western world as a result of reflux oesophagitis and is often sufficient. However, proximal oesophageal tumours most likely presenting as squamous cell carcinomas, require additional surgical access from the neck to remove lymph nodes above the azygos vein entry into the superior vena cava (SVC). This is a standard procedure in Asia where squamous cell carcinomas are more frequent.

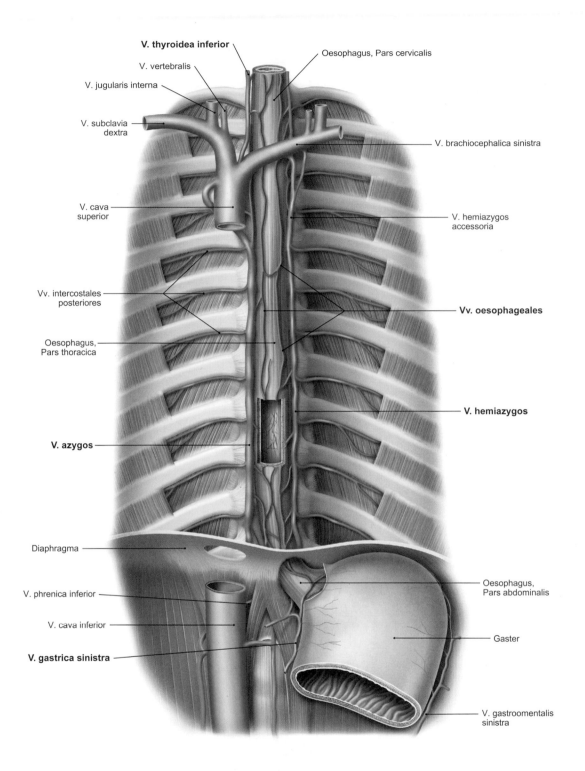

V. thyroidea inferior

V. vertebralis

V. jugularis interna

V. subclavia dextra

Oesophagus, Pars cervicalis

V. brachiocephalica sinistra

V. cava superior

V. hemiazygos accessoria

Vv. intercostales posteriores

Vv. oesophageales

Oesophagus, Pars thoracica

V. hemiazygos

V. azygos

Diaphragma

Oesophagus, Pars abdominalis

V. phrenica inferior

V. cava inferior

Gaster

V. gastrica sinistra

V. gastroomentalis sinistra

Fig. 5.127   Veins of the oesophagus, Vv. oesophageales; ventral view. [S700-L275]

The strong venous plexus in the adventitia is drained via separate veins:

- **Pars cervicalis:** V. thyroidea inferior
- **Pars thoracica:** via the V. azygos and V. hemiazygos in the V. cava superior

- **Pars abdominalis:** the inferior part of the oesophagus has **connections to the portal vein system** via the gastric veins (V. gastrica sinistra). These connections may be utilised in the case of high pressure in the hepatic portal vein (portal hypertension) as **portocaval anastomoses** (→ Fig. 5.128).

Veins of the oesophagus

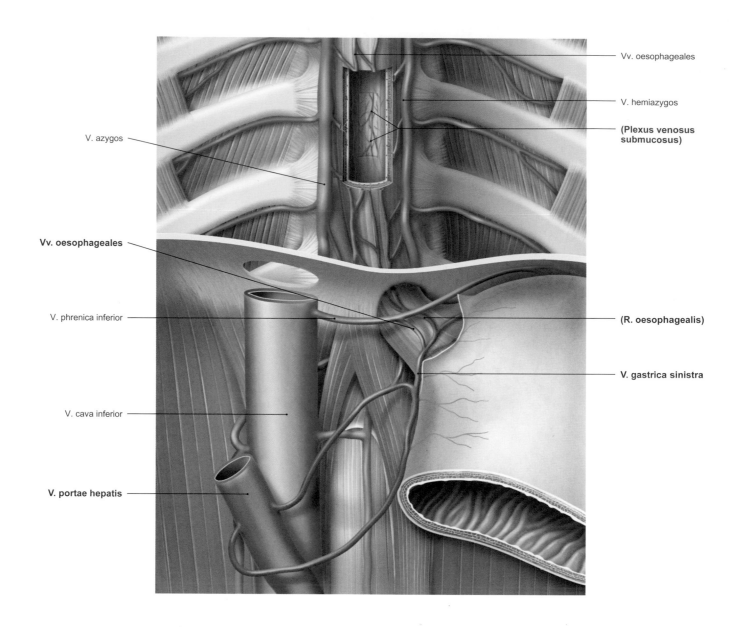

V. azygos

Vv. oesophageales

V. phrenica inferior

V. cava inferior

V. portae hepatis

Vv. oesophageales

V. hemiazygos

(Plexus venosus submucosus)

(R. oesophagealis)

V. gastrica sinistra

Fig. 5.128 **Veins of the oesophagus, Vv. oesophageales, illustrating the portocaval anastomoses between the portal vein, V. portae hepatis and V. cava superior;** ventral view. [S700-L275]
The strong venous plexus in the Tunica adventitia has connections to the submucosal veins (Plexus venosus submucosus). Blood flows cra-

nially via the **V. azygos** (right) and the **V. hemiazygos** (left) to the **V. cava superior.** In the lower parts of the oesophagus, descending via the veins of the lesser curvature of the stomach **(Vv. gastricae dextra and sinistra),** it is also connected to the **V. portae hepatis.**

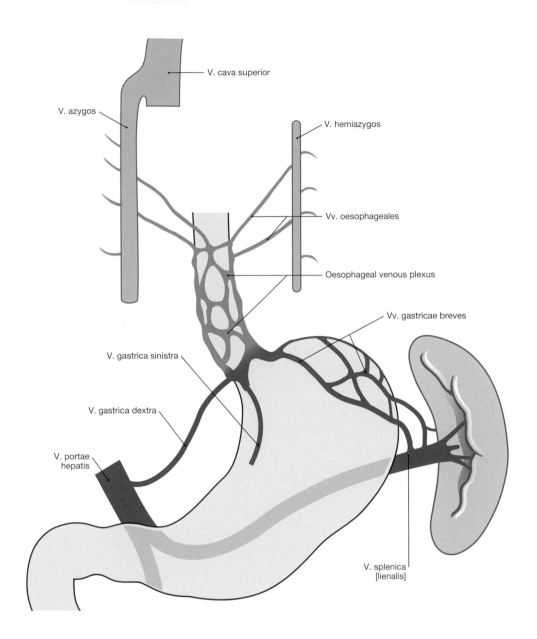

V. cava superior

V. azygos

V. hemiazygos

Vv. oesophageales

Oesophageal venous plexus

Vv. gastricae breves

V. gastrica sinistra

V. gastrica dextra

V. portae hepatis

V. splenica [lienalis]

Fig. 5.129   Veins of the oesophagus, Vv. oesophageales, and portocaval anastomoses; schematic illustration; ventral view. [S700-L126]/[B500]

The submucosal venous plexus in the oesophagus is a component of the angiomuscular closure mechanism of the lower oesophagus (→ Fig. 5.125) and represents a portocaval anastomosis. It connects cranially to the superior vena cava (SVC) and caudally via the Vv. gastrica dextra and sinistra to the hepatic portal vein.

Clinical remarks

If the pressure in the portal vein system rises **(portal hypertension),** e.g. as a result of higher vascular resistance in the liver due to scarred reorganisation (cirrhosis), then blood is directed via collateral circulatory connections of the superior and inferior venae cavae **(portocaval anastomoses).** The clinically most important portocaval anastomoses are the connections via the gastric veins to the oesophagus, since these can cause expansions of the submucosal veins **(oesophageal varices** → Fig. 5.133). Rupture of these varices is associated with a mortality of approximately 50 % and is thus the most frequent cause of death in patients with liver cirrhosis. In the case of a rupture inwards, the stomach is filled with mostly blackened blood; in rarer outward ruptures the blood enters the abdominal cavity.

Caudal oesophageal carcinomas (below the tracheal bifurcation) **metastasise** more frequently to the **liver** than to the lungs due to the venous drainage to the hepatic portal vein.

Oesophagus

Lymph vessels of the oesophagus

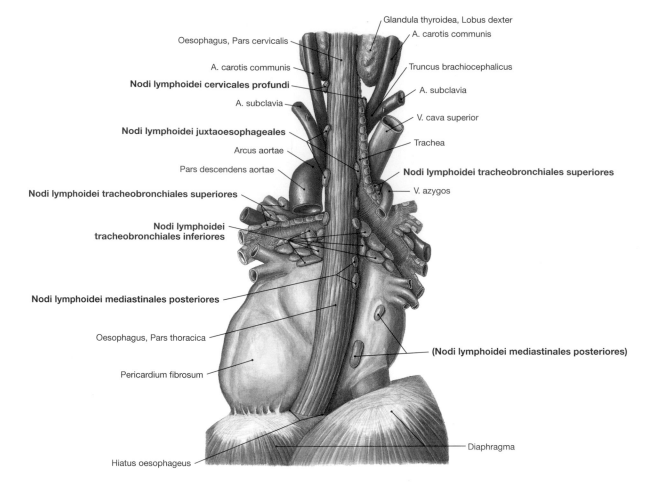

Fig. 5.130 **Lymph nodes, Nodi lymphoidei, of the posterior mediastinum,** dorsal view. [S700]
The lymph of the oesophagus is drained via the lymph nodes which are located directly at the oesophagus (Nodi lymphoidei juxtaoesophageales):
* **Pars cervicalis:** Nodi lymphoidei cervicales profundi

* **Pars thoracica:** Lymph nodes of the mediastinum (Nodi lymphoidei mediastinales posteriores, Nodi lymphoidei tracheobronchiales and paratracheales)
* **Pars abdominalis:** Lymph nodes on the bottom of the diaphragm (Nodi lymphoidei phrenici inferiores) and at the lesser curvature of the stomach (Nodi lymphoidei gastrici).

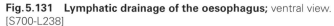

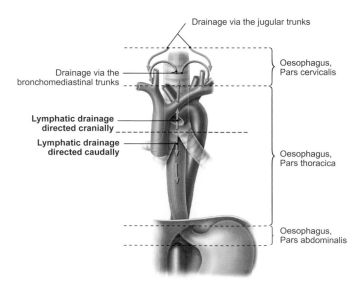

Fig. 5.131 **Lymphatic drainage of the oesophagus;** ventral view. [S700-L238]
The lymph of the cervical part drains via the deep cervical lymph nodes to the **Truncus jugularis.** In the Pars thoracica, there are two flow directions: the top half above the tracheal bifurcation drains upwards into the mediastinal lymph nodes and from there into the **Truncus bronchomediastinalis.** The bottom half below the tracheal bifurcation has connections to the lymph nodes of the abdominal cavity, which also constitute the regional lymph nodes for the Pars abdominalis. From here, the lymph drains via the Nodi lymphoidei coeliaci into the **Truncus intestinalis.**

Clinical remarks

The direction of lymphatic drainage plays a role in the metastasis of **oesophageal and gastric cancers.** Tumours of the lower oesophagus may metastasise into the lymph nodes of the abdomen. Similar drainage areas appear to exist for the venous blood of the oesopha-gus as well, as oesophageal cancer below the tracheal bifurcation causes liver metastases more frequently, while in the case of tumours above the tracheal bifurcation, lung metastases are more common.

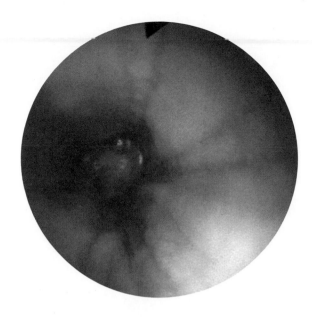

Fig. 5.132 Oesophagus; oesophagoscopy, normal finding. [G159]

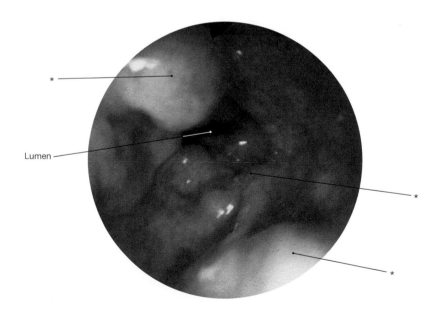

Fig. 5.133 Oesophagus; oesophagoscopy, oesophageal varices in liver cirrhosis. [G159]

* clin.: varices

Clinical remarks

In **portal hypertension,** the dilation of **portocaval anastomoses** involving the veins of the oesophagus may develop into **oesophageal varices.** A rupture of these varices often leads to **life-threatening** **bleeding.** Therefore, oesophageal varices are tethered prophylactically (endoscopic band ligation) or treated with vessel-cauterising substances (sclerotised).

Cross-sectional images

Oesophagus, midsagittal section

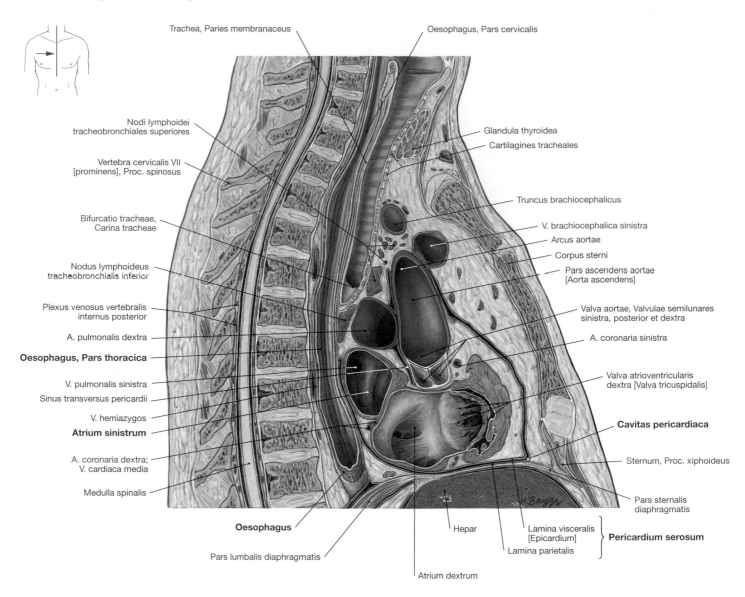

Trachea, Paries membranaceus

Oesophagus, Pars cervicalis

Nodi lymphoidei tracheobronchiales superiores

Glandula thyroidea

Cartilagines tracheales

Vertebra cervicalis VII [prominens], Proc. spinosus

Truncus brachiocephalicus

Bifurcatio tracheae, Carina tracheae

V. brachiocephalica sinistra

Arcus aortae

Corpus sterni

Nodus lymphoideus tracheobronchialis inferior

Pars ascendens aortae [Aorta ascendens]

Plexus venosus vertebralis internus posterior

Valva aortae, Valvulae semilunares sinistra, posterior et dextra

A. pulmonalis dextra

A. coronaria sinistra

Oesophagus, Pars thoracica

V. pulmonalis sinistra

Valva atrioventricularis dextra [Valva tricuspidalis]

Sinus transversus pericardii

V. hemiazygos

Atrium sinistrum

Cavitas pericardiaca

A. coronaria dextra; V. cardiaca media

Sternum, Proc. xiphoideus

Medulla spinalis

Pars sternalis diaphragmatis

Oesophagus

Hepar

Lamina visceralis [Epicardium]

Pericardium serosum

Pars lumbalis diaphragmatis

Lamina parietalis

Atrium dextrum

Fig. 5.134 Cavitas thoracis; midsagittal section; lateral view from the right side. [S700]
This type of sectioning emphasises the proximity of the oesophagus, positioned in the posterior mediastinum, at the left atrium of the heart in the middle mediastinum. Both structures are only separated by the pericardial cavity (Cavitas pericardiaca).

Clinical remarks

The oesophagus is separated from the left atrium of the heart only by the pericardium. Thus, a dilation of the left atrium, e.g. in cases of a mitral valve stenosis, can lead to a compression of the oesophagus, presenting as difficulty in swallowing (**dysphagia**).
In **transoesophageal echocardiography,** the spatial proximity of the oesophagus to the heart is utilised. A depiction of the heart and particularly the heart valves is achieved much more accurately using an ultrasound probe inserted into the oesophagus than through an examination from the outer rib cage.
[G198]

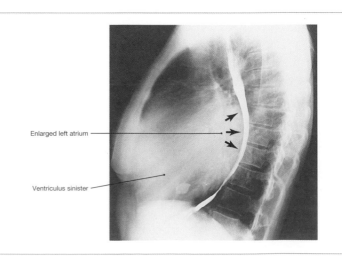

Enlarged left atrium

Ventriculus sinister

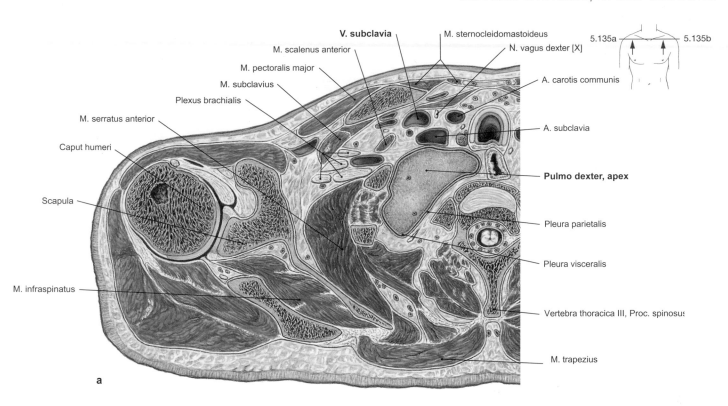

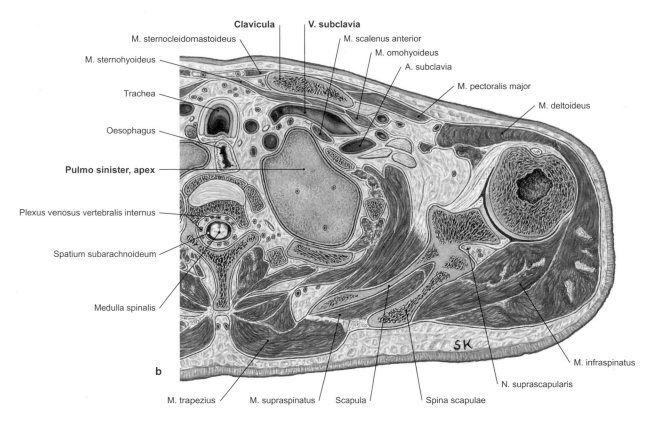

Fig. 5.135a and b   Pleural dome, Cupula pleurae; cross-sections at the level of the shoulder joint; caudal view. [S700-L238]
a Right side.
b Left side.

These sections illustrate that the pleural dome extends behind the neurovascular bundle of the arm above the upper thoracic aperture. As a result, the apex of the lung is positioned directly behind the A. and V. subclavia.

Clinical remarks

When inserting a **central venous catheter** (CVC) into the **V. subclavia,** the extension of the pleural dome must be considered. The cannula is placed just below the anterior convexity of the clavicle, pointing in the direction of the sternoclavicular joint. If the cannula is positioned too steeply, the Cavitas pleuralis may be injured, and an inflow of air into the cavity can result in collapsing of the lung **(pneumothorax).**

Organs of the thoracic cavity

Cavitas thoracis, cross-sections

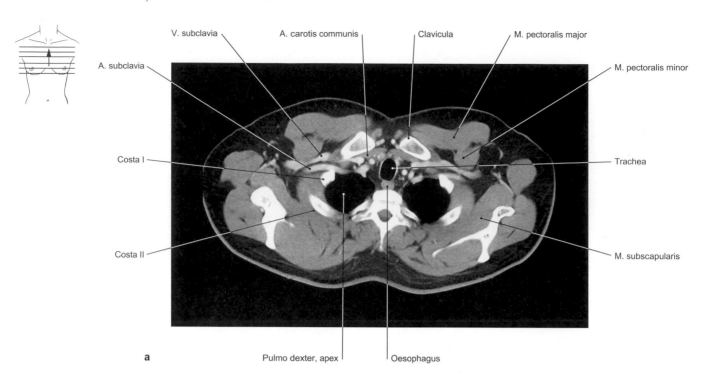

V. subclavia — A. carotis communis — Clavicula — M. pectoralis major

A. subclavia — M. pectoralis minor

Costa I — Trachea

Costa II — M. subscapularis

a — Pulmo dexter, apex — Oesophagus

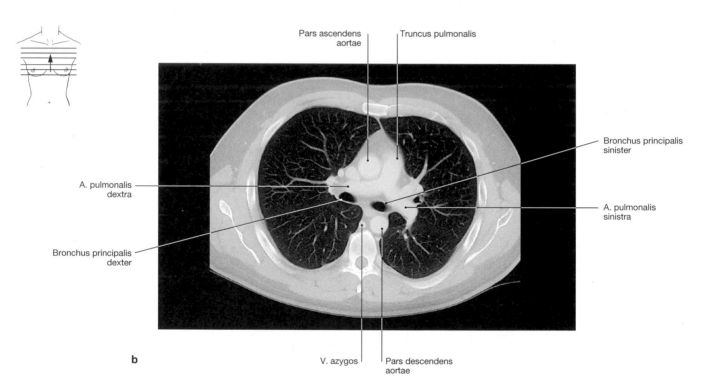

Pars ascendens aortae — Truncus pulmonalis

A. pulmonalis dextra — Bronchus principalis sinister

Bronchus principalis dexter — A. pulmonalis sinistra

b — V. azygos — Pars descendens aortae

Fig. 5.136a and b Upper thoracic aperture; contrast-enhanced CT of the thorax in portal venous phase (46-year-old man). [S700-T832]

a CT at the level of the pleural cupulae.
b CT at the level of the Truncus pulmonalis.

Clinical remarks

Cross-sectional imaging with **computed tomography** (CT) or **magnetic resonance imaging** (MRI) is of great importance in medical diagnostics. According to convention, images are always presented and viewed from a caudal direction.

One of the advantages of **computed tomography (CT)** versus conventional X-ray images is that all the structures are not projected on top of each other as is the case with summation images. All structures are individually recognisable in their spatial distribution on a set of sections with a thickness of a few millimeters. In tomography, the density of pathological structures already provides information regarding the tissue composition.

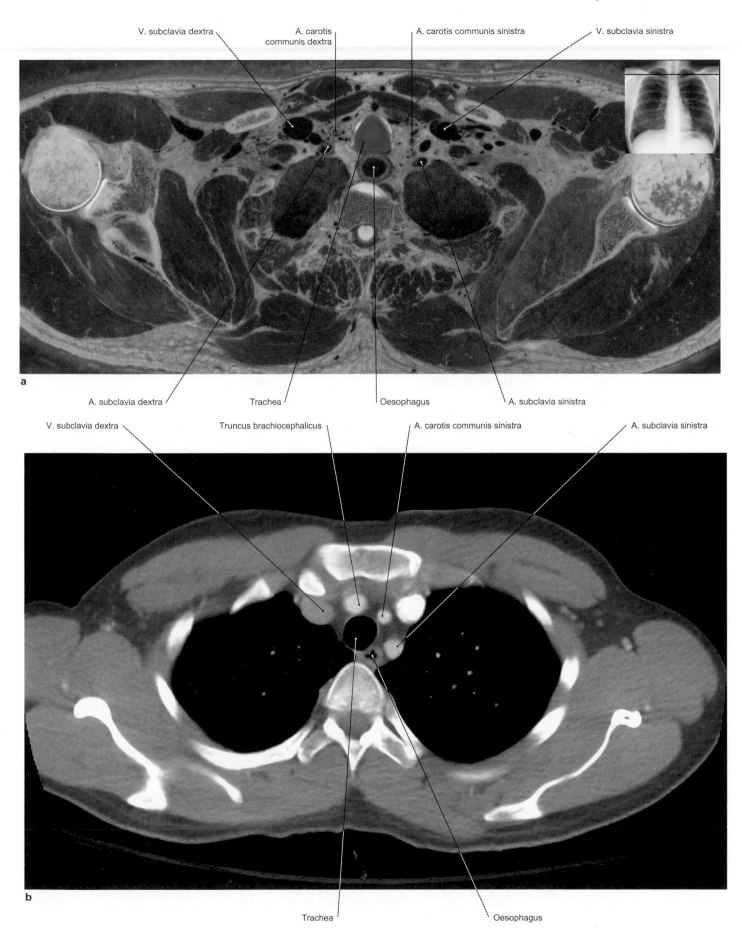

V. subclavia dextra · A. carotis communis dextra · A. carotis communis sinistra · V. subclavia sinistra

A. subclavia dextra · Trachea · Oesophagus · A. subclavia sinistra

a

V. subclavia dextra · Truncus brachiocephalicus · A. carotis communis sinistra · A. subclavia sinistra

b

Trachea · Oesophagus

Fig. 5.137a and b **Upper thoracic aperture**; cross-sections at the level of the second thoracic vertebra; caudal view.
a Photographic representation. [X338]
b CT image of the thorax. [S701-T975]

The cross-sections at the level of the upper margin of the sternum demonstrates that the apex of the lungs reaches above the upper thoracic aperture.

Cavitas thoracis, cross-sections

Organs of the thoracic cavity

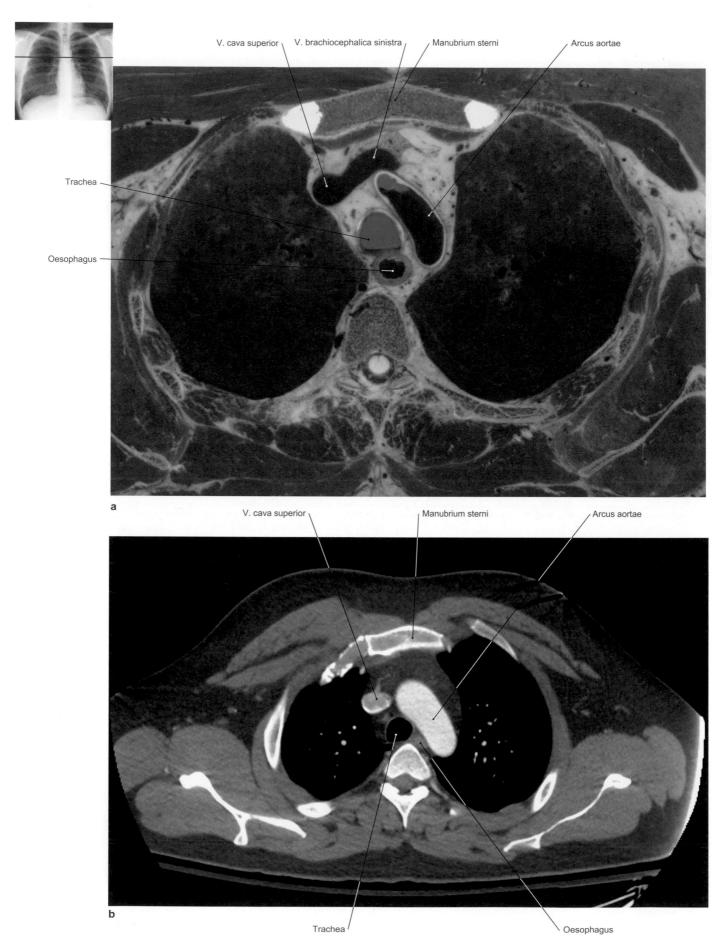

V. cava superior — V. brachiocephalica sinistra — Manubrium sterni — Arcus aortae

Trachea

Oesophagus

a

V. cava superior — Manubrium sterni — Arcus aortae

b

Trachea — Oesophagus

Fig. 5.138a and b   Upper thoracic aperture; cross-sections at the level of the fourth thoracic vertebra; caudal view.
a Photographic representation. [X338]

b CT image of the thorax. [S701-T975]
The cross-section at the level of the Manubrium sterni shows the aortic arch (and the V. brachiocephalica sinistra).

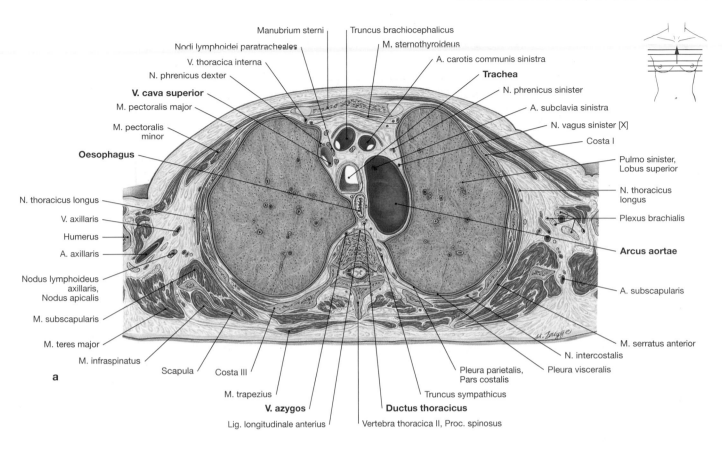

Manubrium sterni
Nodi lymphoidei paratracheales
V. thoracica interna
N. phrenicus dexter
V. cava superior
M. pectoralis major
M. pectoralis minor
Oesophagus
N. thoracicus longus
V. axillaris
Humerus
A. axillaris
Nodus lymphoideus axillaris, Nodus apicalis
M. subscapularis
M. teres major
M. infraspinatus
Scapula
Costa III
M. trapezius
V. azygos
Lig. longitudinale anterius

Truncus brachiocephalicus
M. sternothyroideus
A. carotis communis sinistra
Trachea
N. phrenicus sinister
A. subclavia sinistra
N. vagus sinister [X]
Costa I
Pulmo sinister, Lobus superior
N. thoracicus longus
Plexus brachialis
Arcus aortae
A. subscapularis
M. serratus anterior
N. intercostalis
Pleura visceralis
Pleura parietalis, Pars costalis
Truncus sympathicus
Ductus thoracicus
Vertebra thoracica II, Proc. spinosus

a

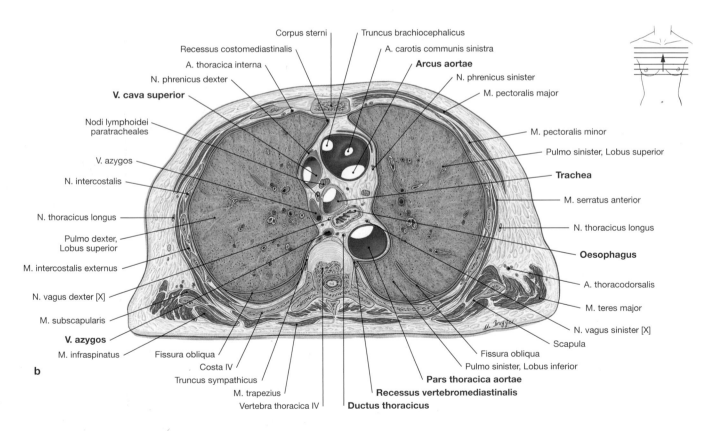

Corpus sterni
Recessus costomediastinalis
A. thoracica interna
N. phrenicus dexter
V. cava superior
Nodi lymphoidei paratracheales
V. azygos
N. intercostalis
N. thoracicus longus
Pulmo dexter, Lobus superior
M. intercostalis externus
N. vagus dexter [X]
M. subscapularis
V. azygos
M. infraspinatus
Fissura obliqua
Costa IV
Truncus sympathicus
M. trapezius
Vertebra thoracica IV

Truncus brachiocephalicus
A. carotis communis sinistra
Arcus aortae
N. phrenicus sinister
M. pectoralis major
M. pectoralis minor
Pulmo sinister, Lobus superior
Trachea
M. serratus anterior
N. thoracicus longus
Oesophagus
A. thoracodorsalis
M. teres major
N. vagus sinister [X]
Scapula
Fissura obliqua
Pulmo sinister, Lobus inferior
Pars thoracica aortae
Recessus vertebromediastinalis
Ductus thoracicus

b

Fig. 5.139a and b Thoracic cavity, Cavitas thoracis; cross-sections at the level of the Arcus aortae; caudal view. [S700]
a Cross-sections at the level of the aortic arch.
b Cross-sections at the level of the lower aortic arch.
In the upper mediastinum, the Arcus aortae is located ventrally and the V. cava superior at the right side of the Arcus aortae. Positioned dorsally

to these blood vessels are the trachea and, to the left, the oesophagus and the Pars thoracica of the aorta. Posteriorly the aorta borders on the Recessus vertebromediastinalis of the Cavitas pleuralis. Directly adjacent to the spine are the V. azygos to the right and the Ductus thoracicus to the left.

Cavitas thoracis, cross-sections

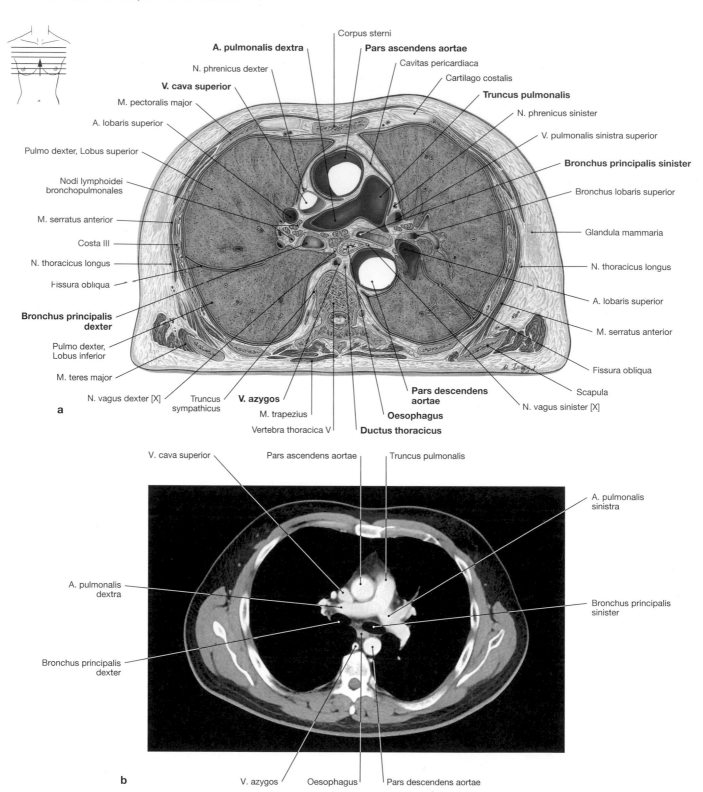

Fig. 5.140a and b   Thoracic cavity, Cavitas thoracis; cross-sections at the level of the ascending aorta and the Truncus pulmonalis; caudal view.
a Cross-sections at the level of the ascending aorta. [S700]
b Contrast-enhanced computed tomography (CT) image of the thorax in portal venous phase at the level of the Truncus pulmonalis. [S700-T832]

Lying at the furthest ventral point in the upper mediastinum is the ascending aorta; behind it to the left is the Truncus pulmonalis which branches into the pulmonary arteries; to the right of the aorta is the V. cava superior. The main bronchi (Bronchi principales) and the oesophagus lie to the posterior of the pulmonary arteries (Aa. pulmonales). The Aorta descendens runs down to the left next to the spine; the V. azygos is truncated to the right in front of the spine.

--- **Clinical remarks** -----------------------------

Using **CT-guided aspiration,** biopsies can even be obtained from individual enlarged lymph nodes. This enables a pathological and microbiological diagnosis.

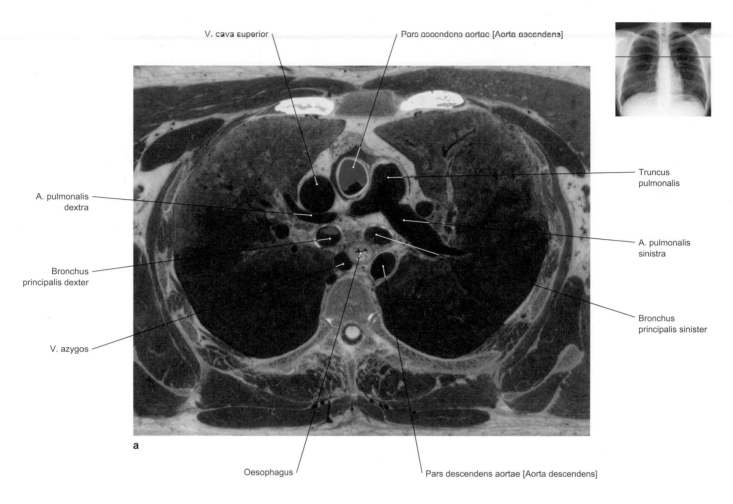

V. cava superior

Pars ascendens aortae [Aorta ascendens]

A. pulmonalis dextra

Bronchus principalis dexter

V. azygos

Truncus pulmonalis

A. pulmonalis sinistra

Bronchus principalis sinister

Oesophagus

Pars descendens aortae [Aorta descendens]

a

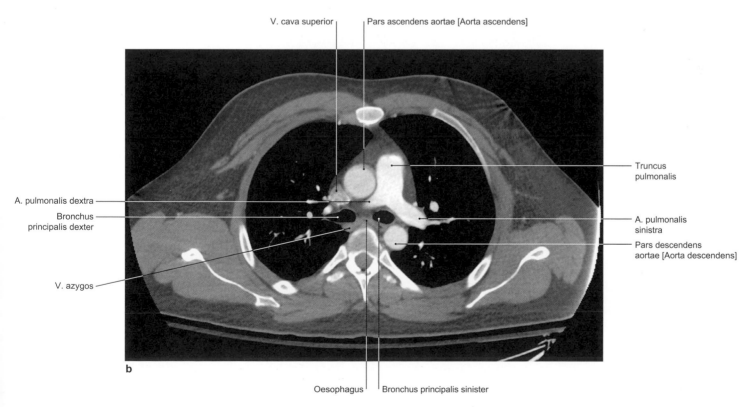

V. cava superior

Pars ascendens aortae [Aorta ascendens]

A. pulmonalis dextra

Bronchus principalis dexter

V. azygos

Truncus pulmonalis

A. pulmonalis sinistra

Pars descendens aortae [Aorta descendens]

b

Oesophagus

Bronchus principalis sinister

Fig. 5.141a and b   Thoracic cavity, Cavitas thoracis; cross-sections at the level of the fifth thoracic vertebra; caudal view.

a Photographic representation. [X338]
b CT image of the thorax. [S701-T975]

Organs of the thoracic cavity

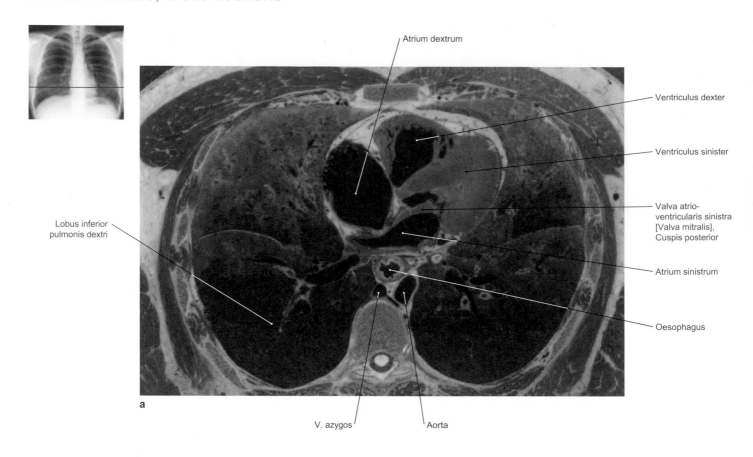

Atrium dextrum

Ventriculus dexter

Ventriculus sinister

Valva atrio-
ventricularis sinistra
[Valva mitralis],
Cuspis posterior

Atrium sinistrum

Oesophagus

Lobus inferior
pulmonis dextri

a

V. azygos

Aorta

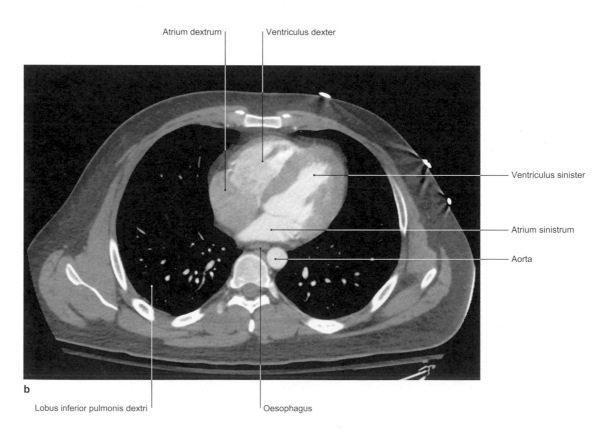

Atrium dextrum

Ventriculus dexter

Ventriculus sinister

Atrium sinistrum

Aorta

b

Lobus inferior pulmonis dextri

Oesophagus

Fig. 5.142 Thoracic cavity, Cavitas thoracis; cross-sections at the level of the seventh thoracic vertebra; caudal view.

a Photographic representation. [X338]
b CT image of the thorax. [S701-T975]

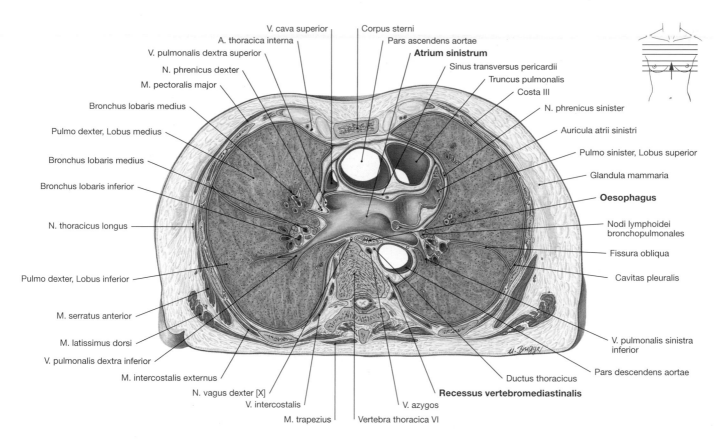

V. cava superior
A. thoracica interna
V. pulmonalis dextra superior
N. phrenicus dexter
M. pectoralis major
Bronchus lobaris medius
Pulmo dexter, Lobus medius
Bronchus lobaris medius
Bronchus lobaris inferior
N. thoracicus longus
Pulmo dexter, Lobus inferior
M. serratus anterior
M. latissimus dorsi
V. pulmonalis dextra inferior
M. intercostalis externus
N. vagus dexter [X]
V. intercostalis
M. trapezius

Corpus sterni
Pars ascendens aortae
Atrium sinistrum
Sinus transversus pericardii
Truncus pulmonalis
Costa III
N. phrenicus sinister
Auricula atrii sinistri
Pulmo sinister, Lobus superior
Glandula mammaria
Oesophagus
Nodi lymphoidei bronchopulmonales
Fissura obliqua
Cavitas pleuralis
V. pulmonalis sinistra inferior
Pars descendens aortae
Ductus thoracicus
Recessus vertebromediastinalis
V. azygos
Vertebra thoracica VI

Fig. 5.143 Thoracic cavity, Cavitas thoracis; cross-sections at the level of the left atrium; caudal view. [S700]

The left atrium (Atrium sinistrum) extends further cranially than the right atrium and is located behind the large vessels. The oesophagus borders directly on the left atrium dorsally.

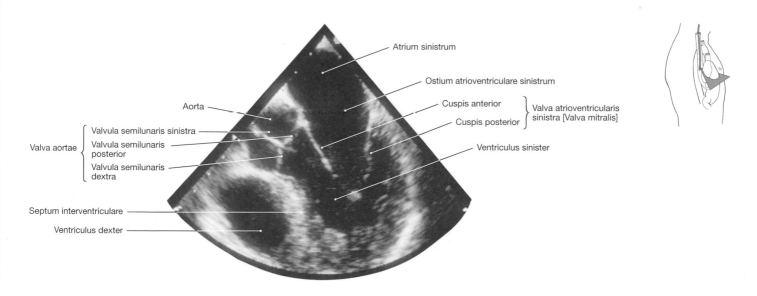

Atrium sinistrum
Ostium atrioventriculare sinistrum
Aorta
Cuspis anterior
Cuspis posterior
Valva atrioventricularis sinistra [Valva mitralis]
Valvula semilunaris sinistra
Valva aortae { Valvula semilunaris posterior
Valvula semilunaris dextra
Ventriculus sinister
Septum interventriculare
Ventriculus dexter

Fig. 5.144 Heart, Cor; ultrasound image of the oesophagus (transoesophageal echocardiography). [S700]

Clinical remarks

When performing a **transoesophageal echocardiography,** the spatial proximity of the oesophagus to the heart is useful (→ Fig. 5.134) An image of the heart and particularly the heart valves is achieved much more accurately using an ultrasound probe inserted into the oesophagus than through an examination from the outside of the rib cage.

Cavitas thoracis, cross-sections

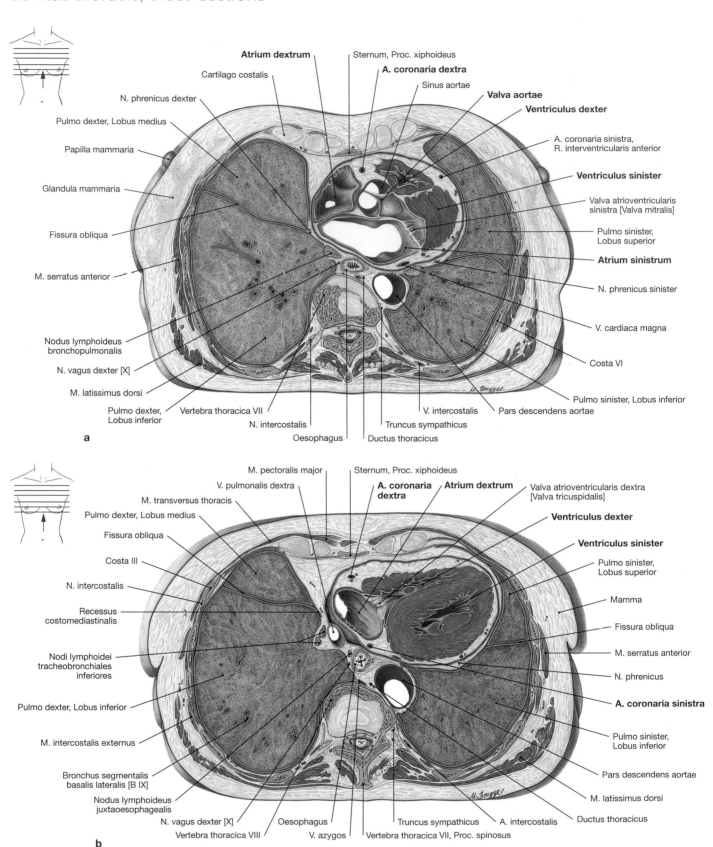

a

Atrium dextrum
Sternum, Proc. xiphoideus
Cartilago costalis
A. coronaria dextra
Sinus aortae
Valva aortae
N. phrenicus dexter
Ventriculus dexter
Pulmo dexter, Lobus medius
A. coronaria sinistra, R. interventricularis anterior
Papilla mammaria
Ventriculus sinister
Glandula mammaria
Valva atrioventricularis sinistra [Valva mitralis]
Pulmo sinister, Lobus superior
Fissura obliqua
Atrium sinistrum
M. serratus anterior
N. phrenicus sinister
V. cardiaca magna
Nodus lymphoideus bronchopulmonalis
Costa VI
N. vagus dexter [X]
M. latissimus dorsi
Pulmo dexter, Lobus inferior
Pulmo sinister, Lobus inferior
Vertebra thoracica VII
V. intercostalis
Pars descendens aortae
N. intercostalis
Truncus sympathicus
Oesophagus
Ductus thoracicus

b

M. pectoralis major
Sternum, Proc. xiphoideus
V. pulmonalis dextra
A. coronaria dextra
Atrium dextrum
Valva atrioventricularis dextra [Valva tricuspidalis]
M. transversus thoracis
Pulmo dexter, Lobus medius
Ventriculus dexter
Fissura obliqua
Ventriculus sinister
Costa III
Pulmo sinister, Lobus superior
N. intercostalis
Mamma
Recessus costomediastinalis
Fissura obliqua
M. serratus anterior
Nodi lymphoidei tracheobronchiales inferiores
N. phrenicus
A. coronaria sinistra
Pulmo dexter, Lobus inferior
Pulmo sinister, Lobus inferior
M. intercostalis externus
Bronchus segmentalis basalis lateralis [B IX]
Pars descendens aortae
M. latissimus dorsi
Nodus lymphoideus juxtaoesophagealis
Ductus thoracicus
N. vagus dexter [X]
Oesophagus
Truncus sympathicus
A. intercostalis
Vertebra thoracica VIII
V. azygos
Vertebra thoracica VII, Proc. spinosus

Fig. 5.145a and b Thoracic cavity, Cavitas thoracis; cross-sections at the level of the aortic valve; caudal view. [S700]
a Cross-sections at the level of the aortic valve.
b Cross-sections at the level below the aortic valve.
These cross-sections show that the middle mediastinum, which contains the heart and the pericardium, extends further to the left side than to the right side. As a result the left lung has a smaller volume. In the pericardium, a thick layer of subepicardial adipose tissue with embedded Aa. coronariae is evident. The margin of the heart (Facies pulmonalis of the heart) at this sectional level is formed by the right atrium on the right side and the left ventricle on the left side. The right ventricle, however, does not confine the margin of the heart but is positioned towards the front (Facies sternocostalis).

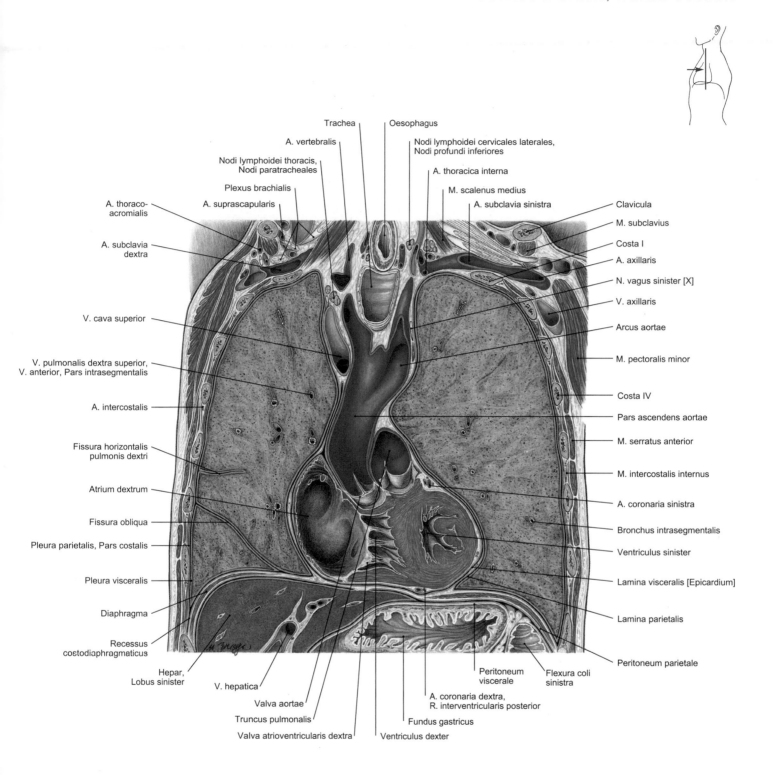

Trachea
Oesophagus
A. vertebralis
Nodi lymphoidei cervicales laterales,
Nodi profundi inferiores
Nodi lymphoidei thoracis,
Nodi paratracheales
A. thoracica interna
Plexus brachialis
M. scalenus medius
A. thoraco-
acromialis
A. suprascapularis
A. subclavia sinistra
Clavicula
M. subclavius
A. subclavia
dextra
Costa I
A. axillaris
N. vagus sinister [X]
V. axillaris
V. cava superior
Arcus aortae
V. pulmonalis dextra superior,
V. anterior, Pars intrasegmentalis
M. pectoralis minor
Costa IV
A. intercostalis
Pars ascendens aortae
M. serratus anterior
Fissura horizontalis
pulmonis dextri
M. intercostalis internus
Atrium dextrum
A. coronaria sinistra
Fissura obliqua
Bronchus intrasegmentalis
Pleura parietalis, Pars costalis
Ventriculus sinister
Pleura visceralis
Lamina visceralis [Epicardium]
Diaphragma
Lamina parietalis
Recessus
costodiaphragmaticus
Peritoneum parietale
Hepar,
Lobus sinister
Peritoneum
viscerale
Flexura coli
sinistra
V. hepatica
A. coronaria dextra,
R. interventricularis posterior
Valva aortae
Truncus pulmonalis
Fundus gastricus
Valva atrioventricularis dextra
Ventriculus dexter

Fig. 5.146 Thoracic cavity, Cavitas thoracis; frontal section at the level of the aortic and pulmonary valves; ventral view. [S700]
The frontal section clearly shows the twisting of the aorta and Truncus pulmonalis after their origin from the two ventricles. From the aorta, beginning at the aortic valve (Valva aortae), the entire ascending part (Pars ascendens) and the Arcus aortae are sectioned here. From the Truncus pulmonalis, however, its origin is only visible just above the pulmonary valve (Valva trunci pulmonalis), because it then passes from the sectional plane to the posterior, where it branches into the two pulmonary arteries (Aa. pulmonales). The right ventricle (Ventriculus dexter) itself, however, is positioned ventral to the sectional plane, while the left ventricle (Ventriculus sinister) is visible.

Cavitas thoracis, frontal section

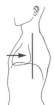

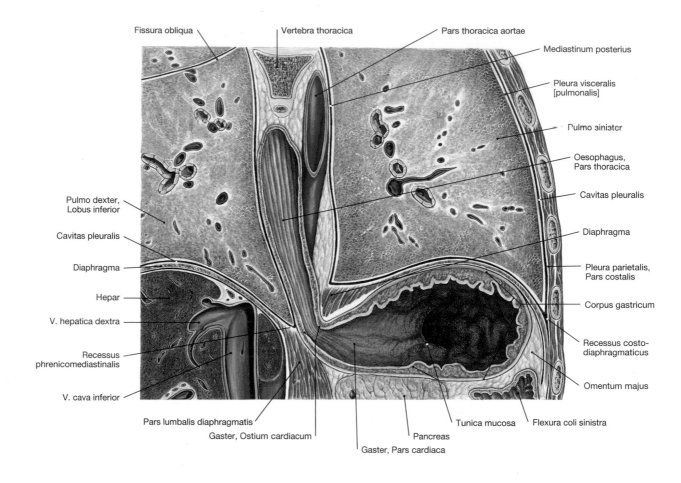

Fissura obliqua

Vertebra thoracica

Pars thoracica aortae

Mediastinum posterius

Pleura visceralis [pulmonalis]

Pulmo sinister

Oesophagus, Pars thoracica

Cavitas pleuralis

Diaphragma

Pleura parietalis, Pars costalis

Corpus gastricum

Recessus costodiaphragmaticus

Omentum majus

Pulmo dexter, Lobus inferior

Cavitas pleuralis

Diaphragma

Hepar

V. hepatica dextra

Recessus phrenicomediastinalis

V. cava inferior

Pars lumbalis diaphragmatis

Gaster, Ostium cardiacum

Gaster, Pars cardiaca

Pancreas

Tunica mucosa

Flexura coli sinistra

Fig. 5.147 Thoracic cavity, Cavitas thoracis; frontal section at the level of the oesophageal hiatus of the diaphragm; ventral view. [S700] The frontal section shows the arrangement of the oesophagus and aorta in the lower mediastinum. The Pars thoracica of the oesophagus lies initially to the right of the Pars thoracica aortae. Before passing through the oesophageal hiatus, the oesophagus runs in front of the aorta. The Pars abdominalis of the oesophagus is very short and transitions into the cardia of the stomach. The mucosal transition between stomach and oesophagus is on a slightly jagged line (Z-line) that is located here relatively widely distal. It is therefore positioned distally to the first gastric mucosal fold in the cardiac notch. Through the notch, the angle of HIS between the cardia of the stomach and the fundus of the stomach is demarcated. The mucosal fold in the angle of HIS contributes to the closure mechanisms of the lower oesophagus.

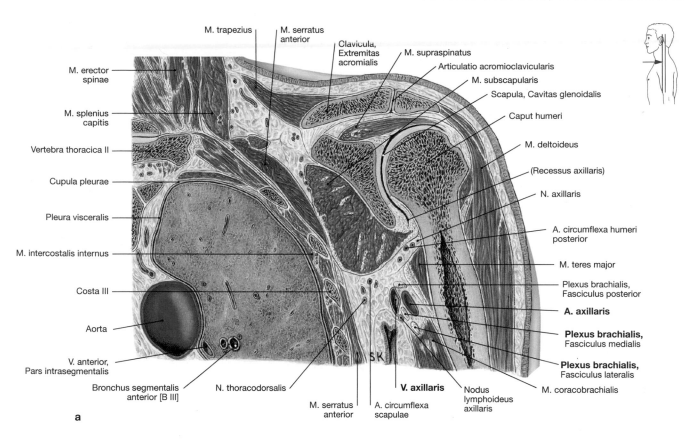

M. trapezius
M. serratus anterior
M. erector spinae
Clavicula, Extremitas acromialis
M. supraspinatus
Articulatio acromioclavicularis
M. subscapularis
Scapula, Cavitas glenoidalis
M. splenius capitis
Caput humeri
Vertebra thoracica II
M. deltoideus
Cupula pleurae
(Recessus axillaris)
N. axillaris
Pleura visceralis
A. circumflexa humeri posterior
M. intercostalis internus
M. teres major
Costa III
Plexus brachialis, Fasciculus posterior
Aorta
A. axillaris
Plexus brachialis, Fasciculus medialis
V. anterior, Pars intrasegmentalis
Plexus brachialis, Fasciculus lateralis
Bronchus segmentalis anterior [B III]
N. thoracodorsalis
V. axillaris
Nodus lymphoideus axillaris
M. coracobrachialis
M. serratus anterior
A. circumflexa scapulae

a

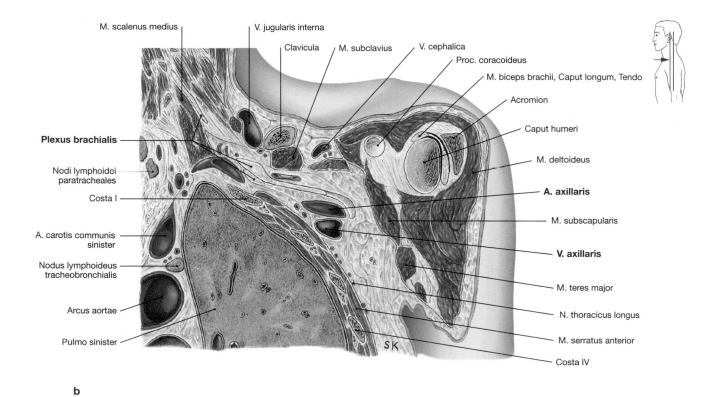

M. scalenus medius
V. jugularis interna
Clavicula
M. subclavius
V. cephalica
Proc. coracoideus
M. biceps brachii, Caput longum, Tendo
Acromion
Plexus brachialis
Caput humeri
Nodi lymphoidei paratracheales
M. deltoideus
Costa I
A. axillaris
A. carotis communis sinister
M. subscapularis
Nodus lymphoideus tracheobronchialis
V. axillaris
Arcus aortae
M. teres major
N. thoracicus longus
Pulmo sinister
M. serratus anterior
Costa IV

b

Fig. 5.148a and b   Thoracic cavity, Cavitas thoracis, armpit, axilla, and shoulder joint, Articulatio humeri; frontal sections at the level of the shoulder joint as well as in front; ventral view. [S700-L238]
a Frontal section at the level of the shoulder joint.

b Frontal section at the level anterior to the shoulder joint.
The illustrations show clearly that ventral of the shoulder joint, the A. and V. axillaris as well as the Plexus brachialis, the neurovascular structures for the arm, are positioned close to the apex of the lung.

Sample exam questions

To check that you are completely familiar with the content of this chapter, sample questions from an oral anatomy exam are listed here.

Indicate the parts of the mediastinum and show the pleural cavities.

- Which organs and neurovascular pathways lie within?
- Which recess does the pleural cavities contain and where is it located?
- Indicate the Ductus thoracicus: how does it run through the Cavitas thoracis?
- Explain the pathway of the azygos system on a dissection.
- Where is the thymus located and what is its function?

Where does the heart project onto the skeleton and which parts of the heart form its borders on the chest X-ray?

- Indicate on a dissection which structures of the heart define its margins on an X-ray.

Explain the construction of the heart valves on a dissection.

- What do they project onto and where does one auscultate for a suspected aortic valve stenosis?

Indicate all important branches of the Aa. coronariae.

- What type of circulation is there in this dissection?
- How are the parts of the cardiac conducting system supplied with blood?

How are the lungs organised and where do the lung lobe boundaries project onto the skeleton?

Explain the functions of the Vasa publica and Vasa privata of the lung.

Which lymphatic drainage systems do the lungs have and which lymph nodes are incorporated into these?

Where are the constrictions of the oesophagus?

How is the oesophagus closed at both ends and what clinical relevance does this have?

Which blood vessels supply the oesophagus and why does this play a role?

- What are oesophageal varices and which anatomical connection can explain their formation?

Describe the lymphatic drainage of the oesophagus on a dissection.

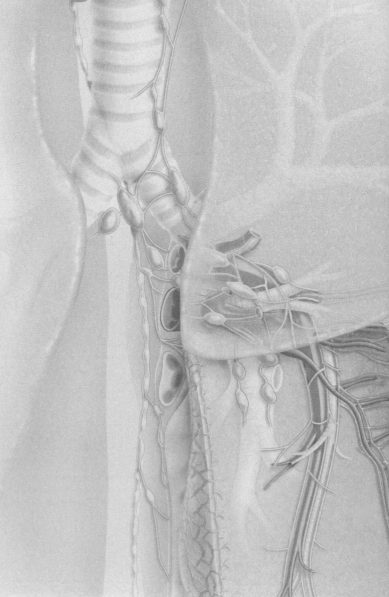

Organs of the abdominal cavity

6

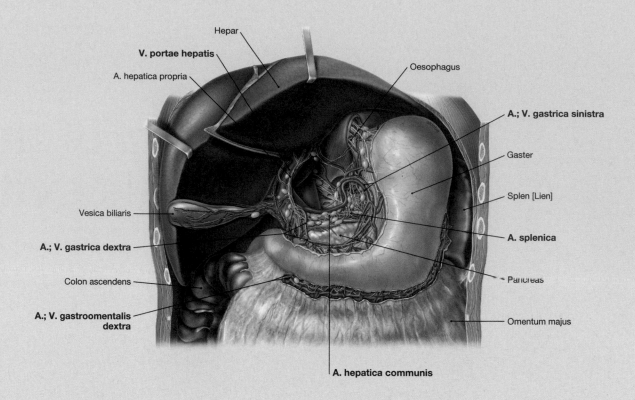

Hepar

V. portae hepatis

A. hepatica propria

Vesica biliaris

A.; V. gastrica dextra

Colon ascendens

A.; V. gastroomentalis dextra

A. hepatica communis

Oesophagus

A.; V. gastrica sinistra

Gaster

Splen [Lien]

A. splenica

Pancreas

Omentum majus

Overview

Opening the abdominal wall reveals a cavity filled with some smooth and some partially solid organs (viscera). In its entirety it is called the 'situs' of the abdominal organs. The inside of the abdominal wall and the surface of the organs are covered with a thin, moist, shiny membrane **(peritoneum).** The lining on the inside of the abdominal wall is referred to as the parietal sheet of the peritoneum, while the visceral sheet covers the various organs. This largest part of the abdominal cavity is therefore known as the peritoneal cavity **(Cavitas peritonealis)** with the retroperitoneal space as a separate flat section behind the parietal peritoneum, which for instance contains the kidneys. The smooth peritoneum guarantees, for instance, that the stomach and intestines change shape during peristalsis so that the intestinal loops can easily move

against each other. The middle transverse part of the large intestine (Colon transversum) divides the peritoneal cavity into an **upper abdominal (epigastric) situs** and a **lower abdominal (hypogastric) situs.**

The situs of the epigastrium (upper abdomen) contains, among other things, the liver (Hepar), with the closely positioned gallbladder (Vesica biliaris), and the pancreas as the biggest glands found in the human body. The stomach (Gaster) nestles up against the liver, which is on the right. On the left, behind the stomach, is the spleen in its own niche. The hypogastrium (lower abdomen) is filled with the loops of the small intestine (Intestinum tenue), which are surrounded and held in place by the large intestine (Intestinum crassum).

Main topics

After working through this chapter, you should be able to:

Peritoneal cavity
- explain the structure of the abdominal cavity with recesses as well as the peritoneal duplications on the dissection;
- explain the neurovascular pathways for all organs, with clinical relevance and organ-specific peculiarities;

Stomach
- show the positional relationships of the stomach to the rest of the epigastric organs and describe its development;

Intestines
- show sections of the small and large intestines on the dissection and explain their structural features;
- describe the origin of the individual intestinal segments, including the boundaries of their areas supplied by neurovascular pathways, and the positional changes they undergo during their development;
- demonstrate the clinical importance of the positional relationships of the appendix with projection onto the body surface;

Liver and gallbladder
- explain the vital importance of the liver and its different functions;
- show the position and projection of the liver and gallbladder and describe their development;
- show the functional structure of the liver, including the liver segments on the dissection and explain their clinical significance;
- describe the opening and closure mechanisms of the common bile duct (Ductus choledochus) and to show the topography of the CALOT's triangle on a dissection;

Pancreas
- explain the vital importance and function of the pancreas;
- show the classification and topography of the pancreas on the dissection, including the gear system, and explain their development, including malformations;

Spleen
- understand the various functions of the spleen and its position and structure.

Clinical relevance

In order not to lose touch with prospective everyday clinical life with so many anatomical details, the following describes a typical case that shows why the content of this chapter is so important.

Colon cancer

Case study
A 63-year-old man visits the family doctor because he has had blood in his stool for several weeks. He also suffers more and more from constipation, which surprises him as he is losing his appetite and doesn't eat much. He mentions that he has lost 5 kg in weight in the last three months.

Result of examination
The physical examination is unremarkable, including the rectal palpation. Bowel sounds are normal and there is no pressure pain on the stomach.

Diagnostic procedure
The blood seepage can be confirmed with a stool test. The colonoscopy conducted by a resident gastroenterologist reveals an ulcerated tumour of 2 cm in diameter in the descending colon; tissue biopsies are taken and sent to the pathology department. Raised levels of the tumour markers CEA and CA 19-9 are found in the blood, typically produced by adenocarcinomas. After admission to a surgical clinic and a computed tomography (CT) of the abdominal and pelvic cavity and skull, diagnostics can exclude metastases.

Diagnosis
Colon cancer (→ Fig. a). Metastases have not been found in the liver, lung and brain. Of all the malignant tumours, colon carcinomas are the most common, along with tumours of the lung, breast and prostate. These can be detected very easily in the early stages through screening with a colonoscopy. The mortality rates have therefore fallen significantly in recent years.

Treatment
The Colon descendens and the Colon sigmoideum, including the lymph nodes along the A. mesenterica inferior, were removed with a hemicolectomy, and sent to the pathology department. The colon can be anastomosed with the rectum, maintaining continence, so that no artificial anus (Anus praeter) is required.

Further developments
On the following day, the patient starts taking in nutrition and is painfree apart from pain where the scar is healing well. Since several lymph nodes are identified as affected by the tumour in the pathological examination, the patient is referred to the ambulatory oncology unit. He there receives intravenous chemotherapy over the next few months on a regular basis which he tolerates very well after initial nausea. Postoperatively, the blood level of the tumour markers is lowered, so that a potential recurrence of the tumour would be indicated by any new increase. After 10 years in complete remission the patient can now be considered as healed.

Dissection lab
The large intestine is found immediately after opening the abdominal cavity

 Here you have to look closely at the interrelated positions of the individual organs to each other.

because it surrounds the small intestine and separates the epigastrium from the hypogastrium. It is divided into several sections: the **caecum (Caecum)** with its **appendix (Appendix vermiformis)** is followed by the colon sections **(Colon ascendens, Colon transversum, Colon descendens and Colon sigmoideum)** and then the **rectum,** and the **anal canal (Canalis analis).** Since the descending colon is shifted to the rear body wall during development, it is located secondarily retroperitoneal. In contrast, the Colon sigmoideum is covered on all sides by the visceral peritoneum and is thus intraperitoneal. For the implementation of a hemicolectomy, knowledge of the neurovascular pathways which supply the individual intestinal segments is essential. This change developmentally affects the left colonic flexure which marks the transition from the transverse colon to the descending colon. The left-sided colon sections (Colon descendens and Colon sigmoideum) are therefore fed by branches from the **A. mesenterica inferior,** which originate from the abdominal part of the aorta and initially run retroperitoneally. The right-sided sections up to the transverse colon, in contrast, are supplied by the **A./V. mesenterica superior.**

 The clinically important anastomosis of the A. mesenterica superior with the A. mesenterica inferior is called RIOLAN 's arcade. You can see it very clearly after preparation of the vascular arcades!

The corresponding vein (V. mesenterica inferior) ascends on the dorsal side of the pancreas and joins the other main veins which then build the **portal vein (V. portae).** Therefore colon tumour cells often metastasise via the venous blood into the liver. The regional lymph nodes along the colon connect to the collecting lymph nodes at the origin of the A. mesenterica inferior **(Nodi lymphoidei mesenterici inferiores).**

 The lymph nodes are seldom easy to find, but their position can be easily tracked along the A. mesenterica.

Back to the clinic
During surgery, the entire A. mesenterica inferior with surrounding lymph nodes can be removed because it only provides the furthest sections of the large intestine. On the other hand, in the case of a tumour in the Colon ascendens, you could not remove the entire A. mesenterica superior, as it also supplies the small intestine and the pancreas.

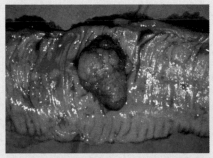

Fig. a Polypous colon carcinoma. [R234]

Development of the epigastric situs

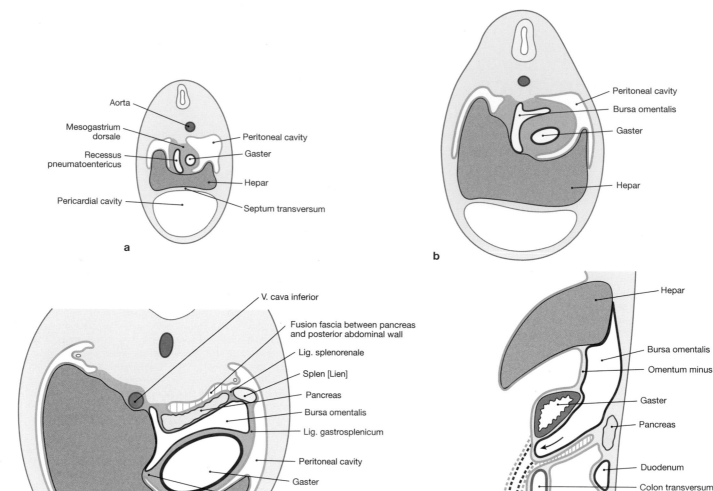

a — Aorta, Mesogastrium dorsale, Recessus pneumatoentericus, Pericardial cavity, Peritoneal cavity, Gaster, Hepar, Septum transversum

b — Peritoneal cavity, Bursa omentalis, Gaster, Hepar

c — V. cava inferior, Fusion fascia between pancreas and posterior abdominal wall, Lig. splenorenale, Splen [Lien], Pancreas, Bursa omentalis, Lig. gastrosplenicum, Peritoneal cavity, Gaster, Omentum minus, Hepar, Lig. coronarium

d — Hepar, Bursa omentalis, Omentum minus, Gaster, Pancreas, Duodenum, Colon transversum, Intestinum tenue, Omentum majus

Fig. 6.1a–d Development of the epigastric situs; peritoneum (green); peritoneum of the Recessus pneumatoentericus and the Bursa omentalis (dark red). [S700-L126]/[B500~T663/L238]
a Cross-section of the epigastrium at the end of the fourth week.
b Cross-section of the epigastrium at the beginning of the fifth week.
c Cross-section of the epigastrium at the beginning of the seventh week.
d Paramedian section of the epigastrium.
The **foregut** predominantly originates from the entoderm and parts of the yolk sac and forms the epithelial tissue of the gastrointestinal tract. In the surrounding mesoderm, crevices are developing which will fuse to form the **abdominal cavity (coelom).** Laterally, the mesoderm of the coelom develops into the somatopleure of the wall of the trunk. Medially, it creates the **splanchnopleure** which covers the outside of the foregut, to become the visceral peritoneum and to coat the abdominal cavity as the parietal peritoneum. The splanchnopleure also generates the smooth musculature and connective tissue of the wall of the gastrointestinal tract. Additionally, the visceral peritoneum forms the mesenteries which serve as attachments and contain the neurovascular structures. The dorsal mesentery connects the foregut with the posterior abdominal wall. In the epigastrium, there is an additional ventral mesentery.
At the beginning of the **fourth week,** the entoderm sprouts develop ventrally from the foregut at the level of the future duodenum, forming the epithelial tissue of the liver, gallbladder, pancreas and bile duct. Finally there is the following redistribution:

1. The **liver** expands into the Mesogastrium ventrale and thereby divides it into a Mesohepaticum ventrale (between the anterior wall of the trunk and the liver) and a Mesohepaticum dorsale (between the liver and the stomach; **a** and **b**). From the Mesohepaticum ventrale the **Lig. coronarium** runs cranially, and the **Lig. falciforme hepatis** caudally. At the caudal aspect is a remnant of the umbilical vein, the **Lig. teres hepatis.** The dorsal mesohepaticum becomes the Omentum minus.
2. In the dorsal mesogastrium a split occurs on the right (Recessus pneumatoentericus) which becomes the **Bursa omentalis (a** and **b).**
3. The **stomach** turns **90° clockwise** (view from above) and thus arrives on the left side of the body in a transverse position **(c).** The Omentum minus also connects the liver and lesser curvature of the stomach in the frontal plane and forms the front wall of the Bursa omentalis to the left posterior to the stomach.
4. In the Mesogastrium dorsale the **pancreas** is formed which shifts retroperitoneally, as well as the **spleen,** which remains intraperitoneally.
5. The Mesogastrium dorsale finally subdivides into a **Lig. gastrosplenicum** (from the greater curvature of the stomach to the spleen) and a **Lig. splenorenale** (from the splenic hilum to the dorsal trunk wall) and forms the remaining parts of the **Omentum majus** (hanging apron-shaped from the greater curvature of the stomach; **d).** This means that the Omentum majus is part of the epigastric situs because of its evolutionary development and its neurovascular pathways.

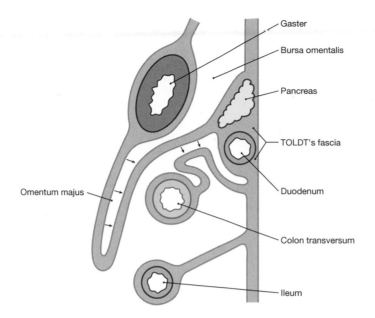

Gaster

Bursa omentalis

Pancreas

TOLDT's fascia

Duodenum

Omentum majus

Colon transversum

Ileum

Fig. 6.2 Repositioning of the epigastric organs from the fifth week; paramedian section of the epigastrium. [S700-L126]/[E347-11] From the fifth week of development, with the rotation of the stomach, the major part of the **duodenum (except for the Pars superior)** and

the **pancreas** move next to the dorsal wall of the trunk, resulting in a **secondary retroperitoneal position**. The visceral peritoneum on the dorsal side of these organs fuses with the parietal peritoneum of the trunk wall to form **TOLDT's fascia**.

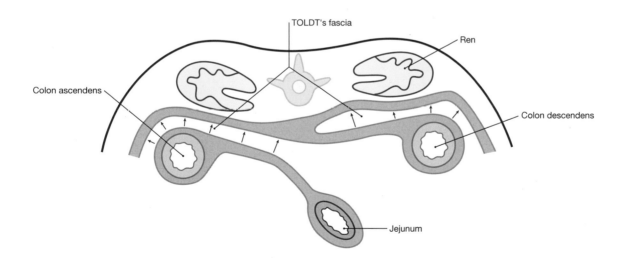

TOLDT's fascia

Ren

Colon ascendens

Colon descendens

Jejunum

Fig. 6.3 Repositioning of epigastric organs at the tenth week; cross-section of the hypogastrium at the level of the Flexura duodenojejunalis. [S700-L126]/[E347-11] During the physiological umbilical herniation and intestinal loop formation, which will be described in more detail as part of the development of the epigastric situs (→ Fig. 6.4), the **Colon ascendens** and **Colon descendens** also assume a **secondary retroperitoneal position**. Both colon parts maintain the position adjacent to the posterior trunk wall and do not develop a distinct mesentery. The fusion of the visceral per-

itoneum with the parietal peritoneum on the inside of the posterior trunk wall forms the **TOLDT's fascia**. **Dissection note:** Secondary retroperitoneal parts of the duodenum, the colon and the pancreas can be bluntly mobilised and detached from the posterior wall of the trunk and the retroperitoneal organs, such as the kidneys and adrenal glands, and the large blood vessels (aorta and the V. cava inferior). This separates the peritoneal linings forming the TOLDT's fascia.

Development of the hypogastric situs

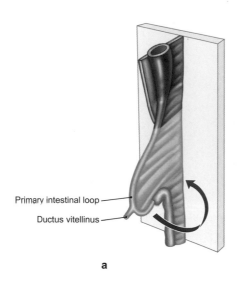

Primary intestinal loop

Ductus vitellinus

a

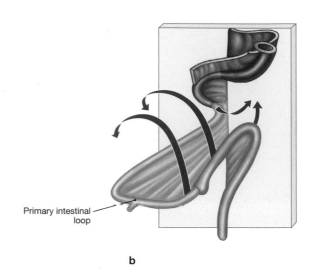

Primary intestinal loop

b

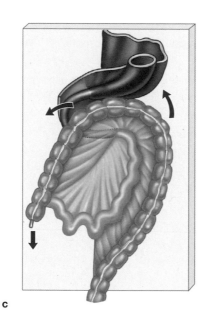

c

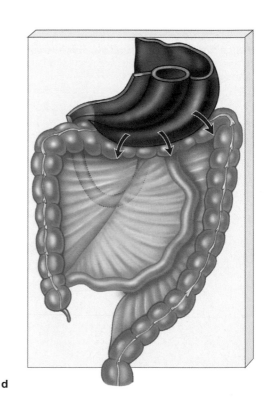

d

Fig. 6.4a–d   Schematic representation of the intestinal rotation.
Intestinal segments and their mesenteries are highlighted in different
colours: stomach and mesogastrium (purple), duodenum and
mesoduodenum (blue), jejunum and ileum with associated mesenteries
(orange), colon and mesocolon (ochre). [S700-L126]/[B500~T663/L238]
The following, partly overlapping, processes occur:

1. Along the length of the intestine, a ventrally pointing sling **(primary
   intestinal loop)** develops. The proximal (upper) crus of this loop develops into the major part of the small intestine, the distal (lower)
   crus develops into the colon, including the Colon transversum. The
   distal colon develops from the rectum and is differentiated in terms
   of its neurovascular pathways.
2. Due to a lack of space, the primary intestinal loop is temporarily
   shifted from the embryo to the umbilical cord **(physiological umbil-**

ical hernia) and remains connected to the yolk sac via the Ductus
vitellinus. If the intestine is not completely shifted back into the embryo, a congenital umbilical hernia **(omphalocele)** remains, which
contains intestinal segments with the mesentery. As this protrudes
through the eventual umbilical ring, it is only covered by amnion and
not abdominal wall musculature.

3. Remnants of the Ductus vitellinus can remain as **MECKEL's diverticulum** in the small intestine.
4. Through longitudinal growth, a **counter-clockwise rotation of the
   intestines of 270°** is induced. As a result, the large intestine surrounds the small intestine as if in a frame.
5. The Colon ascendens and Colon descendens are secondarily shifted
   into a retroperitoneal position. Hereby the embryonic mesocolon
   merges with the Peritoneum parietale (TOLDT's fascia).

Mesoderm

Peritoneum parietale

Digestive tract

Mesenterium

Peritoneum viscerale

Cavitas peritonealis

a

Peritoneum viscerale

Mesenterium

Peritoneum parietale

b

Peritoneum viscerale

Peritoneum parietale

c

Fig. 6.5a–c Schematic illustration of the relative peritoneal positioning; cross-sections; visceral peritoneum in green, parietal peritoneum in purple. [S701-L126]

a Cross-section at the level of the epigastrium. The **visceral peritoneum** covers the surface and the mesenteries of all the viscera within the peritoneal cavity. In contrast, the **parietal peritoneum** lines the inner surface of the wall of the peritoneal cavity. Studies now show that the mesentery forms a continuum, reaching from the mesogastrium to the mesorectum, thus enveloping intra-, retro- and subperitoneal parts of the gastrointestinal tracts.

b Cross-section of an intraperitoneal hollow organ. An **intraperitoneal organ,** such as the stomach, is covered by **visceral peritoneum** on all its surfaces and connects to peritoneal duplications, such as the mesentery, Omentum majus and Omentum minus, as well as the ligaments (→ table below).

c Cross-section of a primary retroperitoneal/subperitoneal organ. Viscera located behind or below the peritoneal cavity are referred to as primary **retroperitoneal** and **subperitoneal viscera**, respectively. These are only covered by **parietal peritoneum** on the anterior or superior aspect, such as the urinary bladder.

Peritoneal duplications	
Structure	**Comment**
Mesenterium	• Dorsal suspension of intra- and retroperitoneal parts of the small and large intestines • Continued peritoneal duplication between the mesogastrium and mesorectum • Contains the neurovascular structures of the intestines
Omentum majus • Lig. gastrocolicum • Lig. gastrosplenicum • Lig. gastrophrenicum • Apron-shaped part	• Apron-shaped duplication comprising several parts • Develops from the dorsal mesogastrium • Contains the neurovascular supply for the greater curvature of the stomach
Omentum minus • Lig. hepatogastricum • Lig. hepatoduodenale	• Develops from the ventral mesogastrium (Mesohepaticum dorsale) • Contains the neurovascular pathways for the lesser curvature of the stomach
Lig. falciforme hepatis	• Develops from the ventral mesogastrium anterior to the liver (Mesohepaticum ventrale) • Contains portacaval anastomoses to the ventral trunk wall
Lig. splenorenale	Develops from the dorsal mesogastrium
Lig. phrenicocolicum	• Develops from the dorsal mesogastrium • Forms the floor of the splenic recess

Clinical remarks

MECKEL's diverticula are common (3 % of the population), and usually occur in the section of the small intestine 100 cm orally of the ileocaecal valve. As they often contain disseminated gastric mucosa, they can simulate the clinical symptoms of appendicitis when inflamed and bleeding. A disruption of the intestinal rotation may lead to **malrotations** (hypo- or hyperrotation). These may cause **twisting of intestinal loops (Volvulus)**, potentially resulting in a bowel obstruction (ileus). If sections of the intestines are hereby shifted into a different, abnor-

mal position, this may complicate the diagnosis for appendicitis. The malrotation may be incomplete (→ Fig. a) or result in the duodenum crossing the Colon transversum ventrally (→ Fig. b). The completely reversed or mirror-image positioning of the organs is referred to as **Situs inversus.**
[S701-L275]

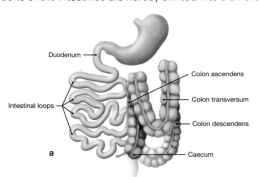

Duodenum

Intestinal loops

Colon ascendens

Colon transversum

Colon descendens

Caecum

a

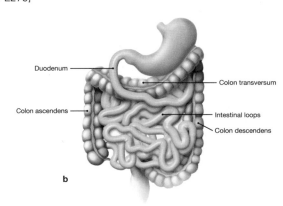

Duodenum

Colon ascendens

Colon transversum

Intestinal loops

Colon descendens

b

Surface anatomy

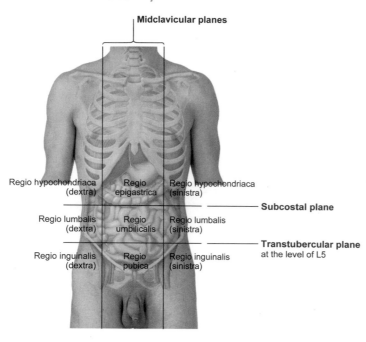

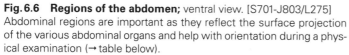

Fig. 6.6 Regions of the abdomen; ventral view. [S701-J803/L275] Abdominal regions are important as they reflect the surface projection of the various abdominal organs and help with orientation during a physical examination (→ table below).

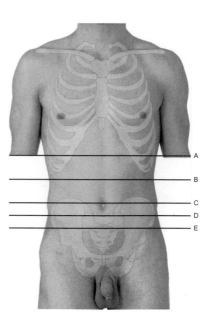

Fig. 6.7 Horizontal planes of the abdomen; ventral view. [S701-J803/L275] Horizontal planes of the abdomen provide helpful orientation for cross-sectional imaging with computed tomography (CT) or magnetic resonance imaging (MRI) (→ table below).

Regions of the abdomen

Region	Projected organs
Right hypochondrium (Regio hypochondriaca dextra)	• Liver (pain with swelling of the liver or fatty liver) • Gallbladder (inflammation of hepatic colic with presence of gall stones)
Epigastrium (upper abdomen) (Regio epigastrica)	• Stomach (gastric ulcer) • Oesophagus (heartburn) • Colon transversum (bloating, obstruction, infarction, inflammation)
Left hypochondrium (Regio hypochondriaca sinistra)	Spleen (splenic rupture, pain with swelling of spleen)
Right flank (Regio lumbalis dextra)	• Right kidney (nephritis, renal colic) • Colon ascendens (bloating, obstruction with pain, infarction, inflammation)
Umbilical region (Regio umbilicalis)	Small intestine (bloating, obstruction with pain, infarction, inflammation)
Left flank (Regio lumbalis sinistra)	• Left kidney (nephritis, renal colic with kidney stones) • Colon ascendens (bloating, obstruction with pain, infarction, inflammation)
Right inguinal region = right groin (Regio inguinalis dextra)	• Appendix vermiformis (appendicitis) • Inguinal canal (inguinal hernia)
Pubic region (Regio pubica)	• Urinary bladder (urinary retention, urinary infection) • Rectum (bloating, obstruction with pain, infarction, inflammation)
Left inguinal region = left groin (Regio inguinalis sinistra)	• Sigmoid colon (bloating, obstruction with pain, infarction, inflammation [particularly also diverticulitis]) • Inguinal canal (inguinal hernia)

Horizontal planes of the abdomen

Plane	Vertebra	Landmark	Anatomical structure
A: Transpyloric plane (ADDISON's plane)	L1	Midway between pubic symphysis and the jugular notch	Pylorus, fundus of gallbladder, Mesocolon transversum, pancreas, Flexura duodenojejunalis, Truncus coeliacus (T12/L1), origin of the hepatic portal vein, A. mesenterica superior, hilum of kidney with A. renalis (L2)
B: Subcostal plane	L2–L3	Inferior border of the 10th rib	A. mesenterica inferior
C: Transumbilical plane	L3–L4	Umbilicus	
Supracristal plane	L4	Iliac crest	Aortic bifurcation (access for lumbar puncture)
D: Transtubercular plane	L5	Tuberculum iliacum	Origin of V. cava inferior
E: Interspinous plane	Midsacrum	Spina iliaca anterior superior	Appendix vermiformis

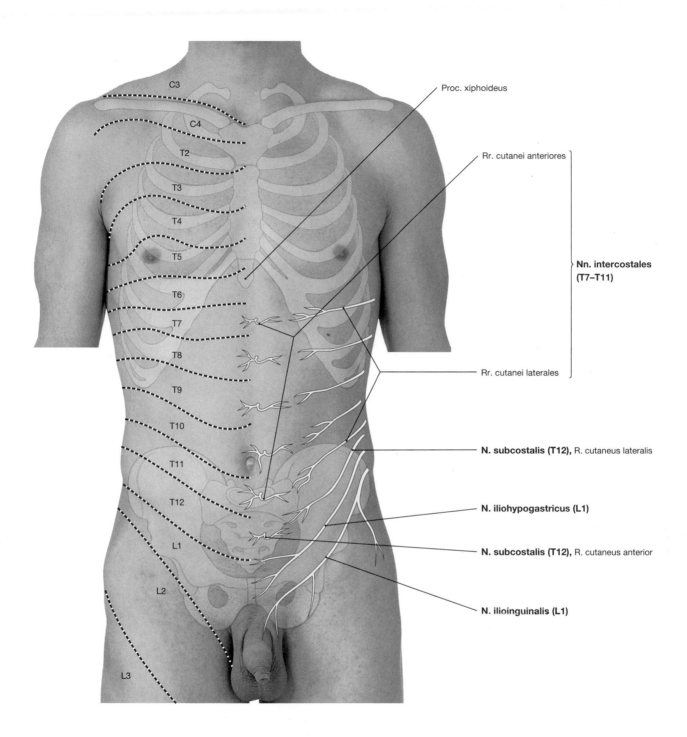

Proc. xiphoideus

Rr. cutanei anteriores

Nn. intercostales (T7–T11)

Rr. cutanei laterales

N. subcostalis (T12), R. cutaneus lateralis

N. iliohypogastricus (L1)

N. subcostalis (T12), R. cutaneus anterior

N. ilioinguinalis (L1)

Fig. 6.8 Cutaneous areas (dermatomes) of the anterior trunk wall with projection of the spinal nerves; ventral view. [S701-J803/L126]
The abdominal wall is innervated by the anterior rami **(Rr. anteriores)** of the **spinal nerves:**
* Intercostal nerves (Nn. intercostales), T7–T11
* N. subcostalis, T12
* N. iliohypogastricus (Plexis lumbalis), T12–L1
* N. ilioinguinalis (Plexus lumbalis), T12–L1.

The **dermatomes** have a belt-shaped pathway and correspond to distinct spinal cord segments. For orientation on the abdominal wall, the following projections are important:
* Umbilicus onto dermatome T10
* Lumbar region onto dermatomes T11/T12
* Groin and pubic regions onto dermatome L1.

6

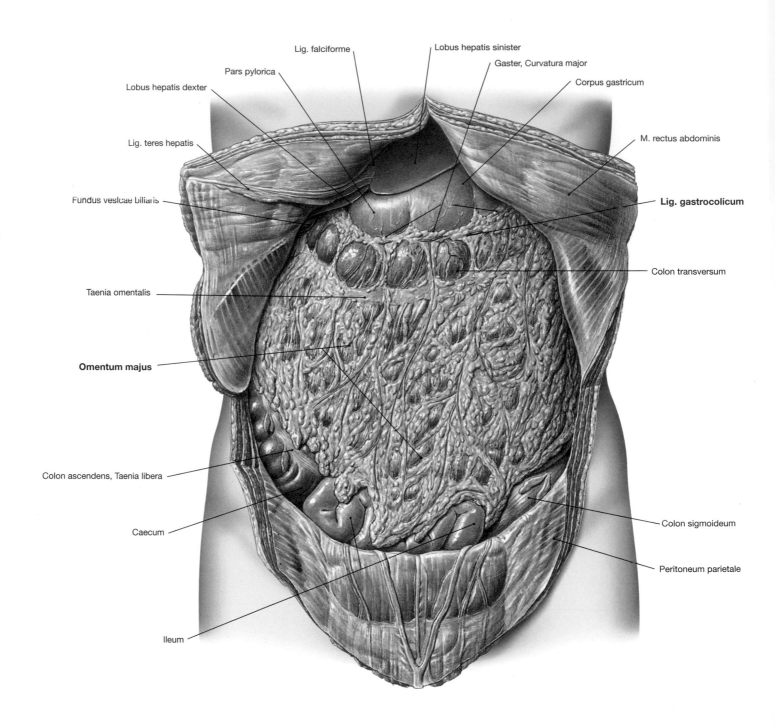

Lig. falciforme

Lobus hepatis sinister

Pars pylorica

Gaster, Curvatura major

Lobus hepatis dexter

Corpus gastricum

Lig. teres hepatis

M. rectus abdominis

Fundus veslcae biliaris

Lig. gastrocolicum

Taenia omentalis

Colon transversum

Omentum majus

Colon ascendens, Taenia libera

Caecum

Colon sigmoideum

Peritoneum parietale

Ileum

Fig. 6.9   Position of the viscera, Situs viscerum, in the epigastrium, and greater omentum, Omentum majus; ventral view. [S700]
Opening the abdominal cavity reveals the diagonally running Colon transversum, which divides the abdomen into an **epigastrium** (so-called glandular stomach) and a **hypogastrium** (so-called intestinal stomach). Here the navel was excised on the left side, in order to prevent an injury of the Lig. teres hepatis, which connects the liver to the anterior trunk wall. The viscera of the hypogastrium are almost completely covered by the **greater omentum (Omentum majus)** which is attached to the greater curvature of the stomach.

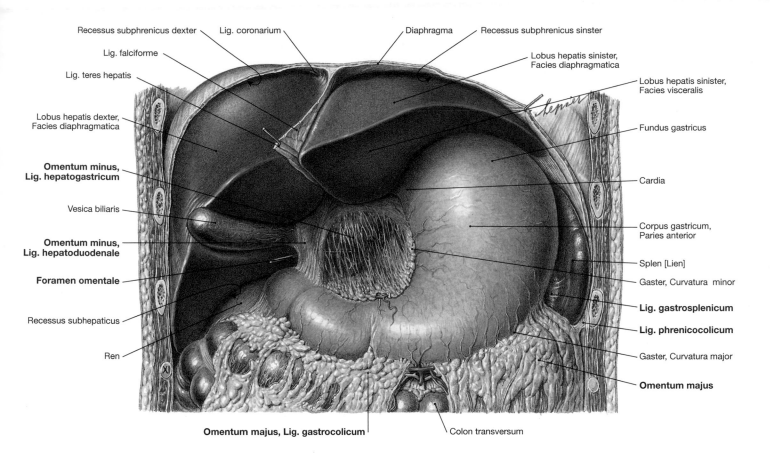

Recessus subphrenicus dexter — Lig. coronarium — Diaphragma — Recessus subphrenicus sinster

Lig. falciforme

Lig. teres hepatis

Lobus hepatis dexter, Facies diaphragmatica

Omentum minus, Lig. hepatogastricum

Vesica biliaris

Omentum minus, Lig. hepatoduodenale

Foramen omentale

Recessus subhepaticus

Ren

Lobus hepatis sinister, Facies diaphragmatica

Lobus hepatis sinister, Facies visceralis

Fundus gastricus

Cardia

Corpus gastricum, Paries anterior

Splen [Lien]

Gaster, Curvatura minor

Lig. gastrosplenicum

Lig. phrenicocolicum

Gaster, Curvatura major

Omentum majus

Omentum majus, Lig. gastrocolicum — Colon transversum

Fig. 6.10 Position of the viscera, Situs viscerum, in the epigastrium; ventral view. The ventral trunk wall and the rostral parts of the diaphragm have been removed. [S700]

If one raises the lower edge of the liver, the lesser omentum (**Omentum minus**) becomes visible. It spans the area between the liver and the lesser curvature of the stomach and the superior part of the duodenum. The lesser omentum is composed of the **Lig. hepatogastricum** and the **Lig. hepatoduodenale,** which guide the Ductus choledochus, the portal vein (V. portae hepatis) and the A. hepatica propria to the

Porta hepatis. Behind the Lig. hepatoduodenale is the entrance of the **Bursa omentalis** (Foramen omentale, marked here by a probe), a shifting space between the stomach and the pancreas, anteriorly confined by the Omentum minus.

The **Omentum majus** is attached to the greater curvature of the stomach and to the Taenia omentalis of the Colon transversum. The spleen sits in a niche on the **Lig. phrenicocolicum** between the left colonic flexure and the diaphragm.

Clinical remarks

For the physical examination of **trauma patients,** it is important to be familiar with the topography of the abdominal situs to exclude internal bleeding after an accident by employing ultrasound (**FAST sonography,** Focused Assessment with Sonography for Trauma). The positioning of the ultrasound probe produces longitudinal and cross-sectional images of the following four regions:

1. Right flank with view of the right-sided **Recessus subphrenicus** and **Recessus subhepaticus** (clinically also known as the hepatorenal recess of MORISON's pouch) surrounding the liver
2. Left flank with view of the left-sided **Recessus subphrenicus** (clin.: KOLLER's pouch) surrounding the spleen
3. Suprapubic region with view of the **Excavatio rectouterina** (pouch of DOUGLAS) in women and the **Excavatio rectovesicalis** (PROUST's space) in men → Fig. 6.19)
4. Infrasternal region with cranial view towards the **pericardium** to rule out a pericardial tamponade.

[S701-L126]

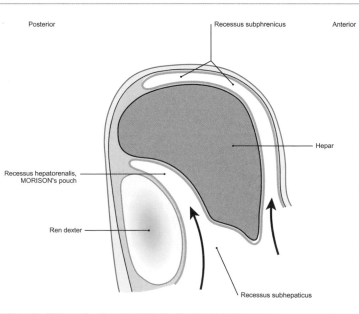

Posterior — Recessus subphrenicus — Anterior

Hepar

Recessus hepatorenalis, MORISON's pouch

Ren dexter

Recessus subhepaticus

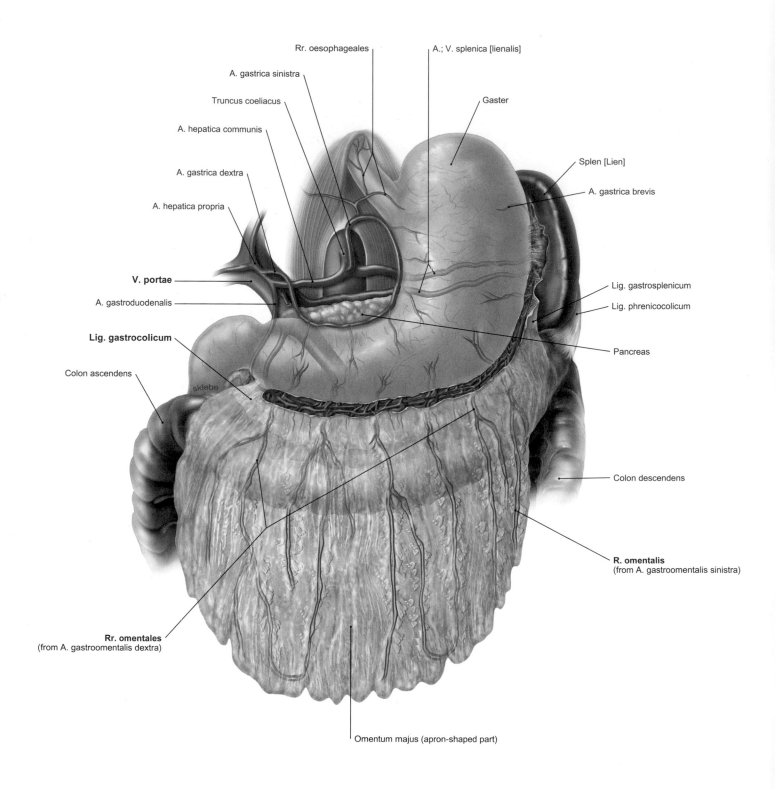

Rr. oesophageales

A. gastrica sinistra

Truncus coeliacus

A. hepatica communis

A. gastrica dextra

A. hepatica propria

V. portae

A. gastroduodenalis

Lig. gastrocolicum

Colon ascendens

sklebe

A.; V. splenica [lienalis]

Gaster

Splen [Lien]

A. gastrica brevis

Lig. gastrosplenicum

Lig. phrenicocolicum

Pancreas

Colon descendens

R. omentalis
(from A. gastroomentalis sinistra)

Rr. omentales
(from A. gastroomentalis dextra)

Omentum majus (apron-shaped part)

Fig. 6.11 Sections and neurovascular pathways of the greater omentum, Omentum majus; semi-schematic representation; ventral view. [S700-L238]/[G1069]

The greater omentum **(Omentum majus)** is divided into a **gastrocolic ligament** (for the Colon transversum), a **Lig. gastrosplenicum** (for the spleen) and a **Lig. gastrosplenicum** (for the posterior abdominal wall). Caudally, these sections continue in an **apron-shaped manner.** The Omentum majus plays a role in the mechanical protection and thermal insulation as well as in the secretion and absorption of the peritoneal fluid; it also has immunological functions, because it is populated by lymphatic tissue.

The greater omentum belongs to the epigastric situs, as it is supplied by the neurovascular pathways of the greater curvature of the stomach. Thereby **five to eight branches (Rr. omentales)** are provided by the **A. gastroomentalis dextra,** while usually only **one branch** is provided by the **A. gastroomentalis sinistra.** The venous branches flow correspondingly into the Vv. gastroomentales on which the Nodi lymphoidei gastroomentales also drain the lymph from the greater omentum.

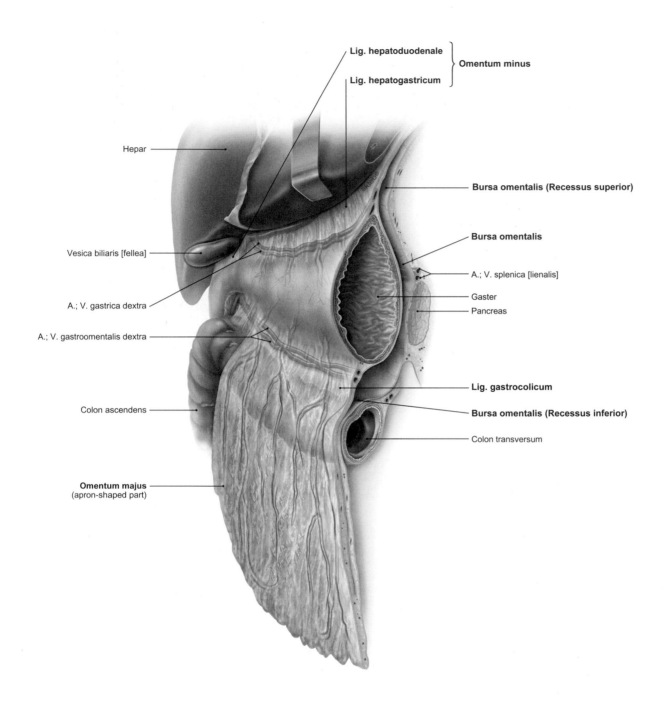

Lig. hepatoduodenale

Lig. hepatogastricum

} Omentum minus

Hepar

Bursa omentalis (Recessus superior)

Bursa omentalis

Vesica biliaris [fellea]

A.; V. splenica [lienalis]

Gaster

A.; V. gastrica dextra

Pancreas

A.; V. gastroomentalis dextra

Lig. gastrocolicum

Colon ascendens

Bursa omentalis (Recessus inferior)

Colon transversum

Omentum majus
(apron-shaped part)

Fig. 6.12 Sections and neurovascular pathways of the greater omentum, Omentum majus; sagittal section of the stomach, pancreas, Colon transversum, Bursa omentalis and Omentum majus; semi-schematic representation; lateral view from the left side. [S700-L238]/[G1069]

The greater omentum **(Omentum majus)** originates with a **Lig. gastrocolicum** from the transverse colon, then runs caudally into the highly variably formed apron-shaped part. The Omentum majus is a peritoneal duplication, which becomes easily recognisable as a lower offshoot

(Recessus inferior) of the **Bursa omentalis** which extends from above into the Lig. gastrocolicum (→ Fig. 6.14). The Bursa omentalis is a protrusion of the peritoneal cavity, extending from the Lig. hepatoduodenale and inserting between the stomach (ventral) and the pancreas (dorsal). Mostly the Recessus inferior does not reach as far as shown here into the apron-shaped part of the Omentum majus.

Epigastric situs with Bursa omentalis

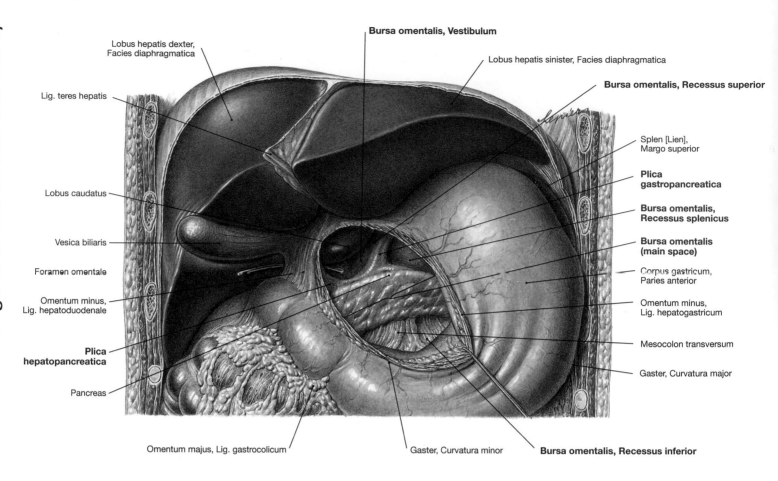

Bursa omentalis, Vestibulum

Lobus hepatis dexter,
Facies diaphragmatica

Lobus hepatis sinister, Facies diaphragmatica

Lig. teres hepatis

Bursa omentalis, Recessus superior

Splen [Lien],
Margo superior

Lobus caudatus

**Plica
gastropancreatica**

Vesica biliaris

**Bursa omentalis,
Recessus splenicus**

Foramen omentale

**Bursa omentalis
(main space)**

Omentum minus,
Lig. hepatoduodenale

Corpus gastricum,
Paries anterior

Omentum minus,
Lig. hepatogastricum

**Plica
hepatopancreatica**

Mesocolon transversum

Pancreas

Gaster, Curvatura major

Omentum majus, Lig. gastrocolicum

Gaster, Curvatura minor

Bursa omentalis, Recessus inferior

Fig. 6.13 Position of the viscera, Situs viscerum, in the epigastrium; ventral view. [S700]
The lesser omentum (Omentum minus) between the liver and the lesser curvature of the stomach has been cut in order to look into the Bursa omentalis.
The **Bursa omentalis** is a shifting space between the stomach and the pancreas, which only communicates with the abdominal cavity via the Foramen omentale which lies behind the Lig. hepatoduodenale. Due to the way it expands, the Bursa omentalis is also referred to as a 'small abdominal cavity' ('lesser sac of the peritoneal cavity').
The Bursa omentalis is divided into four sections:
*   **Foramen omentale:** the entrance to the Bursa omentalis is bordered anteriorly by the Lig. hepatoduodenale, superiorly by the

Lobus caudatus, inferiorly by the Bulbus duodeni and posteriorly by the V. cava inferior.
*   **Vestibulum:** the front of the vestibule is confined by the Omentum minus and reaches behind the liver with a Recessus superior.
*   **Isthmus:** the narrowing between the first and main space is confined by two peritoneal folds, on the right side by the Plica hepatopancreatica which is pushed up by the A. hepatica communis, and on the left side by the Plica gastropancreatica, which marks the pathway of the A. gastrica sinistra.
*   **Main space:** it lies between the stomach (in front) and the pancreas or the Mesocolon transversum (behind). On the left side the Recessus splenicus extends to the hilum of the spleen, and the Recessus inferior extends below the Lig. gastrocolicum to the root of the mesocolon at the Colon transversum.

Borders of the Bursa omentalis		
Orientation	Bordering structure	Recessus
Ventral	Omentum minus, stomach (posterior aspect), Lig. gastrocolicum	–
Dorsal	Pancreas (anterior aspect), aorta with Truncus coeliacus, left kidney (superior pole), left adrenal gland	–
Cranial	Liver (Lobus caudatus), diaphragm	Recessus superior
Caudal	Mesocolon transversum, inferior extension between the layers of the Omentum majus (if not fused)	Recessus inferior
Left	Spleen, Lig. gastrocolicum	Recessus splenicus

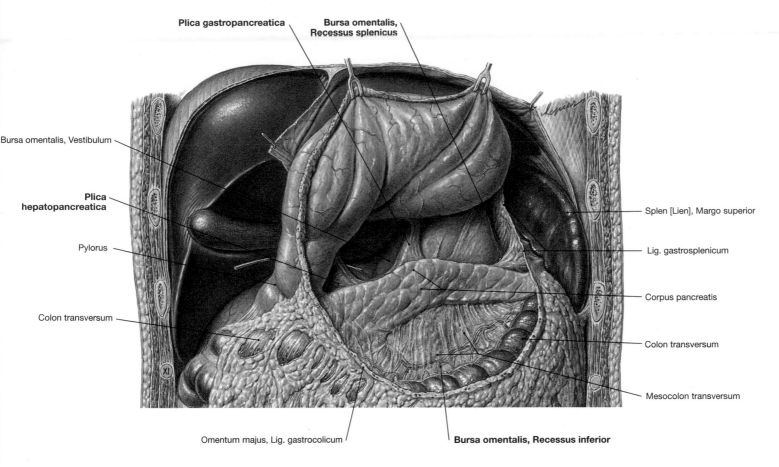

Plica gastropancreatica

Bursa omentalis, Recessus splenicus

Bursa omentalis, Vestibulum

Plica hepatopancreatica

Pylorus

Colon transversum

Omentum majus, Lig. gastrocolicum

Splen [Lien], Margo superior

Lig. gastrosplenicum

Corpus pancreatis

Colon transversum

Mesocolon transversum

Bursa omentalis, Recessus inferior

Fig. 6.14 Position of the viscera, Situs viscerum, in the epigastrium; ventral view. [S700]
The Lig. gastrocolicum has been divided, and the stomach folded back to open up the main space of the Bursa omentalis. The posterior wall of the Bursa omentalis is formed by the pancreas and the Mesocolon transversum. On the left side, it extends into the hilum of the spleen (Recessus splenicus) and downwards to the origin of the mesocolon at the Colon transversum (Recessus inferior).

Clinical remarks

Like other recesses of the peritoneal cavity (→ Fig. a), the Bursa omentalis is of clinical significance due to potential entrapment of intestinal loops **(internal hernias)**, deposition of tumour cells in the case of **peritoneal carcinosis**, or bacterial accumulation in the case of **peritonitis.** During operations in the abdomen, the surgeon therefore inspects the Bursa omentalis, in order to avoid missing any disease.

For **operations** in the epigastrium, e.g. surgical interventions on the pancreas, there are **three access routes** (→ Fig. b) into the Bursa omentalis:

* via the Omentum minus (1; → Fig. 6.13)
* via the Lig. gastrocolicum (2; → Fig. 6.14)
* via the Mesocolon transversum (3).

The illustration (→ Fig. b) below indicates the possible extension of the Recessus inferior of the Bursa omentalis if the two peritoneal layers of the Omentum majus have not fused sufficiently. [S701-L126]

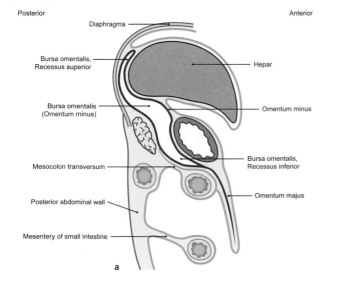

Posterior   Anterior

Diaphragma

Bursa omentalis, Recessus superior

Bursa omentalis (Omentum minus)

Mesocolon transversum

Posterior abdominal wall

Mesentery of small intestine

Hepar

Omentum minus

Bursa omentalis, Recessus inferior

Omentum majus

a

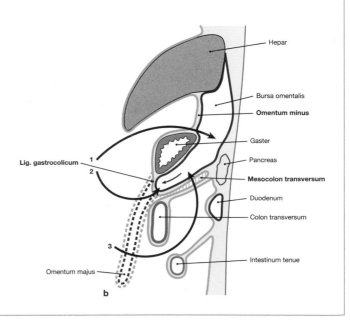

Hepar

Bursa omentalis

Omentum minus

Gaster

Pancreas

Mesocolon transversum

Duodenum

Colon transversum

Intestinum tenue

Lig. gastrocolicum

Omentum majus

b

Hypogastric situs

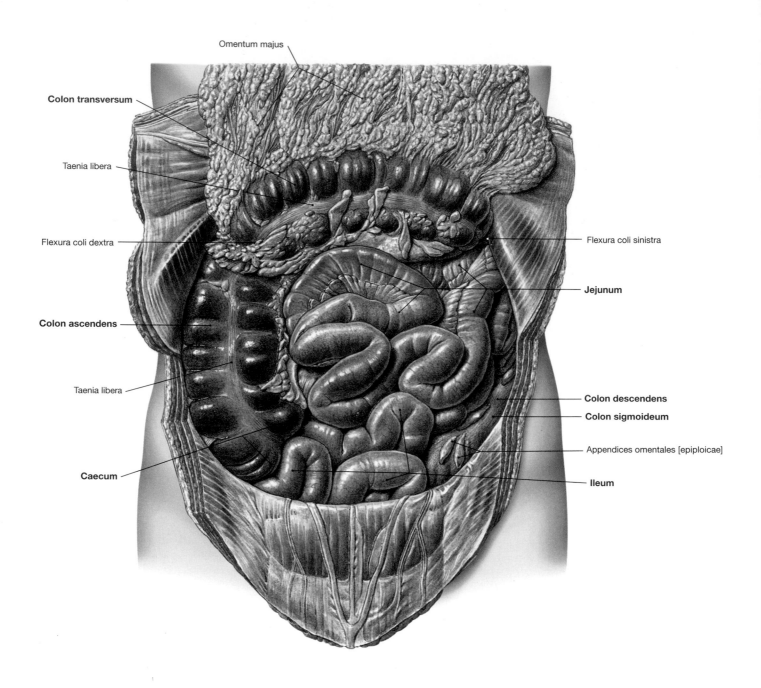

Omentum majus

Colon transversum

Taenia libera

Flexura coli dextra

Flexura coli sinistra

Jejunum

Colon ascendens

Taenia libera

Colon descendens

Colon sigmoideum

Appendices omentales [epiploicae]

Caecum

Ileum

Fig. 6.15 Position of the viscera, Situs viscerum, in the hypogastrium; ventral view. [S700]

The Omentum majus has been folded back cranially to reveal the small and large intestines in the **hypogastrium,** which reveals the intraperitoneal segments: the **jejunum** and **ileum** of the small intestine as well as the **caecum, Colon transversum,** and **Colon sigmoideum** of the large intestine. This figure also shows that the retroperitoneal segments of the colon are shifted to the posterior wall of the trunk to a variable extent. In this case, the **Colon ascendens** is clearly visible, but the **Colon descendens** is shifted further dorsally and is partially covered by the small intestine. The large intestine envelops the bundle of the jejunum and ileum like a frame.

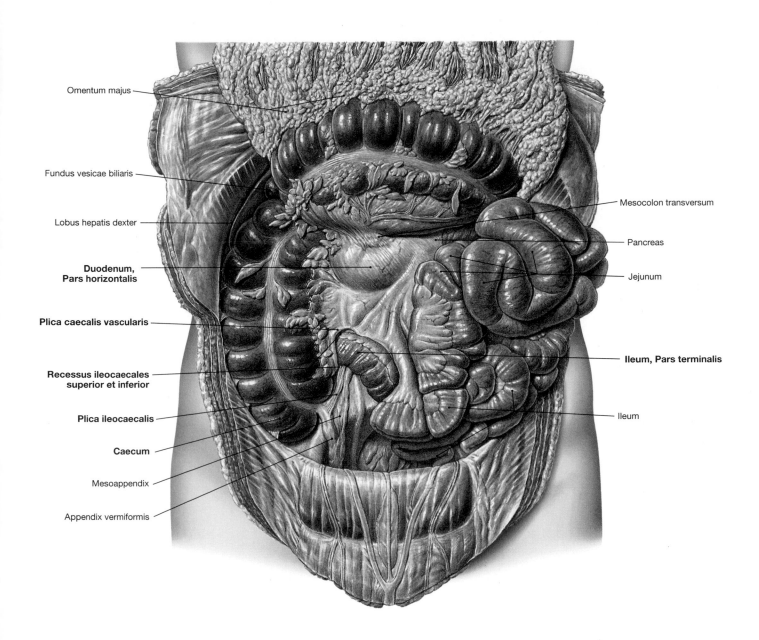

Omentum majus

Fundus vesicae biliaris

Lobus hepatis dexter

**Duodenum,
Pars horizontalis**

Plica caecalis vascularis

**Recessus ileocaecales
superior et inferior**

Plica ileocaecalis

Caecum

Mesoappendix

Appendix vermiformis

Mesocolon transversum

Pancreas

Jejunum

Ileum, Pars terminalis

Ileum

Fig. 6.16 Position of the viscera, Situs viscerum, in the hypogastrium; ventral view. [S700]
The Omentum majus has been folded cranially and the loops of the small intestine have been moved to the left side to make the secondary retroperitoneal Pars horizontalis of the duodenum visible. Between the individual organs, the peritoneal cavity forms bulges **(recesses).** At the junction of the ileum with the caecum, there are two of these spaces.

The **Recessus ileocaecalis superior** is covered by the Plica caecalis vascularis (containing a branch of the A. ileocolica), and the **Recessus ileocaecalis inferior** is covered by the Plica ileocaecalis, located between the ileum and the Appendix vermiformis. In the same way as in the Bursa omentalis and in other recesses, small intestinal loops (internal hernias) can become trapped.

Hypogastric situs with recess of the peritoneal cavity

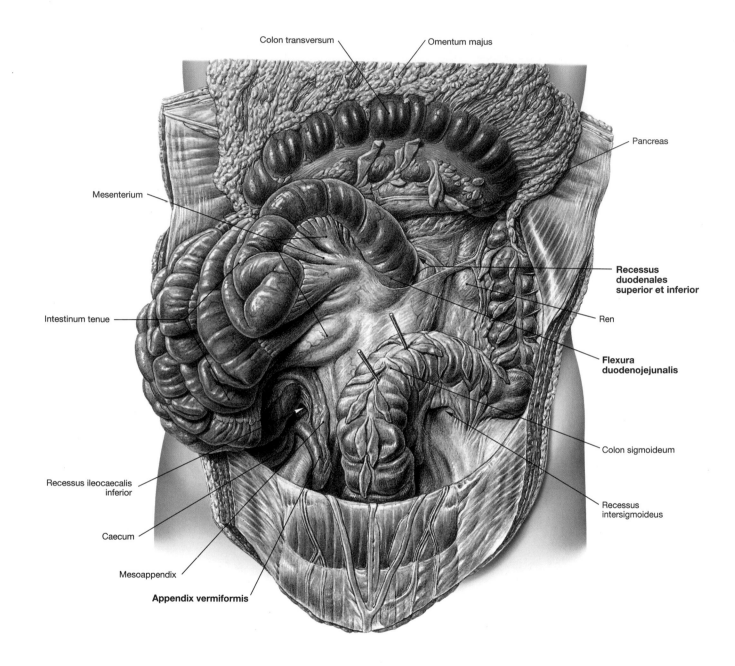

Colon transversum — Omentum majus

Pancreas

Mesenterium

Recessus duodenales superior et inferior

Ren

Intestinum tenue

Flexura duodenojejunalis

Colon sigmoideum

Recessus intersigmoideus

Recessus ileocaecalis inferior

Caecum

Mesoappendix

Appendix vermiformis

Fig. 6.17 Position of the viscera, Situs viscerum, in the hypogastrium; ventral view. [S700]
The Omentum majus has been folded cranially and the loops of the small intestine have been shifted to the right, so that the Flexura duodenojejunalis is visible, in which the retroperitoneal duodenum continues into the intraperitoneal jejunum. This area also contains two recesses: the **Recessus duodenales superior** and **inferior.** In the right hypogastrium, the Appendix vermiformis is visible, the tip of which descends into the small pelvis (descending type).

Clinical remarks

Of all the recesses in the body, small intestinal appendages **(TREITZ hernia)** are most frequently trapped in the Recessus duodenales superior and inferior. This entrapment can cause a blockage (ileus) and bowel infarctions.

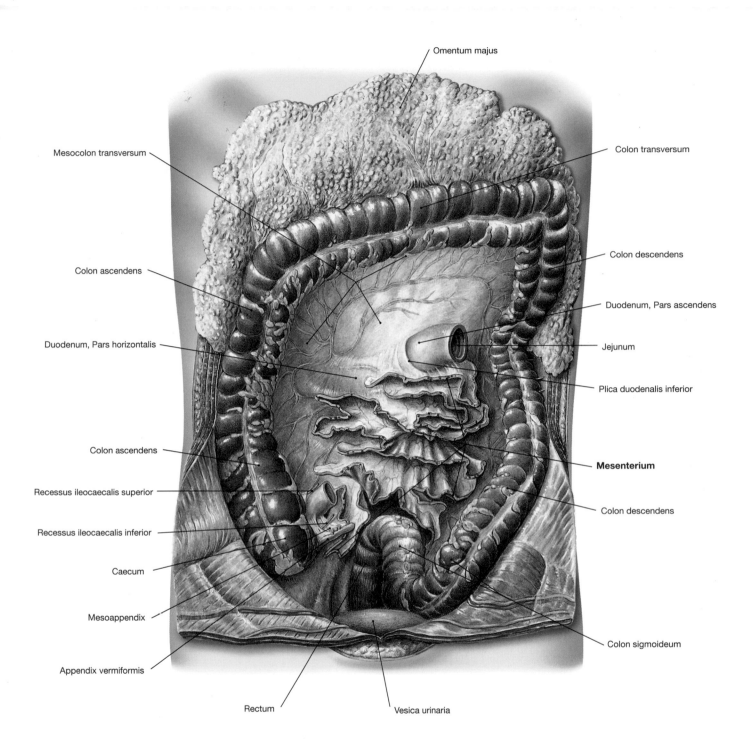

Omentum majus

Mesocolon transversum

Colon transversum

Colon ascendens

Colon descendens

Duodenum, Pars ascendens

Duodenum, Pars horizontalis

Jejunum

Plica duodenalis inferior

Colon ascendens

Mesenterium

Recessus ileocaecalis superior

Colon descendens

Recessus ileocaecalis inferior

Caecum

Mesoappendix

Colon sigmoideum

Appendix vermiformis

Rectum

Vesica urinaria

Fig. 6.18   Mesentery of the small intestine, mesenterium, and large intestine, Intestinum crassum; ventral view. [S700]
The Omentum majus and the Colon transversum have been folded back. The intraperitoneal small intestinal bundle of jejunum and ileum

has been removed at the **mesentery.** The mesentery is a peritoneal duplication which provides a flexible suspension of the small intestine and contains the neurovascular pathways.

Organs of the abdominal cavity

Topography

Secondary retroperitoneal organs

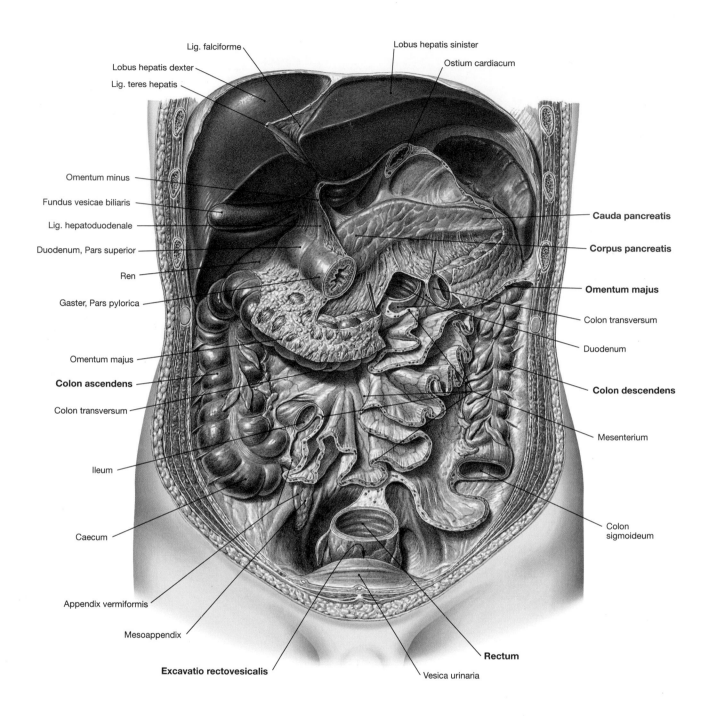

Lig. falciforme
Lobus hepatis dexter
Lig. teres hepatis
Lobus hepatis sinister
Ostium cardiacum

Omentum minus
Fundus vesicae biliaris
Lig. hepatoduodenale
Duodenum, Pars superior
Ren
Gaster, Pars pylorica

Omentum majus
Colon ascendens
Colon transversum

Ileum

Caecum

Appendix vermiformis

Mesoappendix

Excavatio rectovesicalis

Cauda pancreatis
Corpus pancreatis
Omentum majus
Colon transversum
Duodenum
Colon descendens
Mesenterium
Colon sigmoideum

Rectum
Vesica urinaria

Fig. 6.19   Position of the secondary retroperitoneal organs; ventral view. [S700]
The stomach has been removed, the jejunum and ileum were resected at the mesentery, and the Colon transversum and Colon sigmoideum were severed. Most of the secondary retroperitoneal organs are now visible. These include the **duodenum** (except for the Pars superior), **pancreas, Colon ascendens** and **Colon descendens** as well as the **proximal rectum up to the Flexura sacralis.** In front of the rectum, the entrance of the **Excavatio rectovesicalis** can be seen, a recess which is the lowest point of the abdominal cavity in men.

Clinical remarks

In an upright position (seldom in bedridden patients), the most inferior extension of the abdominal cavity, the **Excavatio rectovesicalis** (PROUST's space) in men, and the **Excavatio rectouterina** (pouch of DOUGLAS) in women (→ Fig. 6.20), may collect inflammatory exudate or pus with inflammation in the hypogastrium. An ultrasound may be used to check if the liquid is clear or not.
Ultrasound is also used for rapid exclusion of internal bleeding in **trauma patients (FAST-sonography,** Focused Assessment with

Sonography for Trauma) (Clinical remarks → Fig. 6.10). Placing the ultrasound probe in a horizontal or orientation will offer longitudinal and cross-sectional views of the Excavatio rectouterina (pouch of DOUGLAS) in women and the Excavatio rectovesicalis (PROUST's space) in men to rule out a possible accumulation of blood in these pelvic peritoneal recesses.

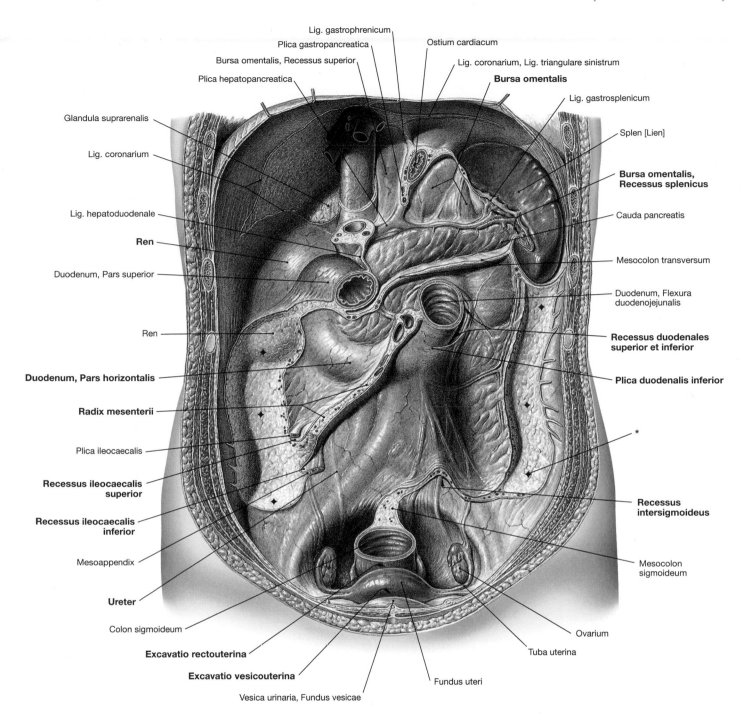

Lig. gastrophrenicum
Plica gastropancreatica
Bursa omentalis, Recessus superior
Plica hepatopancreatica
Glandula suprarenalis
Lig. coronarium
Lig. hepatoduodenale
Ren
Duodenum, Pars superior
Ren
Duodenum, Pars horizontalis
Radix mesenterii
Plica ileocaecalis
Recessus ileocaecalis superior
Recessus ileocaecalis inferior
Mesoappendix
Ureter
Colon sigmoideum
Excavatio rectouterina
Excavatio vesicouterina
Vesica urinaria, Fundus vesicae

Ostium cardiacum
Lig. coronarium, Lig. triangulare sinistrum
Bursa omentalis
Lig. gastrosplenicum
Splen [Lien]
Bursa omentalis, Recessus splenicus
Cauda pancreatis
Mesocolon transversum
Duodenum, Flexura duodenojejunalis
Recessus duodenales superior et inferior
Plica duodenalis inferior
*
Recessus intersigmoideus
Mesocolon sigmoideum
Ovarium
Tuba uterina
Fundus uteri

Fig. 6.20 Dorsal wall of the peritoneal cavity, Cavitas peritonealis, with recess, Recessus, and spleen, Splen [Lien]; ventral view. [S700]

The liver, as well as the small and large intestines have been removed up to the duodenum to expose the back of the peritoneal cavity. On the right kidney and on the Pars horizontalis of the duodenum is the Peritoneum parietale which is easily recognised by its shimmering lustre. The adhesion sites of the secondary retroperitoneal Colon ascendens and Colon descendens lack the coating of the parietal peritoneum.

Peritoneal duplications enclose the contours of the posterior wall of the peritoneal cavity as folds (plicae) and ligaments, forming the various **recesses.** The largest of these recesses is the **Bursa omentalis** (→ Fig. 6.13), of which the sections and offshoots can be seen here. In the area of the Flexura duodenojejunalis, the Plicae duodenales superior and inferior form two recesses, the **Recessus duodenales superior** and **inferior.** There are further recesses at the confluence of the terminal ileum into the caecum **(Recessus ileocaecales superior** and **inferior)** and occasionally below the sigmoid mesocolon **(Recessus intersigmoideus).**

There is a deep peritoneal space anterior to the rectum, which is confined at the ventral side by the uterus. This **Excavatio rectouterina** (pouch of DOUGLAS) is the lowest point of the female peritoneal cavity. The **Excavatio vesicouterina** located ventrally between the urinary bladder and uterus does not go quite as far caudally. The approximately 12–16 cm long **mesentery root (Radix mesenterii),** in which the neurovascular pathways of the small intestine (A./V. mesenterica superior) have been truncated, reaches from the Flexura duodenojejunalis to the right Fossa iliaca. The mesenteric root crosses the Pars horizontalis of the duodenum and the right ureter.

* **TOLDT's fascia;** dorsal of the Colon ascendens and the Colon descendens, which have been removed here. The borders lateral of the Colon ascendens and descendens are the 'white lines of TOLDT' and are created by the lateral reflection of the Peritoneum visceral onto the Peritoneum parietale.

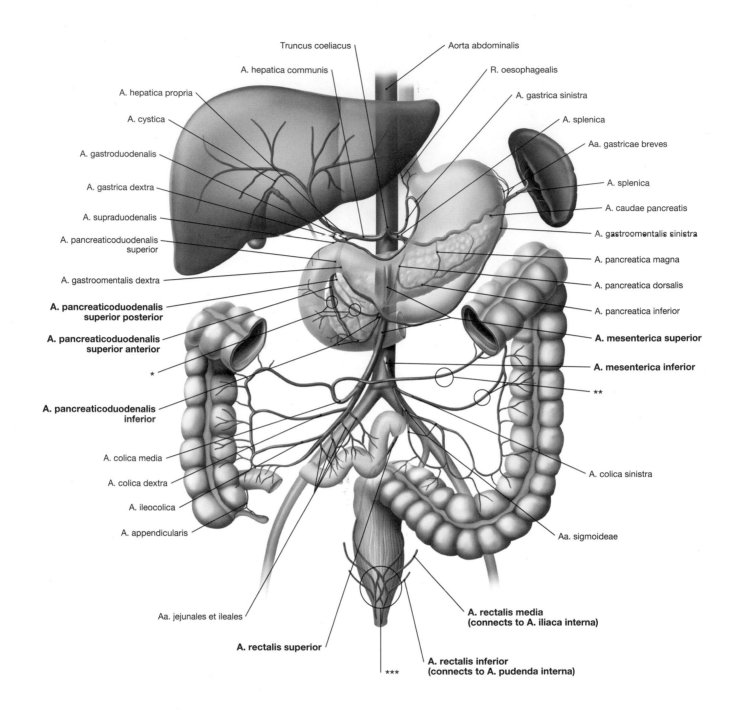

Truncus coeliacus
A. hepatica communis
A. hepatica propria
A. cystica
A. gastroduodenalis
A. gastrica dextra
A. supraduodenalis
A. pancreaticoduodenalis superior
A. gastroomentalis dextra
A. pancreaticoduodenalis superior posterior
A. pancreaticoduodenalis superior anterior
*
A. pancreaticoduodenalis inferior
A. colica media
A. colica dextra
A. ileocolica
A. appendicularis
Aa. jejunales et ileales
A. rectalis superior

Aorta abdominalis
R. oesophagealis
A. gastrica sinistra
A. splenica
Aa. gastricae breves
A. splenica
A. caudae pancreatis
A. gastroomentalis sinistra
A. pancreatica magna
A. pancreatica dorsalis
A. pancreatica inferior
A. mesenterica superior
A. mesenterica inferior
**
A. colica sinistra
Aa. sigmoideae
A. rectalis media (connects to A. iliaca interna)
A. rectalis inferior (connects to A. pudenda interna)
***

Fig. 6.21 Arteries of the abdominal viscera; semi-schematic illustration; ventral view. [S701-L275]/[G1069]

The most important anastomoses are marked with black circles. The three unpaired arteries of the abdominal viscera, which branch off the abdominal aorta, are the Truncus coeliacus, the A. mesenterica superior and the A. mesenterica inferior. The A. mesenterica superior originates directly below the Truncus coeliacus (due to the semi-schematic representation it is not included here). Their individual branches are described on the following pages. The three arteries form **anastomoses** with each other and with branches of the A. iliaca interna, which in the case of an occlusion of one of these vessels can prevent an ischaemic infarction.

Specifically, these are:
- connections between the Truncus coeliacus and the A. mesenterica superior via the Aa. pancreaticoduodenales: **BÜHLER's anastomotic artery** (*)
- connections between the A. mesenterica superior and the A. mesenterica inferior: **RIOLAN's arcade** of the Aa. colicae media and sinistra (**)
- plexus of rectal arteries: this connects the A. rectalis superior from the A. mesenterica inferior with the Aa. rectales media and inferior from the drainage area of the A. iliaca interna (***).

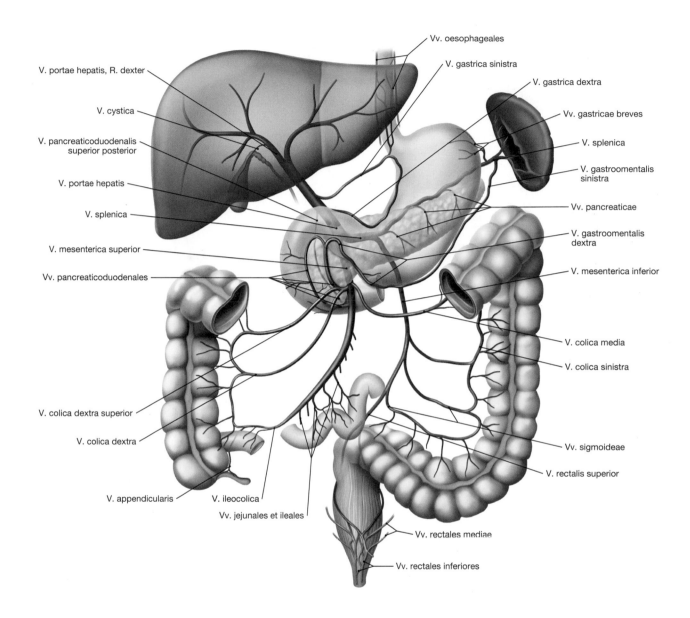

Vv. oesophageales

V. portae hepatis, R. dexter

V. gastrica sinistra

V. gastrica dextra

V. cystica

Vv. gastricae breves

V. pancreaticoduodenalis superior posterior

V. splenica

V. portae hepatis

V. gastroomentalis sinistra

V. splenica

Vv. pancreaticae

V. mesenterica superior

V. gastroomentalis dextra

Vv. pancreaticoduodenales

V. mesenterica inferior

V. colica dextra superior

V. colica media

V. colica dextra

V. colica sinistra

V. appendicularis

Vv. sigmoideae

V. ileocolica

V. rectalis superior

Vv. jejunales et ileales

Vv. rectales mediae

Vv. rectales inferiores

Fig. 6.22 Portal vein, V. portae hepatis, with tributaries; semi-schematic illustration; ventral view. [S701-L275]
The **portal vein** (V. portae hepatis) collects the nutrient-rich blood from the unpaired abdominal organs (stomach, intestines, pancreas, spleen) and takes it to the liver.

The portal vein has three **main tributaries:** behind the head of the pancreas, the V. mesenterica superior merges with the V. splenica to form the V. portae hepatis. The V. mesenterica inferior mostly drains into the V. splenica (70 % of all cases). In addition, some branches lead directly into the portal vein (detailed description → Fig. 6.100).

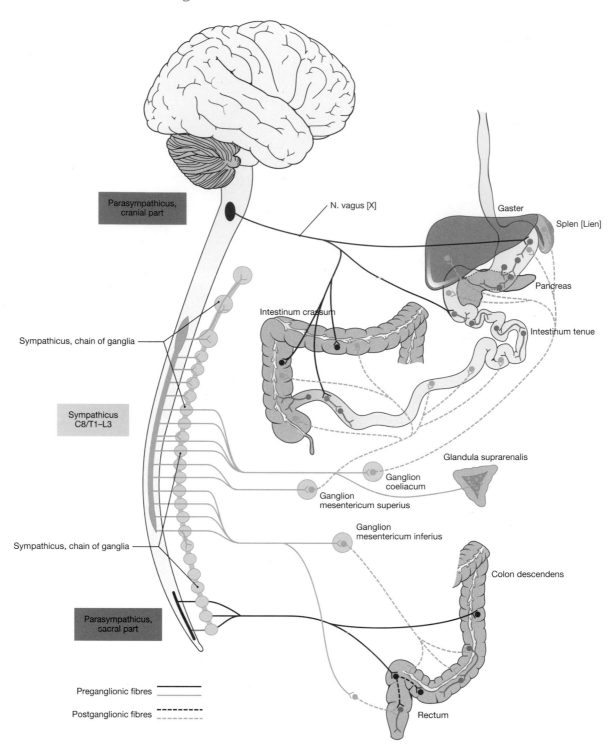

Fig. 6.23 Autonomic innervation of the abdominal organs; schematic drawing. [S700-L126]~[S130-6-L106]

The abdominal organs are autonomically innervated by the **sympathicus** and the **parasympathicus.** The first so-called **preganglionic** neuron is positioned with its nerve cell body in the central nervous system (CNS) and sends its axons as nerve fibres to node-shaped structures **(ganglions),** which are introduced by second **postganglionic** neurons (→ Fig. 12.213, Vol. 3). The **sympathetic ganglia,** located close to the spine **(paravertebral),** form a chain, the sympathetic trunk (Truncus sympathicus), and they also lie on the aorta **(prevertebral),** near the openings of the visceral branches. Conversely, the ganglia of the **parasympathicus** are usually found directly on the effector organs **(close to organs).** The nerves to the abdominal organs form a network on the abdominal aorta **(Plexus aorticus abdominalis)** and reach their target organs mainly as periarterial plexuses embedded in the peritoneal duplications of the mesenteries (→ Fig. 7.10).

*   **Sympathicus**

    Preganglionic neurons: lateral horn of the thoracic and lumbar portions of the spinal cord **(C8–L3) = thoracolumbar** part of the autonomic nervous system.

The nerve fibres for the abdomen are however not switched onto the ganglia of the **sympathicus;** instead they run through the two visceral nerves **(N. splanchnicus major,** T5–T9, and **N. splanchnicus minor,** T10–T11) to the **ganglia of the Plexus aorticus abdominalis,** where they are switched onto the postganglionic neurons.

*   **Parasympathicus**

    Preganglionic neurons: nuclei of the **N. vagus [X]** as well as in the sacral part of the spinal cord **(S2–S4) = craniosacral** part of the autonomic nervous system. Preganglionic neurons for the abdominal organs run with the **N. vagus** and eventually, together with the oesophagus as the **Trunci vagales anterior and posterior,** pass through the diaphragm to the Plexus aorticus abdominalis. The innervation area of the cranial parasympathicus includes all of the epigastric organs and ends in the area of the left colonic flexure (traditionally referred to as the CANNON-BÖHM point). The 'left-sided colon sections' receive their nerve fibres, as do all the pelvic organs, from the sacral parasympathetic trunk (S2–S4), which they exit as the **Nn. splanchnici pelvici,** and are then switched onto postganglionic neurons in the **Plexus hypogastricus inferior** in the area of the rectum.

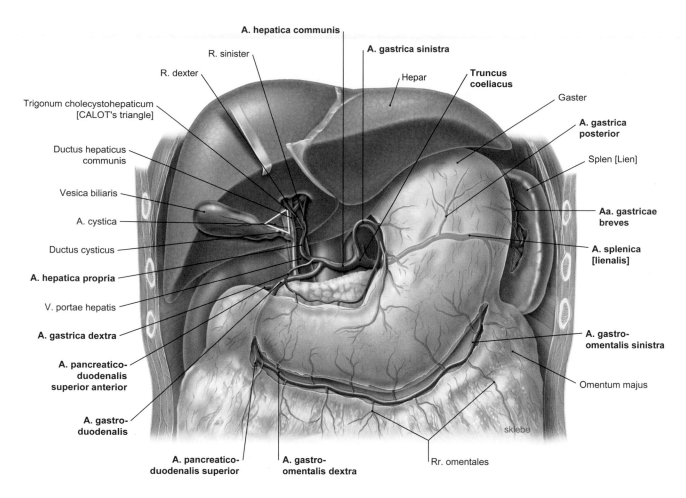

A. hepatica communis

R. sinister

R. dexter

Trigonum cholecystohepaticum
[CALOT's triangle]

Ductus hepaticus
communis

Vesica biliaris

A. cystica

Ductus cysticus

A. hepatica propria

V. portae hepatis

A. gastrica dextra

A. pancreatico-
duodenalis
superior anterior

A. gastro-
duodenalis

A. gastrica sinistra

Hepar

Truncus
coeliacus

Gaster

A. gastrica
posterior

Splen [Lien]

Aa. gastricae
breves

A. splenica
[lienalis]

A. gastro-
omentalis sinistra

Omentum majus

A. pancreatico-
duodenalis superior

A. gastro-
omentalis dextra

Rr. omentales

sklebe

Fig. 6.24 **Branches of the Truncus coeliacus;** semi-schematic illustration; the liver is mobilised upwards; ventral view after removal of the Omentum minus. [S700-L238]/[B500~M282/L132]

The Truncus coeliacus is the first unpaired visceral branch of the abdominal aorta. It has three main branches supplying the epigastric organs (stomach, duodenum, liver, gallbladder, pancreas and spleen). The length of the Truncus coeliacus is highly variable, but without any clinical consequences: e.g. it can be several centimetres in length or very short. Alternatively, distinct branches, such as the A. gastrica sinistra, may originate from the abdominal aorta directly:

- **A. gastrica sinistra:** branches off to the top left, and is usually stronger than the A. gastrica dextra with which it anastomoses along the lesser curvature of the stomach. The A. gastrica sinistra pushes up the Plica gastropancreatica at the rear wall of the bursa omentalis. It then provides the Rr. oesophagealis to the Pars abdominalis of the oesophagus before passing over into the Lig. hepatogastricum of the Omentum minus via the lesser curvature of the stomach. In 10–20 % of all cases, it forms an accessory left hepatic artery for the left lobe of the liver.
- **A. hepatica communis:** turns to the right and subdivides into the:
  - **A. gastroduodenalis:** descends retroperitoneally behind the pylorus or duodenum, bifurcates into the **A. gastroomentalis dextra** of the greater curvature of the stomach as well as of the

Omentum majus, and into the **Aa. pancreaticoduodenales superiores anterior and posterior,** which anastomose (BÜHLER's anastomotic artery) with the A. pancreaticoduodenalis inferior from the A. mesenterica superior and supply the pancreatic head and the duodenum
  - **A. hepatica propria:** constitutes the terminal branch and branches off the **A. gastrica dextra** to the lesser curvature of the stomach. Joining the Lig. hepatoduodenale, it then provides the liver with a R. dexter and a R. sinister to supply the respective functioning parts of the liver. The **A. cystica** to the gallbladder mostly originates from the R. dexter.
- **A. splenica [lienalis]:** passes retroperitoneally to the left side, and runs along the superior border of the pancreas, and provides the following branches on its way to the spleen:
  - Rr. pancreatici to the pancreas
  - A. gastrica posterior to the stomach (in 30–60 % of all cases)
  - A. gastroomentalis sinistra: passes from the left side to the greater curvature of the stomach and anastomoses within the Lig. gastrocolicum with the A. gastroomentalis dextra
  - Aa. gastrici breves: short branches within the Lig. gastrosplenicum to the fundus of the stomach
  - Rr. splenici: terminal branches to the spleen.

Branches of the Truncus coeliacus

Branch	Supply area	Pathway
A. gastrica sinistra	Stomach (lesser curvature), oesophagus (Pars abdominalis), in 10–20 % of the left lobe of the liver	• Plica gastropancreatica • Lig. hepatogastricum
A. hepatica communis	Stomach (lesser and greater curvature), duodenum, pancreas, Omentum majus, liver, gallbladder	• Retroperitoneal • A. hepatica propria in the Lig. hepatoduodenale • A. gastrica dextra in the Lig. hepatogastricum • A. gastroomentalis dextra in the Lig. gastrocolicum
A. splenica	Stomach (rear side, fundus, greater curvature), pancreas, Omentum majus, spleen	• Retroperitoneal • Firstly the A. gastroomentalis sinistra within the Lig. gastrosplenicum, then within the Lig. gastrocolicum

Truncus coeliacus

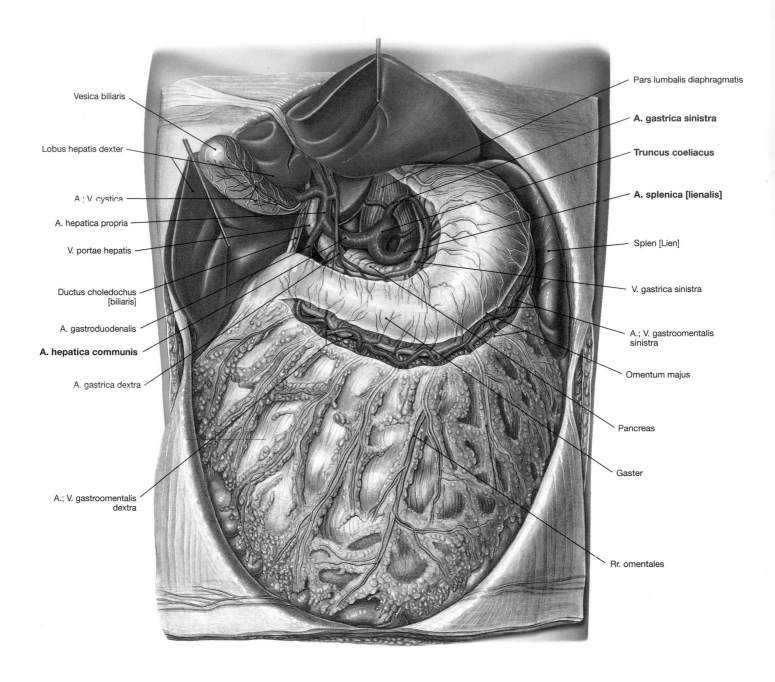

Vesica biliaris

Lobus hepatis dexter

A ; V. cystica

A. hepatica propria

V. portae hepatis

Ductus choledochus [biliaris]

A. gastroduodenalis

A. hepatica communis

A. gastrica dextra

A.; V. gastroomentalis dextra

Pars lumbalis diaphragmatis

A. gastrica sinistra

Truncus coeliacus

A. splenica [lienalis]

Splen [Lien]

V. gastrica sinistra

A.; V. gastroomentalis sinistra

Omentum majus

Pancreas

Gaster

Rr. omentales

Fig. 6.25   Topography of the Truncus coeliacus; ventral view; after removal of the Omentum minus. [S700]

The Truncus coeliacus originates from just below the Hiatus aorticus at the level of the 12th thoracic vertebra as the first unpaired branch of the aorta. In the retroperitoneal space behind the Bursa omentalis, its short (mostly 1–2 cm) trunk divides into the three major arteries:

- The **A. gastrica sinistra** branches off to the top left and emerges on the posterior wall of the Bursa omentalis as the **Plica gastropancreatica** before moving up into the **Lig. hepatogastricum** to the lesser curvature of the stomach.
- The **A. hepatica communis** turns right and forms the **Plica hepatopancreatica** of the Bursa omentalis, before dividing into its main branches:

– The A. hepatica propria provides the A. gastrica dextra and then passes into the **Lig. hepatoduodenale** to the portal vein.

– The A. gastroduodenalis rises retroperitoneally behind the pylorus or duodenum and continues into the Aa. pancreaticoduodenales superiores anterior and posterior.

– The A. gastroomentalis dextra passes into the **Lig. gastrocolicum** of the greater curvature of the stomach.

- The **A. splenica [lienalis]** enters the retroperitoneum on the left side and runs along the superior edge of the pancreas. Their branches supplying the greater curvature of the stomach (A. gastroomentalis sinistra) and the short branches (Aa. gastrici breves) to the fundus of the stomach enter the hilum of the spleen in the **Lig. gastrosplenicum.**

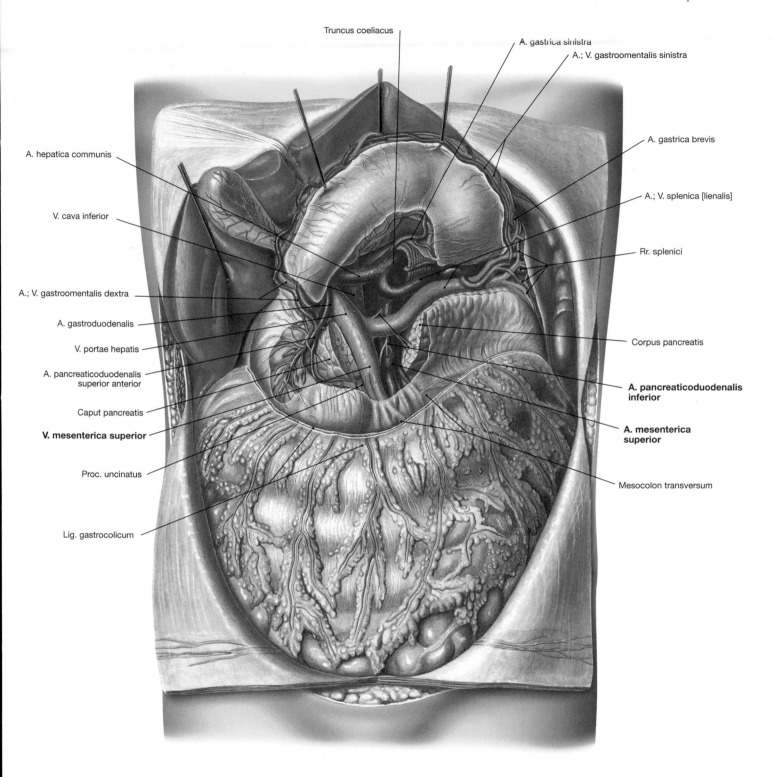

Truncus coeliacus

A. gastrica sinistra

A.; V. gastroomentalis sinistra

A. gastrica brevis

A.; V. splenica [lienalis]

Rr. splenici

Corpus pancreatis

A. pancreaticoduodenalis inferior

A. mesenterica superior

Mesocolon transversum

A. hepatica communis

V. cava inferior

A.; V. gastroomentalis dextra

A. gastroduodenalis

V. portae hepatis

A. pancreaticoduodenalis superior anterior

Caput pancreatis

V. mesenterica superior

Proc. uncinatus

Lig. gastrocolicum

Fig. 6.26 Origin of the A. mesenterica superior and branches of the Truncus coeliacus; ventral view; the stomach is folded back cranially and the pancreas is cut through. [S700]

After its origin from the aorta below the Truncus coeliacus and at the level of the first lumbar vertebra, the **A. mesenterica superior** descends behind the pancreas and enters the mesentery. The pancreas is cut through to show the pathway of the A. and V. mesenterica superior, which are supported by the Proc. uncinatus of the pancreas. As the first branch, the A. mesenterica superior provides the **A. pancreaticoduodenalis inferior** towards the top right. It anastomoses with the **Aa. pancreaticoduodenales superiores anterior and posterior** from

the circulatory area of the Truncus coeliacus. These arteries continue from the A. gastroduodenalis of the A. hepatica propria.

As the stomach is folded back cranially, the vascular arcades on both sides of the curvatures of the stomach are clearly recognisable, and consist of the branches of the Truncus coeliacus.

The **Truncus coeliacus** directly provides the **A. gastrica sinistra** to the lesser curvature of the stomach. It is connected with the **A. gastrica dextra,** which usually branches off from the A. hepatica propria. The **A. gastroomentalis dextra** from the A. gastroduodenalis connects to the greater curvature of the stomach with the **A. gastroomentalis sinistra** from the A. splenica. The **Aa. gastrici breves** also emerge from the A. splenica, turning towards the fundus of the stomach.

Topography

A. mesenterica superior

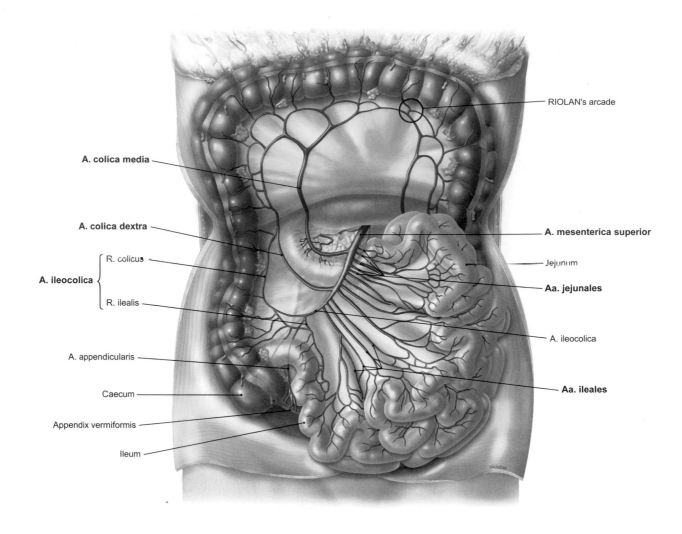

A. colica media

A. colica dextra

A. ileocolica { R. colicus

R. ilealis

A. appendicularis

Caecum

Appendix vermiformis

Ileum

RIOLAN's arcade

A. mesenterica superior

Jejunum

Aa. jejunales

A. ileocolica

Aa. ileales

Fig. 6.27 A. mesenterica superior; ventral view; Colon transversum folded upwards. [S700-L238]

The unpaired A. mesenterica superior originates from the aorta directly below the Truncus coeliacus, initially running retroperitoneally behind the pancreas and then passes into the mesentery. Its branches can be displayed if the mesentery is opened and the adipose tissue between the vascular arcades is removed. It supplies parts of the pancreas and duodenum, the entire small intestine, and the large intestine up to the left colonic flexure (splenic flexure).

Branches of the A. mesenterica superior:
- **A. pancreaticoduodenalis inferior:** branches off to the superior right side; the R. anterior and R. posterior anastomose with the

Aa. pancreaticoduodenales superiores anterior and posterior (BÜHLER's anastomotic artery) (→ Fig. 6.26).
- **Aa. jejunales** (4–5) and **Aa. ileales** (12): directed to the left side
- **A. colica media:** originates from the right side, anastomoses with the A. colica dextra and the A. colica sinistra (RIOLAN's arcade)
- **A. colica dextra:** runs to the Colon ascendens and anastomoses via ascending and descending branches with the A. colica media and the A. ileocolica. Frequently, there is a common stem for both the A. colica media and A. colica dextra.
- **Ileocolic artery:** supplies the distal ileum (R. ilealis), Colon ascendens (R. colicus), caecum (Aa. caecalis anterior and posterior) and Appendix vermiformis (A. appendicularis).

Branches of the A. mesenterica superior		
Branch	**Supply area**	**Pathway**
A. pancreaticoduodenalis inferior	Duodenum, pancreas	Mesenterium
Aa. jejunales and ileales	Jejunum, Ileum	Mesenterium
A. ileocolica, A. colica dextra and A. colica media	Ileum (terminal part), Caecum, Appendix vermiformis, Colon ascendens and Colon transversum	• Mesenterium • Mesocolon • A. appendicularis in the mesentery of the Appendix vermiformis

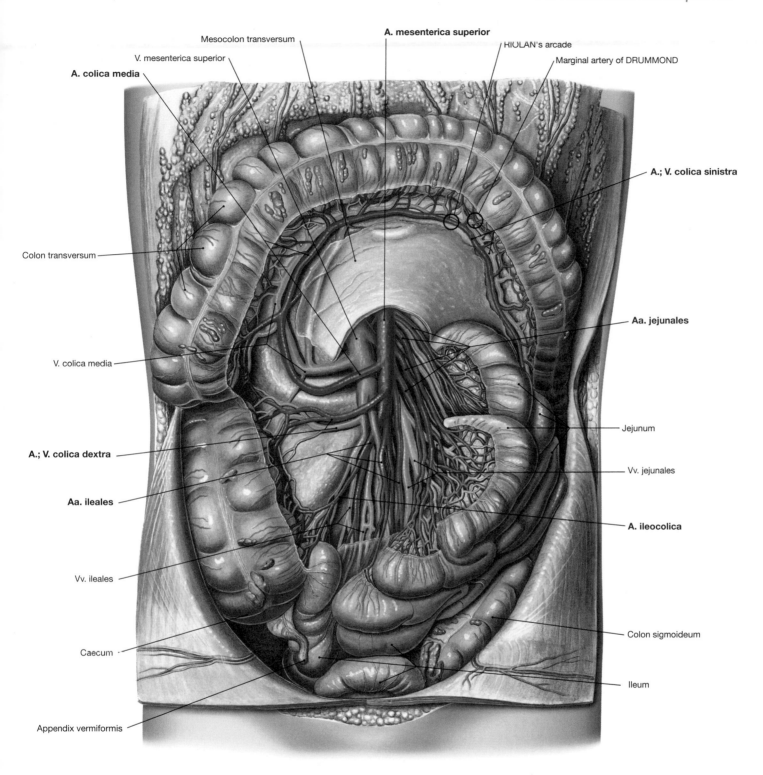

A. colica media

Mesocolon transversum

V. mesenterica superior

A. mesenterica superior

RIOLAN's arcade

Marginal artery of DRUMMOND

A.; V. colica sinistra

Colon transversum

V. colica media

Aa. jejunales

A.; V. colica dextra

Jejunum

Aa. ileales

Vv. jejunales

A. ileocolica

Vv. ileales

Colon sigmoideum

Caecum

Ileum

Appendix vermiformis

Fig. 6.28 Pathway of the A. and V. mesenterica superior; ventral view; after opening of the mesentery with the Colon transversum folded back. [S700]

Within the mesentery, the A. mesenterica superior provides the Aa. jejunales and the Aa. ileales to the left side and the A. colica media, A. colica dextra and A. ileocolica to the right side. All arteries form arcades in the intestines on various branching levels; these enable the movement of the intestinal loops. In the area of the left colonic flexure, the A. colica media forms functionally **important anastomoses (RIOLAN's arcade)** with the A. colica sinistra from the A. mesenterica inferior. This anastomosis may enable a circulatory bypass in case of an arterial occlusion. An anastomosis between both of the two arteries in one of the arcades close to the intestines is occasionally referred to as the marginal artery of DRUMMOND. However, in clinical jargon, all anastomoses in the area of the left colonic flexure are regarded as RIOLAN's arcades.

The venous branches correspond to the arteries.

Clinical remarks

When parts of the colon are surgically removed, such as the Colon ascendens in a **right hemicolectomy,** it is important to keep in mind that besides the large intestine, the A. mesenterica superior also supplies the small intestine and should therefore not be removed completely.

A. mesenterica inferior

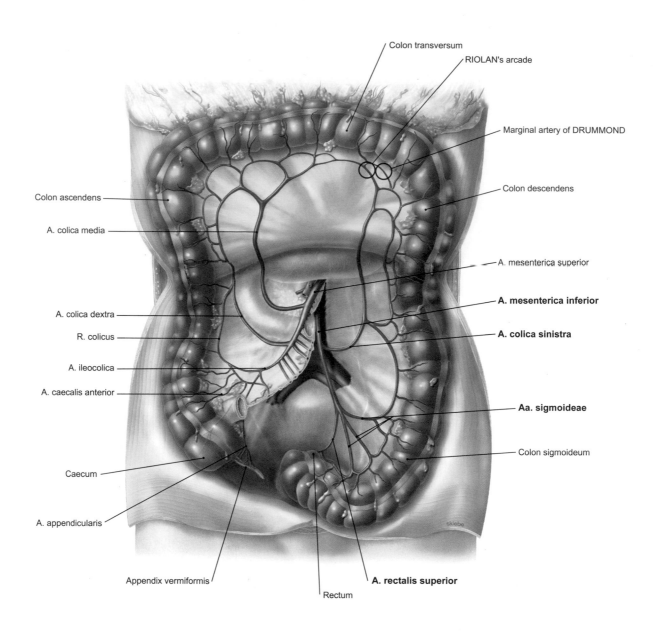

Colon transversum
RIOLAN's arcade
Marginal artery of DRUMMOND
Colon descendens
A. mesenterica superior
A. mesenterica inferior
A. colica sinistra
Aa. sigmoideae
Colon sigmoideum
A. rectalis superior

Colon ascendens
A. colica media
A. colica dextra
R. colicus
A. ileocolica
A. caecalis anterior
Caecum
A. appendicularis
Appendix vermiformis
Rectum

Fig. 6.29   A. mesenterica inferior; ventral view; Colon transversum folded back cranially. [S700-L238]/[G1069]
The unpaired A. mesenterica inferior branches off the aorta to the left, approximately 5 cm above its bifurcation, and then runs retroperitoneally. It supplies the Colon descendens and the upper rectum.

Branches of the A. mesenterica inferior:
*   **A. colica sinistra:** ascends along the Colon descendens, anastomoses with the A. colica media from the A. mesenterica superior (RIOLAN's arcade)
*   **Aa. sigmoideae:** several branches to the Colon sigmoideum
*   **A. rectalis superior:** enters the mesorectum from cranial and supplies the rectum and the upper anal canal (Zona columnaris). Here it mainly feeds the cavernous body (Corpus cavernosum recti), a part of the continence organ.

Branches of the A. mesenterica inferior		
Branch	**Supply area**	**Pathway**
A. colica sinistra	Colon descendens and Colon transversum	Mesocolon
Aa. sigmoideae	Colon sigmoideum	Mesocolon
A. rectalis superior	• Rectum • Anal canal (Zona columnaris)	• Retroperitoneal • Mesorectum

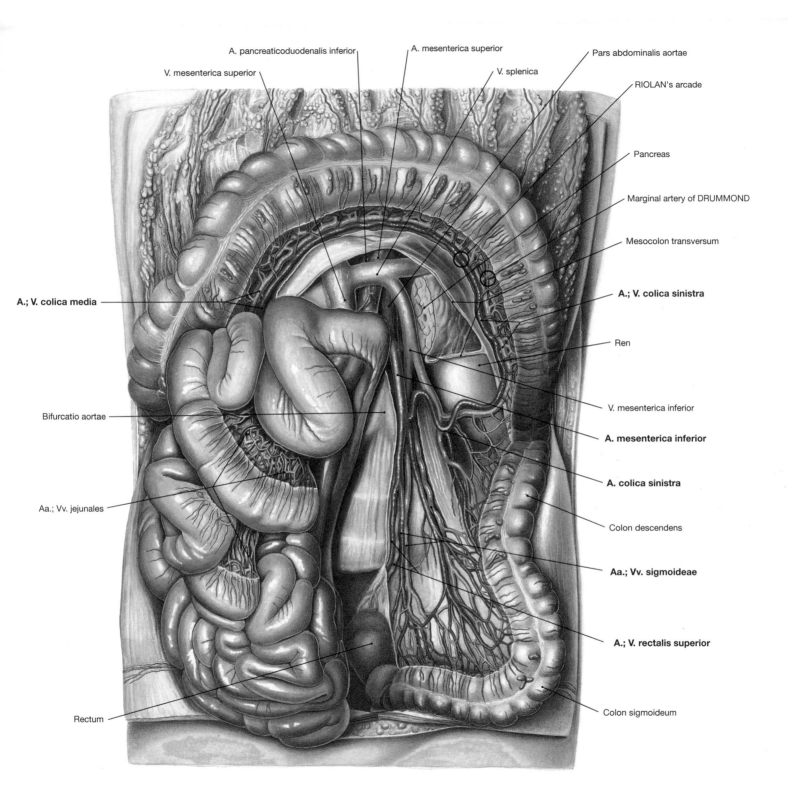

A. pancreaticoduodenalis inferior

V. mesenterica superior

A. mesenterica superior

V. splenica

Pars abdominalis aortae

RIOLAN's arcade

Pancreas

Marginal artery of DRUMMOND

Mesocolon transversum

A.; V. colica sinistra

Ren

V. mesenterica inferior

A. mesenterica inferior

A. colica sinistra

Colon descendens

Aa.; Vv. sigmoideae

A.; V. rectalis superior

Colon sigmoideum

A.; V. colica media

Bifurcatio aortae

Aa.; Vv. jejunales

Rectum

Fig. 6.30   Pathway of the A. and V. mesenterica inferior in the retroperitoneum; ventral view; Colon transversum folded back and small intestinal loops shifted to the right. [S700]
From its origin above the bifurcation of the aorta, the A. mesenterica inferior descends into the retroperitoneum and firstly provides the A. colica sinistra to the left, then several Aa. sigmoideae and finally the (unpaired) A. rectalis superior.

The A. colica sinistra ascends the Colon descendens, forms arcades and anastomoses with the A. colica media from the A. mesenterica superior **(RIOLAN 's arcade).** Occasionally, the connection in one of the arcades near the intestines is referred to as the marginal artery of DRUMMOND.

Neurovascular pathways in the mesenteries

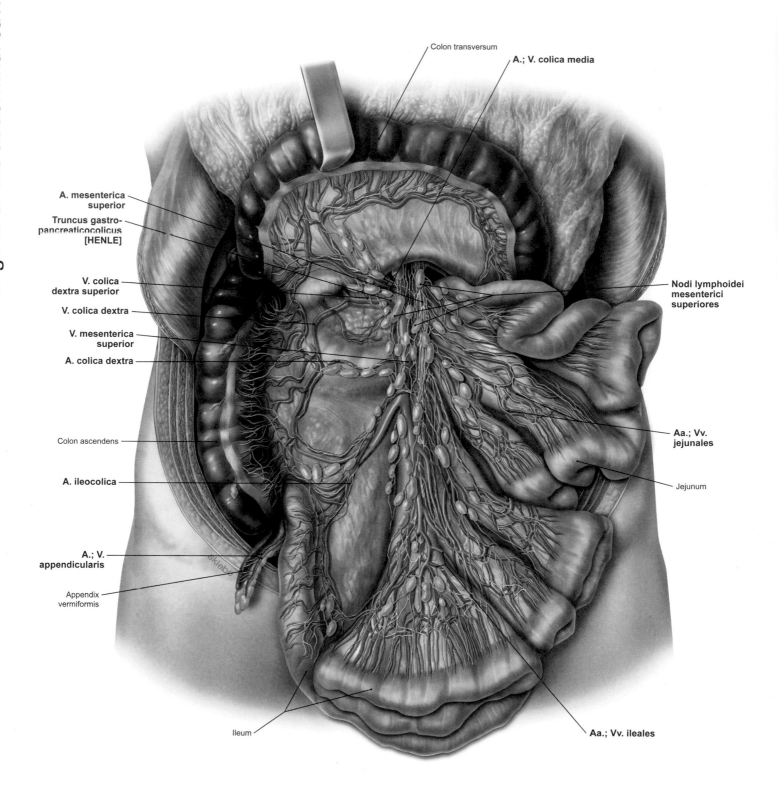

Colon transversum

A.; V. colica media

A. mesenterica superior

Truncus gastro-pancreaticocolicus [HENLE]

V. colica dextra superior

V. colica dextra

V. mesenterica superior

A. colica dextra

Colon ascendens

A. ileocolica

A.; V. appendicularis

Appendix vermiformis

Nodi lymphoidei mesenterici superiores

Aa.; Vv. jejunales

Jejunum

Aa.; Vv. ileales

Ileum

Fig. 6.31 Pathway of the A. and V. mesenterica superior and con-comitant lymphatic pathways and autonomic nerves in the mes-entery; view from ventral; Colon transversum folded back cranially and small intestinal loops shifted to the left. [S700-L238]/[Q300]

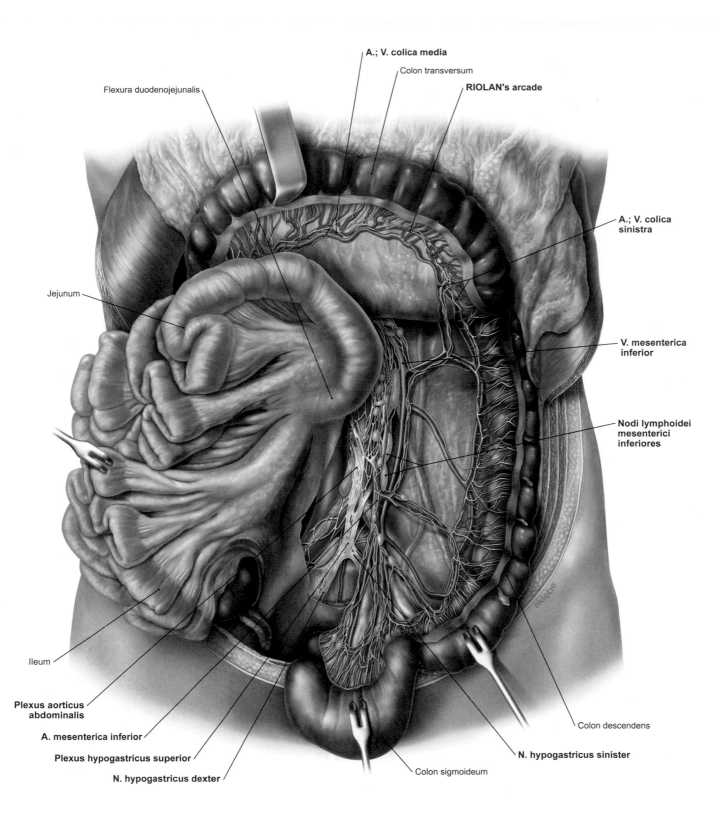

A.; V. colica media

Colon transversum

RIOLAN's arcade

Flexura duodenojejunalis

A.; V. colica sinistra

Jejunum

V. mesenterica inferior

Nodi lymphoidei mesenterici inferiores

Ileum

Colon descendens

Plexus aorticus abdominalis

A. mesenterica inferior

N. hypogastricus sinister

Plexus hypogastricus superior

Colon sigmoideum

N. hypogastricus dexter

Fig. 6.32 Pathway of the A. and V. mesenterica inferior and concomitant lymphatic pathways and autonomic nerves in the retroperitoneal space; view from ventral; Colon transversum folded back cranially and the small intestinal loops shifted to the right. [S700-L238]/[Q300]

The lymphatic pathways and autonomic nerves (Plexus aorticus abdominalis) of the Pars abdominalis aortae are also shown. The autonomic nerves continue from the **Plexus hypogastricus superior** to both sides as **N. hypogastricus dexter and sinister** into the small pelvis.

Stomach

Projection of the stomach

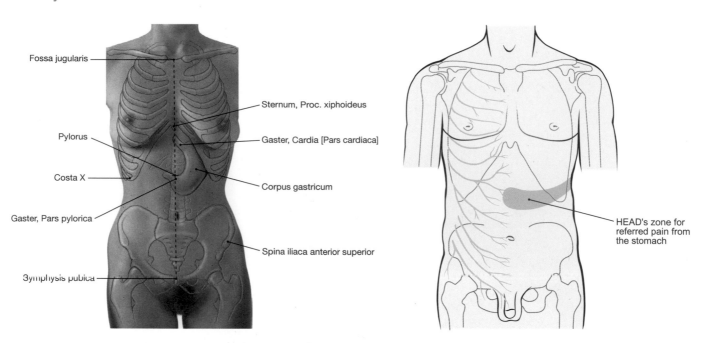

Fig. 6.33 Projection of the stomach, Gaster, onto the ventral trunk wall; ventral view. [S700]

The entrance of the stomach (cardia) projects approximately to the height of the tenth thoracic vertebra and ventrally below the xiphoid process of the breastbone. The caudal portion of the body of the stomach is relatively variable at the level of the second to third lumbar vertebrae. Conversely, the pylorus is relatively consistently found at the midpoint of a line between the pubic symphysis (Symphysis pubica) and the jugular fossa (Fossa jugularis). This central point projects approximately to the first lumbar vertebra.

Fig. 6.34 Zone of referred pain (HEAD's zone) of the stomach, schematic drawing; ventral view. [S700-L126]/[G1071]

The organ-related area for referred pain or the **HEAD's zone** of the stomach is represented by the dermatome T8, where pain perceptions related to stomach diseases are projected. This is because the afferent nerve fibres from the stomach converge at the spinal cord level with those from the eighth cutaneous area, so it is not possible to differentiate between them.

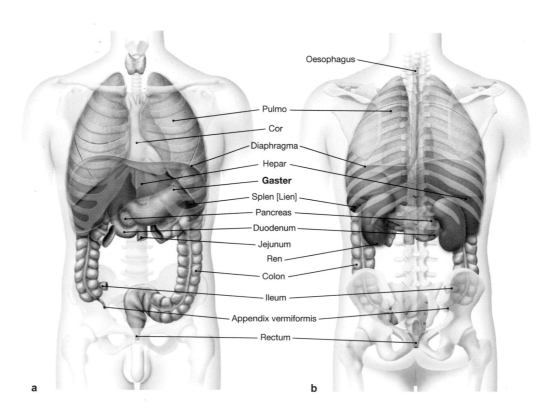

Fig. 6.35a and b Projection of inner organs onto the body surface. [S700-L275]

a Ventral view.
b Dorsal view.

The stomach is positioned **intraperitoneally** in the left epigastrium between the left lobe of the liver and the spleen. The stomach is mostly covered by the left costal arch but a small area is directly adjacent to the ventral abdominal wall. This area is clinically relevant since PEG (**p**ercutaneous **e**ndoscopic **g**astrostomy) tubes can be placed here for parenteral nutrition.

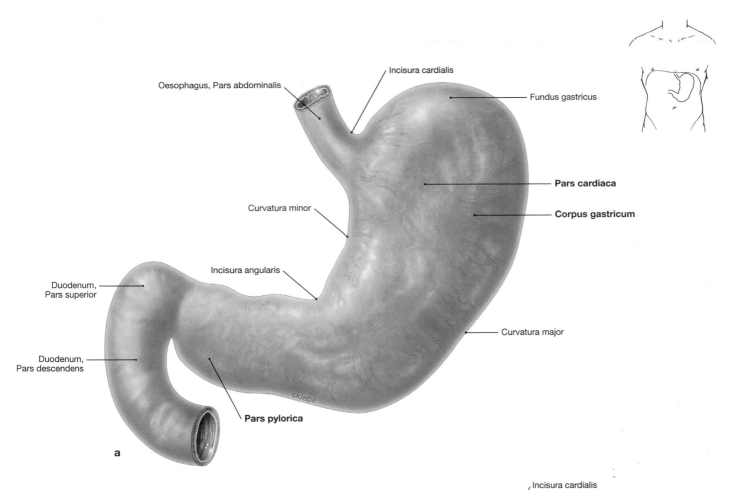

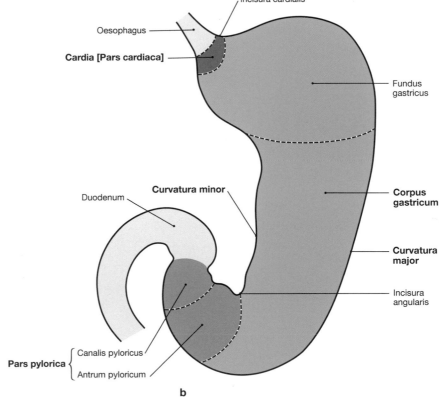

Fig. 6.36a and b   Stomach, Gaster.
a Ventral view. [S700-L238]
b Schematic illustration. [S700-L126]/[B500]
The stomach is divided into three parts:

* **Pars cardiaca:** stomach entrance
* **Corpus gastricum:** main part with Fundus gastricus above
* **Pars pylorica:** pylorus, which continues in the Antrum pyloricum and the Canalis pyloricus, which is surrounded by the M. sphincter pyloricus.

The stomach has an anterior and posterior wall (Paries anterior and posterior). The lesser curvature (Curvatura minor) is to the right, the greater curvature (Curvatura major) is to the left. On the lesser curvature there is a notch (Incisura angularis), where the Pars pylorica begins. The greater curvature also starts with a recess (Incisura cardialis) which is responsible for the formation of the angle of HIS between the stomach and the oesophagus. Internally, this angle corresponds to a mucosal fold which, in addition to the oesophageal sphincter, is responsible for the closure of the stomach.

Clinical remarks

If the angle of HIS is lost, e.g. due to faulty attachment in the diaphragm (axial hiatus hernia), this may lead to reflux of gastric juices with inflammation of the oesophagus **(reflux oesophagitis).** If drug therapy to reduce acid production with proton pump blockers fails, an operation is needed to improve the closure by looping the fundus of the stomach around the oesophagus (NISSEN's fundoplication).

Musculature of the stomach

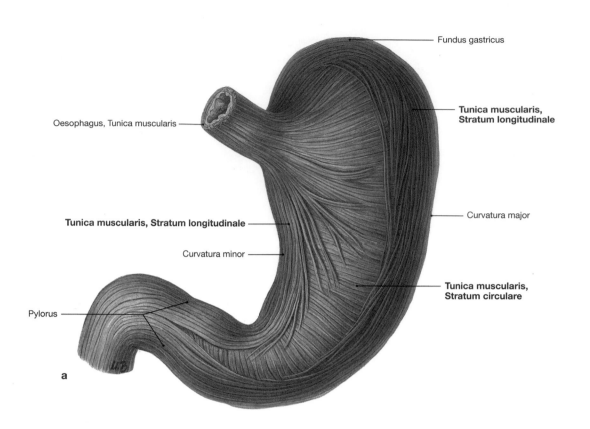

Fundus gastricus

Oesophagus, Tunica muscularis

Tunica muscularis, Stratum longitudinale

Tunica muscularis, Stratum longitudinale

Curvatura minor

Pylorus

Curvatura major

Tunica muscularis, Stratum circulare

a

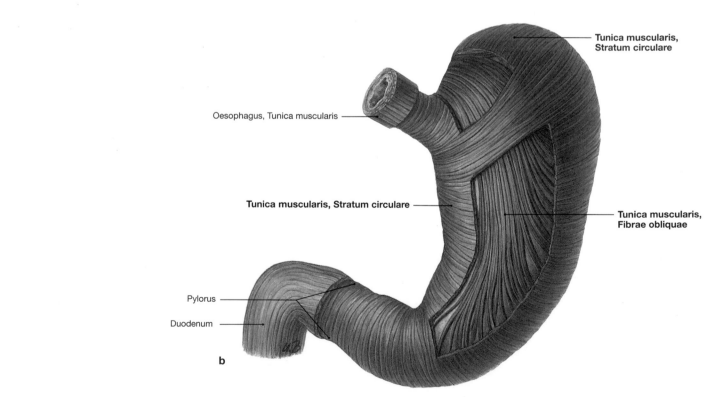

Tunica muscularis, Stratum circulare

Oesophagus, Tunica muscularis

Tunica muscularis, Stratum circulare

Tunica muscularis, Fibrae obliquae

Pylorus

Duodenum

b

Fig. 6.37a and b   Muscle layers of the stomach, Gaster; ventral view. [S700]
a Outer muscle layers.
b Inner muscle layers.
The wall of the stomach comprises three muscle layers (Tunica muscularis); however, these are not consistently found throughout the stomach. The external longitudinal muscular layer (Stratum longitudinale) is adjacent to the circular muscular layer (Stratum circulare). Muscle fibres (Fibrae obliquae) run obliquely at its deepest point; in the lesser curvature, however, these are absent.

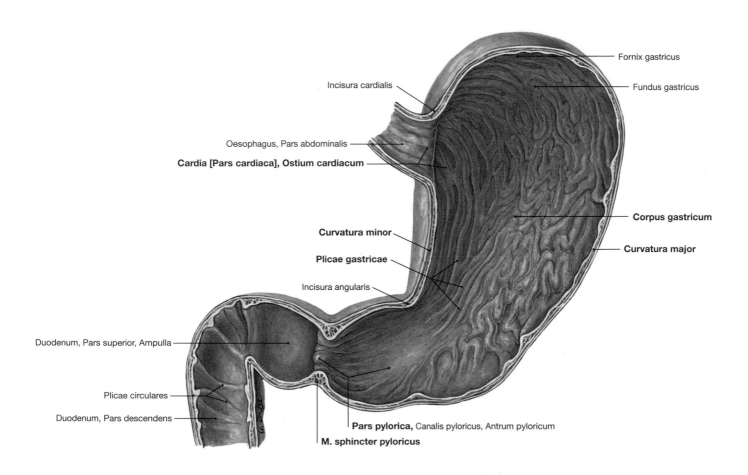

Fornix gastricus

Incisura cardialis

Fundus gastricus

Oesophagus, Pars abdominalis

Cardia [Pars cardiaca], Ostium cardiacum

Corpus gastricum

Curvatura minor

Curvatura major

Plicae gastricae

Incisura angularis

Duodenum, Pars superior, Ampulla

Plicae circulares

Duodenum, Pars descendens

Pars pylorica, Canalis pyloricus, Antrum pyloricum

M. sphincter pyloricus

Fig. 6.38   Stomach, Gaster, and duodenum; ventral view. [S700]
The gastric mucous membrane has a characteristic **surface** which can
expand. Macroscopically, however, only the **gastric folds (Plica gastricae)** are visible, and these run lengthways (gastric canal). With a magni-

fying glass, small, slightly elevated **polygonal areas (Areae gastricae)**
are visible on these folds (→ Fig. 6.39). At the exit of the stomach (pylorus) the circular muscular layer is thickened to form the pyloric sphincter muscle (M. sphincter pyloricus).

Structure of the wall of the stomach

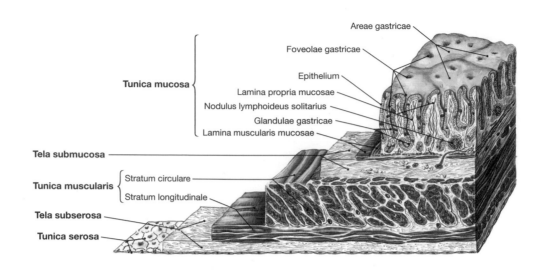

Tunica mucosa {
- Areae gastricae
- Foveolae gastricae
- Epithelium
- Lamina propria mucosae
- Nodulus lymphoideus solitarius
- Glandulae gastricae
- Lamina muscularis mucosae

Tela submucosa

Tunica muscularis {
- Stratum circulare
- Stratum longitudinale

Tela subserosa

Tunica serosa

Fig. 6.39   Structure of the wall of the stomach, Gaster; microscopic view. [S700]
Similar to the whole of the intestines, the wall of the stomach comprises an inner mucosal layer (Tunica mucosa) which is separated from the muscular layer (Tunica muscularis, → Fig. 6.37) by a layer of loose connective tissue (Tela submucosa). As an intraperitoneal organ, the stomach is covered on its outer surface by visceral peritoneum (Peritoneum viscerale), which forms a Tunica serosa.

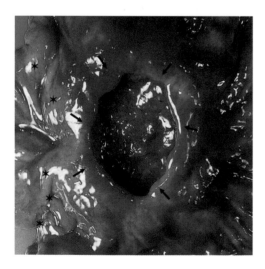

Fig. 6.40   Gastric ulcer, Ulcus ventriculi. [R235]
Gastric ulcers are sores which can affect the entire mucous membrane of the stomach.
Asterisks mark the pylorus ring, and arrows mark the edges of the ulcer.

Clinical remarks

More than 80 % of all gastric and duodenal ulcers are caused by the bacterium *Helicobacter pylori*. In addition, increased gastric acid production or a reduced formation of mucus, e. g. after taking painkillers containing the active substance acetylsalicylic acid, promote the formation of gastric ulcers. Accordingly, treatment involves eliminating bacteria with antibiotics, along with inhibiting the secretion of gastric acid. In the case of complications, surgical treatment is indicated. Complications may include a perforation into adjacent organs or the abdominal cavity, resulting in life-threatening peritonitis, or the erosion of a gastric artery (→ Fig. 6.42), leading to heavy bleeding.

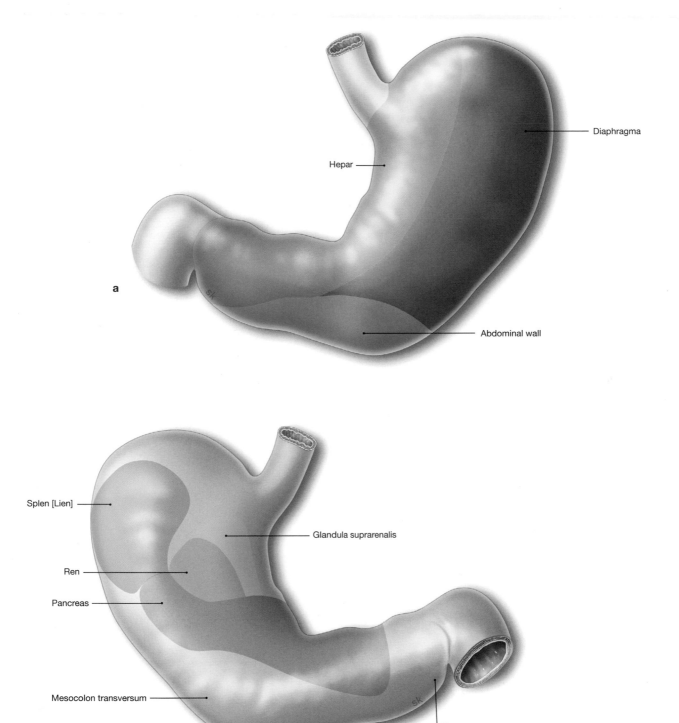

Diaphragma

Hepar

a

Abdominal wall

Splen [Lien]

Glandula suprarenalis

Ren

Pancreas

Mesocolon transversum

Hepar

b

Fig.6.41a and b   Contact areas, Facies, of the stomach with adja-cent organs. [S700-L238]
a Contact areas of the anterior wall of the stomach: liver, diaphragm, abdominal wall.

b Contact areas of the posterior wall of the stomach: spleen, kid-ney, adrenal gland, pancreas, Mesocolon transversum.
The stomach can move relatively easily compared to its adjacent or-gans. Contact areas are also heavily dependent on the extent to which the stomach is filled.

Clinical remarks

The contact areas have a certain clinical relevance, as gastric ulcers or gastric tumours may lead to a **perforation in adjacent organs,** which can lead to organ damage or it may complicate the removal of tumours.

Organs of the abdominal cavity

Stomach

Arteries of the stomach

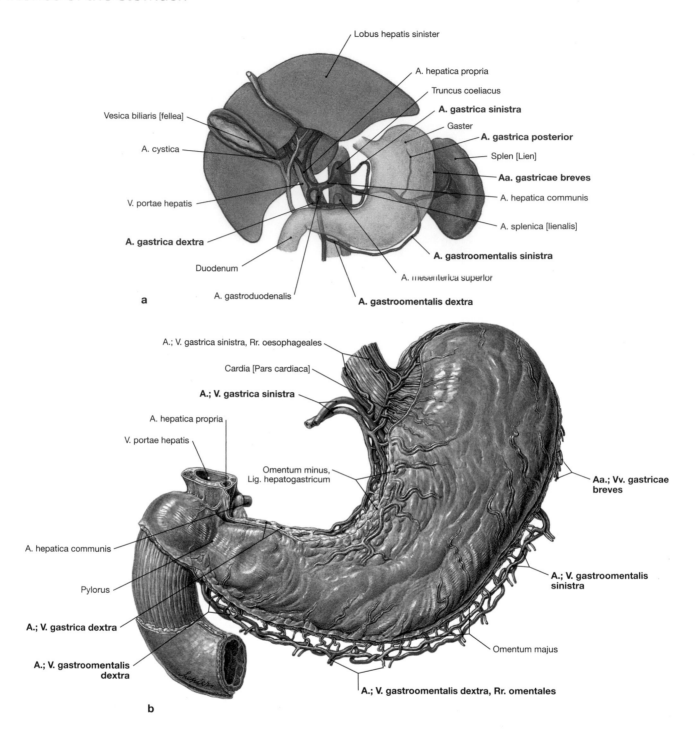

Lobus hepatis sinister

A. hepatica propria

Truncus coeliacus

A. gastrica sinistra

Gaster

A. gastrica posterior

Splen [Lien]

Aa. gastricae breves

A. hepatica communis

A. splenica [lienalis]

A. gastroomentalis sinistra

A. mesenterica superior

A. gastroomentalis dextra

Vesica biliaris [fellea]

A. cystica

V. portae hepatis

A. gastrica dextra

Duodenum

A. gastroduodenalis

a

A.; V. gastrica sinistra, Rr. oesophageales

Cardia [Pars cardiaca]

A.; V. gastrica sinistra

A. hepatica propria

V. portae hepatis

Omentum minus,
Lig. hepatogastricum

A. hepatica communis

Pylorus

A.; V. gastrica dextra

**A.; V. gastroomentalis
dextra**

**Aa.; Vv. gastricae
breves**

**A.; V. gastroomentalis
sinistra**

Omentum majus

A.; V. gastroomentalis dextra, Rr. omentales

b

Fig. 6.42a and b   Arteries of the stomach, Gaster, ventral view.
[S700]
a Schematic diagram.
b Pathway at the curvatures of the stomach.

The three main branches of the Truncus coeliacus (A. gastrica sinistra, A. hepatica communis, A. splenica) give rise to a total of six gastric arteries (→ table below).

Arteries of the stomach	
Supply area	**Arteries**
Lesser curvature	• A. gastrica sinistra (directly from the Truncus coeliacus) • A. gastrica dextra (from the A. hepatica propria)
Greater curvature	• A. gastroomentalis sinistra (from the A. splenica) • A. gastroomentalis dextra (from the A. gastroduodenalis of the A. hepatica communis) The vessels also supply the Omentum majus!
Fundus	Aa. gastricae breves (branch off from the A. splenica in the area of the hilum of the spleen)
Posterior side	A. gastrica posterior (present in 30–60 % of cases, originates behind the stomach from the A. splenica)

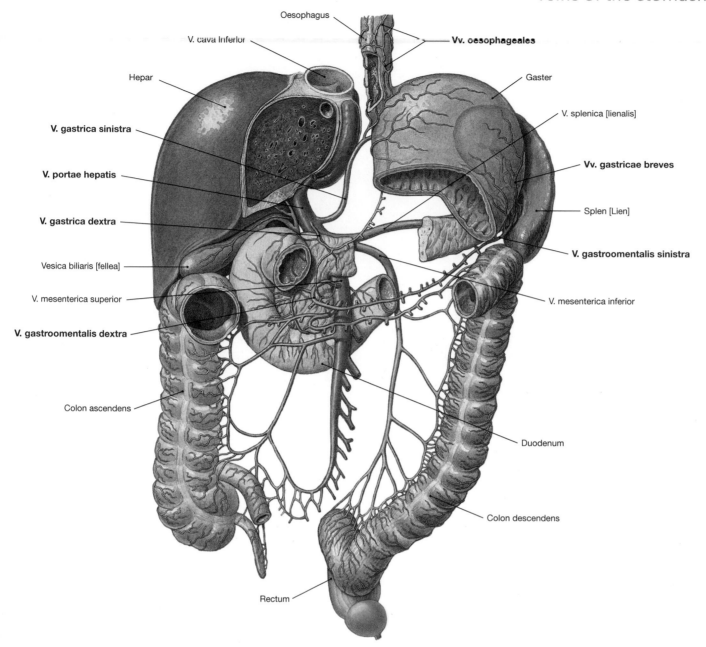

Oesophagus

V. cava inferior

Hepar

V. gastrica sinistra

V. portae hepatis

V. gastrica dextra

Vesica biliaris [fellea]

V. mesenterica superior

V. gastroomentalis dextra

Colon ascendens

Rectum

Vv. oesophageales

Gaster

V. splenica [lienalis]

Vv. gastricae breves

Splen [Lien]

V. gastroomentalis sinistra

V. mesenterica inferior

Duodenum

Colon descendens

Fig. 6.43   Veins of the stomach, Gaster, with reference to the portal vein, V. portae hepatis; ventral view. [S700]
The veins correspond to the arteries, but the veins at the lesser curvature enter directly into the portal vein, whereas the veins at the greater curvature drain into the larger branches of the portal vein. (→ table below).

Veins of the stomach	
Area of venous drainage	**Veins**
Lesser curvature	• V. gastrica sinistra • V. gastrica dextra Drainage into the V. portae hepatis: these veins anastomose via the Vv. oesophageales with the azygos system and thereby with the V. cava superior!
Greater curvature	• V. gastroomentalis sinistra (to V. splenica) • V. gastroomentalis dextra (to the V. mesenterica superior)
Fundus	Vv. gastricae breves (to V. splenica)
Posterior side	V. gastrica posterior (present in 30–60 %, to V. splenica)

Clinical remarks

Increased pressure in the portal vein (portal hypertension), e.g. in the case of cirrhosis of the liver, may lead to development of **portocaval anastomoses** via the Vv. oesophageales. These may become enlarged **(oesophageal varices)** and cause life-threatening internal bleeding if they rupture (→ Fig. 5.133).

Organs of the abdominal cavity

Stomach

Lymph vessels of the stomach

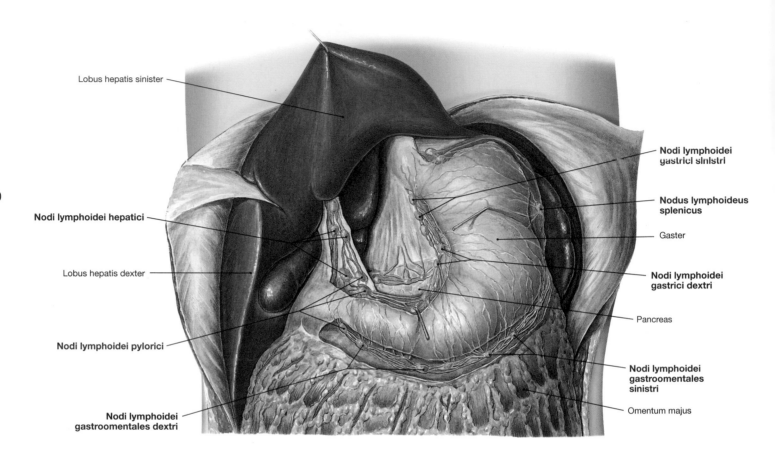

Lobus hepatis sinister

Nodi lymphoidei hepatici

Lobus hepatis dexter

Nodi lymphoidei pylorici

Nodi lymphoidei
gastroomentales dextri

Nodi lymphoidei
gastrici sinistri

Nodus lymphoideus
splenicus

Gaster

Nodi lymphoidei
gastrici dextri

Pancreas

Nodi lymphoidei
gastroomentales
sinistri

Omentum majus

**Fig. 6.44   Lymph vessels and lymph nodes of the stomach,
Gaster, and liver, Hepar;** ventral view. [S700]
The lymph vessels and lymph nodes of the stomach run alongside both
curvatures and the **pylorus:** the **Nodi lymphoidei gastrici** are located
on the lesser curvature, at the greater curvature the **Nodi lymphoidei**

splenici are located cranially and the **Nodi lymphoidei gastroomentales** caudally. The **Nodi lymphoidei pylorici** in the pyloric area are
connected to the Nodi lymphoidei hepatici of the hepatic porta.
There are three large lymphatic drainage areas with three distinct subsequent stations (→ Fig. 6.45).

Clinical remarks

The lymphatic drainage stations (→ Fig. 6.46) of the stomach are of
clinical relevance in the **surgical treatment of stomach cancer.** The
lymph nodes of the first and second stations are usually removed

along with the stomach. If lymph nodes of the third station are also
affected by metastatic cancer cells, curative therapy is not possible.
In this case the patient is spared the removal of the stomach.

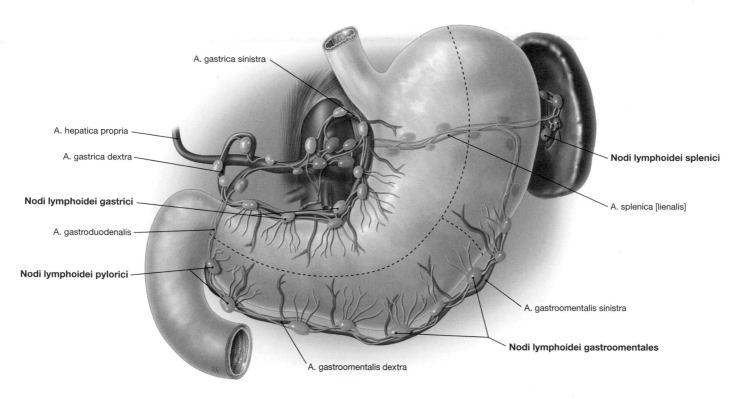

A. gastrica sinistra

A. hepatica propria

A. gastrica dextra

Nodi lymphoidei gastrici

A. gastroduodenalis

Nodi lymphoidei pylorici

Nodi lymphoidei splenici

A. splenica [lienalis]

A. gastroomentalis sinistra

Nodi lymphoidei gastroomentales

A. gastroomentalis dextra

Fig. 6.45 Drainage areas of the lymph and regional lymph nodes of the stomach, Gaster; ventral view. [S700-L238]/[B500]
There are **three large drainage pathways** of the lymph **(zones of lymphatic drainage),** shown here with dotted lines:

- **Cardiac area** and **lesser curvature:** Nodi lymphoidei gastrici
- **Upper left quadrant:** Nodi lymphoidei splenici
- **Lower two-thirds of the greater curvature and pylorus:** Nodi lymphoidei gastroomentales and Nodi lymphoidei pylorici.

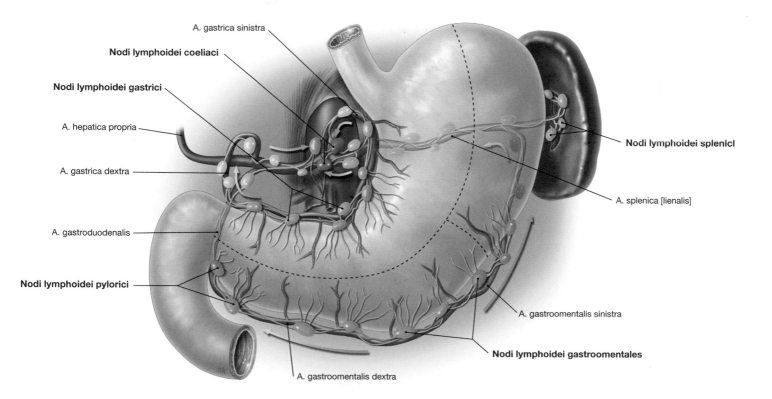

A. gastrica sinistra

Nodi lymphoidei coeliaci

Nodi lymphoidei gastrici

A. hepatica propria

A. gastrica dextra

A. gastroduodenalis

Nodi lymphoidei pylorici

Nodi lymphoidei splenici

A. splenica [lienalis]

A. gastroomentalis sinistra

Nodi lymphoidei gastroomentales

A. gastroomentalis dextra

Fig. 6.46 Lymphatic drainage stations of the stomach, Gaster; ventral view. [S700-L238]
In the three major drainage areas, there is a **series of three interconnected stations:**

- First station (green): lymph nodes along the curvatures (→ Fig. 6.45)
- Second station (yellow): lymph nodes along the branches of the Truncus coeliacus
- Third station (blue): lymph nodes at the opening of the Truncus coeliacus (Nodi lymphoidei coeliaci); from there, the lymph is collected via the Truncus intestinalis into the Ductus thoracicus.

6

Organs of the abdominal cavity

Autonomic innervation of the stomach

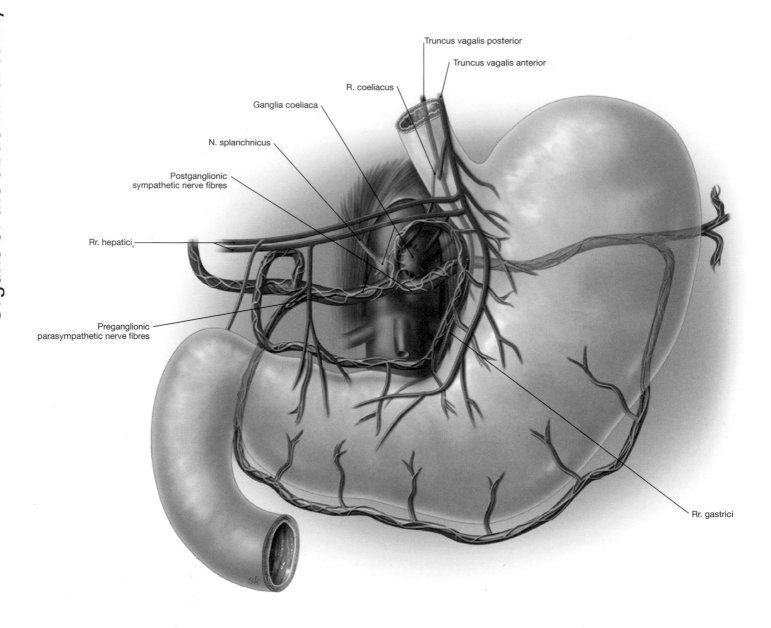

Truncus vagalis posterior

Truncus vagalis anterior

R. coeliacus

Ganglia coeliaca

N. splanchnicus

Postganglionic sympathetic nerve fibres

Rr. hepatici

Preganglionic parasympathetic nerve fibres

Rr. gastrici

Fig. 6.47 Autonomic innervation of the stomach, Gaster;
semi-schematic illustration. Sympathetic innervation (green), parasympathetic innervation (purple). [S700-L238]~[B500]
Preganglionic **parasympathetic fibres** (Rr. gastrici) reach the stomach as Trunci vagales anterior and posterior, descending along the oesophagus and running along the lesser curvature. As a result of the gastric rotation during development, the Truncus vagalis anterior is predominantly derived from the N. vagus [X] on the left, and the Truncus vagalis posterior from the N. vagus [X] on the right. The Pars pylorica is reached through its own branches (Rr. hepatici), which also derive from the va-

gal trunks. Postganglionic neurons are mostly in the stomach wall. The **parasympatheticus promotes** gastric acid production and the peristalsis of the stomach.
Preganglionic **sympathetic fibres** pass as Nn. splanchnici major and minor on both sides through the diaphragm and reach the Ganglia coeliaca at the opening of the Truncus coeliacus, where they are switched to postganglionic neurons. These reach the different sections of the stomach as periarterial nerve plexuses. The sympatheticus works in an antagonistic way to the parasympathicus by **curbing** the gastric acid secretion, peristalsis and circulation.

Clinical remarks

A former treatment for patients with peptic ulcers was to sever the entire N. vagus [X] below the diaphragm **(total vagotomy)** or its branches to the stomach **(selective vagotomy)** to reduce the production of gastric acid. However, since it has become possible to

block acid with medication and to stop the causally involved *Helicobacter pylori* bacteria with antibiotics, this procedure has become significantly less important.

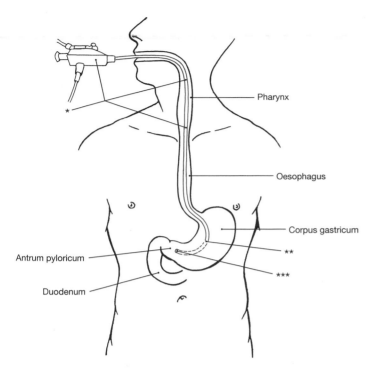

Pharynx

Oesophagus

Corpus gastricum

**

***

Antrum pyloricum

Duodenum

Fig. 6.48 Technique of the oesophagoscopy and gastroscopy.
[S700]

*   gastroscope
** gastroscope, tip in the Corpus gastricum (→ Fig. 6.49a)
*** gastroscope, tip in the Antrum pyloricum (→ Fig. 6.49b)

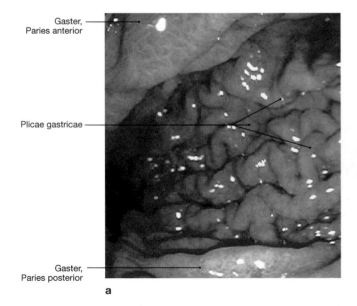

Gaster,
Paries anterior

Plicae gastricae

Gaster,
Paries posterior

a

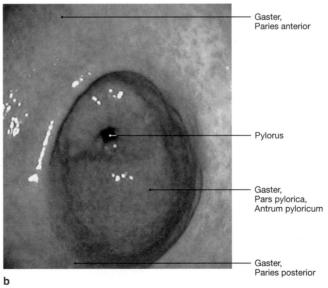

Gaster,
Paries anterior

Pylorus

Gaster,
Pars pylorica,
Antrum pyloricum

Gaster,
Paries posterior

b

Fig. 6.49a and b Stomach, Gaster; gastroscopy; view from cranial.
[S700-T901]

a View from the Corpus gastricum with pronounced longitudinal folds of the mucosa (Plicae gastricae).
b View from the Antrum pyloricum with a largely smooth mucosa.

Clinical remarks

Gastroscopy enables the **inspection** of the stomach lining. Pathological findings, such as erosive gastric lesions or ulcers (→ Fig. 6.40) require tissue **biopsies** for further pathological diagnostics to distinguish between a benign peptic ulcer and a gastric carcinoma.

Organs of the digestive system

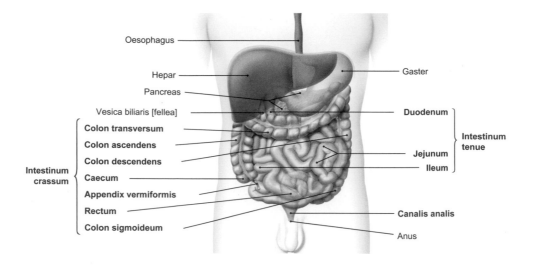

Fig. 6.50 Organs of the digestive system; ventral view. [S700-L275]
The digestive system is made up of organs forming a unit, all of which
serve the digestion and regulate each other for this purpose. The exact
understanding of this regulation process is only possible after the additional study of microscopic anatomy, since individual organs create hormones and chemical messengers, which partly make it possible for the
organs to communicate and coordinate with each other via the blood.
The apparent autonomy suggested by the macroscopic demarcation of
the individual organs is therefore conditional.

The digestive system includes the oral cavity, the **hollow organs,**
which are connected to it, and reaches up to the Canalis analis:
● pharynx
● oesophagus
● stomach (Gaster)
● small intestine (Intestinum tenue)
● large intestine (Intestinum crassum).
Also included in the digestive system are the **accessory glands** of the
gastrointestinal tract:
● liver (Hepar)
● gallbladder (Vesica biliaris)
● pancreas.

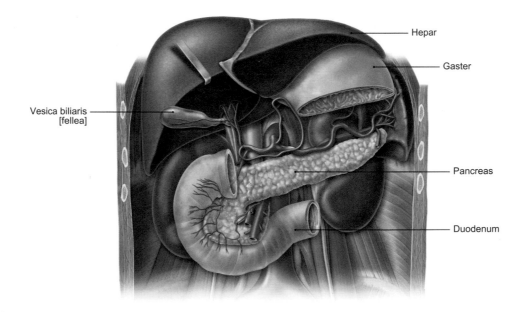

Fig. 6.51 Organs of the epigastrium, semi-schematic illustration;
ventral view. [S700-L238]
The stomach, small intestine, liver, gallbladder and pancreas very mark-
edly communicate with each other in the digestive process. This recip-
rocal regulation largely occurs via hormones and chemical messengers,
and complements the control of the central nervous system by parasympathetic nerves, which also promote digestion. The **parasympathetic system** is already activated by the sight, smell and taste of food
and often by the sheer thought of food. Filling of the **stomach** stimulates the formation of gastric acid. When the acidified stomach contents with their nutrients are passed into the first section of the **small**

intestine (duodenum), this stimulates the release of hormones from
the intestinal mucosa. This induces the delivery of bile from the **gallbladder** and the secretion of digestive juice from the **pancreas.**
Through the ductal systems, bile and pancreatic juice are directly added
to the food bolus in the duodenum and facilitate the digestion and absorption of nutrients. The nutrients are transported to the liver via the
portal vein, as well as the lymph vessel system and the blood. The liver
finally produces chemical messengers that generate a feeling of satiety
in the brain. Hormones are also produced by the intestinal mucosa and
stimulate the afferent nerve fibres of the N. vagus [X]. Coupled with the
gastric stretch receptors, this leads to the cessation of food intake.

Organs of the abdominal cavity

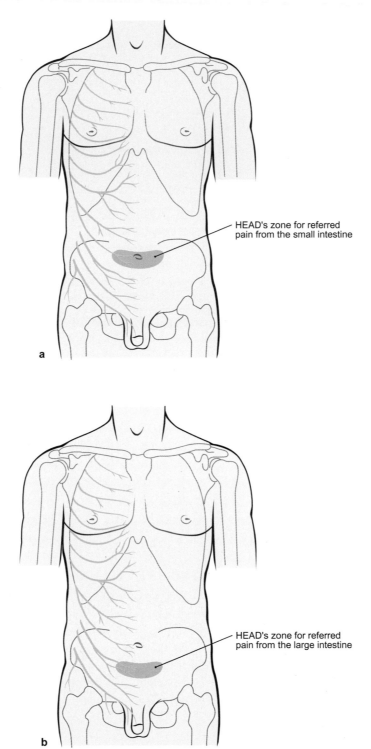

HEAD's zone for referred
pain from the small intestine

HEAD's zone for referred
pain from the large intestine

a

b

Fig. 6.52a and b   Referred pain areas (HEAD's zones) of the small and large intestines, schematic representation; ventral view. [S700-L126]/[G1071]

a HEAD's zone of the small intestine in dermatome T10.
b HEAD's zone of the small intestine in dermatome T11.

The body surface is innervated segmentally by afferent neurons from individual spinal cord segments. These areas are known as cutaneous areas or **dermatomes.** In the spinal cord segments, the afferent neurons of the surface of the body converge with those of the internal or-

gans, so that irritation of the organs often leads to discomfort (paraesthesia) and pain which are perceived on the surface of the body in the corresponding dermatomes. We call this projected or referred pain. These organ-related cutaneous areas are the **HEAD's zones.** The referred pain areas of the small and large intestines should only be understood as maximal points and they often overlap, which makes it impossible to make precise distinctions between the individual intestinal sections.

Organs of the abdominal cavity

Structure of the small intestine and projection of the duodenum

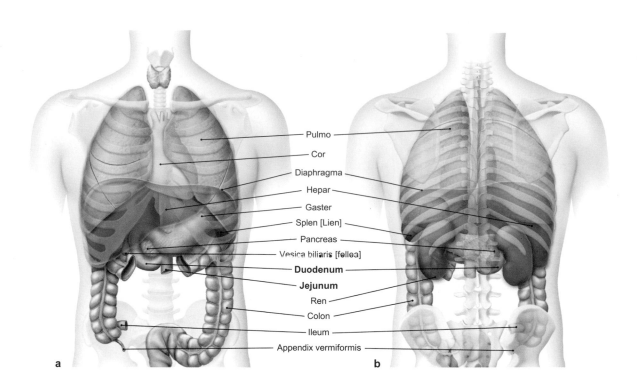

Pulmo
Cor
Diaphragma
Hepar
Gaster
Splen [Lien]
Pancreas
Vesica biliaris [fellea]
Duodenum
Jejunum
Ren
Colon
Ileum
Appendix vermiformis

a   b

Fig. 6.53a and b   Projection of the duodenum onto the body surface. Jejunum and ileum have been completely removed. [S700-L275]
a Ventral view.
b Dorsal view.

The small intestine is usually 3 m in length (4–6 m) and has three parts:
- **duodenum:** 25–30 cm
- **jejunum:** two-fifths of the total length
- **ileum:** three-fifths of the total length.

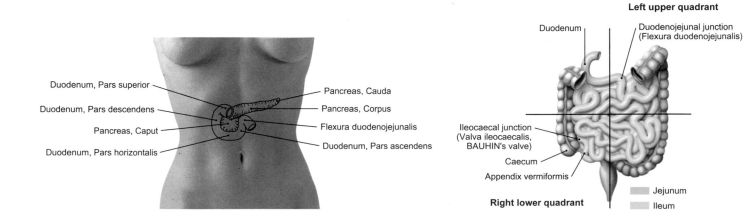

Duodenum, Pars superior
Duodenum, Pars descendens
Pancreas, Caput
Duodenum, Pars horizontalis

Pancreas, Cauda
Pancreas, Corpus
Flexura duodenojejunalis
Duodenum, Pars ascendens

Duodenum

Left upper quadrant
Duodenojejunal junction
(Flexura duodenojejunalis)

Ileocaecal junction
(Valva ileocaecalis,
BAUHIN's valve)
Caecum
Appendix vermiformis

Right lower quadrant

Jejunum
Ileum

Fig. 6.54   Projection of the duodenum and pancreas onto the ventral trunk wall. [S700]
The **intraperitoneal Pars superior** of the duodenum projects onto the level of the first lumbar vertebra. All **other parts** are located **secondarily retroperitoneally** and encompass the head of the pancreas in a C-shaped manner. The head of the pancreas is adjacent to the Pars descendens of the duodenum. The Pars horizontalis runs diagonally at the level of the third lumbar vertebra and continues in the Pars ascendens up to the Flexura duodenojejunalis at the level of the second lumbar vertebra. This flexure marks the transition to the intraperitoneal jejunum.

Fig. 6.55   Projection of jejunum and ileum in the abdominal cavity; ventral view. The Colon transversum has been removed extensively. [S701-L275]
The **duodenum** begins at the pylorus of the stomach and extends to the **Flexura duodenojejunalis**. The Pars superior typically projects onto the first lumbar vertebra and the **Flexura duodenojejunalis** onto the second lumbar vertebra.
In contrast, the **intraperitoneal convolute of the jejunum and ileum** are not easily subdivided macroscopically and reach distally to the Valva ileocaecalis (BAUHIN's valve) at the transition to the colon. Intestinal loops of the jejunum are mostly located in the epigastrium and those of the ileum in the hypogastrium.

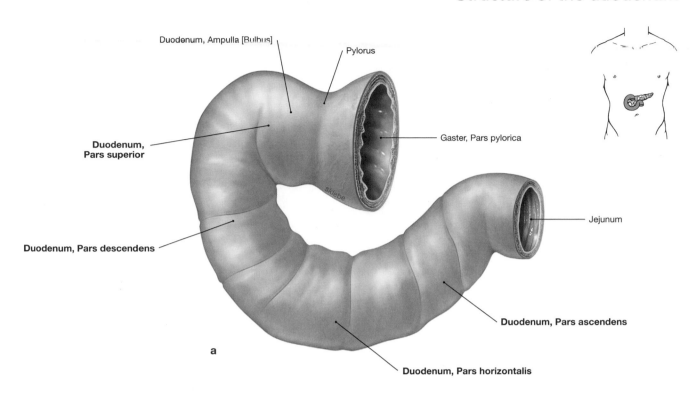

Duodenum, Ampulla [Bulbus]

Pylorus

Duodenum,
Pars superior

Gaster, Pars pylorica

Duodenum, Pars descendens

Jejunum

Duodenum, Pars ascendens

a

Duodenum, Pars horizontalis

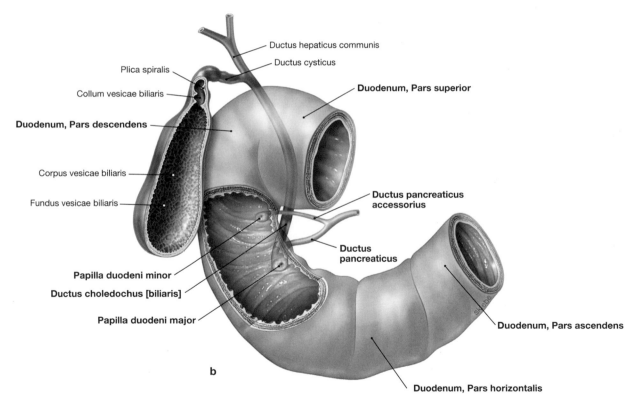

Ductus hepaticus communis

Ductus cysticus

Plica spiralis

Collum vesicae biliaris

Duodenum, Pars superior

Duodenum, Pars descendens

Corpus vesicae biliaris

Ductus pancreaticus
accessorius

Fundus vesicae biliaris

Ductus
pancreaticus

Papilla duodeni minor

Ductus choledochus [biliaris]

Papilla duodeni major

Duodenum, Pars ascendens

b

Duodenum, Pars horizontalis

Fig. 6.56a and b   Parts of the duodenum, ventral view.
a   Display in isolation. [S700-L238]
b   Display together with the extrahepatic bile ducts. [S700-L238]/
[G1060-002]
The duodenum is divided into **four parts:**
* Pars superior
* Pars descendens
* Pars horizontalis
* Pars ascendens.
The **Pars superior** is the only intraperitoneal part and its wide proximal
lumen is referred to as the duodenal ampulla (Bulbus duodeni).

The excretory duct of the pancreas (Ductus pancreaticus, duct of WIR-
SUNG) enters the **Pars descendens** of the duodenum, usually along
with the common bile duct (Ductus choledochus) on a mucosal papilla
(Papilla duodeni major, Papilla VATERI) which is found 8–10 cm distal to
the pylorus. Usually, 2 cm proximal to the latter, a Papilla duodeni minor
is found, into which the Ductus pancreaticus accessorius (SANTORINI's
duct) empties its secretion.
The **Pars horizontalis** crosses the spine, and then crosses over into
the **Pars ascendens.**

Structure of the wall of the small intestine

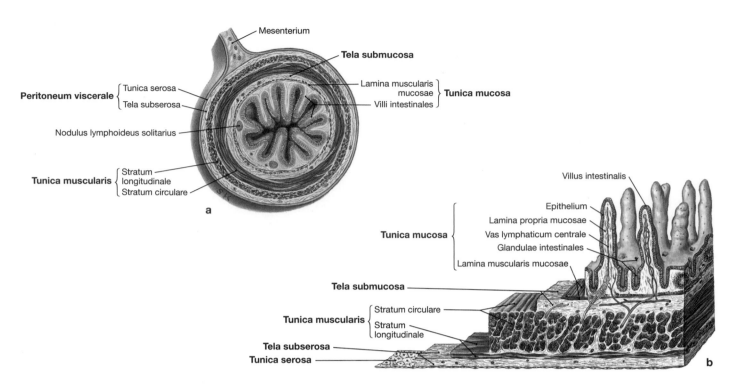

Fig. 6.57a and b   Structure of the wall of the small intestine, Intestinum tenue; cross-section. [S700-L238]
a Cross-section.
b Microscopic view.
Similar to other parts of the intestines, the wall of the small intestine consists of an inner mucosal layer **(Tunica mucosa)** with intestinal villi (Villi intestinales), which become visible with magnification. Separated by a loose connective tissue layer **(Tela submucosa),** the muscular lay-

er **(Tunica muscularis)** follows, consisting of an internal circular muscle layer (Stratum circulare) and an external longitudinal muscle layer (Stratum longitudinale). The intraperitoneal parts (Pars superior of the duodenum, jejunum and ileum) are covered on the outside by visceral peritoneum (Peritoneum viscerale), which forms a **Tunica serosa.** In contrast, the retroperitoneal parts of the duodenum are anchored by the **Tunica adventitia** in the connective tissue of the retroperitoneal space.

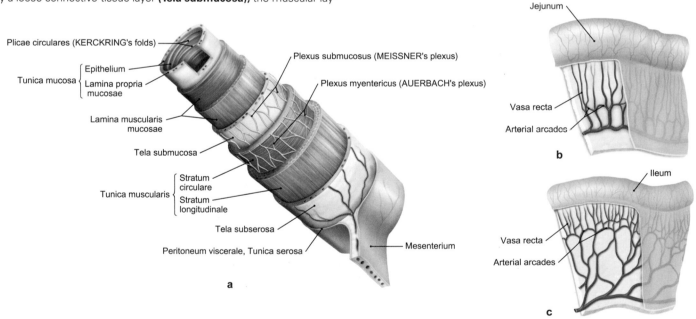

Fig. 6.58a–c   Structure of the wall of the small intestine, Intestinum tenue; with arterial supply, schematic illustration. [S701-L275]
a Layers of the intestinal wall with mesentery.
b Arterial arcades of the jejunum.
c Arterial arcades of the ileum.

The arteries to the jejunum and ileum branch out from the A. mesenterica superior, travel within the mesenteries to the intestines and branch out within the Tela subserosa (or subserosa) **(a)**. Arterial arcades of the jejunum **(b)** have a larger diameter and are therefore stronger, with bigger vascular arches, compared to the ileum **(c)**. The straight terminal arteries (Vasa recta) are also longer in the jejunum.

Clinical remarks

The straight arteries distal of the arcades do not communicate with each other and are therefore terminal arteries. Thus, the occlusion of these terminal arteries through an **embolus,** a torsion **(volvolus)** and an internal or external **hernia** results in ischaemia and potentially necrosis of the intestinal wall.

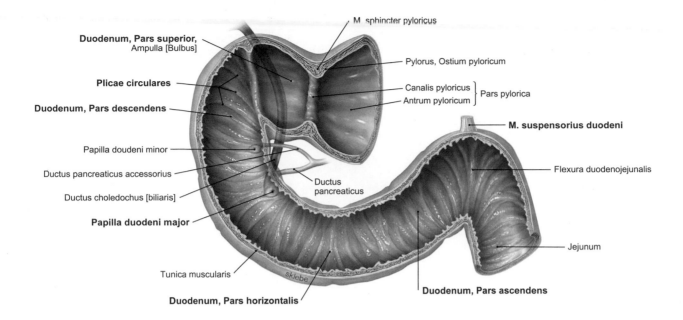

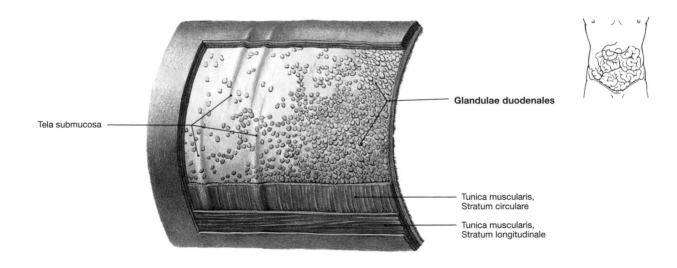

Fig. 6.59 Inner surface of the duodenum; frontal section; ventral view. [S700-L238]

The inner surface of the duodenum, as well as of the remaining small intestine is raised with **circular folds (Plicae circulares, KERCKRING's valves).** The duodenum is divided into four parts: 1. Pars superior, 2. Pars descendens, 3. Pars horizontalis, 4. Pars ascendens. In the Pars descendens is the **Papilla duodeni major (Papilla VATERI)** as a conflu-

ence of the Ductus pancreaticus (duct of WIRSUNG) and Ductus choledochus, which together usually form the Ampulla hepatopancreatica. The Pars ascendens is attached with smooth muscle **(M. suspensorius duodeni, muscle of TREITZ)** and dense **connective tissue (Lig. suspensorium duodeni)** at the point where the A. mesenterica superior leaves the aorta, before the duodenum in the Flexura duodenojejunalis passes over into the intraperitoneal jejunum.

Fig. 6.60 Structure of the wall of the duodenum with Glandulae duodenales; view from outside. [S700]

The mucous-producing Glandulae duodenales (BRUNNER's glands) lie in the Tela submucosa. These allow a clear identification of the duodenum (with a microscope!).

Clinical remarks

The muscle of TREITZ defines the boundary between **upper and lower gastrointestinal bleeding (GI-bleeding).** The suspension of the Pars ascendens of the duodenum near the A. mesenterica superior and distal of the Flexura duodenojejunalis prevents the reflux of intestinal content as well as blood. This demarcation is of clinical relevance since the origin of intestinal haemorrhage has different causes and requires different diagnostic steps. With an **upper GI**

bleed the blood is usually discoloured and very dark due to contact with gastric acid. Therefore, in this case, gastroduodenal imaging (gastroduodenoscopy) would be used for clarification. With **lower GI bleeding** on the other hand, the blood is light red. If the subsequent colonoscopy provides no clue to the source of the bleeding, an endoscopy of the entire intestine can be performed by swallowing a tablet-sized video capsule.

Intestines

Duodenum, imaging

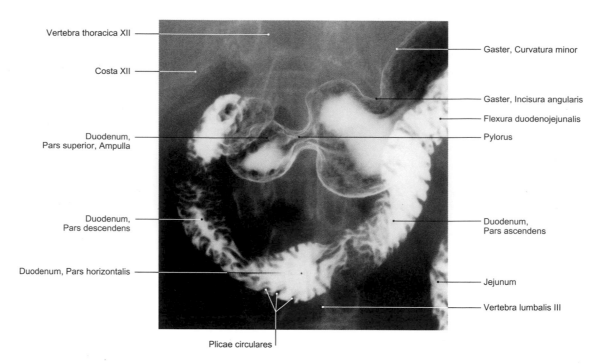

Vertebra thoracica XII

Costa XII

Duodenum,
Pars superior, Ampulla

Duodenum,
Pars descendens

Duodenum, Pars horizontalis

Plicae circulares

Gaster, Curvatura minor

Gaster, Incisura angularis

Flexura duodenojejunalis

Pylorus

Duodenum,
Pars ascendens

Jejunum

Vertebra lumbalis III

Fig. 6.61 Duodenum; X-ray with an anteroposterior (AP) projection after oral application of a contrast agent; patient in upright position; ventral view. [S700-T893]

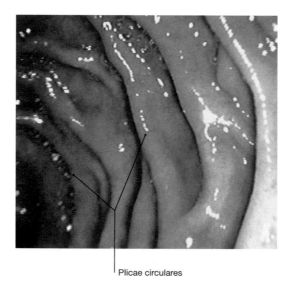

Plicae circulares

Fig. 6.62 Duodenum; endoscopic image. [S700-T901]
Here the circular **mucosal folds (Plicae circulares, KERCKRING's valves)** are clearly visible.

Clinical remarks

Like the stomach, the duodenum is often the location for ulcers **(Ulcera duodeni),** which are clinically not easily differentiated from gastric ulcers (→ Fig. 6.40). Malignant tumours, however, are rare in the duodenum.

For the evaluation of these diseases, there are various diagnostic options. **X-ray contrast imaging** has become less relevant in recent years, as it is inferior to an **upper endoscopy** (duodenoscopy), which includes inspecting the mucous membrane as well as allowing a biopsy to be taken.

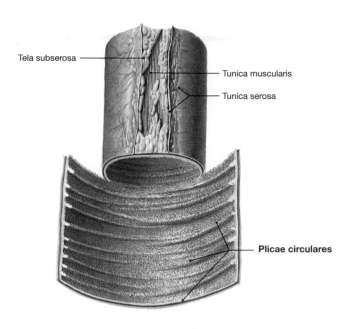

Tela subserosa

Tunica muscularis

Tunica serosa

Plicae circulares

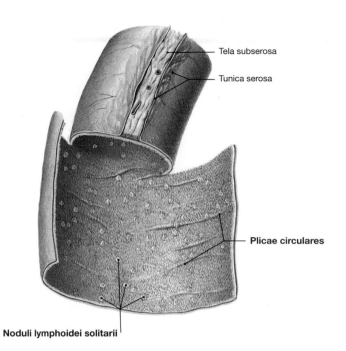

Tela subserosa

Tunica serosa

Plicae circulares

Noduli lymphoidei solitarii

Fig. 6.63 Section of the jejunum. [S700]
The structure of the jejunum is very similar to the duodenum but does not contain the **Glandulae duodenales (BRUNNER's glands).**

Fig. 6.64 Section of the proximal ileum. [S700]
There are far fewer **circular folds (Plicae circulares, KERCKRING's valves)** in the ileum compared to the upper small intestine.

Noduli lymphoidei aggregati

Plicae circulares

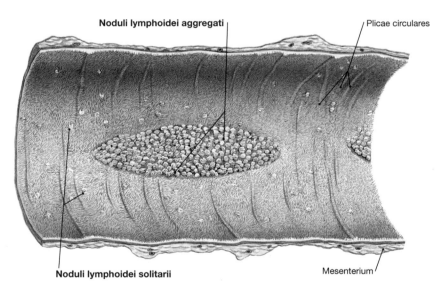

Noduli lymphoidei solitarii

Mesenterium

Fig. 6.65 Section of the ileum. [S700]
The large number of lymph follicles that serve the immune system is characteristic. These are either found individually in the Tela submucosa (Noduli lymphoidei solitarii; → Fig. 6.64) or in groups (Noduli lymphoidei aggregati, **PEYER's patches),** formed within the mucosa.

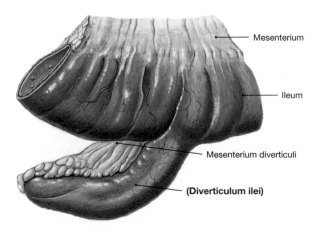

Mesenterium

Ileum

Mesenterium diverticuli

(Diverticulum ilei)

Fig. 6.66 MECKEL's diverticulum, Diverticulum ilei. [S700]
In up to 3 % of people, one can find a diverticulum, mostly in the 100 cm long ileocaecal valve located opposite the mesenteric root; this is the developmental remnant of the embryological Ductus vitellinus (Ductus omphaloentericus; → Fig. 6.4).
MECKEL's diverticula can contain disseminated gastric mucosa and can simulate the clinical symptoms of appendicitis when inflamed and bleeding.

Organs of the abdominal cavity

Projection of the large intestine

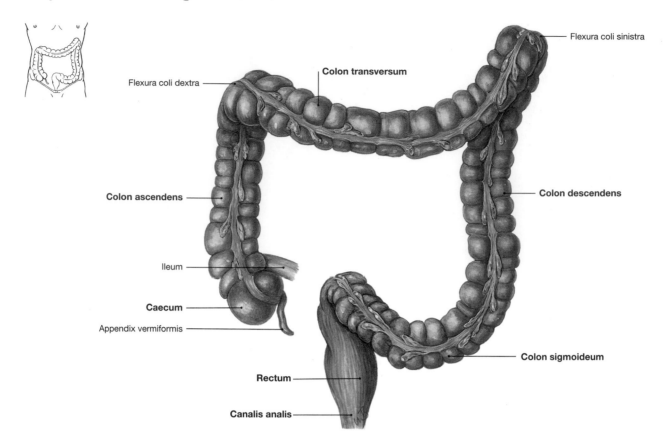

Fig. 6.67   Structure of the large intestine, Intestinum crassum; ventral view. [S700]

The Intestinum crassum is about 1–1.5 m long and consists of **four parts:**

- caecum with Appendix vermiformis
- colon with Colon ascendens, Colon transversum, Colon descendens, and Colon sigmoideum
- rectum
- Canalis analis (anal canal).

The Canalis analis is dealt with as part of the pelvic organs (→ Chapter 7).

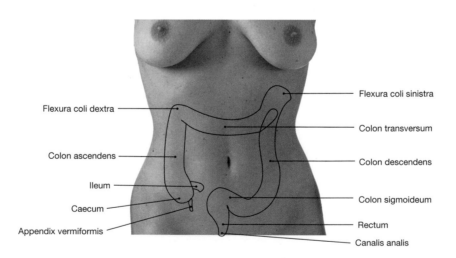

Fig. 6.68   Projection of the large intestine, Intestinum crassum, onto the ventral trunk wall. [S700]

The **caecum with the Appendix vermiformis, Colon transversum, and Colon sigmoideum** are positioned **intraperitoneally,** and each has its own respective mesentery. The caecum and the Appendix vermiformis can also lie retroperitoneally (Caecum fixum) when a mesentery is missing. The **Colon ascendens, Colon descendens** and most of the **rectum** are usually secondary **retroperitoneal organs,** and the distal rectum and the **Canalis analis** are **subperitoneal.** The projection and the length of the individual segments of the Intestinum crassum are highly variable and the retroperitoneal segments are often inconsistently fused with the posterior trunk wall. Due to the position of the liver on the right side, the splenic or left colonic flexure (Flexura coli sinistra) is generally positioned further cranially than the hepatic or right colonic flexure (Flexura coli dextra; → Fig. 6.85).

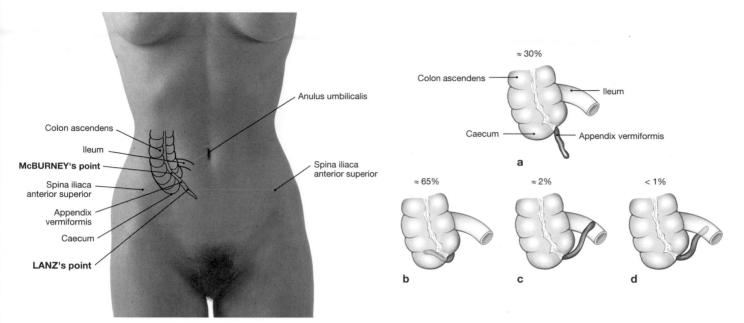

Fig. 6.69 Projection of the caecum and the appendix, Appendix vermiformis, onto the ventral trunk wall. [S700]
The base of the Appendix vermiformis projects onto the **McBURNEY's point** (the transition between the lateral third and the medial two-thirds on a line connecting the umbilicus with the Spina iliaca anterior superior). The tip of the pendulous appendix projects onto the **LANZ's point** (marked on the line connecting both of the two Spinae iliacae anteriores superiores, one third of the distance from the right spine); 30 %; → Fig. 6.70 and → Fig. 6.71).

Fig. 6.70a–d Positional variants of the Appendix vermiformis; ventral view. [S700-L126]
a Descending into the lesser pelvis (pendulous).
b Retrocaecal (most frequently!).
c Praeileal.
d Retroileal.

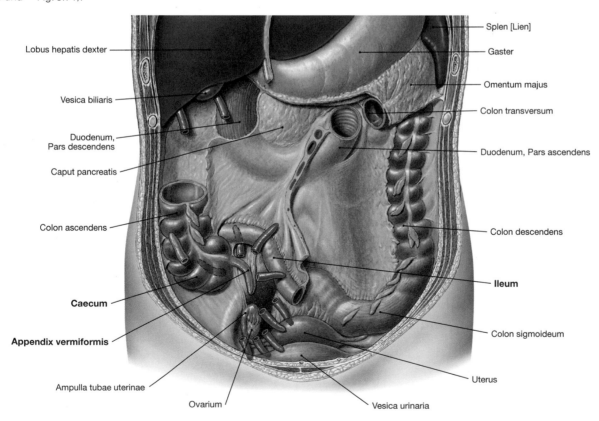

Fig. 6.71 Positional variants of the Appendix vermiformis; ventral view. [S700]

Clinical remarks

It is often difficult to diagnose **appendicitis,** as pain in the right hypogastrium can be a result of enteritis, or can be caused in women by inflammation of the ovaries and FALLOPIAN tubes. Tenderness upon manual pressure at McBURNEY's point or the LANZ's point can therefore be an important diagnostic sign.

Intestines

Structure of the large intestine

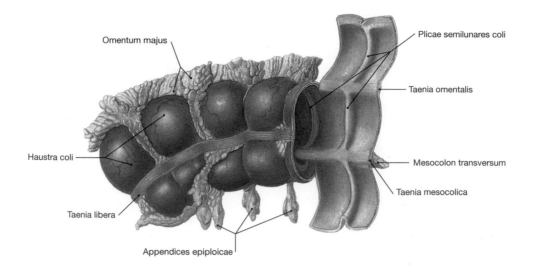

Fig. 6.72 **Structural features of the large intestine, Intestinum crassum, with the Colon transversum as an example;** ventral caudal view. [S700]

The large intestine of the colon has four characteristic differences to the small intestine:

- **Larger diameter** (it is 'thick', while the small intestine is 'thin'): however, the diameter is highly variable – from 2.5 cm in the Colon sigmoideum up to 7.5 cm in the caecum.
- **Taenia:** the longitudinal muscle layer is reduced to three bands. Of these the Taenia libera is visible, while the Mesocolon transversum

is attached to the Taenia mesocolica and the Omentum majus is attached to the Taenia omentalis.

- **Haustra** and **Plicae semilunares:** the haustra of the colon (Haustra coli) are pouches caused by the sacculations on the inside, which look like halfmoon-shaped folds (Plicae semilunares).
- **Appendices epiploicae:** tags caused by the adipose tissue contained in the Tela subserosa.

These structural features apply to all parts of the Intestinum crassum apart from the Appendix vermiformis, rectum and Canalis analis. These sections have no taenia, haustra and omental appendices.

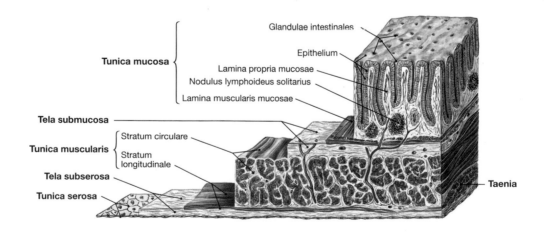

Fig. 6.73 **Structure of the wall of the large intestine, Intestinum crassum;** microscopic view. [S700]

Similar to the other parts of the intestines, the wall of the Intestinum crassum consists of an inner mucosal layer **(Tunica mucosa)** which, in contrast to the duodenum, has no mucosal villi. Separated by a loose connective tissue layer **(Tela submucosa),** the muscular layer **(Tunica muscularis)** is divided into an internal circular muscle layer **(Stratum circulare)** and an external longitudinal muscle layer **(Stratum longitu-**

dinale). However, the longitudinal layer is not continuous but is reduced to three bands **(taeniae).** The intraperitoneal segments (caecum with appendix, Colon transversum, and Colon sigmoideum) are covered on the outside by visceral peritoneum (Peritoneum viscerale), forming a **Tunica serosa.** In contrast, the retroperitoneal parts (Colon ascendens, Colon descendens, and upper rectum) are anchored by the **Tunica adventitia** in the connective tissue of the retroperitoneal space.

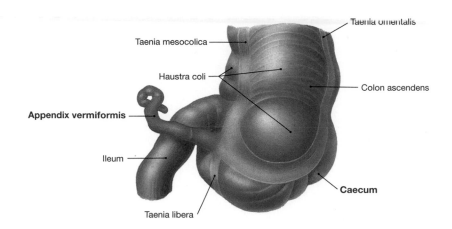

Taenia omentalis
Taenia mesocolica
Haustra coli
Colon ascendens
Appendix vermiformis
Ileum
Caecum
Taenia libera

Fig. 6.74 Caecum with Appendix vermiformis and terminal ileum, Pars terminalis ilei; dorsal view. [S700]
The **caecum** is approximately 7 cm long. The 8–9 cm long Appendix vermiformis is attached to the caecum and usually has its own mesoap-pendix (not shown here), with the supplying neurovascular pathways. The diameter of the appendix is 0.5 cm. The taenia of the colon converge at the appendix to form a continuous longitudinal muscle layer.

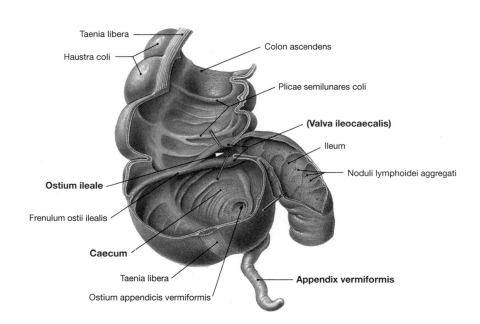

Taenia libera
Haustra coli
Colon ascendens
Plicae semilunares coli
(Valva ileocaecalis)
Ileum
Noduli lymphoidei aggregati
Ostium ileale
Frenulum ostii ilealis
Caecum
Taenia libera
Appendix vermiformis
Ostium appendicis vermiformis

Fig. 6.75 Caecum with Appendix vermiformis and terminal ileum, Pars terminalis ilei; ventral view; after removal of the anterior parts of the wall. [S700]
The caecum joins the terminal ileum and is separated by the **ileocaecal valve** (BAUHIN's valve). Inside, the two lips of the valve are raised by Papilae ileales and together they border the opening (ileal orifice). Later-ally, the lips continue into the Frenulum ostii ilealis. The terminal ileum contains aggregations of lymph follicles (Noduli lymphoidei aggregati) which are referred to as **PEYER's patches** and serve the immune system. The appendix also contains many lymph follicles and serves the immune system.

Clinical remarks

Appendicitis is a common disease in the second and third decades of life. It is an inflammation, mostly caused by the obstruction of the lumen of the appendix by faeces, or (rarely) by other foreign bodies with a resulting transmural inflammation due to intestinal microorganisms. This can result in perforation with a life-threatening perito-nitis. Apart from its role in the absorption of vitamin B_{12} and bile acids, the terminal ileum is particularly important due to its immunological functions. It is often affected by **CROHN's disease,** a chronic bowel disease with an autoimmune component, which can also lead to anaemia due to a vitamin B_{12} deficiency.

Intestines

Topography of the small and large intestines

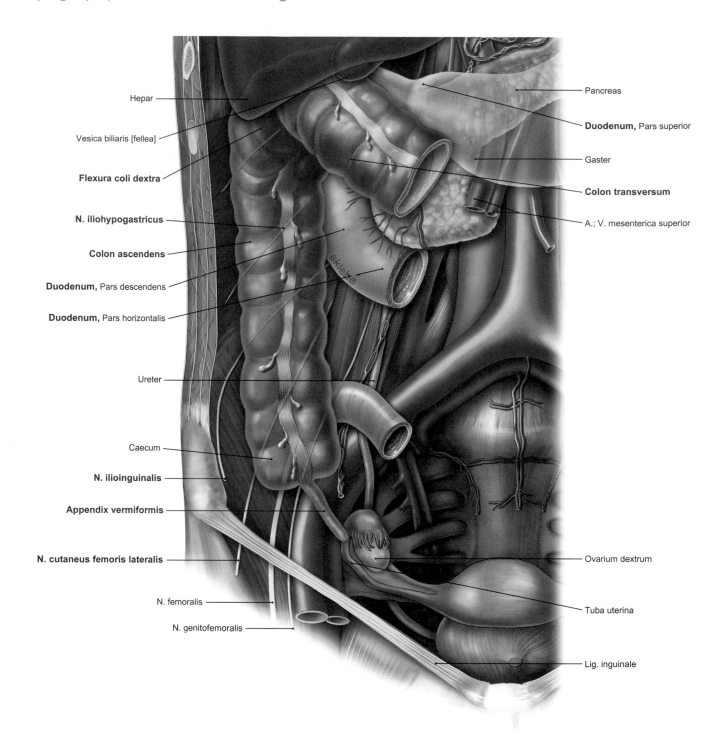

Hepar

Vesica biliaris [fellea]

Flexura coli dextra

N. iliohypogastricus

Colon ascendens

Duodenum, Pars descendens

Duodenum, Pars horizontalis

Ureter

Caecum

N. ilioinguinalis

Appendix vermiformis

N. cutaneus femoris lateralis

N. femoralis

N. genitofemoralis

Pancreas

Duodenum, Pars superior

Gaster

Colon transversum

A.; V. mesenterica superior

Ovarium dextrum

Tuba uterina

Lig. inguinale

Fig. 6.76 Topography of the duodenum and the 'right-sided' parts of the colon (caecum with Appendix vermiformis, Colon ascendens and transversum); semi-schematic representation; after removal of the small intestine, ventral view. [S700-L238]
Topography of the parts of the small intestine:
The **Pars superior** of the duodenum is located behind the gallbladder and has direct contact with the visceral surface of the liver. The **Pars descendens** is directly adjacent to the right kidney and adrenal glands, but it is separated by the capsules enveloping the kidneys. The head of the pancreas nestles medially on the Pars descendens. The **Pars horizontalis** crosses the spine below the head of the pancreas. It also crosses over the Aorta abdominalis and the V. cava inferior as well as the right Vasa testicularia/ovarica and the right ureter. The **Pars ascendens** ascends to the Flexura duodenojejunalis and thereby covers the

left kidney with the left ureter and the left Vasa testicularia/ovarica (not shown).
Topography of the 'right-sided' parts of the large intestine:
The **caecum and Appendix vermiformis** are positioned ventrally to the M. psoas major and thus cover different nerves of the Plexus lumbalis and the right Vasa testicularia/ovarica. In the pelvic position illustrated here, the appendix can come in close proximity to the right ovary and FALLOPIAN tube (Tuba uterina). The **Colon ascendens** then ascends to the right colonic flexure and crosses the N. cutaneus femoris lateralis as well as the N. ilioinguinalis and the N. iliohypogastricus. The right **colonic flexure (Flexura coli dextra)** touches the inferior surface of the liver and is therefore referred to as the 'hepatic' flexure; it comes into contact with the fundus of the gallbladder and is located ventral to the right kidney and lateral to the Pars descendens of the duodenum.

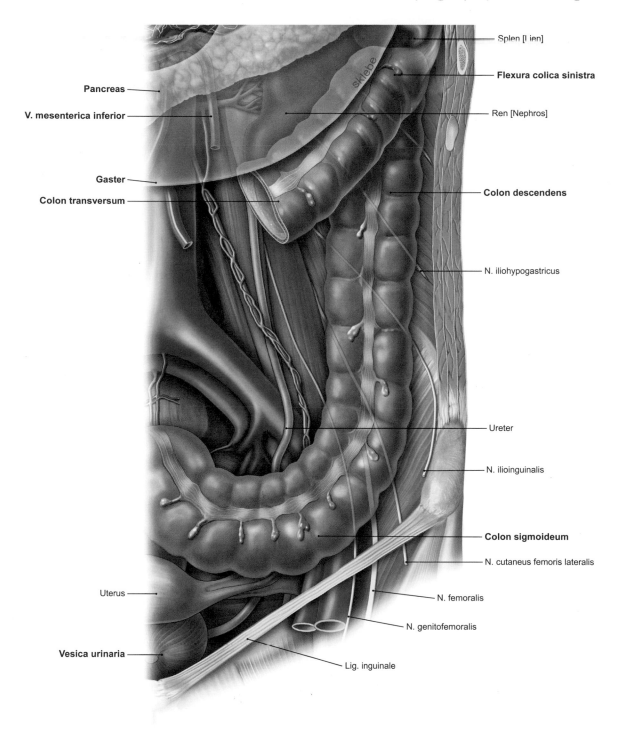

Pancreas

V. mesenterica inferior

Gaster

Colon transversum

Uterus

Vesica urinaria

Splen [Lien]

Flexura colica sinistra

Ren [Nephros]

Colon descendens

N. iliohypogastricus

Ureter

N. ilioinguinalis

Colon sigmoideum

N. cutaneus femoris lateralis

N. femoralis

N. genitofemoralis

Lig. inguinale

Fig. 6.77 Topography of the 'left-sided' parts of the large intestine (Colon descendens and Colon sigmoideum) semi-schematic representation; after removal of most of the small intestine, ventral view. [S700-L238]

The **Colon transversum** passes caudal to the stomach to the left colonic flexure. It is positioned ventral of the Pars descendens of the duodenum and the head of the pancreas, ventral to the small intestinal loops of the jejunum and ileum and ventral to the Flexura duodenojejunalis. The **left colonic flexure (Flexura coli sinistra)** touches the vis-

ceral surface of the spleen and is therefore also called the 'splenic flexure'. Dorsal from these are the left kidney and the tail of the pancreas (Cauda pancreatis). The **Colon descendens** descends ventrally of the left kidney and crosses the nerves of the left Plexus lumbalis. The **Colon sigmoideum** turns to the right and crosses the nerves of the lumbar plexus, the left ureter and the Vasa testicularia/ovarica as well as the Vasa iliaca externa and interna. In the pelvis it touches the surface of the urinary bladder (Vesica urinaria) and, in women, it touches the uterus with its appendages (ovaries and FALLOPIAN tubes).

Organs of the abdominal cavity

Arteries of the small intestine

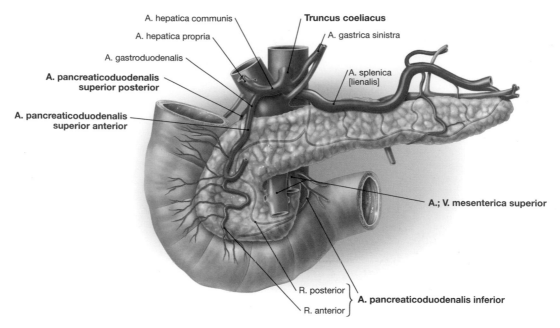

Fig. 6.78 **Arteries of the duodenum;** ventral view. [S700-L238]
The blood supply of the duodenum is accomplished ventrally and dorsally through a double arterial arch. This is fed cranially by the **Aa. pancreaticoduodenales superiores anterior and posterior**, supplied

from the Truncus coeliacus, and caudally by the **A. pancreaticoduodenalis inferior** (R. anterior and R. posterior) from the A. mesenterica superior. The connection between the cranial and caudal arcades is referred to as **BÜHLER's anastomotic artery**.

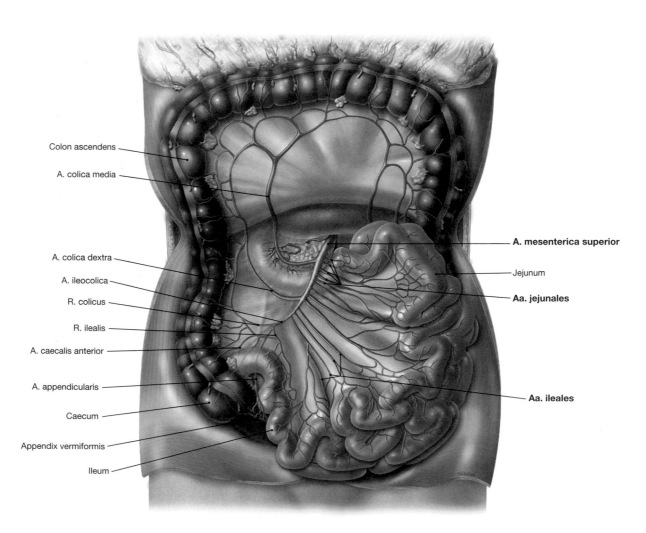

Fig. 6.79 **Arteries of the jejunum and ileum;** ventral view; Colon transversum folded back. [S700-L238]
The intraperitoneal convolute of the jejunum and ileum is supplied by the A. mesenterica superior, of which the branches (usually four to five)

Aa. jejunales and 12 **Aa. ileales** are distributed within the mesentery of the small intestine (→ Fig. 6.27).

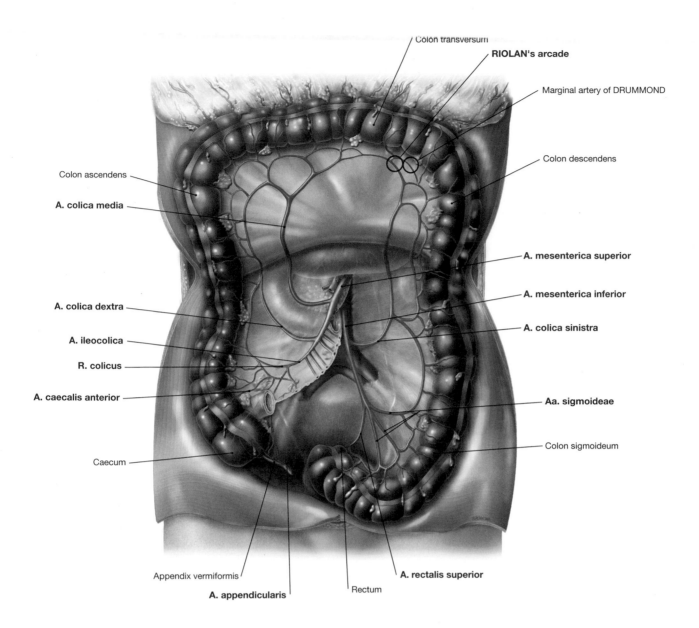

Colon transversum
RIOLAN's arcade
Marginal artery of DRUMMOND
Colon descendens
Colon ascendens
A. colica media
A. mesenterica superior
A. mesenterica inferior
A. colica dextra
A. colica sinistra
A. ileocolica
R. colicus
A. caecalis anterior
Aa. sigmoideae
Colon sigmoideum
Caecum
Appendix vermiformis
A. appendicularis
Rectum
A. rectalis superior

Fig. 6.80 Arteries of the large intestine, Intestinum crassum; ventral view; Colon transversum folded back. [S700-L238]/[G1069]

- **Caecum and Appendix vermiformis: A. ileocolica** with a R. ilealis to the terminal ileum (anastomoses with the last A. ilealis) and a R. colicus (connected with the A. colica dextra). Then the artery divides into an A. caecalis anterior and an A. caecalis posterior on both sides of the caecum and into the A. appendicularis, which runs inside the mesoappendix and supplies the Appendix vermiformis.
- **Colon ascendens and Colon transversum: A. colica dextra** and **A. colica media** (from the A. mesenterica superior) anastomose with each other. The A. colica media is connected to the A. colica sinistra **(RIOLAN's arcade).** Occasionally, the connection in one of

the arcades close to the intestines is referred to as the marginal artery of DRUMMOND.

- **Colon descendens and Colon sigmoideum: A. colica sinistra** and **Aa. sigmoideae** from the A. mesenterica inferior. The A. rectalis superior, also derived from the A. mesenterica inferior, supplies the upper rectum.

Note: Due to their **developmental origins,** all areas supplied by neurovascular pathways **switch** at the **left colonic flexure.** Regarding the arteries: the **A. mesenterica superior** supplies the Colon ascendens and Colon transversum, and the **A. mesenterica inferior** supplies the Colon descendens.

Clinical remarks

The short connections between the A. colica media and the A. colica sinistra, which clinically are collectively referred to as **RIOLAN's arcade,** play a role in circulatory disorders, e.g. in arteriosclerosis or in the case of an embolism (displaced blood clot). Similar connections exist in the area of the duodenum and the rectum (→ Fig. 6.21). Even

the complete occlusion of one of the three unpaired abdominal arteries (Truncus coeliacus, A. mesenterica superior and A. mesenterica inferior) can largely be compensated for without intestinal infarction. Circulatory disorders of the intestines are usually characterised by abdominal pain which occurs after a meal (postprandial pain).

Veins of the small and large intestines

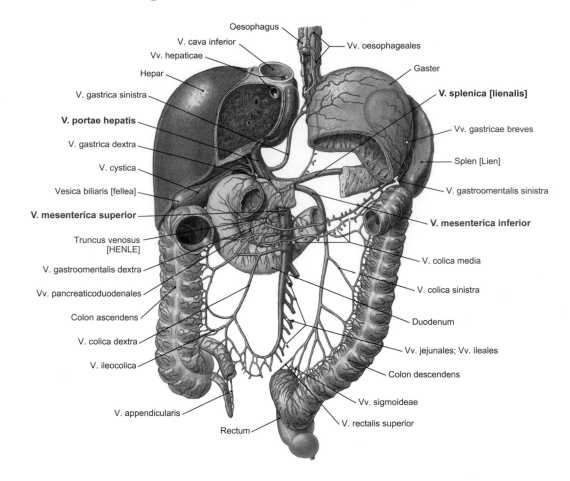

Fig. 6.81 Veins of the small intestine, Intestinum tenue, and the large intestine, Intestinum crassum; ventral view. [S700]
The veins correspond to the arteries and all flow into the three **major tributaries of the portal vein:** behind the Caput pancreatis, the V. mesenterica superior merges with the V. splenica to form the V. portae hepatis. The V. mesenterica inferior usually drains into the V. splenica

(70 % of all cases) or into the V. mesenterica superior (30 %). For the branches of the V. mesenterica superior and inferior → Fig. 6.100.
Note: Based on **developmental origins,** the neurovascular pathways of the **left colonic flexure** vary proximally and distally. Regarding the veins: the **V. mesenterica superior** drains blood from the Colon ascendens and Colon transversum, the **V. mesenterica inferior** from the Colon descendens.

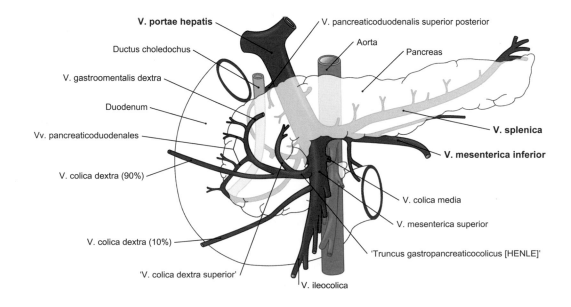

Fig. 6.82 Tributaries of the V. mesenterica superior; schematic illustration, view from ventral. [S700-L303]~[G1072]
The V. gastroomentalis dextra typically collects blood from the Vv. pancreaticoduodenales, the V. colica dextra and a vein from the right colon-

ic flexure, prior to connecting to the V. mesenterica superior. This venous trunk is commonly referred to as the **venous trunk of HENLE (Truncus gastropancreaticocolicus HENLE).** In contrast, the V. colica media joins as a separate vessel.

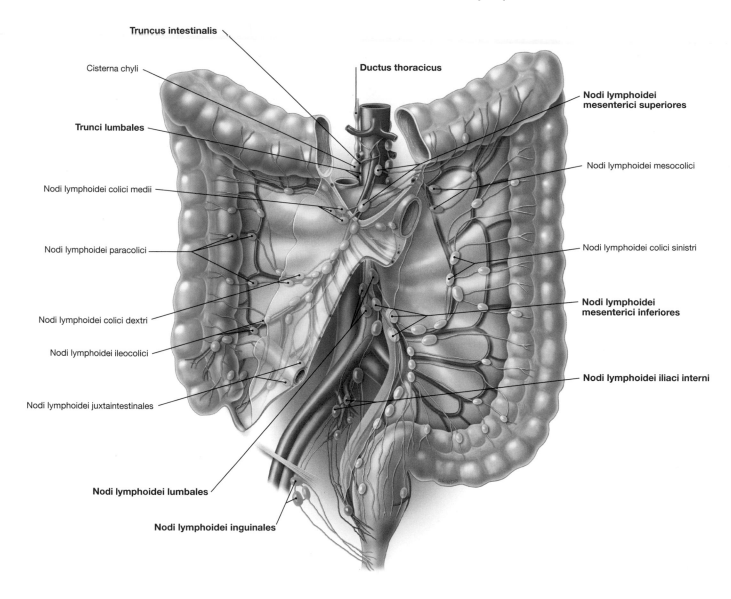

Truncus intestinalis

Cisterna chyli

Ductus thoracicus

Nodi lymphoidei
mesenterici superiores

Trunci lumbales

Nodi lymphoidei mesocolici

Nodi lymphoidei colici medii

Nodi lymphoidei paracolici

Nodi lymphoidei colici sinistri

Nodi lymphoidei
mesenterici inferiores

Nodi lymphoidei colici dextri

Nodi lymphoidei ileocolici

Nodi lymphoidei iliaci interni

Nodi lymphoidei juxtaintestinales

Nodi lymphoidei lumbales

Nodi lymphoidei inguinales

Fig. 6.83 Lymph vessels and regional lymph nodes of the small intestine, Intestinum tenue, and the large intestine, Intestinum crassum. The distinct groups of lymph nodes (a total of 100 to 200 lymph nodes) are coloured differently according to their drainage areas. [S700-L238]~[G1073]

The **Nodi lymphoidei juxtaintestinales** are positioned directly adjacent to the small intestine; next to the large intestine are the **Nodi lymphoidei paracolici.** The lymph flows via various lymph node stations along the vascular arcades (e.g. **Nodi lymphoidei colici dextri, colici medii, colici sinistri, ileocolici, mesocolici**) in two separate drainage systems:

- Lymph from the entire **small intestine** as well as the **caecum, Colon ascendens, and Colon transversum** drains into the **Nodi lymphoidei mesenterici superiores** at the origin of the A. mesenterica superior, where it continues via the Truncus intestinalis into the Ductus thoracicus (green).

- Lymph from the **Colon descendens, Colon sigmoideum, and proximal rectum** reaches the **Nodi lymphoidei mesenterici inferiores** at the origin of the A. mesenterica inferior (yellow) and from there within the retroperitoneal para-aortic lymph nodes (Nodi lymphoidei lumbales, grey) and into the Trunci lumbales (grey).

The **distal rectum** and the **anal canal** also connect to the drainage area of the Trunci lumbales. The first lymph node stations, however, are the **Nodi lymphoidei iliaci interni** (pink), and the **Nodi lymphoidei inguinales** (turquoise) for the terminal parts of the anal canal, respectively.

Note: Due to their **developmental origins,** all neurovascular pathways switch at the **left colonic flexure.** The **Nodi lymphoidei mesenterici superiores** are the regional lymph nodes for the Colon ascendens and Colon transversum, whereas the **Nodi lymphoidei mesenterici inferiores** drain the Colon descendens.

Clinical remarks

Lymphatic drainage plays a clinically important role in the staging of colon carcinomas and the therapeutic approach depends on the stage of the disease. In the case of a tumour located in the Colon ascendens or the Colon transversum, lymph node metastases should be anticipated in the area draining to the Nodi lymphoidei

mesenterici superiores. However, in the case of a tumour in the Colon descendens, the lymph nodes in the drainage area for the inferior mesenteric lymph nodes are relevant. These frequently connect to other retroperitoneal lymph nodes due to the retroperitoneal pathway of the concomitant A. mesenterica inferior.

Innervation of the small and large intestines

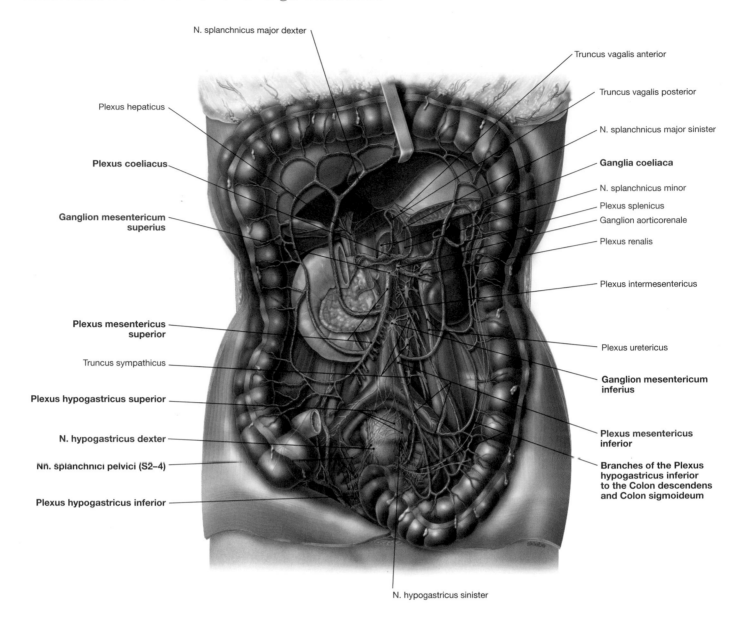

Fig. 6.84 Autonomic innervation of the small intestine, Intestinum tenue, and the large intestine, Instestinum crassum; ventral view. [S700-L238]

On the anterior side of the aorta, the autonomic sympathetic (green) and parasympathetic (purple) nerve fibres generate a plexus **(Plexus aorticus abdominalis),** which forms its own plexuses around the openings of the aortic branches, and these nerve fibres accompany the respective blood vessels to their target organs. The small and large intestines are innervated by fibres derived from the plexus around the three unpaired visceral branches of the aorta **(Plexus coeliacus, Plexus mesenterici superior and inferior).**

The perikarya of the **preganglionic sympathetic neurons** are located in the lateral horns of the spinal cord (for the small intestine and large intestine proximal of the left colonic flexure in T5–T12 and for the distal large intestine in L1–L2). Their axons reach the Truncus sympathicus and continue without synapsing via the Nn. splanchnici major and minor to the aortic plexus, where they synapse in the eponymous ganglia **(Ganglion coeliacum, Ganglion mesenterica superius and inferius)** onto postganglionic neurons, of which the axons reach the respective intestinal areas along with the branches of the respective arteries.

The **preganglionic parasympathetic neurons** of the **Nn. vagi [X]** descend along the oesophagus as the Trunci vagales anterior and posterior, traverse the diaphragm and travel to the autonomic nerve plexuses

of the abdominal aorta without synapsing to reach the walls or areas of their target organs, within which the postganglionic neurons lie. The supply area of the Nn. vagi [X] ends in the Plexus mesentericus superior and thereby in the area of the left colonic flexure (traditionally known as the CANNON-BÖHM point).

By contrast, the Colon descendens is supplied by the **sacral part of the parasympathicus** of which the preganglionic neurons are located within the sacral spinal cord (S2–S4). They emerge from the spinal nerves as Nn. splanchnici pelvici and synapse in the Plexus hypogastricus inferior in the area of the rectum onto postganglionic neurons. Only a minor portion of the postganglionic nerve fibres ascend to the Plexus mesentericus inferior (not shown); most postganglionics reach the Colon descendens as direct branches.

The **parasympathicus promotes,** and the **sympathicus inhibits** peristalsis and blood flow to the bowel.

Note: Due to their **developmental origins,** all neurovascular pathways switch at the **left colonic flexure.** Regarding the autonomic nerves: the **Plexus mesentericus superior** innervates the Colon ascendens and Colon transversum, while the **Plexus mesentericus inferior** and **Plexus hypogastricus inferior** innervate the Colon descendens and Colon sigmoideum. The origin of the parasympathetic neurons switches from the cranial part (N. vagus) to the sacral part (Nn. splanchnici pelvici).

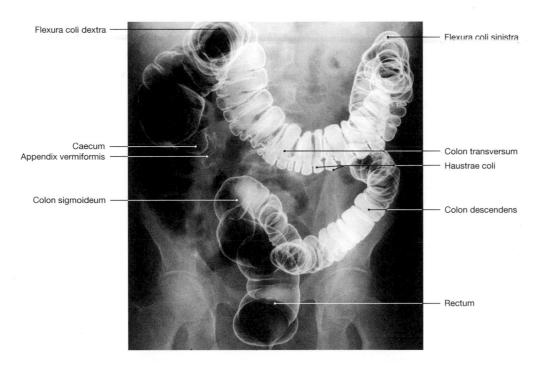

Flexura coli dextra

Caecum
Appendix vermiformis

Colon sigmoideum

Flexura coli sinistra

Colon transversum
Haustrae coli

Colon descendens

Rectum

Fig. 6.85   Large intestine, Intestinum crassum; X-ray in anteroposterior (AP) projection after filling it with contrast agent and air (double contrast method). In the X-ray image various positional variants of the Colon transversum can be verified (→ Fig. 6.86). [S700]

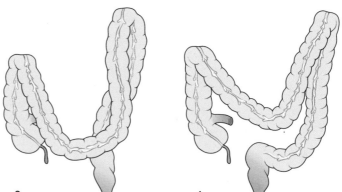

a   b   c   d

Fig. 6.86a–d   Positional variants of the transverse colon, Colon transversum; ventral view. [S700-L126]

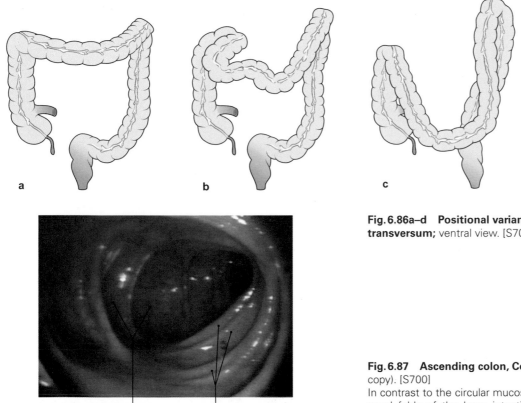

Haustrae coli   Plicae semilunares coli

Fig. 6.87   Ascending colon, Colon ascendens; colonoscopy (endoscopy). [S700]
In contrast to the circular mucosal folds of the small intestine, the mucosal folds of the large intestine are crescent-shaped (Plicae semilunares).

Clinical remarks

Malignant tumours of the colon **(colon carcinomas)** are among the most common malignancies in both men and women, and therefore contribute substantially to the causes of death in the Western world. These deaths could largely be prevented by taking suitable precautions. The diagnosic method of choice for the evaluation of colon cancers is the colonoscopy, and screening is therefore recommended at regular intervals in preventative medicine. In addition to the inspection of the mucosa, a colonoscopy also allows for the sampling of biopsies for a definitive diagnosis by a pathologist. The importance of radiological contrast-imaging has declined. However, in the case of an occluded lumen, e.g. due to a stenosing tumour, or a submucosal disease process which is endoscopically not accessible, radiological imaging can reveal characteristic changes of shape and position of the lumen which also give a relatively reliable diagnosis.

Projection of the liver and gallbladder

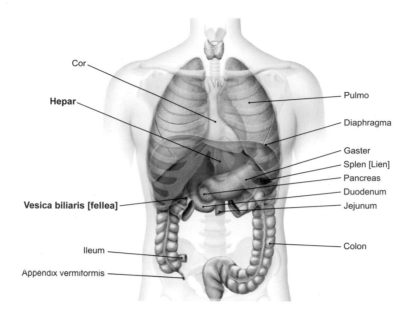

Fig. 6.88   Projection of the internal organs onto the body surface; ventral view. [S700-L275]

The liver and gallbladder are located **intraperitoneally** in the right upper abdomen. The upper margin of the liver projects to the right on the fourth intercostal space (ICS), and on the left somewhat deeper onto the fifth rib. The fundus of the gallbladder projects onto the right midclavicular line at the level of the ninth rib. The left lobe of the liver is located in the left epigastrium (approximately up to the left midclavicular line) where it is anterior to the stomach. Its position depends on breathing (lowers on breathing in, rises on breathing out) because its surface area grows with the diaphragm. Therefore, its position is also dependent on the size of the lungs. Because of the domed shape of the diaphragm, the anterior and posterior sides of the liver are partially covered by the pleural cavity (→ Fig. 6.148). The lower margin of the liver in normal anatomy aligns with the costal margin in the midclavicular line, so that it is not possible to palpate the liver.

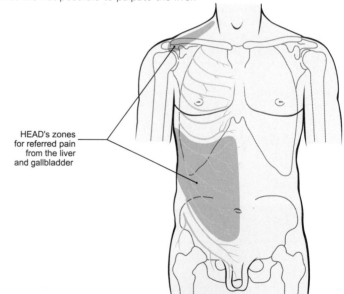

Fig. 6.89   Zones of referred pain, HEAD's zones of the liver and gallbladder, schematic drawing; ventral view. [S700-L126]/[G1071]

The organ-related areas for referred pain or **HEAD's zones** for the liver and gallbladder project into the dermatomes (cutaneous areas) T8–T11 of the right side of the body. Dermatome C4 in the area of the right shoulder is also a HEAD's zone of the liver and gallbladder, because the N. phrenicus from the Plexus cervicalis is usually fed by the C4, and its terminal branch (R. phrenicoabdominalis) on the right side also provides sensory innervation to the peritoneum on the surface of the liver and gallbladder.

Clinical remarks

Inflammatory conditions of the liver and gallbladder (hepatitis or cholecystitis) or a diagnostically investigated **liver biopsy** may cause referred pain in the right shoulder.

Assessing the size of the liver always forms part of a complete physical examination, as its consistency and size can provide the first evidence of abnormal changes, e.g. **hepatic steatosis** (in diabetes mellitus, alcohol abuse), **inflammation** (hepatitis) due to hepatitis viruses, alcohol abuse or **liver cirrhosis** as the pathological terminal stage in most chronic liver diseases. The inferior margin of the liver is determined by palpation during inhalation and the superior margin of the liver is assessed by tapping (percussion) on the chest. As a rule of thumb, the liver should not extend beyond 12 cm in its craniocaudal diameter in the right midclavicular line.
[S701-J803/L126]

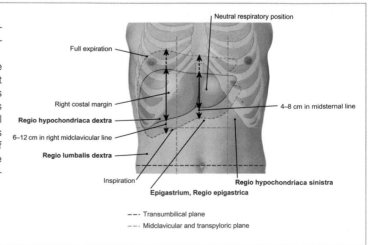

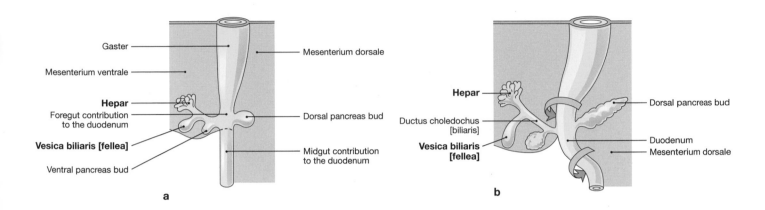

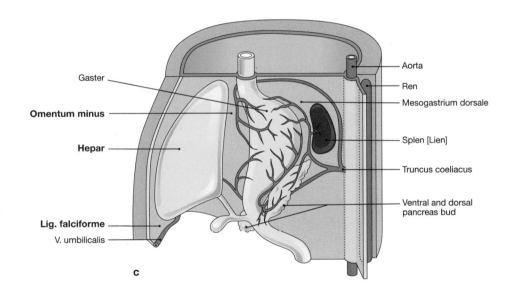

Fig. 6.90a–c   Developmental stages of the liver, Hepar, and gall-bladder, Vesica biliaris, in the fourth to fifth week. [E347-09]
a Development of liver and gallbladder in week 4.
b Further development of liver and gallbladder during intestinal rotation.
c Repositioning of the liver into the Mesogastrium ventrale.
The epithelial tissues of the liver and the gallbladder derive from the entoderm of the foregut at the level of the future duodenum. In the fourth week (from the 22nd day onwards) the entoderm forms a thickening **(hepatic diverticulum)** which divides into a superior liver primordium and an inferior primordium for the bile duct system **(a** and **b).** The

epithelium of the liver system grows in the connective tissue of the Septum transversum, in which islets of haematopoiesis develop. This places the connective tissue components and the regional blood vessels (sinusoids) within the liver system. The liver then moves into the Mesogastrium ventrale **(c),** thereby dividing it into a Mesohepaticum ventrale and a Mesohepaticum dorsale (→ Fig. 6.1). The Mesohepaticum ventrale develops into the **Lig. falciforme hepatis** and connects to the anterior trunk wall. The Mesohepaticum dorsale becomes the **Omentum minus,** connecting the liver with the stomach and the duodenum.

Liver, overview

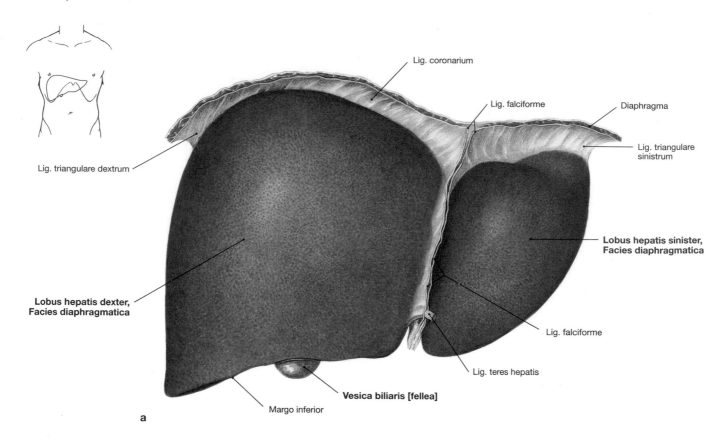

Lig. coronarium

Lig. falciforme

Diaphragma

Lig. triangulare sinistrum

Lig. triangulare dextrum

Lobus hepatis sinister, Facies diaphragmatica

Lobus hepatis dexter, Facies diaphragmatica

Lig. falciforme

Lig. teres hepatis

Vesica biliaris [fellea]

Margo inferior

a

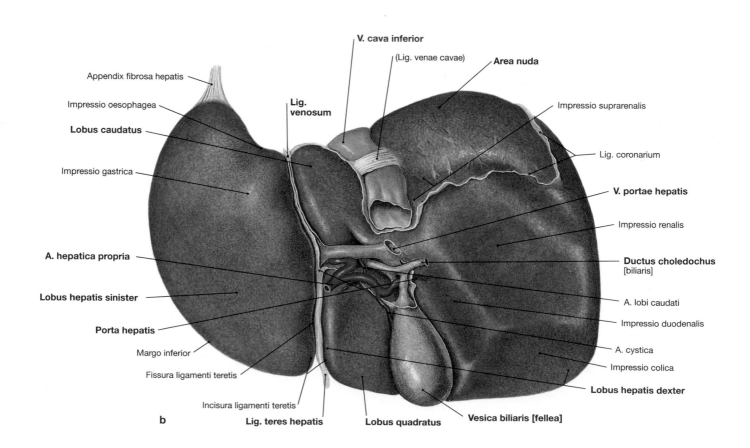

V. cava inferior

(Lig. venae cavae)

Area nuda

Appendix fibrosa hepatis

Impressio oesophagea

Lig. venosum

Impressio suprarenalis

Lobus caudatus

Lig. coronarium

Impressio gastrica

V. portae hepatis

Impressio renalis

A. hepatica propria

Ductus choledochus [biliaris]

Lobus hepatis sinister

A. lobi caudati

Porta hepatis

Impressio duodenalis

Margo inferior

A. cystica

Fissura ligamenti teretis

Impressio colica

Incisura ligamenti teretis

Lobus hepatis dexter

b

Lig. teres hepatis

Lobus quadratus

Vesica biliaris [fellea]

Fig. 6.91a and b   Liver, Hepar. For a description → Fig. 6.92. [S700]   **a** Ventral view.
b Dorsocaudal view.

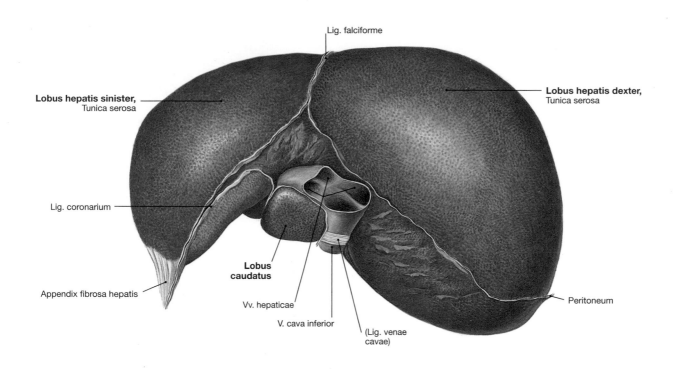

Lig. falciforme

Lobus hepatis sinister, Tunica serosa

Lobus hepatis dexter, Tunica serosa

Lig. coronarium

Lobus caudatus

Appendix fibrosa hepatis

Vv. hepaticae

V. cava inferior

(Lig. venae cavae)

Peritoneum

Fig. 6.92 Liver, Hepar; cranial view. [S700]

The liver is the largest gland (1,200–1,800 g) and the main metabolic organ of the body. The Facies diaphragmatica lies adjacent to the diaphragm and the Facies visceralis with the anterior lower margin (Margo inferior) points towards the abdominal viscera (→ Fig. 6.91).

The **Facies diaphragmatica** has partially grown into the diaphragm and is not covered with visceral peritoneum **(Area nuda).** The liver is divided into a large right lobe and a small left lobe **(Lobus dexter and Lobus sinister),** separated at the front by the **Lig. falciforme.** This continues cranially into the **Lig. coronarium,** which ends on the right and left in a **Lig. triangulare** connected to the diaphragm. The left Lig. triangulare passes into the pointed Appendix fibrosa hepatis. Below, the **Lig. teres hepatis** (a remnant from the fetal circulation of the V. umbilicalis) joins with the falciform ligament. Both bands reach the ventral trunk wall.

On the **Facies visceralis,** the Fissura ligamenti teretis hepatis continues to the hilum of the liver (Porta hepatis), into which the neurovascular pathways of the liver (V. portae hepatis, A. hepatica propria, Ductus

hepaticus communis) enter and exit. The **Lig. venosum (ARANTII,** a remnant of the fetal circulatory Ductus venosus) is shown cranially. On the right side of the Porta hepatis, the V. cava inferior is located in a superior groove, and the **gallbladder (Vesica biliaris)** is embedded in the inferior fossa for the gallbladder (Fossa vesicae biliaris). The Lig. teres hepatis, Lig. venosum, V. cava inferior and gallbladder delineate two rectangular areas on both sides of the Porta hepatis at the inferior side of the right hepatic lobe, the ventral **Lobus quadratus** and the dorsal **Lobus caudatus.** The liver is not covered by peritoneum in four larger areas: Area nuda, the hilum of the liver, the bed of the gallbladder, and the groove of the V. cava inferior.

In living patients the liver is malleable and adjusts to the shape of the surrounding organs. In a fixed state the organs leave marks (impressions), which are regarded as fixation artefacts and are without significance. However, they provide information about the positioning of the liver.

Liver and gallbladder

Structure of the liver

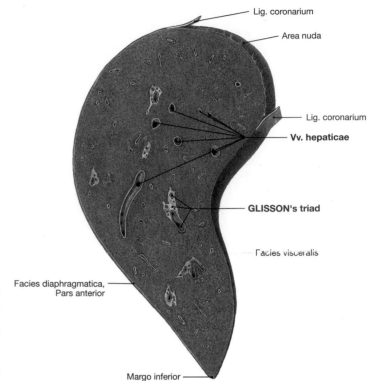

Fig. 6.93 Liver, Hepar; sagittal section through the right liver lobe. [S700]
The entry and exit of the vascular and bile duct structures at the **Porta hepatis (V. portae hepatis, A. hepatica propria, Ductus hepaticus communis)** branch out surrounded by connective tissue into the parenchyma of the liver and form the **GLISSON's triad** (→ Fig. 6.94) in the periportal field.
The **liver veins (Vv. hepaticae)** and their tributaries, which take the blood from the liver into the V. cava inferior run separately from the vessels of the GLISSON's triad.

Fig. 6.94 Lobular structure of the hepatic parenchyma; schematic representation of a histological section. [S700-L126]/[S133]
The hepatic parenchyma is divided into liver lobules which are made up of radially arranged trabeculae of **hepatocytes.** The almost hexagonal **classic hepatic lobule** is surrounded by **portal tracts** at three to six corners. The portal tract contains the **GLISSON's triad** (A./V. interlobularis, Ductus bilifer interlobularis which is embedded in connective tissue. The blood vessels constitute the terminal branches of the A. hepatica propria/portal vein, while the interlobular bile duct forms the beginning of the bile duct system, which unites at the hilum of the liver with the Ductus hepaticus communis. In the centre of the liver lobule is the **V. centralis.** The blood from the peripheral lobular arteries and veins, which enter the liver sinusoids between the liver trabeculae, is collected by the central lobular veins and drained via the Vv. sublobulares into the liver veins (Vv. hepaticae). This allows the hepatocytes to extract nutrients and waste products to be eliminated from the blood and to secrete synthesised substances, such as plasma proteins, into the blood. The bile flows between the liver cells to the portal fields. The bile duct is thereby located in the centre of the triangular **portal lobule,** while the three corners are formed by the central veins. The **acinus of the liver** is rhomboid and bordered by two portal fields and two central lobular veins. Oxygen and nutrient supply is best along the connection between adjacent portal fields, so that the hepatocytes in the different zones of the acinus can take on different roles.

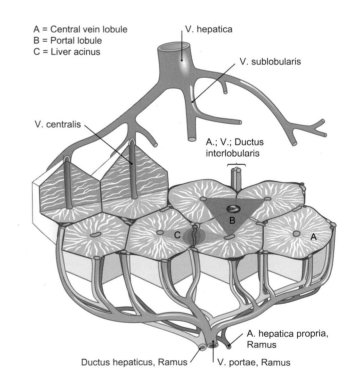

A = Central vein lobule
B = Portal lobule
C = Liver acinus

Clinical remarks

The blood flow in the liver lobes is extremely important for the liver function. In the case of **liver cirrhosis,** the lobular structure is destroyed by nodular connective tissue remodelling, and the blood flow is compromised. The high parenchymal resistance in the liver results in an increased blood pressure in the portal vein **(portal hypertension).** As a result, the formation of collateral circulations **(portocaval anastomoses)** may occur (→ Fig. 6.102).

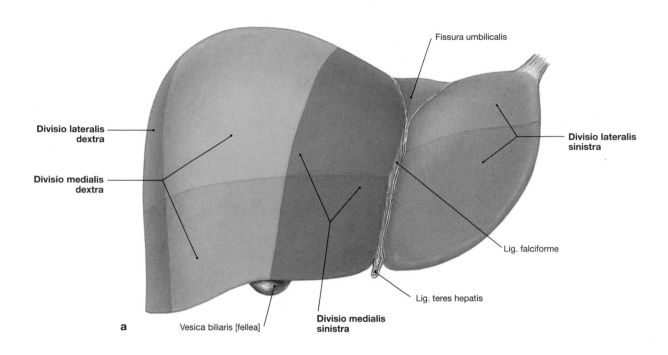

Fissura umbilicalis

Divisio lateralis
dextra

Divisio medialis
dextra

Divisio lateralis
sinistra

Lig. falciforme

Lig. teres hepatis

a   Vesica biliaris [fellea]   **Divisio medialis
sinistra**

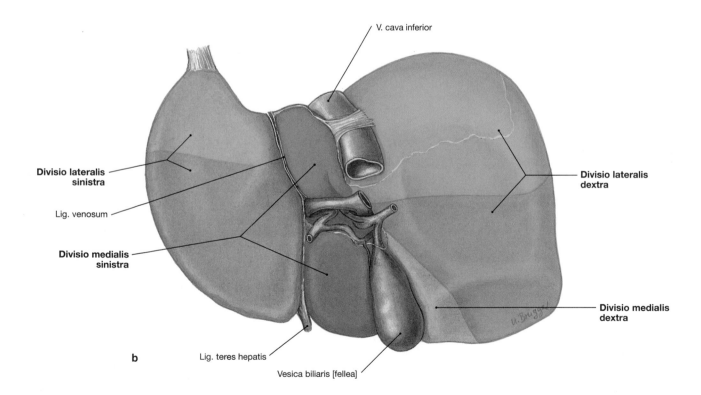

V. cava inferior

Divisio lateralis
sinistra

Lig. venosum

**Divisio medialis
sinistra**

Divisio lateralis
dextra

**Divisio medialis
dextra**

b   Lig. teres hepatis

Vesica biliaris [fellea]

Fig. 6.95a and b   Segments of the liver, Hepar. Segments of the liver lobes are highlighted in colour. [S700]
a Ventral view.
b Dorsal view.
The **three** almost vertically oriented **hepatic veins** (Vv. hepaticae; → Fig. 6.96) divide the liver into **four adjacent divisions.** The **Divisio lateralis sinistra** corresponds to the left anatomical lobe of the liver and thus reaches the Lig. falciforme hepatis, behind the left hepatic

vein. The extended **Divisio medialis sinistra** lies between the Lig. falciforme and the gallbladder, at the level of the V. hepatica intermedia. Then to the right, the **Divisio medialis dextra** and the **Divisio lateralis dextra** follow, separated by the right hepatic vein; but without any visible landmark on the outer surface. The neurovascular pathways of the **portal triad** organise these liver segments into **eight functional** and clinically very important **liver segments** (→ Fig. 6.96) which are indicated here with different colours.

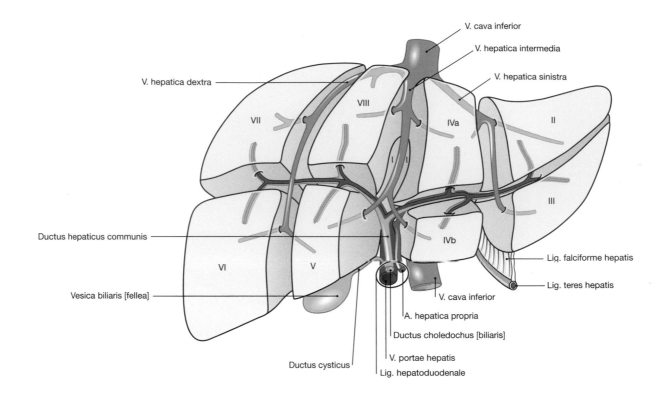

I	Lobus caudatus	V	Segmentum anterius mediale dextrum
II	Segmentum posterius laterale sinistrum	VI	Segmentum anterius laterale dextrum
III	Segmentum anterius laterale sinistrum	VII	Segmentum posterius laterale dextrum
IV (a/b)	Segmentum mediale sinistrum	VIII	Segmentum posterius mediale dextrum

Fig. 6.96 Schematic illustration of the liver segments and their relationship with the regional vessels and bile ducts; ventral view. [S700-L126]/[B500~M282/L132]

The liver is divided into **eight functional segments** which are each supplied by a branch of the portal triad (V. portae hepatis, A. hepatica propria, Ductus hepaticus communis) and are therefore functionally independent. Two segments at a time are loosely combined to four adjacent divisions of the liver via the three vertically running hepatic veins (→ Fig. 6.95). The original association of a segment IX with the Lobus caudatus was abandoned.

Functionally it is important that the **segments II to IV** are supplied by the left branches of the portal triad and are thus combined into a functional **left liver lobe,** while the **segments V to VIII** are dependent on the branches of the blood vessels on the right and represent the functional **right liver lobe.** As a result, the border between the functional right and left liver lobes is located in the sagittal plane between the V. cava inferior and the gallbladder **(V. cava-gallbladder plane)** and not at the level of the Lig. falciforme hepatis. The **segment I (Lobus caudatus)** is regularly supplied from the branches on both sides and is not seen as part of the two functioning liver lobes.

Clinical remarks

The liver segments are of great clinical significance in **visceral surgery.** Resection of distinct parts of the liver with little loss of blood is possible when segmental borders are maintained. Thus, pathologies such as liver metastases can be treated by the surgical resection of individual segments in different parts of the liver without compromising the liver function as a whole. Ligation of the individual branches of the hepatic vessels and the ensuing discolouration of the affected segment due to lack of perfusion enables the surgeon to identify each segment.
[S008-3-P498]

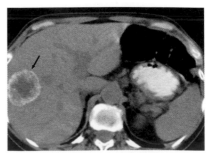

Abdominal CT showing liver with metastasis (arrow)

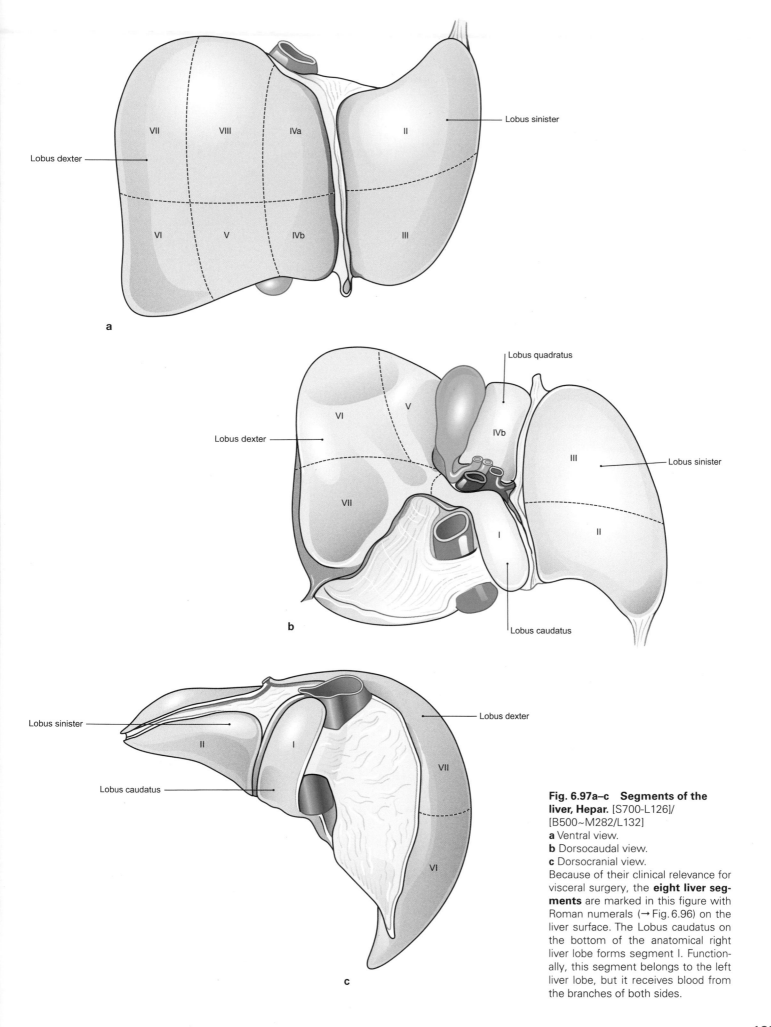

Fig. 6.97a–c   Segments of the liver, Hepar. [S700-L126]/[B500~M282/L132]
a Ventral view.
b Dorsocaudal view.
c Dorsocranial view.
Because of their clinical relevance for visceral surgery, the **eight liver segments** are marked in this figure with Roman numerals (→ Fig. 6.96) on the liver surface. The Lobus caudatus on the bottom of the anatomical right liver lobe forms segment I. Functionally, this segment belongs to the left liver lobe, but it receives blood from the branches of both sides.

Organs of the abdominal cavity

Arteries of the liver and gallbladder

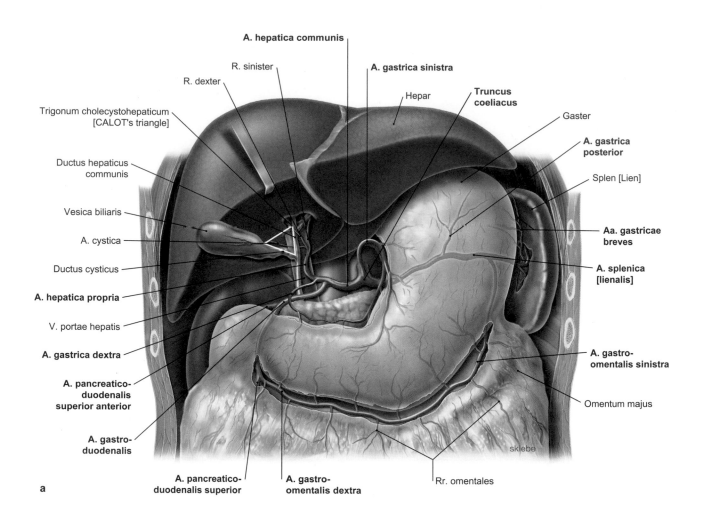

A. hepatica communis

R. sinister

A. gastrica sinistra

R. dexter

Hepar

Truncus coeliacus

Trigonum cholecystohepaticum [CALOT's triangle]

Gaster

A. gastrica posterior

Ductus hepaticus communis

Splen [Lien]

Vesica biliaris

Aa. gastricae breves

A. cystica

A. splenica [lienalis]

Ductus cysticus

A. hepatica propria

V. portae hepatis

A. gastrica dextra

A. gastro-omentalis sinistra

A. pancreatico-duodenalis superior anterior

Omentum majus

A. gastro-duodenalis

A. pancreatico-duodenalis superior

A. gastro-omentalis dextra

Rr. omentales

sklebe

a

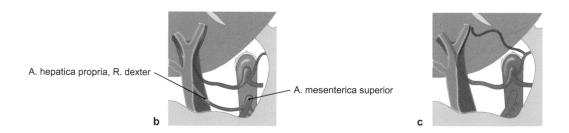

A. hepatica propria, R. dexter

A. mesenterica superior

b

c

Fig. 6.98a–c Arteries of the liver, Hepar, and gallbladder, Vesica biliaris. a [S700-L238]/[B500], b, c [S700-L281]

a Textbook case of hepatic blood supply (≈ 50 %).

b A. mesenterica superior contributes to the blood supply of the right liver lobe (≈ 10–20 %).

c A. gastrica sinistra contributes to the blood supply of the left liver lobe (10–20 %).

Besides the V. portae hepatis, which provides 75 % of the blood flow to the liver and carries nutrient-rich blood, the **A. hepatica propria** provides 25 % of the blood flow to the liver and carries oxygen-rich blood. The A. hepatica propria is the continuation of the A. hepatica commu-

nis, a main branch of the Truncus coeliacus. Rarely, the A. hepatica communis originates from the A. mesenterica superior (1.5–4 %). After providing the A. gastrica dextra, the A. hepatica propria runs within the Lig. hepatoduodenale along with the V. portae hepatis and the Ductus choledochus to the Porta hepatis. There it is typically divided into a R. dexter and a R. sinister for the two lobes of the liver. The **A. cystica** originates from the R. dexter and supplies the gallbladder. In 10–20 % of all cases, the A. mesenterica superior contributes to the blood supply of the right liver lobe **(b)**, and the A. gastrica sinistra contributes to the supply of the left liver lobe **(c)**.

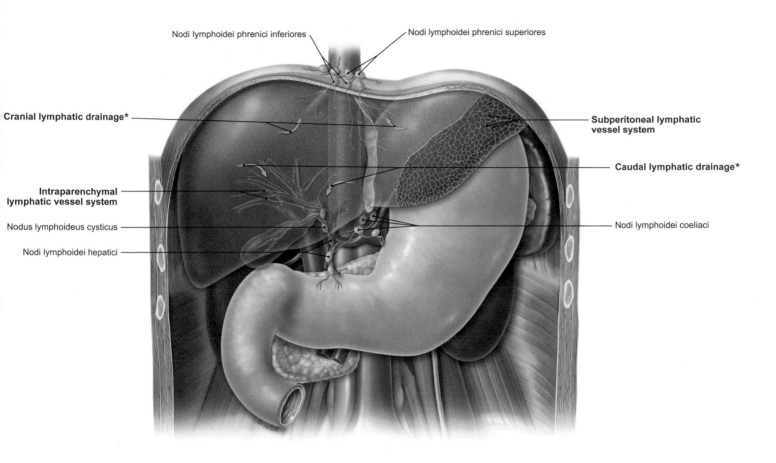

Nodi lymphoidei phrenici inferiores

Nodi lymphoidei phrenici superiores

Cranial lymphatic drainage*

Subperitoneal lymphatic vessel system

Caudal lymphatic drainage*

Intraparenchymal lymphatic vessel system

Nodus lymphoideus cysticus

Nodi lymphoidei hepatici

Nodi lymphoidei coeliaci

Fig. 6.99   Lymph vessels and lymph nodes of the liver and bile duct system. [S700-L238]

The **liver** has **two lymph vessel systems:**
- the subperitoneal system on the surface of the liver
- the intraparenchymal system that follows the structures in the portal triad to the hilum of the liver.

Corresponding to the regional lymph nodes, there are **two major lymphatic drainage routes:**
- **caudally to the hilum of the liver** (most important with 80 % of the lymph volume) via the Nodi lymphoidei hepatici to the hepatic porta (→ Fig. 6.44) and from there via the Nodi lymphoidei coeliaci to the intestinal trunk
- **cranially through the diaphragm** via the Nodi lymphoidei phrenici inferiores and superiores into the Nodi lymphoidei mediastinales an-

teriores and posteriores which drain into the Trunci bronchomediastinales; using this pathway, liver carcinomas may metastasise into thoracic lymph nodes.

There are also **two further routes** of lesser importance:
- to the anterior trunk wall via lymph vessels in the Lig. teres hepatis to the inguinal and axillary lymph nodes
- to the stomach and pancreas from the left lobe of the liver.

The **gallbladder** usually has its own Nodus lymphoideus cysticus in the area of the neck, which drains into the lymph nodes at the hilum of the liver (predominantly caudally).

For the autonomic innervation of the liver and gallbladder → Fig. 6.144

* The arrows depict the direction of lymphatic drainage from the liver parenchyma cranially or caudally.

Clinical remarks

Malignancies of the liver and gallbladder rarely metastasise to the ventral wall of the trunk, and confer a poor prognosis. It may lead to a painless, progressively growing tumour in the umbilicus **(Sister MARY JOSEPH node)**. The relevance of this rare phenomenon lies in the fact that a diagnosis can be assumed on an inspection of the patient. As with the VIRCHOW's node in the left supraclavicular area, it is necessary to be familiar with the lymphatic drainage pathways to establish the primary disease and the origin.

Veins of the liver and gallbladder

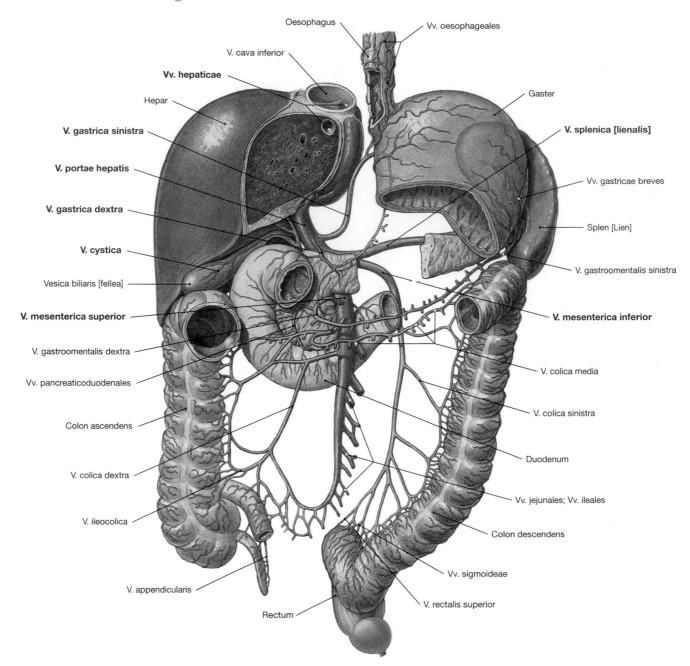

Oesophagus

V. cava inferior

Vv. hepaticae

Hepar

V. gastrica sinistra

V. portae hepatis

V. gastrica dextra

V. cystica

Vesica biliaris [fellea]

V. mesenterica superior

V. gastroomentalis dextra

Vv. pancreaticoduodenales

Colon ascendens

V. colica dextra

V. ileocolica

V. appendicularis

Rectum

Vv. oesophageales

Gaster

V. splenica [lienalis]

Vv. gastricae breves

Splen [Lien]

V. gastroomentalis sinistra

V. mesenterica inferior

V. colica media

V. colica sinistra

Duodenum

Vv. jejunales; Vv. ileales

Colon descendens

Vv. sigmoideae

V. rectalis superior

Fig. 6.100   Veins of the liver, Hepar, and the gallbladder, Vesica biliaris; ventral view. [S700]

The liver has an incoming and an outgoing venous system. The **V. portae hepatis** collects the nutrient-rich blood from the unpaired abdominal organs (stomach, intestines, pancreas, spleen) and feeds this blood, along with the arterial blood from the A. hepatica communis, into the sinusoids of the liver lobules. Three **Vv. hepaticae** (→ Fig. 6.96) transport the blood from the liver to the V. cava inferior. Only the Lobus caudatus connects via short liver veins directly to the V. cava inferior.

The portal vein has three main tributaries: behind the Caput pancreatis, the V. mesenterica superior merges with the V. splenica to form the V. portae hepatis. The V. mesenterica inferior drains into the V. splenica (in 70 % of all cases) or into the V. mesenterica superior (30 %). The length of the hepatic portal vein is about 8 cm before it divides into the right (1–2 cm) and left (3–4 cm) main branches.

Branches of the V. splenica (collecting blood from the spleen and from parts of the stomach and pancreas):

- Vv. gastricae breves
- V. gastroomentalis sinistra
- Vv. pancreaticae (from the tail and body of the pancreas).

Branches of the V. mesenterica superior (collecting blood from parts of the stomach and pancreas, from the entire small intestine, the Colon ascendens, and Colon transversum):

- V. gastroomentalis dextra with Vv. pancreaticoduodenales
- Vv. pancreaticae (from the neck and body of the pancreas)
- Vv. jejunales und ileales
- V. ileocolica
- V. colica dextra
- V. colica media.

Branches of the V. mesenterica inferior (collecting blood from the Colon descendens and the upper rectum):

- V. colica sinistra
- Vv. sigmoideae
- V. rectalis superior: the vein is connected to the V. rectalis media and the V. rectalis inferior, which count as a drainage area of the V. cava inferior.

In addition, there are **veins** which drain **directly into the portal vein** once the main venous branches have merged:

- V. cystica (from the gallbladder)
- Vv. paraumbilicales (via veins in the Lig. teres hepatis from the abdominal wall around the umbilicus)
- Vv. gastricae dextra and sinistra (from the lesser curvature of the stomach)
- V. pancreaticoduodenalis superior posterior.

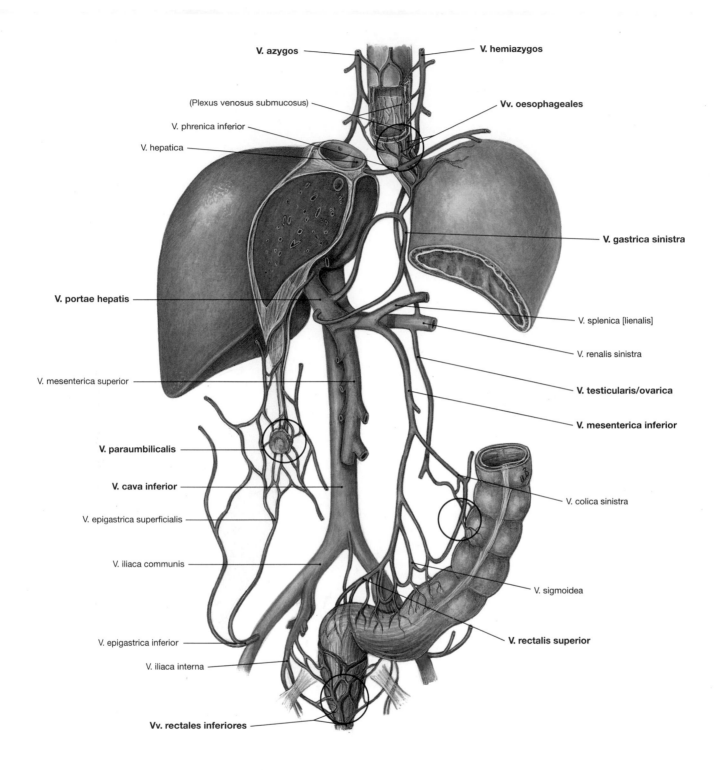

V. azygos

V. hemiazygos

(Plexus venosus submucosus)

Vv. oesophageales

V. phrenica inferior

V. hepatica

V. gastrica sinistra

V. portae hepatis

V. splenica [lienalis]

V. renalis sinistra

V. mesenterica superior

V. testicularis/ovarica

V. mesenterica inferior

V. paraumbilicalis

V. cava inferior

V. colica sinistra

V. epigastrica superficialis

V. iliaca communis

V. sigmoidea

V. epigastrica inferior

V. iliaca interna

V. rectalis superior

Vv. rectales inferiores

Fig. 6.101   Portocaval anastomoses (connections between V. portae hepatis and V. cava superior/inferior). Tributaries to the V. cava superior/inferior (blue) and the V. portae hepatis (purple). [S700] There are four possible collateral circulations via portocaval anastomoses (marked with black circles), through which the blood from the portal vein can bypass the liver on its way to the heart:

- Vv. gastricae dextra and sinistra via oesophageal veins and azygos veins to the V. cava superior. Hereby, enlarged (dilated) submucosal veins of the oesophagus **(oesophageal varices)** can occur.

- Vv. paraumbilicales via the veins of the ventral trunk wall (deep: Vv. epigastricae superior and inferior; superficial: V. thoracoepigastrica and V. epigastrica superficialis) to the Vv. cavae inferior and superior. Extension of the superficial veins may lead to **Caput medusae.**
- V. rectalis superior via veins of the distal rectum and the V. iliaca interna to the V. cava inferior.
- retroperitoneal anastomoses via the V. mesenterica inferior to the V. testicularis/ovarica with connection to the V. cava inferior.

6

Liver cirrhosis

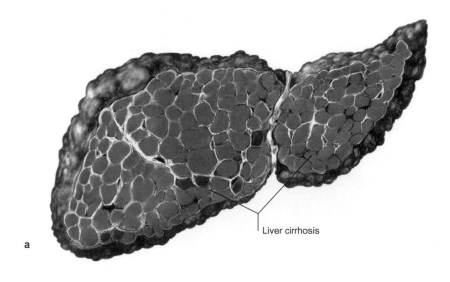

Liver cirrhosis

a

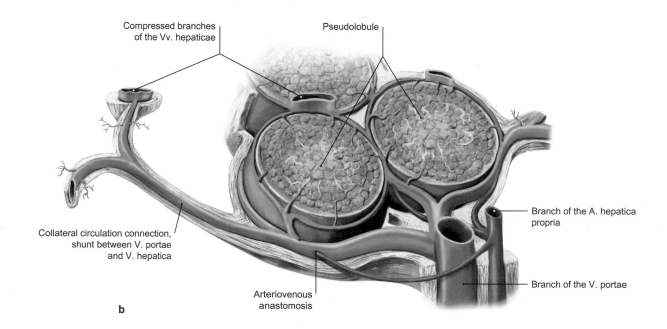

Compressed branches
of the Vv. hepaticae

Pseudolobule

Collateral circulation connection,
shunt between V. portae
and V. hepatica

Arteriovenous
anastomosis

Branch of the A. hepatica
propria

Branch of the V. portae

b

Fig. 6.102a and b Morphological changes to the liver in liver cirrhosis. [S701-L266]
a Macroscopically visible node formation; frontal section through the liver.

b Formation of pseudonodules; schematic representation, partly with microscopic view.

Clinical remarks

Cirrhosis is the end stage of many chronic liver diseases, when the liver is not acutely destroyed as, for instance, in the case of poisoning with a deathcap mushroom, but 'scarred' due to slowly progressing inflammation or persistent damage caused by connective tissue remodeling. Globally, liver cirrhosis is most frequently caused by viral hepatitis (hepatitis B, C and D), whereas in the industrialised world it is usually caused metabolically through an alcohol-induced hepatitis or increasingly also by hepatic steatosis in diabetes mellitus or obesity (adipositas). The scarring is already macroscopically visible in the formation of **nodules** on the liver surface. Histologically, the nodular structure of the liver parenchyma is abrogated. Remodeling of the liver parenchymal tissue with increased connective tissue results in the formation of **pseudonodules** and compression of veins, causing high parenchymal resistance and stasis of blood flow in the portal vein.

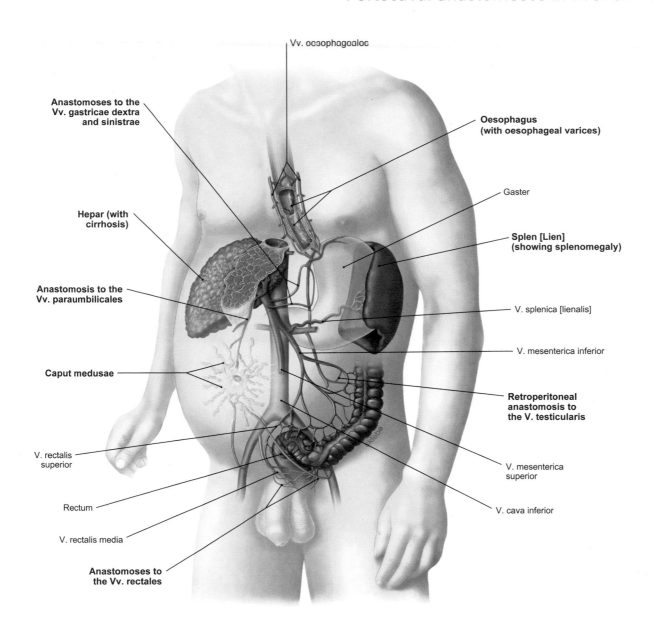

Vv. oesophagoaloc

Anastomoses to the
Vv. gastricae dextra
and sinistrae

Hepar (with
cirrhosis)

Anastomosis to the
Vv. paraumbilicales

Caput medusae

V. rectalis
superior

Rectum

V. rectalis media

Anastomoses to
the Vv. rectales

Oesophagus
(with oesophageal varices)

Gaster

Splen [Lien]
(showing splenomegaly)

V. splenica [lienalis]

V. mesenterica inferior

Retroperitoneal
anastomosis to
the V. testicularis

V. mesenterica
superior

V. cava inferior

**Fig. 6.103 Symptoms of portocaval anastomoses with cirrhosis
of the liver;** schematic illustration, ventral view from the left side.
[S701-L238]

Clinical remarks

In the case of liver cirrhosis, the high parenchymal resistance causes
stasis in the V. portae hepatis (→ Fig. 6.102), resulting in high blood
pressure in the portal vein circulation **(portal hypertension).** As a
result, pre-existing connections in tributaries of the Vv. cavae superi-
or and inferior **(portocaval anastomoses)** can open or recanalise.
Clinically important are the connections to the **oesophageal veins**
because rupture of oesophageal varices may result in a **life-threat-**
ening haemorrhage, the most common cause of death in patients
with liver cirrhosis. The connections to superficial veins of the ventral
trunk wall are only of diagnostic value. Although the **Caput medusae**
is rare, the appearance is so characteristic that liver cirrhosis cannot
be overlooked! In contrast, the retroperitoneal connections and
anastomoses between the veins of the rectum are not clinically significant.

Organs of the abdominal cavity

Liver, imaging

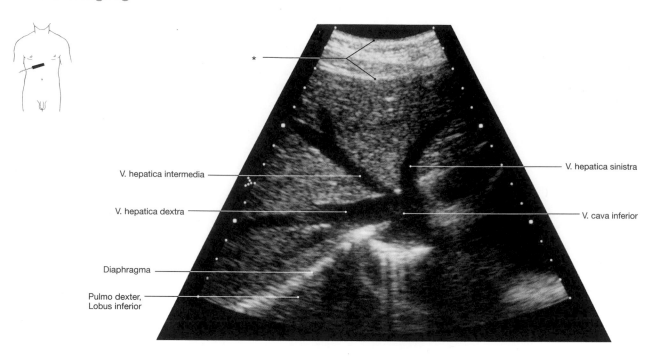

V. hepatica intermedia

V. hepatica dextra

Diaphragma

Pulmo dexter,
Lobus inferior

V. hepatica sinistra

V. cava inferior

Fig. 6.104 Confluence of the Vv. hepaticae into the V. cava inferior; ultrasound image; caudal view. [S700-T894]

* abdominal wall

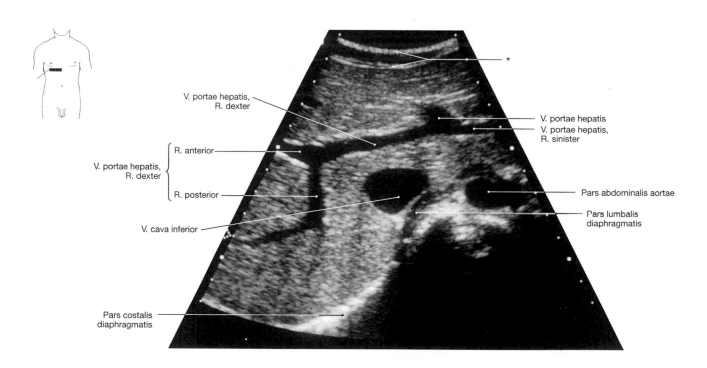

V. portae hepatis,
R. dexter

V. portae hepatis,
R. dexter { R. anterior

R. posterior

V. cava inferior

Pars costalis
diaphragmatis

V. portae hepatis

V. portae hepatis,
R. sinister

Pars abdominalis aortae

Pars lumbalis
diaphragmatis

Fig. 6.105 Liver, Hepar, and V. portae hepatis; presentation of the branches of the portal vein; ultrasound image; caudal view.
[S700-T894]

* abdominal wall

Clinical remarks

An **ultrasound examination** of the liver is a standard diagnostic tool used by specialists in internal medicine and by radiologists. It permits noninvasive investigation of the liver parenchyma whereby echo-dense steatosis (low echo) or fibrosis (increased echo) can be detected in hepatitis or liver cirrhosis. Focal tumours or cysts can also be captured. When ultrasound findings are unclear, liver biopsies (→ Fig. 6.106, → Fig. 6.107) or a laparoscopic examination of the liver (→ Fig. 6.109) will subsequently be carried out for further clarification.

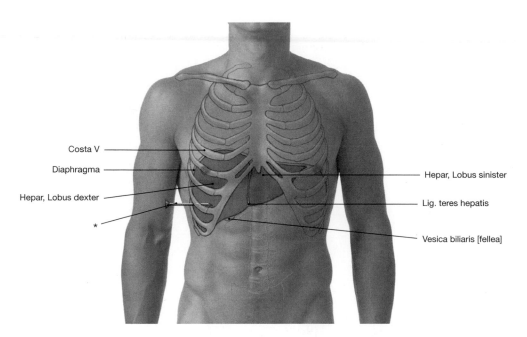

Fig. 6.106   Projection of the liver, Hepar, and gallbladder, Vesica biliaris, onto the ventral trunk wall in mid-respiratory position. [S700]

* position of the needle during puncture biopsy of the liver

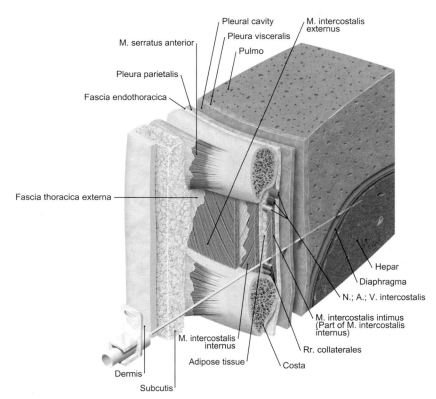

Fig. 6.107   Layers of the chest wall and liver, Hepar; frontal section; puncture biopsy of the liver. [S700-L127]
The biopsy is carried out using ultrasound technology during expiration through one of the lower intercostal spaces, otherwise there is the danger of causing a pneumothorax, as the liver is covered from above by the pleural cavity. In order to preserve the intercostal neurovascular structures, the puncture is always made at the superior costal margin. As the peritoneum covering the liver capsule is innervated by the N. phrenicus (C3–C5) from the Plexus cervicalis, patients often feel a **referred pain** in the area of the right shoulder.

Clinical remarks

A liver biopsy is often performed to determine the nature of **ambiguous tumours,** or the staging of a **hepatitis** or **liver cirrhosis,** respectively. A definitive diagnosis by a pathologist is however only possible with a tissue biopsy.

Structure of the gallbladder and extrahepatic bile ducts

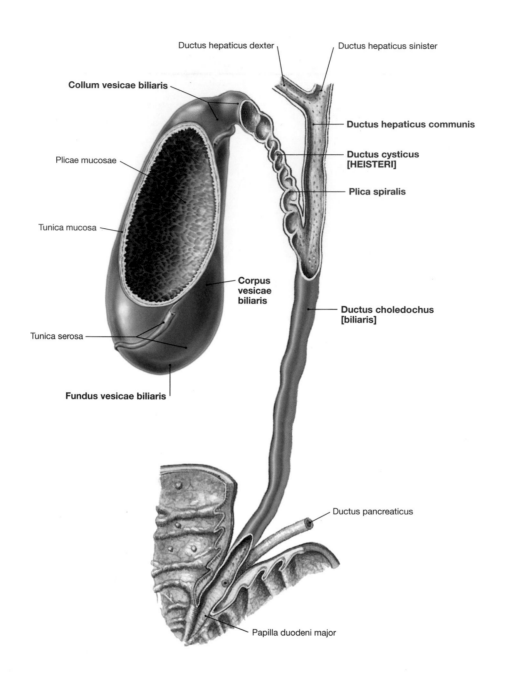

Ductus hepaticus dexter

Ductus hepaticus sinister

Collum vesicae biliaris

Ductus hepaticus communis

Plicae mucosae

Ductus cysticus [HEISTERI]

Tunica mucosa

Plica spiralis

Corpus vesicae biliaris

Ductus choledochus [biliaris]

Tunica serosa

Fundus vesicae biliaris

Ductus pancreaticus

Papilla duodeni major

Fig. 6.108   Gallbladder, Vesica biliaris, and extrahepatic bile ducts; ventral view. [S700-L238]
The gallbladder usually holds approximately 40–70 ml of bile. It consists of a **body (Corpus vesicae biliaris)** with a fundus and a **neck section (Collum vesicae biliaris).** At the terminal end of the neck is the **excre-** tory cystic duct **(Ductus cysticus),** which is closed by a **spiral fold (Plica spiralis HEISTERI),** before fusing with the common hepatic duct (Ductus hepaticus communis) to form the common bile duct (Ductus choledochus).

Clinical remarks

Inflammation of the gallbladder (cholecystitis) is a serious condition because the infection can quickly spread via the blood and cause a life-threatening **sepsis.** According to current recommendations, the therapy of choice is the surgical removal of the gallbladder **(chol-** **ecystectomy)** within 24 hours of diagnosis. This surgery is performed laparoscopically and opening the abdominal wall is thus avoided. As this intervention is frequently performed, we give all the necessary information in this part of the chapter!

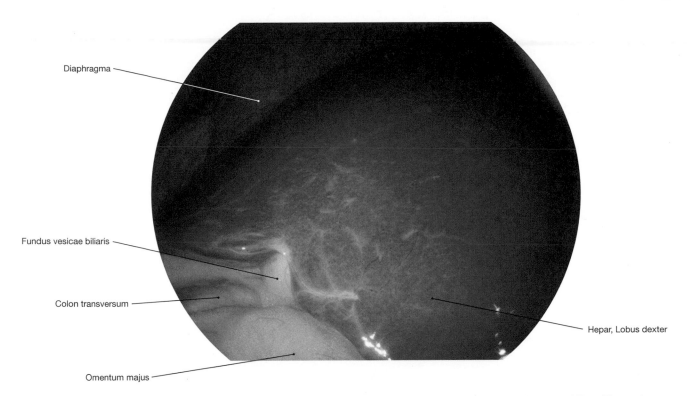

Diaphragma

Fundus vesicae biliaris

Colon transversum

Omentum majus

Hepar, Lobus dexter

Fig. 6.109   Gallbladder, Vesica biliaris, and liver, Hepar; laparoscopy; oblique caudal view from the left side. [S700-T894]

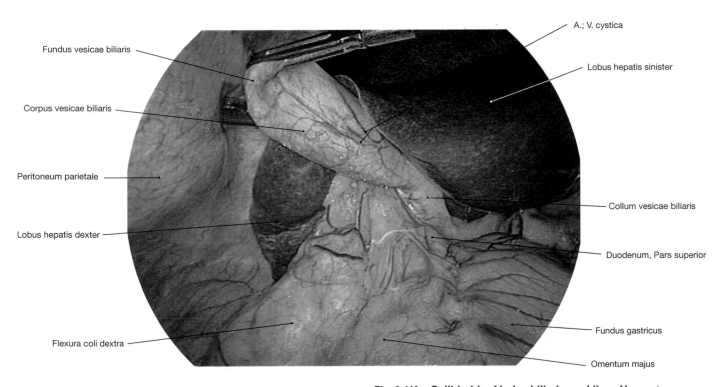

Fundus vesicae biliaris

Corpus vesicae biliaris

Peritoneum parietale

Lobus hepatis dexter

Flexura coli dextra

A.; V. cystica

Lobus hepatis sinister

Collum vesicae biliaris

Duodenum, Pars superior

Fundus gastricus

Omentum majus

Fig. 6.110   Gallbladder, Vesica biliaris, and liver, Hepar; laparoscopy; ventral view. [S700-T894]

Clinical remarks

A **laparoscopy** enables the diagnostic imaging and resection of the gallbladder, without the need for any surgical opening of the abdominal wall. Using a laparoscope and one or two additional entrance ports for light sources, camera, or biopsy instruments, the entire abdominal cavity can be inspected. A further indication for a laparosco-py is the assessment of the liver for a targeted biopsy. If imaging methods (→ Fig. 6.104, → Fig. 6.105) and the blind liver puncture (→ Fig. 6.106, → Fig. 6.107) are not successful, laparoscopically targeted biopsies can be taken.

Liver and gallbladder

Extrahepatic bile ducts

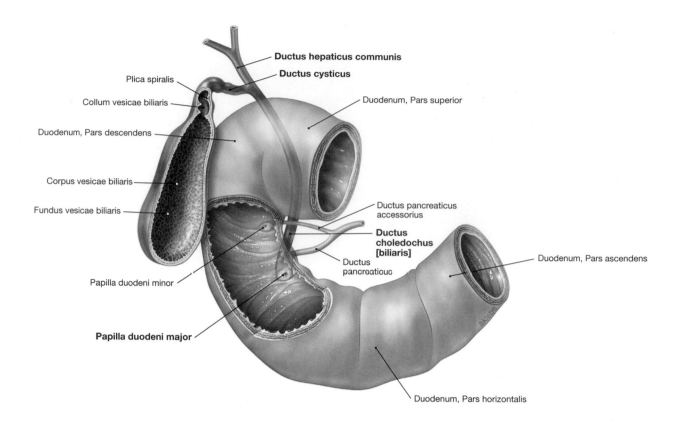

Fig. 6.111   Gallbladder, Vesica biliaris, extrahepatic bile ducts and duodenum; ventral view. [S700-L238]/[G1060-002]
The Ductus hepaticus communis is formed in the liver by unifying two regional bile ducts (Ductus hepatici dexter and sinister). It receives the **Ductus cysticus** of the gallbladder in the Lig. hepatoduodenale, transitioning into the Ductus choledochus. The Ductus cysticus is about 3 mm wide and 2–4 cm long.

The **Ductus choledochus** is usually 6 cm long and 0.4–0.9 cm in diameter. It firstly runs ventrally of the portal vein in the Lig. hepatoduodenale, then behind the superior part of the duodenum to reach the Pars descendens of the duodenum via the head of the pancreas. It usually connects with the Ductus pancreaticus and culminates in a small mucosal papilla, **Papilla duodeni major (Papilla VATERI).**

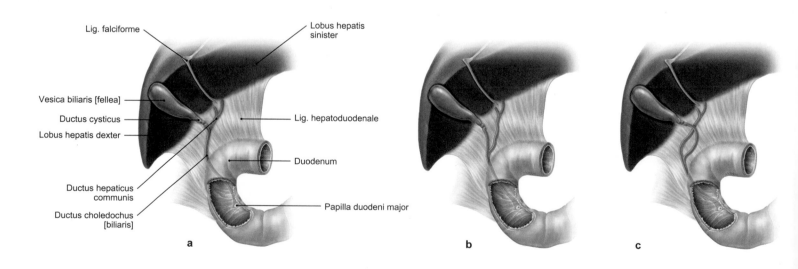

Fig. 6.112a–c   Variants of bile ducts with the merging of the Ductus hepaticus communis and Ductus cysticus. [S700-L238]

a High junction.
b Low junction.
c Low junction with a crossover.

Clinical remarks

The variability of the bile ducts must be borne in mind for the diagnosis and treatment of **gallstones (cholecystolithiasis)** and during the surgical **removal of the gallbladder (cholecystectomy).** For diagnostic evaluation, endoscopic X-ray contrast imaging (endoscopic retrograde cholangiopancreatography, ERCP) is often used. A Ductus choledochus with an extended diameter beyond 1 cm is suggestive of **cholestasis.**

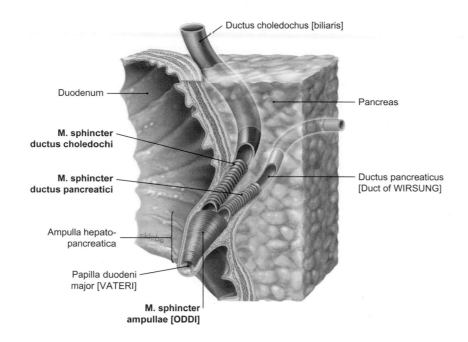

Ductus choledochus [biliaris]

Duodenum

Pancreas

M. sphincter ductus choledochi

M. sphincter ductus pancreatici

Ductus pancreaticus [Duct of WIRSUNG]

Ampulla hepato-pancreatica

Papilla duodeni major [VATERI]

M. sphincter ampullae [ODDI]

Fig. 6.113   Ampulla hepatopancreatica at the junction of the Ductus choledochus and Ductus pancreaticus; semi-schematic illustration; ventral view. [S700-L238]/[(B500~M282/L132)/H230-001]
Typically (in 60 % of cases) the Ductus choledochus joins with the Ductus pancreaticus to the **Ampulla hepatopancreatica,** which flows into the duodenum at the **Papilla duodeni major (Papilla VATERI).** The papilla is 8–10 cm away from the pylorus of the stomach and is located in the dorsomedial wall in the middle third of the Pars descendens of the duodenum.

On the Papilla duodeni major, underneath the mucous membrane, there is a sphincter system. The smooth muscles of the excretory ducts continue on the ampulla. The circular muscle fibres of the Ductus choledochus form a smooth M. sphincter ductus choledochi. Correspondingly, there is a M. sphincter ductus pancreatici. The distal sections of the sphincters include the ampulla and its junction as the **M. sphincter ampullae (ODDI).**

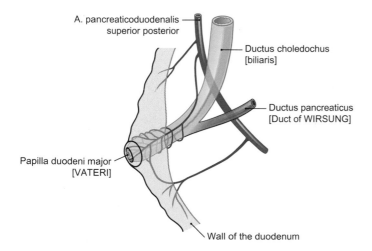

A. pancreaticoduodenalis superior posterior

Ductus choledochus [biliaris]

Ductus pancreaticus [Duct of WIRSUNG]

Papilla duodeni major [VATERI]

Wall of the duodenum

Fig. 6.114   Arterial blood supply of the Ampulla hepatopancreatica and the Ductus choledochus; schematic drawing; ventral view. [S700-L126]/[G1069]
The Ductus choledochus is supplied by fine branches of the **A. cystica** and the R. dexter of the **A. hepatica propria** as well as by ascending branches of the **A. gastroduodenalis.** The distal third of the Ductus choledochus, including the Ampulla hepatopancreatica, receives blood from the **A. pancreaticoduodenalis superior posterior.**

Clinical remarks

The common terminal path of the Ductus choledochus and Ductus pancreaticus is clinically highly relevant. **Gallstones** from the gallbladder **(cholecystolithiasis)** can spontaneously exit and obstruct the Papilla duodeni major. This can lead to a **backflow of bile (cholestasis),** which is most commonly associated with a painful swelling of the gallbladder. The fundus of the gallbladder projects onto the ninth rib on the right side. Due to deposits of the bile pigment bilirubin in the connective tissue, there is a yellowing of the sclera of the eye and skin **(jaundice).** In this case, the gallstone must be removed endoscopically. Due to the good blood supply in the area of the Papilla duodeni major, strong bleeding may occur. In the case of cholestasis, a **pancreatic cancer** in the area of the pancreatic head should also always be excluded. Here the enlargement of the gallbladder is not associated with inflammation and is therefore mostly painless.

CALOT's triangle

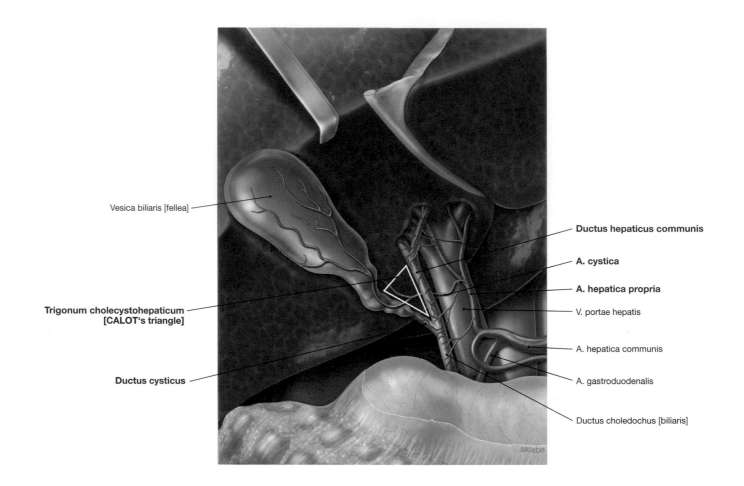

Vesica biliaris [fellea]

Trigonum cholecystohepaticum
[CALOT's triangle]

Ductus cysticus

Ductus hepaticus communis

A. cystica

A. hepatica propria

V. portae hepatis

A. hepatica communis

A. gastroduodenalis

Ductus choledochus [biliaris]

Fig. 6.115 CALOT's triangle, Trigonum cholecystohepaticum; caudal view. [S700-L238]/[S124]
The Ductus cysticus, the Ductus hepaticus communis, and the inferior area of the liver together form the **Trigonum cholecystohepaticum,** also referred to as **CALOT's triangle.** In 75 % of all cases, the A. cystica originates in the area of this triangle from the R. dexter of the A. hepatica propria and runs posteriorly through this triangle to reach the Ductus cysticus and the neck of the gallbladder.

Boundaries of CALOT's triangle	
Directions	**Bordering structure**
Cranial	Inferior margin of the liver
Right	Ductus cysticus
Left	Ductus hepaticus communis

Clinical remarks

If gallstones repeatedly lead to an **inflammation of the gallbladder (cholecystitis),** it is usually indicated to surgically remove the **gallbladder (cholecystectomy). CALOT's triangle** is an important landmark with the surgical removal of the gallbladder. Prior to removal of the gallbladder, all structures are identified before the A. cystica and the Ductus cysticus are ligated. This way, the risk of an accidental ligation of the Ductus choledochus with subsequent backflow of the bile (cholestasis) is reduced.

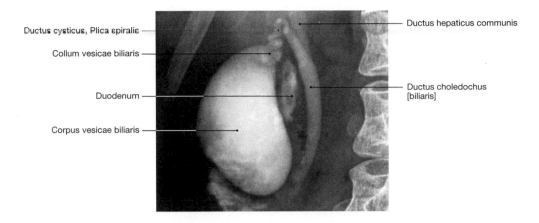

Ductus cysticus, Plica spiralis

Collum vesicae biliaris

Duodenum

Corpus vesicae biliaris

Ductus hepaticus communis

Ductus choledochus [biliaris]

Fig. 6.116   Gallbladder, Vesica biliaris, and extrahepatic bile ducts;
X-ray in anteroposterior (AP) projection after application of contrast
agent; patient in upright position; ventral view. [S700]

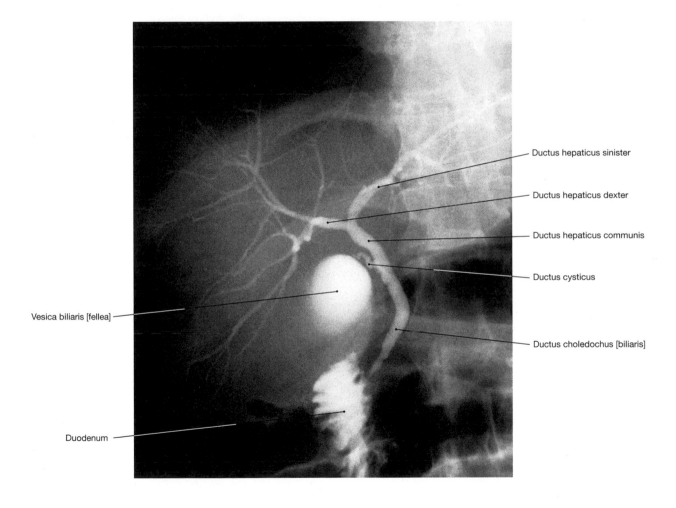

Ductus hepaticus sinister

Ductus hepaticus dexter

Ductus hepaticus communis

Ductus cysticus

Vesica biliaris [fellea]

Ductus choledochus [biliaris]

Duodenum

Fig. 6.117   Gallbladder, Vesica biliaris, as well as intra- and extra-hepatic bile ducts; X-ray in anteroposterior (AP) projection after appli-cation of contrast agent; patient in upright position; ventral view. [S700]

Clinical remarks

Radiography after intravenous application of contrast agent allows the visualisation of the gallbladder and bile ducts, including the detection of noncalcified gallstones. Malignant tumours of the bile ducts (cholangiocarcinoma) or the pancreas (pancreatic carcinoma) may cause cholestasis which appears as dilation of the bile ducts.

Projection of the pancreas

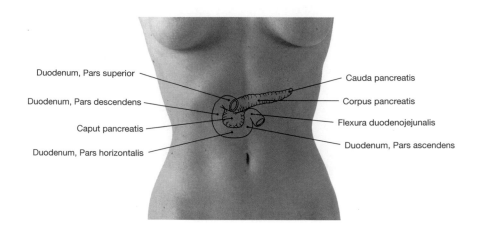

Fig. 6.118   Projection of the pancreas and duodenum onto the ventral trunk wall. [S700]
The pancreas is in a **secondary retroperitoneal** position and projects approximately onto the first to second lumbar vertebrae. The head (Caput pancreatis) is adjacent to the Pars descendens of the duodenum and continues as the body of the pancreas (Corpus pancreatis), which crosses the spine to continue as the tail of the pancreas (Cauda pancreatis), which then reaches up to the hilum of the spleen.

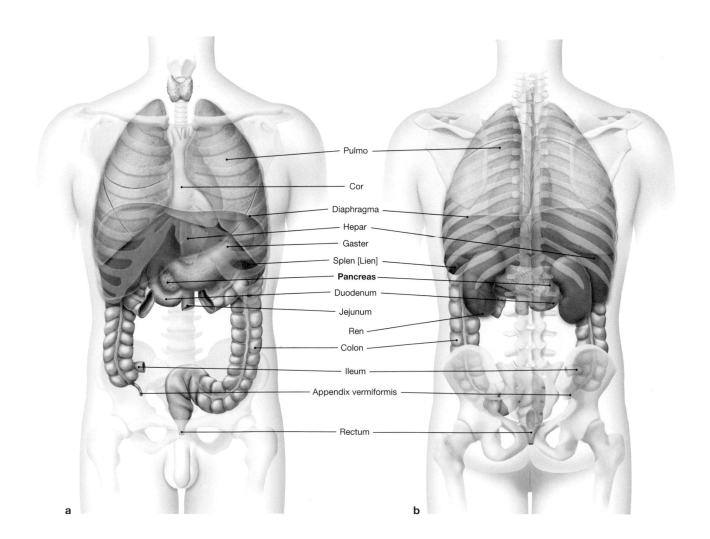

a

b

Fig. 6.119a and b   Projection of inner organs onto the body surface. [S700-L275]

a Ventral view.
b Dorsal view.

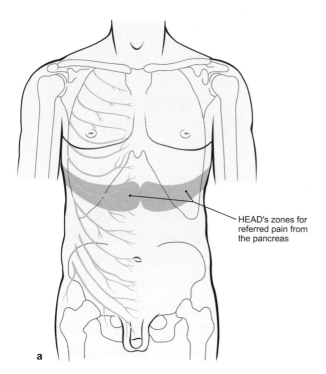

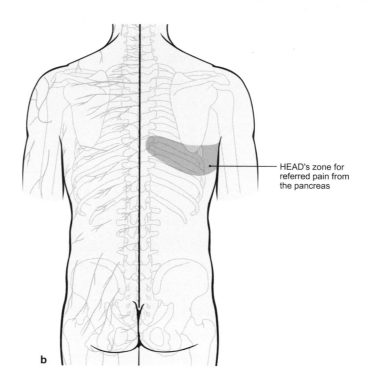

HEAD's zones for referred pain from the pancreas

HEAD's zone for referred pain from the pancreas

Fig. 6.120a and b   HEAD's zone of the pancreas, schematic drawing. [S700-L126]/[G1071]
a Ventral view.
b Dorsal view.
The organ-related area or the **HEAD's zone** of the pancreas is usually not exactly localised. If pain occurs in a defined area, in diseases of the pancreas, it is often projected into the **T8 dermatome** (cutaneous area). This is because in the corresponding spinal cord segment, afferent neurons from the pancreas converge with those of the body surface, so that in cases of (mostly inflammatory) diseases of the pancreas, pain is perceived on the body surface in the T8 dermatome. We therefore talk about referred pain. A special feature of the pancreas is that the pain is also projected dorsally onto the same dermatome due to the retroperitoneal position of the organ.

Clinical remarks

Inflammation of the pancreas (pancreatitis) is most commonly related to a gallstone blocking the papillae and causing a backflow of pancreatic secretions or with alcohol abuse. It is typically associated with belt-like radiating pain.

Pancreatic carcinomas may cause pain radiating to the back. The retroperitoneal position of the pancreas allows infiltrative tumour growth to aortic autonomic nerve plexuses (Plexus aorticus abdominalis). This should be considered with presentation of back pain.

Development

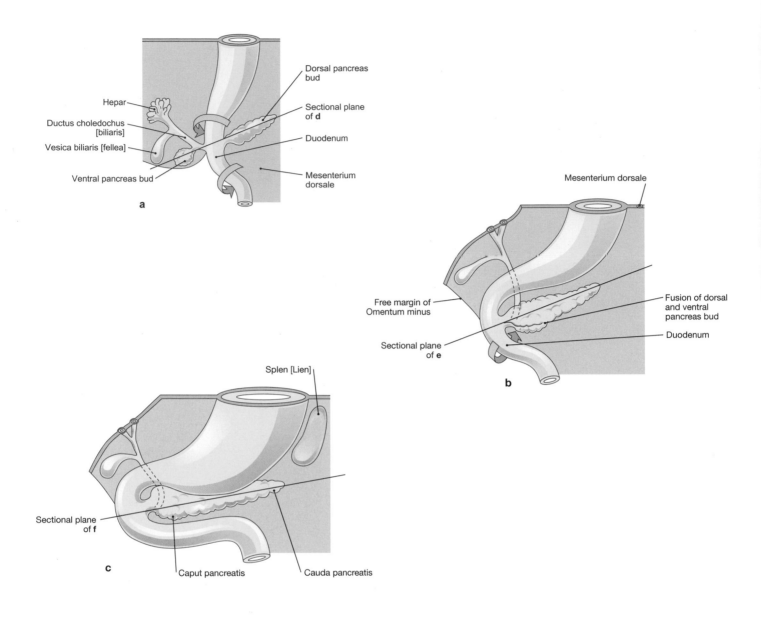

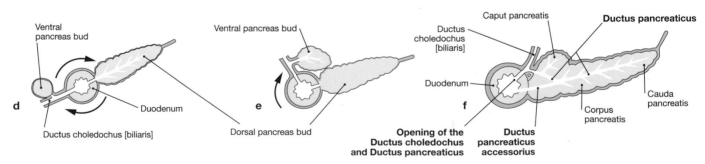

Fig. 6.121a–f Developmental stages of the pancreas in the fifth to eighth week. [E347-09]

a–c Ventral view

d–f Schematic cross-sections through the duodenum and pancreatic system: rotations marked by arrows.

On the 28th day, a ventral and a dorsal pancreatic bud emerge from the entoderm of the foregut **(a, d)**, inferior to the primordium of the liver and gallbladder at the level of the duodenum. The ventral pancreatic bud

folds dorsally **(b, e)** and fuses, together with the excretory ducts, with the dorsal pancreatic bud **(c, f)** in the sixth–seventh week.

The excretory duct of the pancreas is formed by the union of the distal dorsal Ductus pancreaticus and the ventral Ductus pancreaticus and enters the Papilla duodeni major. The proximal portion of the dorsal Ductus pancreaticus develops (in 6 % of all cases) into the Ductus pancreaticus accessorius which joins the duodenum at the Papilla duodeni minor.

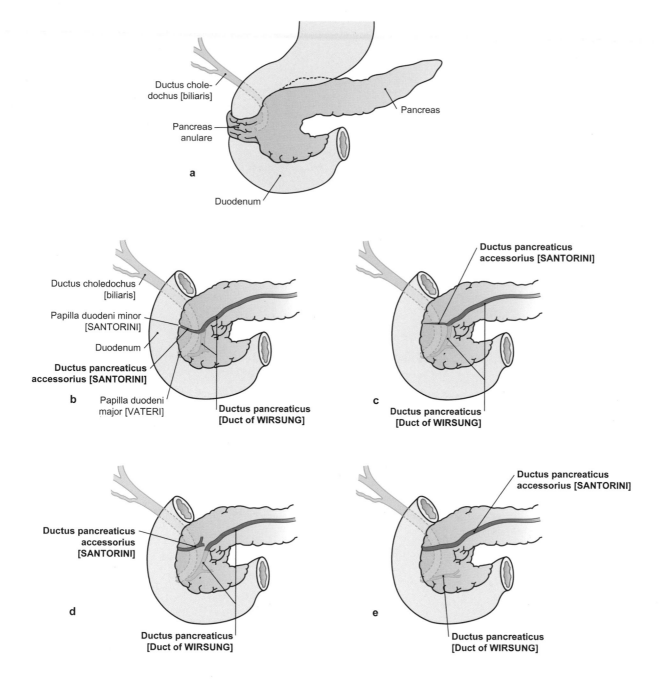

Fig. 6.122a–e Malformations of pancreatic development; schematic illustration, ventral view. [S700-L126]/[G1069]
a A ring-shaped formation of the pancreas system around the descending part of the duodenum **(Pancreas anulare),** which can lead to passage disorders of the food bolus.

b and **c** Normal union of the pancreatic ducts, whereby the Ductus pancreaticus accessorius (in b) is stenosed at its opening into the duodenum.
d and **e** Incomplete union of the excretory ducts **(Pancreas divisum)** with the Ductus pancreaticus and Ductus pancreaticus accessorius remaining separate, independently discharging into the duodenum.

Clinical remarks

If the pancreatic parenchyma grows as a circular gland around the duodenum **(Pancreas anulare),** an ileus with vomiting may occur which is particularly evident in newborns. The symptoms often occur only when switching from milk to solid foods. In this case, the duodenum has to be severed and sewn back into place next to the pancreatic duct system.

If the fusion of both pancreatic buds is incomplete **(Pancreas divisum),** the dorsal Ductus pancreaticus may constitute the main excretory duct (10 % of all cases) which may cause repetitive pancrea-

titis due to a stasis of secretions. In cases of recurring inflammation, a diagnosis of a Pancreas divisum needs to be considered after ruling out gallstones and alcohol abuse as the cause.

If the fusion of the two Ductus pancreatici does not take place, an obstruction of the Papilla duodeni major by a **gallstone (cholelithiasis)** may stop the flow of pancreatic secretions via the Papilla duodeni minor. With a Pancreas divisum – in addition to the **bile backflow (cholestasis)** – the pancreas may also become severely inflamed **(pancreatitis).**

Structure and topographical relationships of the pancreas

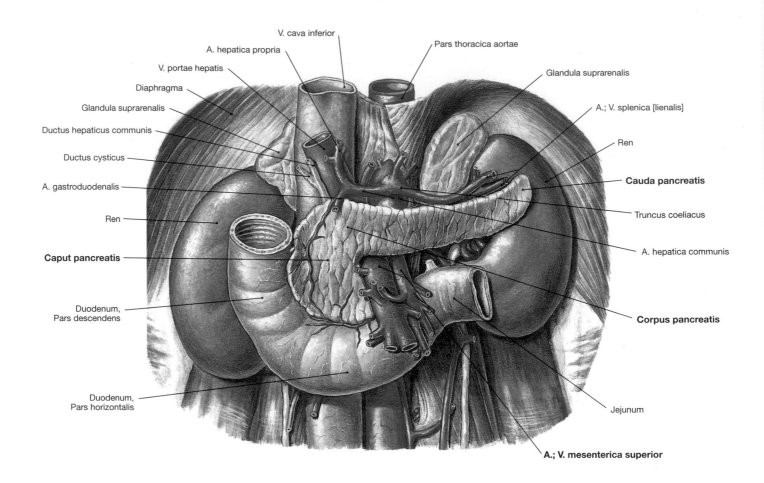

V. cava inferior

A. hepatica propria

V. portae hepatis

Diaphragma

Glandula suprarenalis

Ductus hepaticus communis

Ductus cysticus

A. gastroduodenalis

Ren

Caput pancreatis

Duodenum, Pars descendens

Duodenum, Pars horizontalis

Pars thoracica aortae

Glandula suprarenalis

A.; V. splenica [lienalis]

Ren

Cauda pancreatis

Truncus coeliacus

A. hepatica communis

Corpus pancreatis

Jejunum

A.; V. mesenterica superior

Fig. 6.123   Retroperitoneal organs of the epigastrium: pancreas, duodenum and, on both sides, the kidney, Ren, and adrenal gland, Glandula suprarenalis; ventral view. [S700]

The pancreas is in a **secondary retroperitoneal** position. The head of the pancreas **(Caput pancreatis)** lies on the descending part of the duodenum and has a dorsal uncinate process **(Proc. uncinatus),** which comprises the A. and V. mesenterica superior. The horizontal part of the duodenum is positioned caudally.

To the left side, the head of the pancreas continues above a short (1.5–2 cm) neck **(Collum pancreatis),** ventral to the A./V. mesenterica superior in the body **(Corpus pancreatis),** which crosses the spine. The subsequent tail of the pancreas **(Cauda pancreatis)** passes on the dor-

sal side of the left colonic flexure in front of the left kidney and extends to the hilum of the spleen.

The pancreas has an anterior and a posterior surface (Facies anterior and Facies posterior), which are separated from each other by the blunt upper and lower margins (Margo superior and Margo inferior). The anterior aspect of the pancreas is covered by the parietal peritoneum and forms the posterior wall of the Bursa omentalis. The posterior aspect of the pancreas is fused to the original parietal peritoneum of the posterior abdominal wall, because the pancreas was repositioned into the retroperitoneal space during its development. The fusion area presents during dissection as fascia (TOLDT's fascia, → Fig. 6.20).

Clinical remarks

The close positional relationships of the head of the pancreas, the A./V. mesenterica superior and the portal vein bears the risk of injury to the vessels during **endoscopic examination of the Papilla duodeni major,** a procedure performed to remove a gallstone or to per-

form contrast-imaging of the bile and pancreatic ducts (ERCP, endoscopic retrograde cholangiopancreatography). In most cases this can only be resolved with emergency surgery.

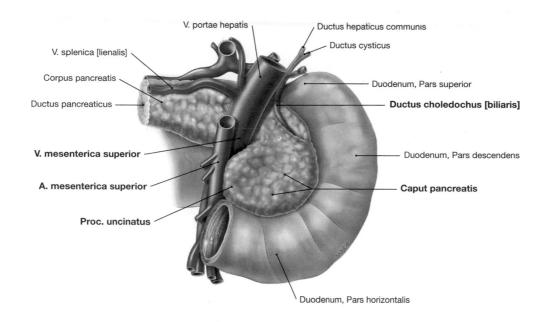

V. portae hepatis
Ductus hepaticus communis
V. splenica [lienalis]
Ductus cysticus
Corpus pancreatis
Duodenum, Pars superior
Ductus pancreaticus
Ductus choledochus [biliaris]
V. mesenterica superior
Duodenum, Pars descendens
A. mesenterica superior
Caput pancreatis
Proc. uncinatus
Duodenum, Pars horizontalis

Fig. 6.124 Pancreas and duodenum; dorsal view. [S700-L238]
The figure illustrates the **Caput pancreatis** located in the C-shaped descending part of the duodenum where it is obliquely pierced by the common bile duct (Ductus choledochus) on its pathway to the Papilla duodeni major. Dorsally, the uncinate process **(Proc. uncinatus)** of the pancreatic head comprises the A./V. mesenterica superior.

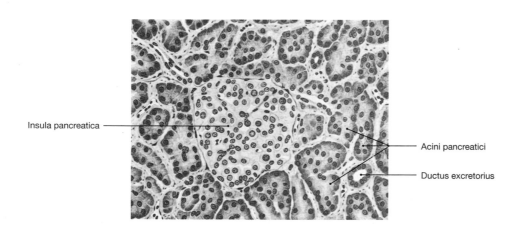

Insula pancreatica
Acini pancreatici
Ductus excretorius

Fig. 6.125 Structure of the pancreas; microscopic view. [R252]
The pancreas is a mixed exocrine and endocrine gland. The **exocrine** part uses its tail end (acini) to produce digestive enzymes which are provided as precursors via the system of ducts into the intestinal lumen. The **endocrine** part form the islets of LANGERHANS (Insulae pan-creaticae) which are embedded in the parenchyma of the exocrine part, especially in the tail of the pancreas. Besides other hormones, the islets produce insulin and glucagon, which are secreted into the blood and serve to regulate the blood glucose level.

Clinical remarks

The function of the pancreas explains why destructive tissue damage (necrosis), e.g. with inflammation **(pancreatitis),** can cause **indigestion,** diarrhoea and in cases of very extensive damage (loss of 80–90 % of the tissue), **diabetes mellitus,** due to insufficient insulin production.

Pancreas

Excretory ducts of the pancreas

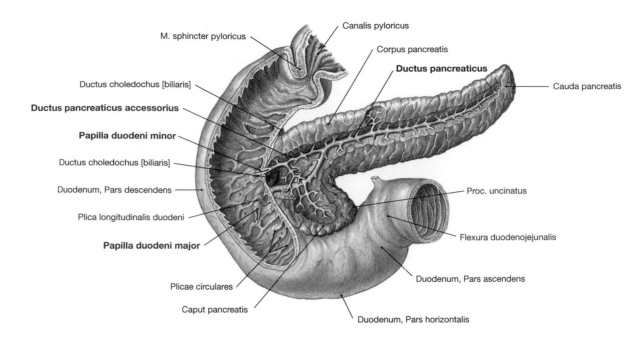

M. sphincter pyloricus

Canalis pyloricus

Corpus pancreatis

Ductus pancreaticus

Ductus choledochus [biliaris]

Ductus pancreaticus accessorius

Papilla duodeni minor

Ductus choledochus [biliaris]

Duodenum, Pars descendens

Plica longitudinalis duodeni

Papilla duodeni major

Plicae circulares

Caput pancreatis

Cauda pancreatis

Proc. uncinatus

Flexura duodenojejunalis

Duodenum, Pars ascendens

Duodenum, Pars horizontalis

Fig. 6.126 Excretory duct system of the pancreas; ventral view; Ductus pancreaticus after partial resection of the pancreas and duodenum. [S700]
The main **excretory duct (Ductus pancreaticus [Duct of WIRSUNG])** fuses with the terminal segment of the Ductus choledochus in 60 % of all cases to form the **Ampulla hepatopancreatica** which then flows via the Papilla duodeni major (Papilla VATERI) into the Pars descendens of the duodenum. Developmentally (→ Fig. 6.121), an accessory duct **(Ductus pancreaticus accessorius [Ductus SANTORINI])** exists in 65 % of all cases opening separately on the duodenum 2 cm proximal to the Papilla duodeni major.

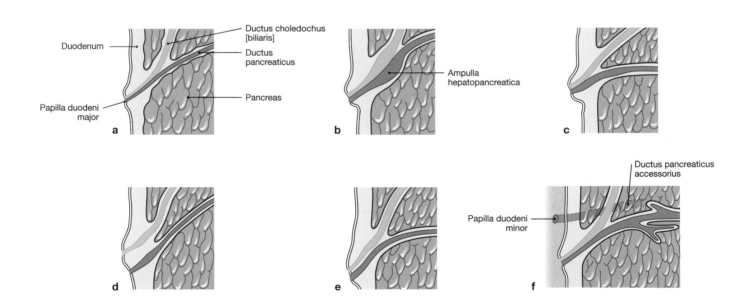

Duodenum

Ductus choledochus [biliaris]

Ductus pancreaticus

Pancreas

Papilla duodeni major

a

Ampulla hepatopancreatica

b

c

d

e

Ductus pancreaticus accessorius

Papilla duodeni minor

f

Fig. 6.127a–f Variants of the junction of the Ductus pancreaticus and Ductus choledochus. [S700-L126]
a Long common portion.
b Ampullary dilation of the terminal part (60 % of all cases), → Fig. 6.113.
c Short common portion.
d Separate openings.
e Unified opening with septation of the common duct.
f Additional duct (Ductus pancreaticus accessorius, in 65 % of all cases).

Clinical remarks

The variation in the fusion of the excretory ducts has an impact on the **progression of pancreatic diseases.** In addition to alcohol abuse, damage to the Papilla duodeni major by gallstones is the most common cause of inflammation of the pancreas (pancreatitis), which is caused by a backflow of secretions with autodigestion. A Ductus pancreaticus accessorius with a separate opening can then prove to be useful when it communicates with the main duct, enabling an outflow of the digestive secretions.

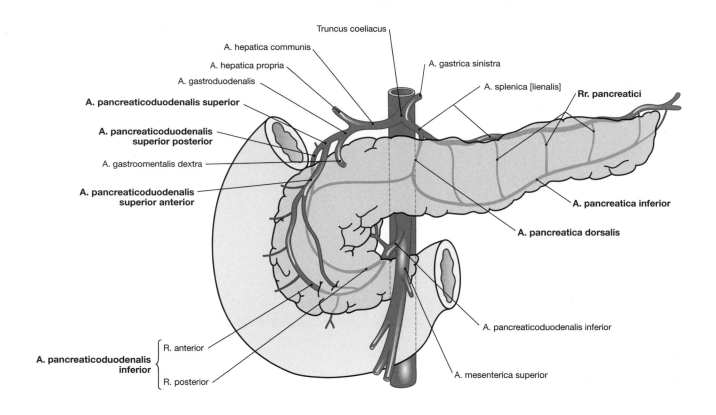

Truncus coeliacus

A. hepatica communis

A. hepatica propria

A. gastroduodenalis

A. gastrica sinistra

A. pancreaticoduodenalis superior

A. splenica [lienalis]

Rr. pancreatici

A. pancreaticoduodenalis superior posterior

A. gastroomentalis dextra

A. pancreaticoduodenalis superior anterior

A. pancreatica inferior

A. pancreatica dorsalis

A. pancreaticoduodenalis inferior

A. pancreaticoduodenalis inferior { R. anterior / R. posterior }

A. mesenterica superior

Fig. 6.128 Arteries of the pancreas; schematic illustration, ventral view. [S700-L126]/[G1069]

The pancreas is supplied by **two separate arterial systems,** for the pancreatic head and for the pancreatic body and tail areas, respectively.

- **Head and collum:** double arterial arches from the Aa. pancreaticoduodenales superiores anterior and posterior (from the A. gastroduodenalis) and from the A. pancreaticoduodenalis inferior with a R. anterior and a R. posterior (from the A. mesenterica superior). Thus its supply is ensured from the drainage areas of the Truncus coeliacus and A. mesenterica superior.

- **Body and tail:** Rr. pancreatici from the A. splenica, which form the A. pancreatica dorsalis behind the pancreas and the A. pancreatica inferior at the inferior border of the gland. The A. pancreatica inferior is usually connected with the posterior vascular arcades of the pancreatic head, so that there is a marked redundancy of the supply.

The **veins** of the pancreas correspond to the arteries and drain via the V. mesenterica superior and the V. splenica into the V. portae hepatis (→ Fig. 6.100).

Arteries of the pancreas	
Supply area	**Arteries**
Caput pancreatis, Collum pancreatis	- A. pancreaticoduodenalis superior (provided by the A. gastroduodenalis, drainage via the Truncus coeliacus) - A. pancreaticoduodenalis inferior (provided by the A. mesenterica superior)
Corpus pancreatis, Cauda pancreatis	Rr. pancreatici of the A. splenica

Clinical remarks

This **substantial arterial blood supply** via two arteries of the Truncus coeliacus and additionally by the A. mesenterica superior explains why infarctions of this vital gland are rare.

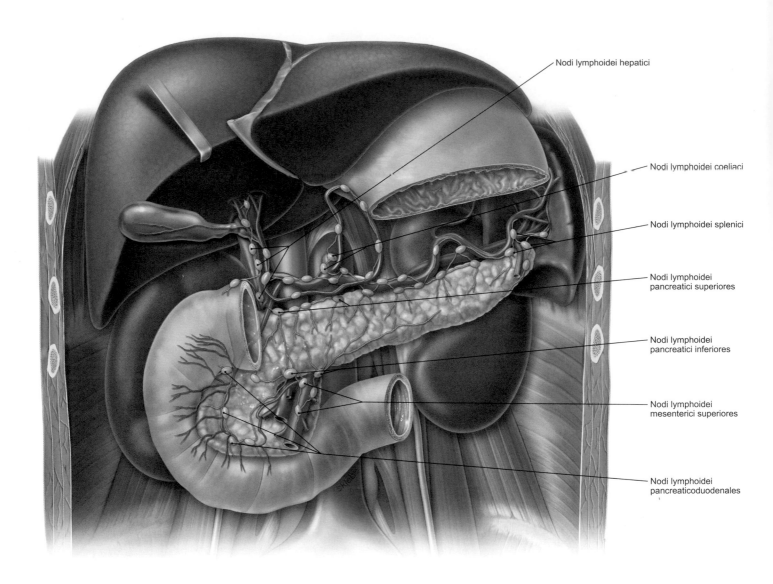

Nodi lymphoidei hepatici

Nodi lymphoidei coeliaci

Nodi lymphoidei splenici

Nodi lymphoidei pancreatici superiores

Nodi lymphoidei pancreatici inferiores

Nodi lymphoidei mesenterici superiores

Nodi lymphoidei pancreaticoduodenales

Fig. 6.129 Lymph vessels and lymph nodes of the pancreas; ventral view. [S700-L238]

The different parts of the pancreas have separate regional lymph nodes:
* **Head and collum: Nodi lymphoidei pancreaticoduodenales anteriores and posteriores** along the eponymous arteries (Aa. pancreaticoduodenales superiores anterior and posterior)

* **Body: Nodi lymphoidei pancreatici superiores and inferiores** along the A. and V. splenica
* **Tail:** Nodi lymphoidei splenici.

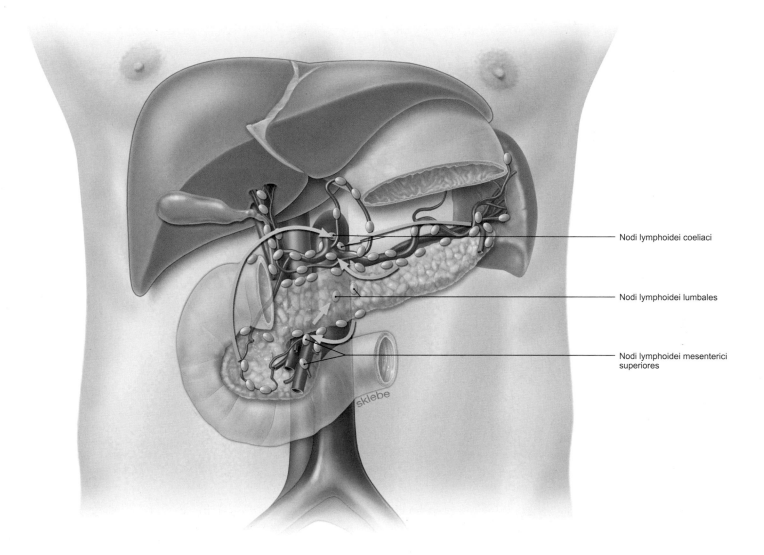

Nodi lymphoidei coeliaci

Nodi lymphoidei lumbales

Nodi lymphoidei mesenterici superiores

Fig. 6.130 Lymphatic drainage of the pancreas; ventral view. [S700-L238]
The regional groups of lymph nodes are strongly connected with each other and with lymph nodes in the surrounding area:
- **Head and collum:** The Nodi lymphoidei pancreaticoduodenales drain via the Nodi lymphoidei hepatici to the **Nodi lymphoidei coeliaci** or directly to the **Nodi lymphoidei mesenterici superiores.** The other connection is made via the **Trunci intestinales** to the Ductus thoracicus.

- **Body and tail:** The regional lymph nodes at the upper edge of the gland are the Nodi lymphoidei pancreatici; conversely, for the tail area, these are the Nodi lymphoidei splenici. These are connected via lymph vessels along the A. and V. splenica to the **Nodi lymphoidei coeliaci.** From the inferior margin of the gland, the Nodi lymphoidei pancreatici are connected to the **Nodi lymphoidei mesenterici superiores.** Due to the retroperitoneal position, there are also connections to the **retroperitoneal Nodi lymphoidei lumbales.** Drainage is then carried out via the **Trunci lumbales.**

Clinical remarks

Based on the various pathways of lymphatic drainage, cases of **pancreatic carcinoma** usually present with extensive **lymph node me-** tastases at the time of diagnosis. Because they cannot be completely removed, curative surgery is seldom achievable.

Innervation of the pancreas

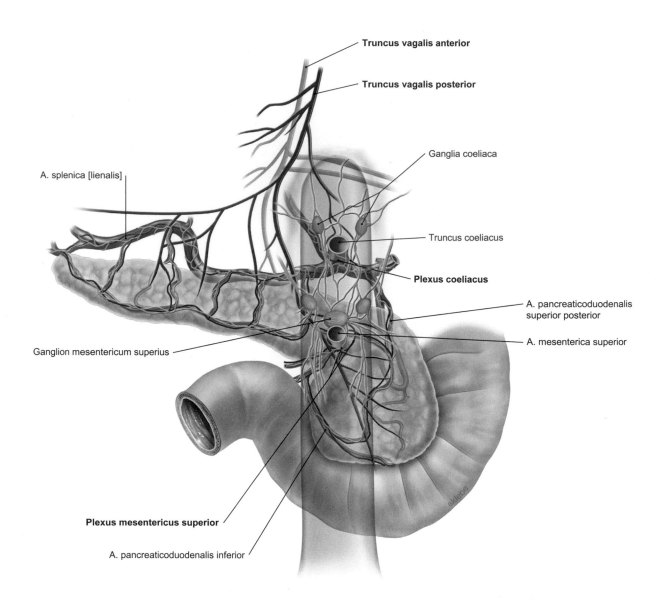

Truncus vagalis anterior

Truncus vagalis posterior

Ganglia coeliaca

A. splenica [lienalis]

Truncus coeliacus

Plexus coeliacus

A. pancreaticoduodenalis
superior posterior

A. mesenterica superior

Ganglion mesentericum superius

Plexus mesentericus superior

A. pancreaticoduodenalis inferior

Fig. 6.131 Autonomic innervation of the pancreas; schematic illustration, dorsal view. [S700-L238]
The pancreas is sympathetically and parasympathetically innervated. The **parasympathicus** promotes the release of the digestive secretions and insulin formation, and the **sympathicus** inhibits these functions. The sympathetic postganglionic neurons and the parasympathetic preganglionic nerve fibres reach the pancreas from the **Plexus coeliacus** predominantly via perivascular plexuses. Particularly for the head area, nerve fibres from the **Truncus vagalis posterior** and occasionally from the **Truncus vagalis anterior** go directly to the gland. Synaptic switching of the parasympathetic fibres is performed by microscopically small ganglia, which are partially embedded in the pancreas.

Clinical remarks

The close proximity of the pancreas to the autonomic nerve plexus on the aorta (Plexus aorticus abdominalis) explains why **pancreatic carcinomas** only become symptomatic after having infiltrated the nerve plexus, which may cause intense **back pain.** It also confers a poor prognosis because complete surgical removal of the tumour is impossible in this case.

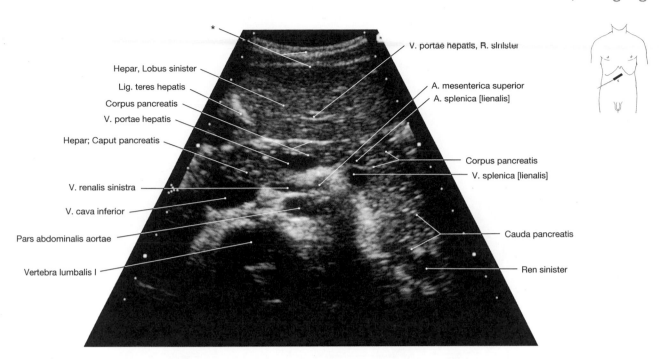

Fig. 6.132 Pancreas; ultrasound image; oblique caudal view; with deep inspiration. [S700-T894]

Ultrasound examination of the pancreas is often unsatisfactory due to its retroperitoneal position, in which the view is often obstructed by the air-filled intestines.

* abdominal wall

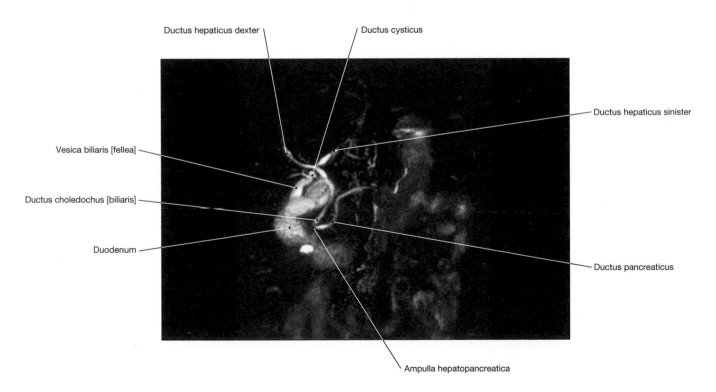

Fig. 6.133 Pancreas and bile ducts; endoscopic retrograde cholangiopancreatography (ERCP); ventral view. [S700-T832]

To visualise the duct systems on an X-ray, the excretory duct of the pancreas and the Ductus choledochus were filled with contrast medium from the Papilla duodeni major via an endoscope.

Clinical remarks

Imaging of the pancreas is often carried out in the first instance by ultrasound examination, e.g. to assess a swelling of the organ possibly indicating pancreatitis. If this is not clear due to impedance from air-filled lungs, computed tomography (CT) becomes necessary. By using ERCP, for example, a Pancreas divisum can be diagnosed as the cause of recurrent pancreatitis. Discontinued ducts may indicate malignant pancreatic tumours.

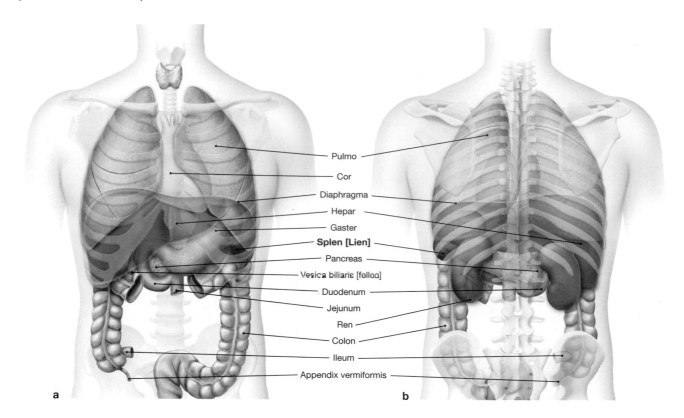

Fig. 6.134a–c   Projection of inner organs onto the body surface.
[S700-L275]
a Ventral view.
b Dorsal view.
c View from the left side.
The spleen is located **intraperitoneally** in the left upper abdomen. Its longitudinal axis projects along the pathway of the 10th rib. Therefore, a normal-sized spleen cannot be palpated under the costal arch. Due to the large contact area with the diaphragm, the position of the spleen is highly dependent on breathing. The spleen lies in the so-called **splenic niche,** which is confined inferiorly by the Lig. phrenicocolicum between the left colonic flexure and the diaphragm (→ Fig. 6.10).

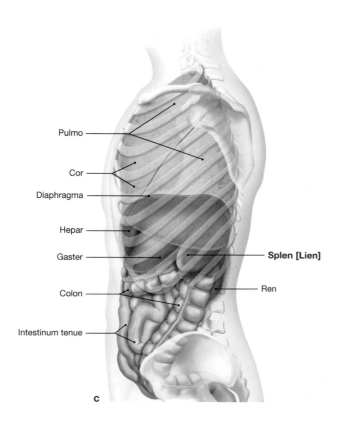

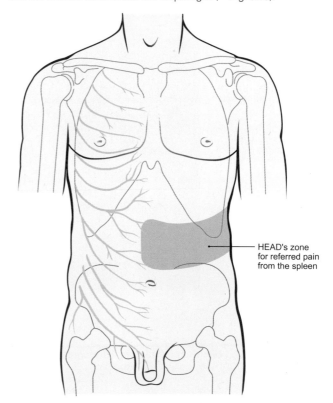

Fig. 6.135   HEAD's zone of the spleen; schematic drawing; ventral view. [S700-L126]/[G1071]
The organ-specific skin area or the **HEAD's zone** of the spleen is not clearly bordered and projects into dermatomes (cutaneous areas) T8–T9 of the left upper abdomen. This is because afferent neurons from the spleen converge with those from the body surface in the corresponding spinal cord segments, so if there is swelling or rupture of the spleen, pain is perceived on the body surface in dermatomes T8 and T9. Hence we talk about referred pain.

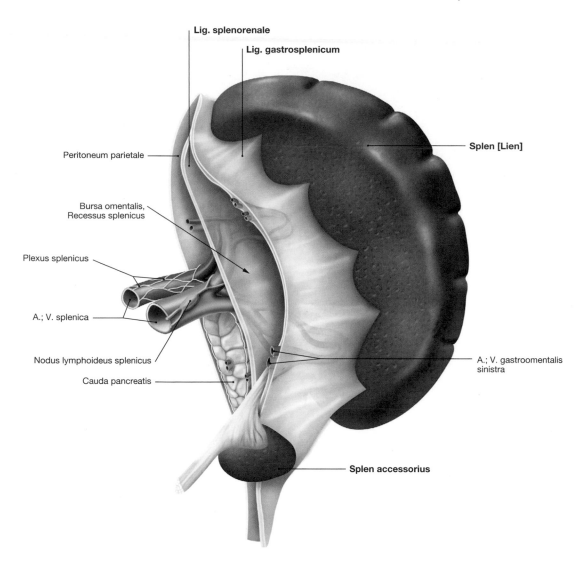

Lig. splenorenale

Lig. gastrosplenicum

Peritoneum parietale

Bursa omentalis,
Recessus splenicus

Plexus splenicus

A.; V. splenica

Nodus lymphoideus splenicus

Cauda pancreatis

Splen [Lien]

A.; V. gastroomentalis
sinistra

Splen accessorius

Fig. 6.136   Peritoneal duplications of the spleen in the Lig. splenorenale; spleen folded back laterally; ventromedial view. [S700-L275]
The spleen is anchored to its surroundings by two **peritoneal duplications,** both of which insert at the Hilum splenicum. Coming from the stomach is the **gastrosplenic ligament,** which then continues as the **Lig.**

splenorenale to the posterior trunk wall. Between these two peritoneal duplications, the Recessus splenicus of the omental bursa extends up to the hilum of the spleen. Posterior to the Lig. splenorenale, and therefore retroperitoneally, the neurovascular pathways (A. splenica with the autonomic Plexus splenicus, V. splenica and the lymph vessels of the Nodi lymphoidei splenici) reach the spleen cranially of the tail of the pancreas.

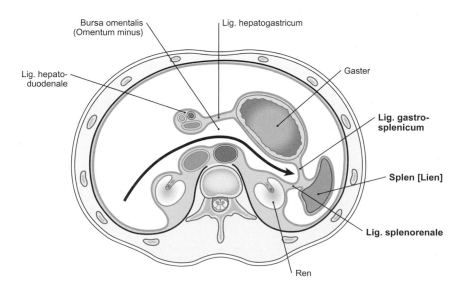

Bursa omentalis
(Omentum minus)

Lig. hepatogastricum

Lig. hepato-
duodenale

Gaster

Lig. gastro-
splenicum

Splen [Lien]

Lig. splenorenale

Ren

Fig. 6.137   Peritoneal duplications of the spleen; schematic drawing of a cross-section; caudal view. [S701-L126]
With its Recessus splenicus, the Bursa omentalis (arrow) reaches the hilum of the spleen. The Recessus splenicus is bordered by the ventral

(Lig. gastrosplenicum) and the dorsal (Lig. splenorenale) peritoneal duplications, which anchor the spleen.

Structure of the spleen

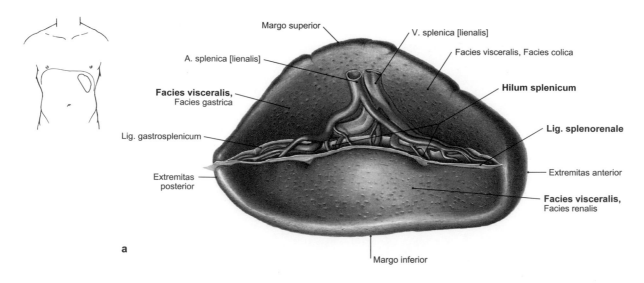

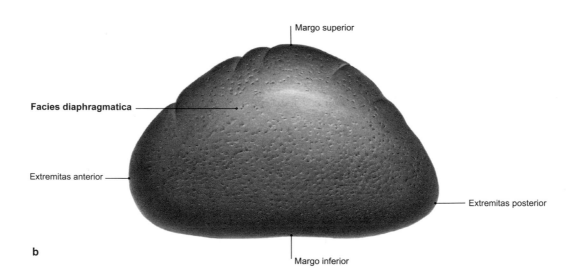

Fig. 6.138a and b   Spleen, Splen [Lien]. [S700]
a Medial ventral view.
b Lateral cranial view.
The spleen is a **secondary lymphatic organ** and plays a role in the immune system as well as in filtering of the blood. It weighs 150 g, is 11 cm long, 7 cm wide and 4 cm deep. It has a convex side, **Facies diaphragmatica,** running along the diaphragm, and a concave side, **Facies** **visceralis,** facing the intestines. This lies adjacent to the left kidney, the left colonic flexure and the stomach. The edge facing upwards (Margo superior) between the two areas is usually notched, while the bottom edge (Margo inferior) is rather smooth. Blood vessels enter and exit through the Hilum splenicum. The branching pattern of the blood vessels results in segmentation of the spleen, which cannot however be outlined on the surface.

Clinical remarks

Since the spleen sits relatively far cranially in the left upper abdomen and projects onto the 10th rib, it is also completely covered by the ribs during inspiration. In the course of pathological alteration, such as a malignant transformation of white blood cells in **leukaemia** or **lymphoma,** as well as in viral infections, such as **infectious mononu-** cleosis ('kissing disease', because asymptomatic carriers transfer it in their saliva), the spleen can become massively enlarged (splenomegaly) and weigh several kilograms, and can then appear as a mass when examining the left upper abdomen.

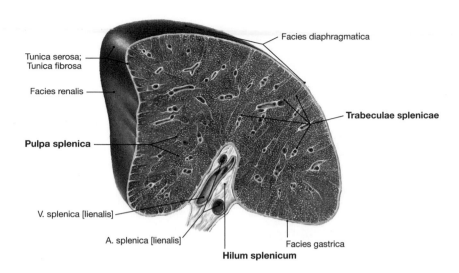

Facies diaphragmatica

Tunica serosa;
Tunica fibrosa

Facies renalis

Trabeculae splenicae

Pulpa splenica

V. splenica [lienalis]

A. splenica [lienalis]

Facies gastrica

Hilum splenicum

Fig. 6.139 Spleen, Splen [Lien]; cross-section through the hilum; medial cranial view. [S700]
The spleen is surrounded by a fixed capsule, from which trabeculations of connective tissue run into the parenchyma (Pulpa splenica). In these trabeculae run larger branches of the A. and V. splenica. The Pulpa splenica consists of the blood-filled **red pulp** and disseminated 'white' nodules which are collectively referred to as **white pulp.** The white pulp contains lymphatic tissue.

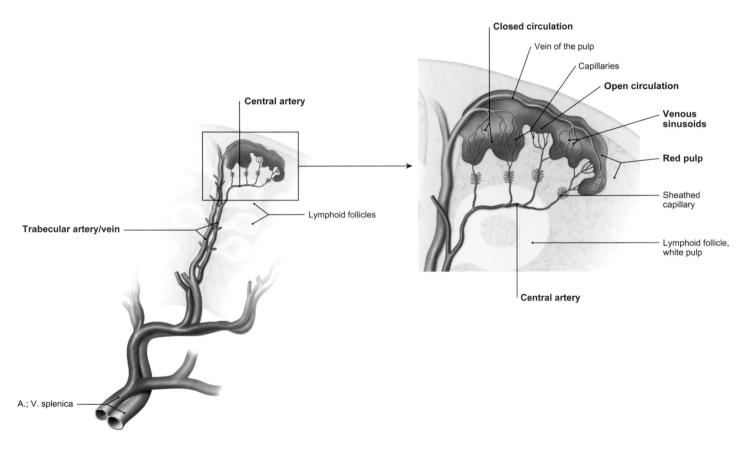

Central artery

Closed circulation

Vein of the pulp

Capillaries

Open circulation

Venous sinusoids

Red pulp

Sheathed capillary

Lymphoid follicles

Trabecular artery/vein

Lymphoid follicle, white pulp

Central artery

A.; V. splenica

Fig. 6.140 Parenchyma and blood vessel system of the spleen; schematic representation. [S700-L275]
The **parenchyma of the spleen (Pulpa splenica)** consists of a basic fibrous framework into which blood from blood vessels of the 'open' circulatory system flows. This **red pulp** helps with the breakdown of red blood cells (erythrocytes) and the storage of platelets (thrombocytes) and, along with the liver, is responsible for the formation of the blood in the fetal period. Stored in the red pulp there are white nodules which are visible microscopically as **white pulp.** Within the white pulp there is lymphatic tissue, which on the one hand forms a lymphatic follicle and on the other hand forms periarterial lymphatic sheaths (PALS).
The pathway and the branching patterns of the blood vessels are functionally and clinically significant: **A. splenica** and **V. splenica** branch off in the hilum, and their branches penetrate through the trabeculae of connective tissue **(trabecular arteries and veins)** into the parenchyma. Since the terminal branches of the A. splenica do not anastomose with each other, they form functional terminal arteries and subdivide the spleen into segments. From the trabecular arteries, vessels branch off surrounded by lymphocytes of the white pulp and are therefore known as **central arteries.** They branch off in a brush-like manner and lead into capillaries. They either terminate as open vessels with the blood flowing into the connective tissue mesh of the red pulp **(open circulation)** or pass directly into **venous sinusoids (closed circulation).** The blood cells, which pass via the open circulation into the red pulp, have to re-enter the circulatory system between the endothelial cells in the wall of the sinusoids. Thus 'old' or pathologically altered red blood cells (erythrocytes) can be intercepted and filtered out. From the sinusoids, the blood passes via the pulp veins back into the trabecular veins and thus to the V. splenica.

Neurovascular pathways of the spleen

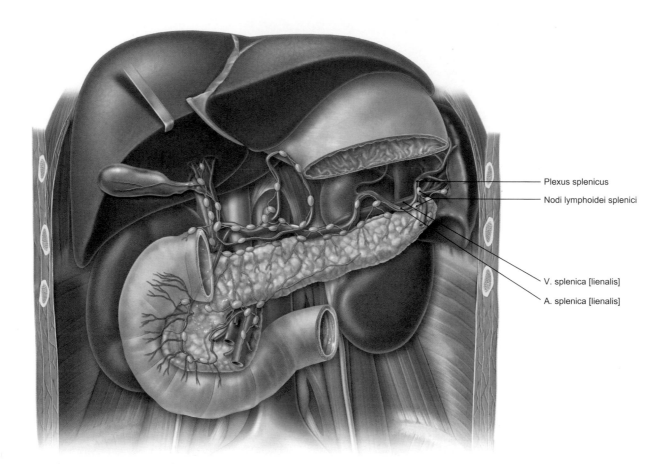

Plexus splenicus

Nodi lymphoidei splenici

V. splenica [lienalis]

A. splenica [lienalis]

Fig. 6.141   Neurovascular pathways of the spleen, Splen [Lien]; ventral view. [S700-L238]

The spleen has its own neurovascular pathways which enter and exit at the hilum. After exiting the Truncus coeliacus, the **A. splenica** turns to the left and passes retroperitoneally at the upper edge of the pancreas to the spleen. In doing so, it is accompanied by autonomic nerve fibres of the **Plexus splenicus** (not shown here, → Fig. 6.136). At the hilum it divides into two to three main branches and then up to six terminal branches. Before branching off, in 30–60 % of cases, it provides a A. gastrica posterior to the posterior side of the stomach. Then at the

hilum, the A. gastroomentalis sinistra and the Aa. gastricae breves branch off to the stomach.

The **V. splenica** usually passes along the dorsal side of the pancreas up to the neck section where it connects to the portal vein with the V. mesenterica superior. In the majority of all cases (70 %), the V. mesenterica inferior is incorporated on the way. The **Nodi lymphoidei splenici** at the hilum are not only the regional lymph nodes for the spleen, but also for the tail of the pancreas and the upper part of the greater curvature of the stomach. They drain via the Nodi lymphoidei coeliaci to the Trunci intestinales.

Clinical remarks

In the case of a surgical **removal of the spleen (splenectomy),** the A. and V. splenica are also removed. Since the spleen can store large quantities of platelets, the formation of **blood clots** must be pre-

vented before surgery to mitigate the increased risk of stroke or heart attack.

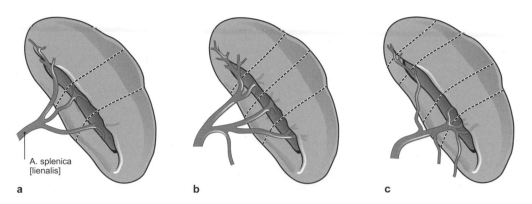

a   b   c

Fig. 6.142a–c   Segments of the spleen, Splen [Lien]; schematic illustration of three, four or five segments; ventral view. [S700-L126]

The terminal branches of the A. splenica are functional terminal arteries and divide the spleen variably in **three to six tapered segments.**

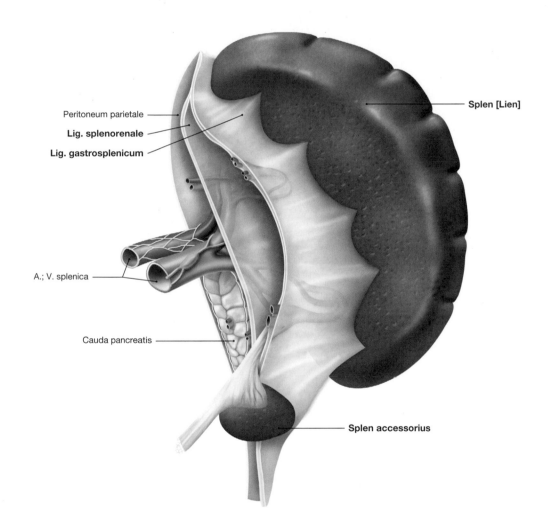

Peritoneum parietale

Lig. splenorenale

Lig. gastrosplenicum

Splen [Lien]

A.; V. splenica

Cauda pancreatis

Splen accessorius

Fig. 6.143   Accessory spleen in the Lig. splenorenale; spleen folded back; ventral view. [S700-L275]

In 5–30 % of cases (< 15 % in large real-world studies), an **accessory spleen** occurs as an independent organ, usually close to the hilum and embedded into one of the peritoneal duplications.

Clinical remarks

Abdominal traumas may cause a **splenic rupture,** which can lead to life-threatening bleeding. Here the spleen segments are significant: in particular, vertical tears which incorporate multiple segments, bleed heavily; conversely, horizontal tears bleed relatively little, since the splenic arteries are functionally terminal arteries. The segmental structure also explains why **infarctions of the spleen** usually expand in a wedge shape between the borders of the segments.

An accessory spleen may be clinically significant after the surgical **removal of the spleen (splenectomy),** and its presence should be noted. If the spleen has to be removed due to a traumatic rupture, the accessory spleen can take on its function and no compromise to the immune system occurs. If a splenectomy is therapeutically indicated, e.g. with anaemia due to genetically modified red blood cells being broken down too quickly, the accessory spleen should also be removed, otherwise the symptoms may persist.

Topography of the epigastric organs with neurovascular pathways

Organs of the abdominal cavity

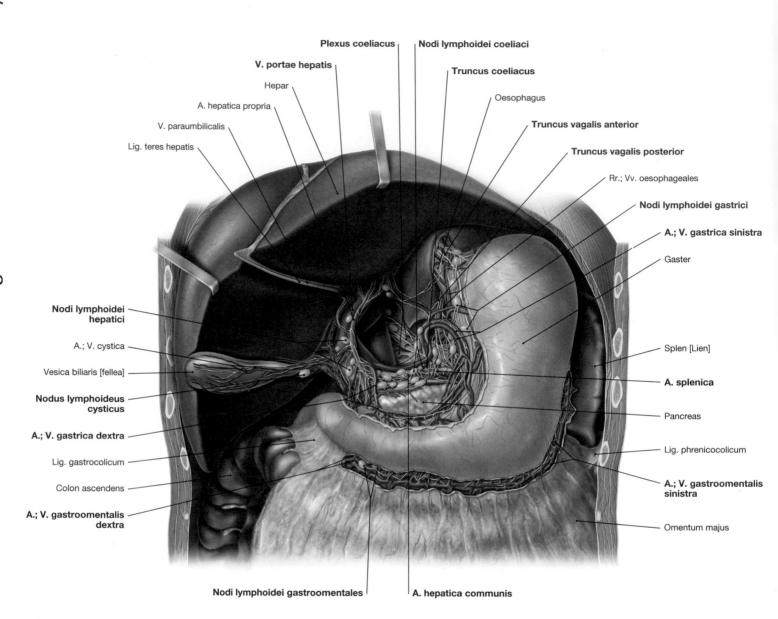

Plexus coeliacus

V. portae hepatis

Hepar

A. hepatica propria

V. paraumbilicalis

Lig. teres hepatis

Nodi lymphoidei coeliaci

Truncus coeliacus

Oesophagus

Truncus vagalis anterior

Truncus vagalis posterior

Rr.; Vv. oesophageales

Nodi lymphoidei gastrici

A.; V. gastrica sinistra

Gaster

Nodi lymphoidei hepatici

A.; V. cystica

Vesica biliaris [fellea]

Nodus lymphoideus cysticus

A.; V. gastrica dextra

Lig. gastrocolicum

Colon ascendens

A.; V. gastroomentalis dextra

Splen [Lien]

A. splenica

Pancreas

Lig. phrenicocolicum

A.; V. gastroomentalis sinistra

Omentum majus

Nodi lymphoidei gastroomentales

A. hepatica communis

Fig. 6.144 Situs of the epigastric organs; the liver has been mobilised upwards, the Omentum minus has been removed and the Lig. gastrocolicum has been cut open to display the neurovascular pathways; ventral view. [S700-L238]/[Q300]

This view is very useful for the dissection of the epigastric organs, as it also shows all their neurovascular pathways. First, the liver has to be mobilised upwards in order to remove the Omentum minus. By doing this, the branches of the **Truncus coeliacus** and the tributaries to the **V. portae hepatis** become visible. The **A. hepatica communis** turns to the right, the **A. splenica** to the left. The **A. gastrica sinistra** turns cranially to reach the lesser curvature of the stomach. Usually it is divided into two trunks and anastomoses with the **A. gastrica dextra.** The accompanying veins drain directly into the portal vein. The fine branches of the A. gastrica sinistra supply the Pars abdominalis of the oesophagus and here, the left lobe of the liver with an additional branch, occurring in 10–20 % of cases. The **Aa./Vv. gastroomentales dextra and sinistra** are connected to the greater curvature of the stomach.

The illustration also shows the lymph vessels and autonomic nerves, which are often not clearly displayed in dissections. On the lesser curvature of the stomach are located the **Nodi lymphoidei gastrici,** of which the collectors are clearly visible where they are connected with the **Nodi lymphoidei coeliaci** at the opening of the Truncus coeliacus. These collecting lymph nodes also drain the **Nodi lymphoidei hepatici** and the **Nodus lymphoideus cysticus** at the neck of the gallbladder. From the autonomic network around the Truncus coeliacus **(Plexus coeliacus),** the autonomic nerve fibres of the sympathicus and parasympathicus join the blood vessels and reach their target organs as a perivascular plexus. Preganglionic sympathetic neurons pass as the **Nn. splanchnici major and minor** through the diaphragm and are synaptically interconnected in the **Ganglia coeliaca.** Conversely, the parasympathetic neurons reach the Plexus coeliacus via the **Trunci vagales anterior and posterior,** which together with the oesophagus pass through the diaphragm and run along the lesser curvature of the stomach.

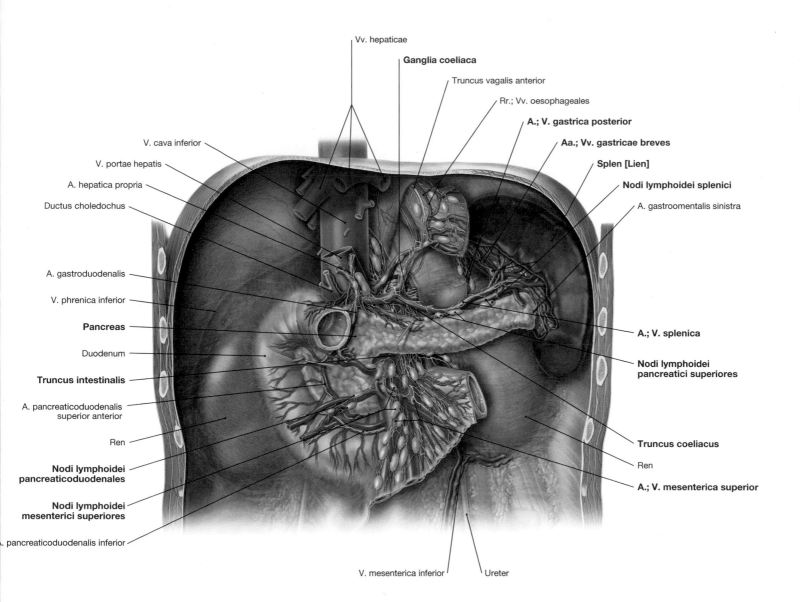

Vv. hepaticae

Ganglia coeliaca

Truncus vagalis anterior

Rr.; Vv. oesophageales

A.; V. gastrica posterior

Aa.; Vv. gastricae breves

Splen [Lien]

Nodi lymphoidei splenici

A. gastroomentalis sinistra

V. cava inferior

V. portae hepatis

A. hepatica propria

Ductus choledochus

A. gastroduodenalis

V. phrenica inferior

Pancreas

Duodenum

Truncus intestinalis

A. pancreaticoduodenalis superior anterior

Ren

Nodi lymphoidei pancreaticoduodenales

Nodi lymphoidei mesenterici superiores

A. pancreaticoduodenalis inferior

A.; V. splenica

Nodi lymphoidei pancreatici superiores

Truncus coeliacus

Ren

A.; V. mesenterica superior

V. mesenterica inferior

Ureter

Fig. 6.145 Situs of the epigastric organs with depiction of the re-troperitoneal organs; the liver has been removed completely as well as most of the stomach, to show the retroperitoneal organs and the neurovascular pathways of the epigastrium. The mesentery has been cut at the root and resected with the small intestinal loops of the jeju-num and ileum; ventral view. [S700-L238]/[Q300]

Of the intraperitoneal epigastric organs, only the spleen has been left. This makes the pancreas and also the duodenum visible. The branches of the **A. splenica** leading to the stomach **(A. gastrica posterior, A. gastroomentalis sinistra and Aa. gastricae breves)** can be recog-nised. The **A. gastrica sinistra** branches out to the oesophagus, into

which the **Trunci vagales anterior and posterior** enter into the abdom-inal cavity (Cavitas abdominalis). The **A. gastroduodenalis** branches off from the **A. hepatica communis,** and as its terminal branch, connects the A. pancreaticoduodenalis superior anterior with the A. pancreati-coduodenalis inferior from the A. mesenterica superior. The **A. and V. mesenterica superior** run behind the neck of the pancreas, and en-ter the mesentery. They are accompanied by the **Nodi lymphoidei mesenterici superiores,** of which the collectors join the **Trunci intesti-nales** along the Truncus coeliacus, as do the corresponding lymph ves-sels. With the Trunci lumbales, these form the **Ductus thoracicus.**

Abdomen and pelvis, median section

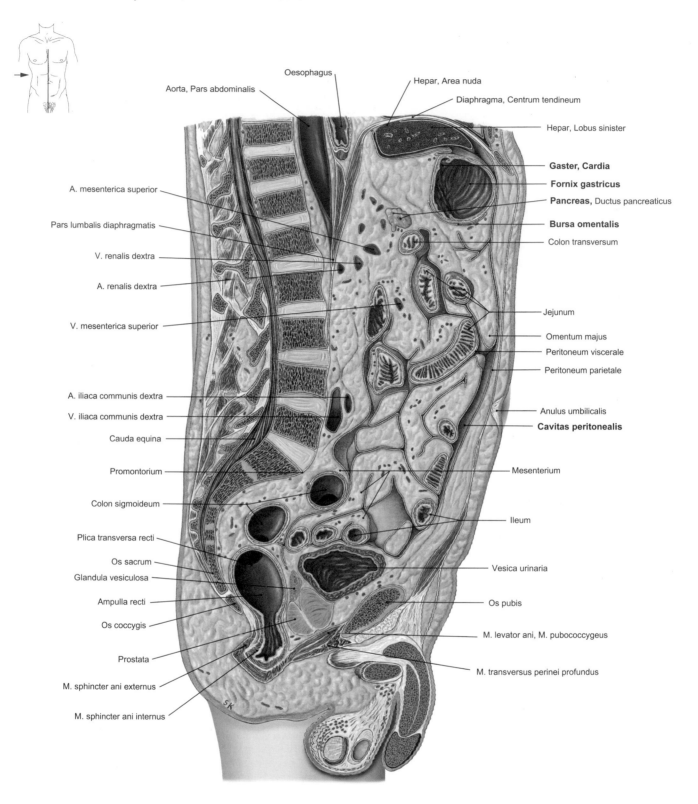

Oesophagus

Aorta, Pars abdominalis

Hepar, Area nuda

Diaphragma, Centrum tendineum

Hepar, Lobus sinister

A. mesenterica superior

Gaster, Cardia

Fornix gastricus

Pancreas, Ductus pancreaticus

Pars lumbalis diaphragmatis

Bursa omentalis

Colon transversum

V. renalis dextra

A. renalis dextra

V. mesenterica superior

Jejunum

Omentum majus

Peritoneum viscerale

Peritoneum parietale

A. iliaca communis dextra

V. iliaca communis dextra

Anulus umbilicalis

Cavitas peritonealis

Cauda equina

Promontorium

Mesenterium

Colon sigmoideum

Ileum

Plica transversa recti

Os sacrum

Vesica urinaria

Glandula vesiculosa

Ampulla recti

Os pubis

Os coccygis

M. levator ani, M. pubococcygeus

Prostata

M. transversus perinei profundus

M. sphincter ani externus

M. sphincter ani internus

Fig. 6.146 Abdomen and pelvis of a man; median section; view from the right side. [S700-L238]

It is clear from the illustration that the peritoneal cavity (Cavitas peritonealis) is not a wide, empty space but instead is made up of small recesses which are spread out between the intraperitoneal organs. The omental bursa between the stomach and the pancreas is also only a narrow, peritoneum-lined gap. A large part of the abdomen is taken up by the mesentery, where very large amounts of adipose tissue can be stored.

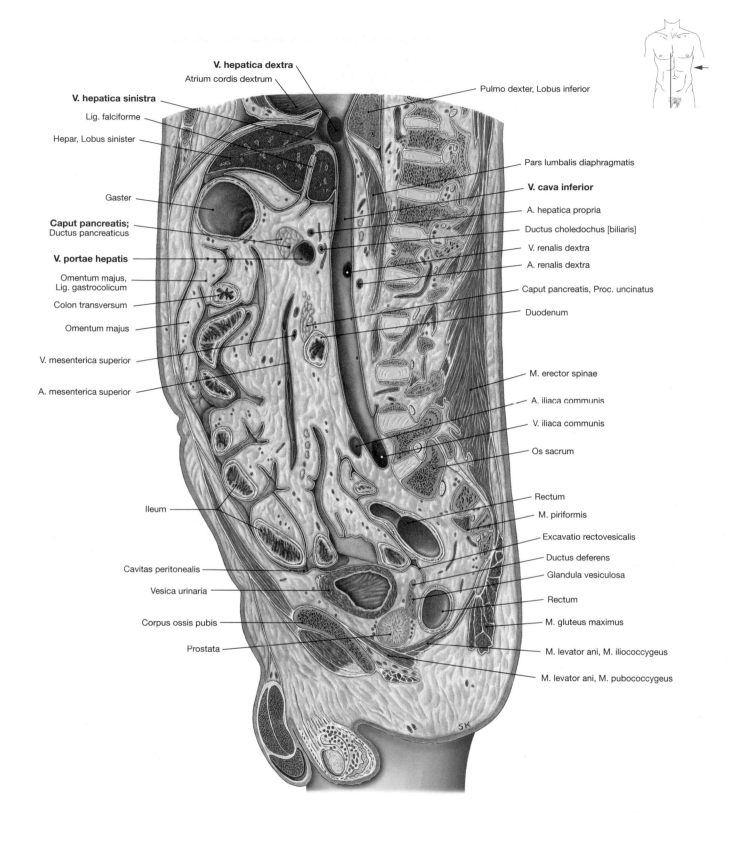

V. hepatica dextra
Atrium cordis dextrum

V. hepatica sinistra
Lig. falciforme
Hepar, Lobus sinister
Gaster
Caput pancreatis;
Ductus pancreaticus
V. portae hepatis
Omentum majus,
Lig. gastrocolicum
Colon transversum
Omentum majus
V. mesenterica superior
A. mesenterica superior
Ileum
Cavitas peritonealis
Vesica urinaria
Corpus ossis pubis
Prostata

Pulmo dexter, Lobus inferior
Pars lumbalis diaphragmatis
V. cava inferior
A. hepatica propria
Ductus choledochus [biliaris]
V. renalis dextra
A. renalis dextra
Caput pancreatis, Proc. uncinatus
Duodenum
M. erector spinae
A. iliaca communis
V. iliaca communis
Os sacrum
Rectum
M. piriformis
Excavatio rectovesicalis
Ductus deferens
Glandula vesiculosa
Rectum
M. gluteus maximus
M. levator ani, M. iliococcygeus
M. levator ani, M. pubococcygeus

Fig. 6.147 Abdomen and pelvis of a man; sagittal section; view from the left side. [S700-L238]
The sectional plane runs paramedially to the right at the level of the V. cava inferior. Thus, the confluence of the Vv. hepaticae, which drain the venous blood from the liver, is clearly visible. The V. portae hepatis, which takes the nutrient-rich blood of the unpaired abdominal organs to the liver, comes from its main veins behind the head of the pancreas.

Abdomen and pelvis, frontal section

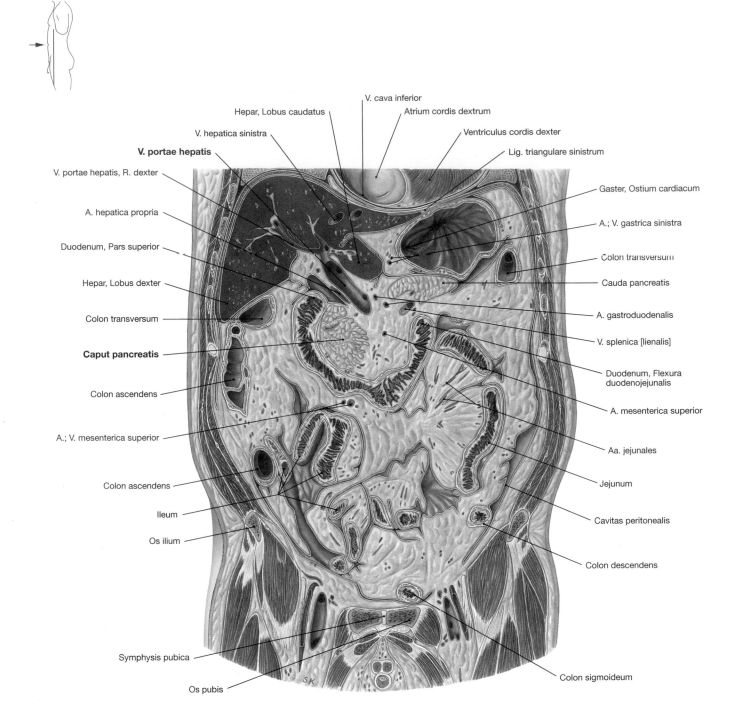

V. cava inferior

Hepar, Lobus caudatus

Atrium cordis dextrum

V. hepatica sinistra

Ventriculus cordis dexter

V. portae hepatis

Lig. triangulare sinistrum

V. portae hepatis, R. dexter

Gaster, Ostium cardiacum

A. hepatica propria

A.; V. gastrica sinistra

Duodenum, Pars superior

Colon transversum

Hepar, Lobus dexter

Cauda pancreatis

Colon transversum

A. gastroduodenalis

Caput pancreatis

V. splenica [lienalis]

Colon ascendens

Duodenum, Flexura duodenojejunalis

A.; V. mesenterica superior

A. mesenterica superior

Colon ascendens

Aa. jejunales

Ileum

Jejunum

Os ilium

Cavitas peritonealis

Colon descendens

Symphysis pubica

Os pubis

Colon sigmoideum

Fig. 6.148 Abdomen and pelvis of a man; frontal section through the posterior part; ventral view. [S700-L238]

This frontal section passes through the V. portae hepatis, which passes above the head of the pancreas (Caput pancreatis) to the hilum of the liver and there divides into its right and left branches.

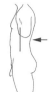

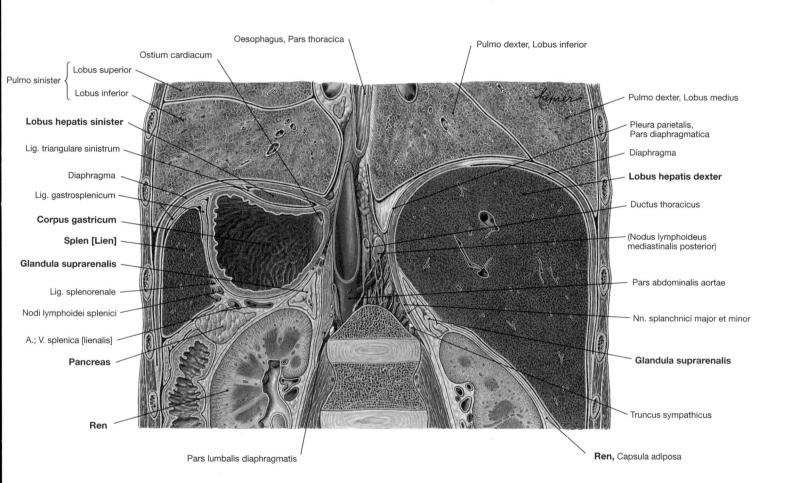

Oesophagus, Pars thoracica

Ostium cardiacum

Pulmo sinister { Lobus superior

Lobus inferior

Lobus hepatis sinister

Lig. triangulare sinistrum

Diaphragma

Lig. gastrosplenicum

Corpus gastricum

Splen [Lien]

Glandula suprarenalis

Lig. splenorenale

Nodi lymphoidei splenici

A.; V. splenica [lienalis]

Pancreas

Ren

Pars lumbalis diaphragmatis

Pulmo dexter, Lobus inferior

Pulmo dexter, Lobus medius

Pleura parietalis,
Pars diaphragmatica

Diaphragma

Lobus hepatis dexter

Ductus thoracicus

(Nodus lymphoideus
mediastinalis posterior)

Pars abdominalis aortae

Nn. splanchnici major et minor

Glandula suprarenalis

Truncus sympathicus

Ren, Capsula adiposa

Fig. 6.149 Abdominal cavity, Cavitas abdominalis, and thoracic cavity, Cavea thoracis; frontal section at the level of the kidneys; dorsal view. [S700]
The section shows the positions of the individual epigastric organs in relation to each other. The right upper abdomen is completely filled by the right lobe of the liver (Lobus hepatis dexter), which is caudally in contact with the right kidney (Ren) and the right adrenal gland (Glandula suprarenalis). On the left side, the cranial part of the left hepatic lobe covers the stomach (Gaster) which, in turn, is in contact with the spleen on the left and caudally with the left kidney, the left adrenal gland and the pancreas. The tail of the pancreas extends to the spleen.

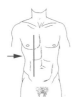

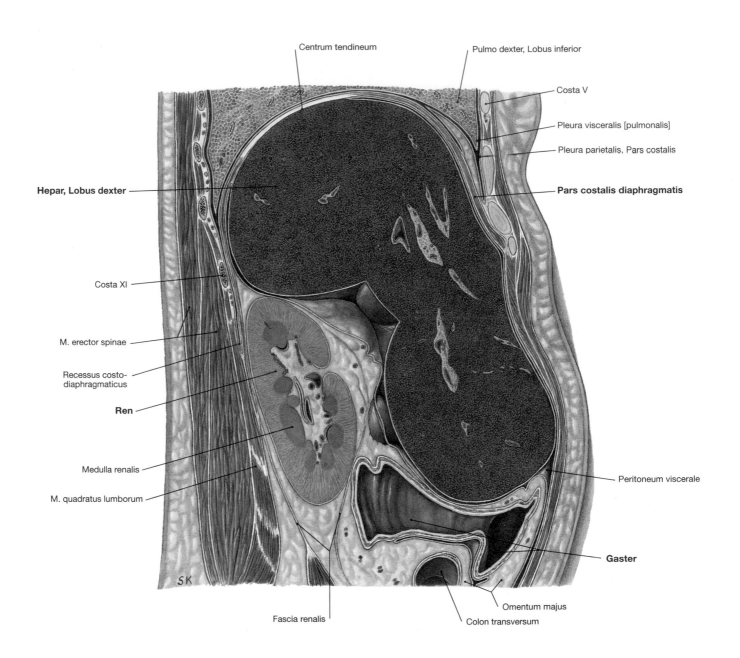

Centrum tendineum

Pulmo dexter, Lobus inferior

Costa V

Pleura visceralis [pulmonalis]

Pleura parietalis, Pars costalis

Hepar, Lobus dexter

Pars costalis diaphragmatis

Costa XI

M. erector spinae

Recessus costo-
diaphragmaticus

Ren

Medulla renalis

M. quadratus lumborum

Peritoneum viscerale

Gaster

Omentum majus

Fascia renalis

Colon transversum

SK

Fig. 6.150 Abdomen; sagittal section through the right upper abdomen at the level of the kidney; view from the right side. [S700-L238] In the right upper abdomen is the right lobe of the liver (Hepar, Lobus dexter), spreading out over the underside of the diaphragm. The right kidney (Ren) is positioned dorsally below the liver (Hepar) in the retroperitoneal space, and ventrally thereof the Pars pylorica of the stomach (Gaster) in the intraperitoneal cavity.

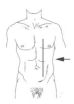

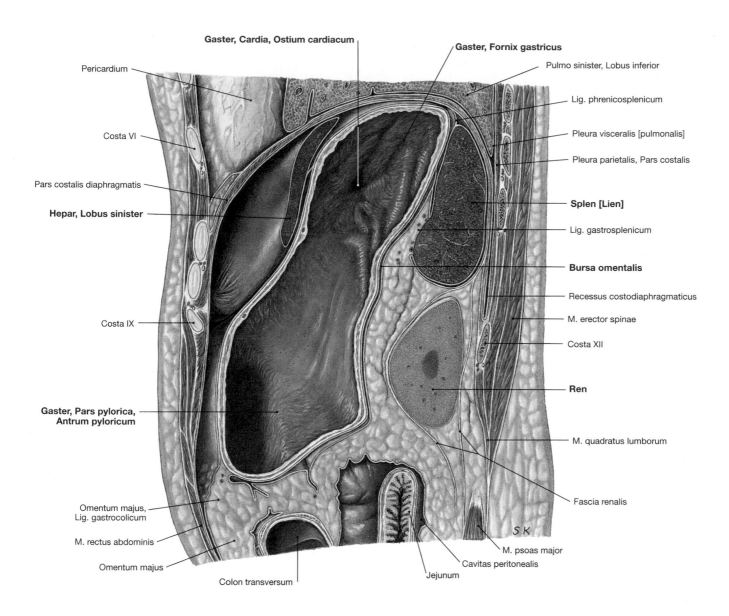

Gaster, Cardia, Ostium cardiacum

Gaster, Fornix gastricus

Pericardium

Pulmo sinister, Lobus inferior

Lig. phrenicosplenicum

Costa VI

Pleura visceralis [pulmonalis]

Pleura parietalis, Pars costalis

Pars costalis diaphragmatis

Hepar, Lobus sinister

Splen [Lien]

Lig. gastrosplenicum

Bursa omentalis

Recessus costodiaphragmaticus

Costa IX

M. erector spinae

Costa XII

Ren

Gaster, Pars pylorica, Antrum pyloricum

M. quadratus lumborum

Fascia renalis

Omentum majus, Lig. gastrocolicum

M. rectus abdominis

S K

M. psoas major

Omentum majus

Cavitas peritonealis

Jejunum

Colon transversum

Fig. 6.151 Abdomen; sagittal section through the left upper abdomen at the level of the spleen; view from the left side. [S700-L238] The stomach (Gaster) occupies the majority of the left upper abdomen. Ventrally it is covered by the left lobe of the liver (Hepar, Lobus sinister) and dorsally it has extensive contact with the spleen (Splen) and the left kidney (Ren), which is located in the retroperitoneal space. The Bursa omentalis forms a small recess, lined with peritoneum, behind the stomach.

Epigastrium, cross-sections

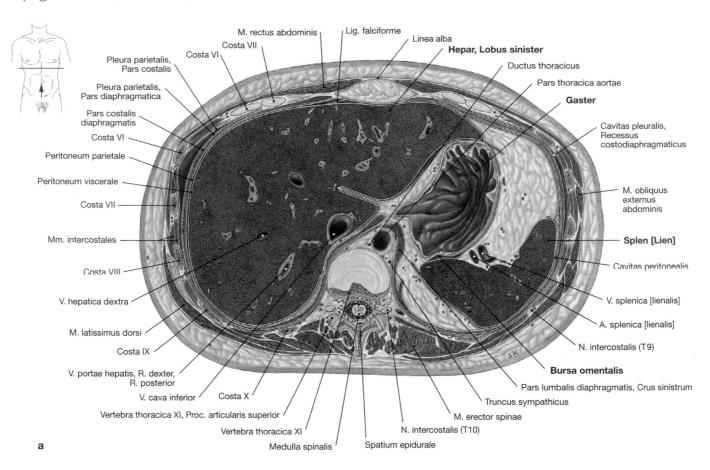

M. rectus abdominis
Costa VII
Costa VI
Lig. falciforme
Linea alba
Hepar, Lobus sinister
Ductus thoracicus
Pars thoracica aortae
Gaster
Pleura parietalis, Pars costalis
Pleura parietalis, Pars diaphragmatica
Pars costalis diaphragmatis
Costa VI
Peritoneum parietale
Peritoneum viscerale
Costa VII
Mm. intercostales
Costa VIII
V. hepatica dextra
M. latissimus dorsi
Costa IX
V. portae hepatis, R. dexter, R. posterior
V. cava inferior
Costa X
Vertebra thoracica XI, Proc. articularis superior
Vertebra thoracica XI
Medulla spinalis
Spatium epidurale
N. intercostalis (T10)
M. erector spinae
Truncus sympathicus
Pars lumbalis diaphragmatis, Crus sinistrum
Bursa omentalis
N. intercostalis (T9)
A. splenica [lienalis]
V. splenica [lienalis]
Cavitas peritonealis
Splen [Lien]
M. obliquus externus abdominis
Cavitas pleuralis, Recessus costodiaphragmaticus

a

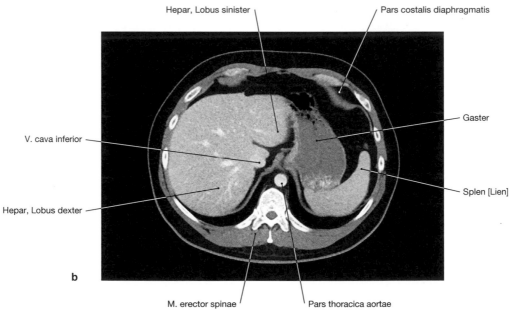

Hepar, Lobus sinister
Pars costalis diaphragmatis
V. cava inferior
Gaster
Hepar, Lobus dexter
Splen [Lien]
M. erector spinae
Pars thoracica aortae

b

Fig. 6.152a and b Abdominal cavity, Cavitas abdominalis; caudal view.
a Cross-section at the level of the 11th thoracic vertebra. [S700-L238]
b Corresponding computed tomographic (CT) cross-section. [S700-T832]

The liver (Hepar) occupies the whole right upper abdomen and with its left lobe extends left to reach the front of the stomach (Gaster). Behind the stomach is the Bursa omentalis, lined by peritoneum. The spleen is truncated in the left upper abdomen.

Clinical remarks

Sectional diagnostic imaging, e.g. by **computed tomography** (CT), has now become a routine imaging procedure. Without the use of a contrast agent, it allows for the presentation of the soft tissue and is not as susceptible to interference as ultrasound, for example by air-filled intestinal loops. Therefore CT scans are carried out for further diagnostic clarification, or for the planning of surgery. Generally, CT scans are **always shown from a caudal view.** Therefore, it is always advisable to also look at anatomical cross-sectional images from a caudal view.

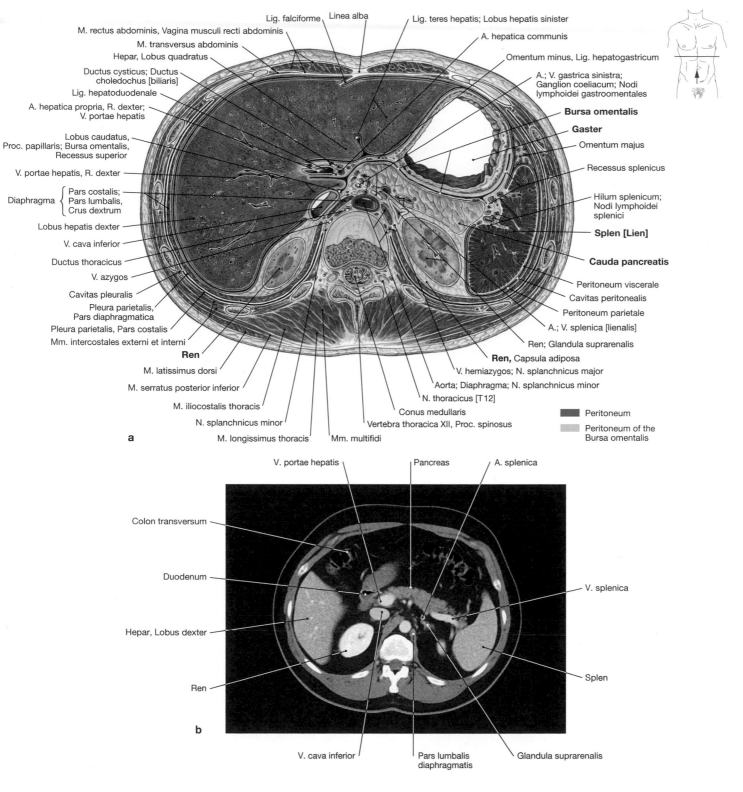

Lig. falciforme Linea alba
M. rectus abdominis, Vagina musculi recti abdominis
M. transversus abdominis
Hepar, Lobus quadratus
Ductus cysticus; Ductus choledochus [biliaris]
Lig. hepatoduodenale
A. hepatica propria, R. dexter; V. portae hepatis
Lobus caudatus, Proc. papillaris; Bursa omentalis, Recessus superior
V. portae hepatis, R. dexter
Diaphragma { Pars costalis; Pars lumbalis, Crus dextrum
Lobus hepatis dexter
V. cava inferior
Ductus thoracicus
V. azygos
Cavitas pleuralis
Pleura parietalis, Pars diaphragmatica
Pleura parietalis, Pars costalis
Mm. intercostales externi et interni
Ren
M. latissimus dorsi
M. serratus posterior inferior
M. iliocostalis thoracis
N. splanchnicus minor
M. longissimus thoracis Mm. multifidi

Lig. teres hepatis; Lobus hepatis sinister
A. hepatica communis
Omentum minus, Lig. hepatogastricum
A.; V. gastrica sinistra; Ganglion coeliacum; Nodi lymphoidei gastroomentales
Bursa omentalis
Gaster
Omentum majus
Recessus splenicus
Hilum splenicum; Nodi lymphoidei splenici
Splen [Lien]
Cauda pancreatis
Peritoneum viscerale
Cavitas peritonealis
Peritoneum parietale
A.; V. splenica [lienalis]
Ren; Glandula suprarenalis
Ren, Capsula adiposa
V. hemiazygos; N. splanchnicus major
Aorta; Diaphragma; N. splanchnicus minor
N. thoracicus [T 12]
Conus medullaris
Vertebra thoracica XII, Proc. spinosus

Peritoneum
Peritoneum of the Bursa omentalis

a

V. portae hepatis   Pancreas   A. splenica

Colon transversum

Duodenum

Hepar, Lobus dexter

Ren

V. splenica

Splen

b

V. cava inferior   Pars lumbalis diaphragmatis   Glandula suprarenalis

Fig. 6.153a and b   Abdominal cavity, Cavitas abdominalis; caudal view.
a Cross-section at the level of the first lumbar vertebra. [S700]
b Corresponding computed tomographic (CT) cross-section. [S700-T832]

At the level of the first lumbar vertebra, the posterior poles of the kidneys (Renes) and the pancreas have also been truncated. The pancreas is located posterior to the stomach (Gaster), separated by the Bursa omentalis, and extends to the left side to reach the hilum of the spleen (Splen).

Clinical remarks

For the examination of the pancreas, ultrasound imaging is often not very informative due to the air-filled intestinal loops, and requires CT scans for clarification. These CT scans, e.g. in cases of inflammation **(pancreatitis),** often reveal an oedematous and cystic swelling of the organ, and they can be consulted to evaluate progression.

Organs of the abdominal cavity

Epigastrium, cross-sections

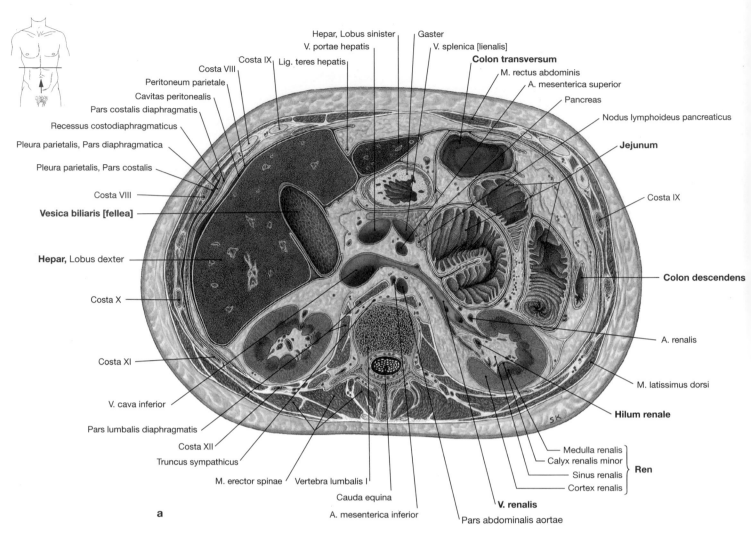

Hepar, Lobus sinister
Gaster
V. portae hepatis
V. splenica [lienalis]
Costa IX
Lig. teres hepatis
Colon transversum
Costa VIII
M. rectus abdominis
Peritoneum parietale
A. mesenterica superior
Cavitas peritonealis
Pancreas
Pars costalis diaphragmatis
Nodus lymphoideus pancreaticus
Recessus costodiaphragmaticus
Jejunum
Pleura parietalis, Pars diaphragmatica
Pleura parietalis, Pars costalis
Costa VIII
Costa IX
Vesica biliaris [fellea]
Hepar, Lobus dexter
Colon descendens
Costa X
A. renalis
Costa XI
M. latissimus dorsi
V. cava inferior
Hilum renale
Pars lumbalis diaphragmatis
Medulla renalis
Costa XII
Calyx renalis minor
Truncus sympathicus
Sinus renalis } **Ren**
M. erector spinae
Vertebra lumbalis I
Cortex renalis
Cauda equina
V. renalis
A. mesenterica inferior
Pars abdominalis aortae

a

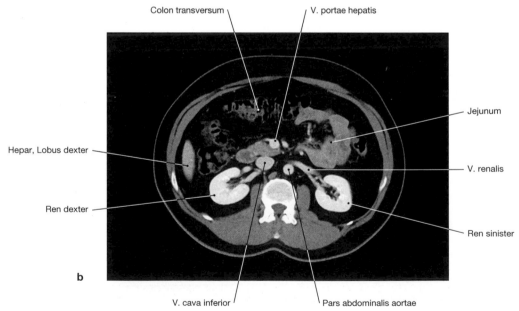

Colon transversum
V. portae hepatis
Jejunum
Hepar, Lobus dexter
V. renalis
Ren dexter
Ren sinister
b
V. cava inferior
Pars abdominalis aortae

Fig. 6.154a and b   Abdominal cavity, Cavitas abdominalis; caudal view.
a Cross-section at the level of the first lumbar vertebra. [S700-L238]
b Corresponding computed tomographic (CT) cross-section. [S700-T832]

The hilum of the kidney (Ren) is typically at the level of the first to second lumbar vertebrae (recognisable at the opening of the left V. renalis). On the lower margin of the liver (Hepar), the gallbladder (Vesica biliaris) is truncated. In the left upper abdomen, portions of the small intestinal loops (jejunum) and portions of the large intestine (Colon transversum and Colon descendens) are visible.

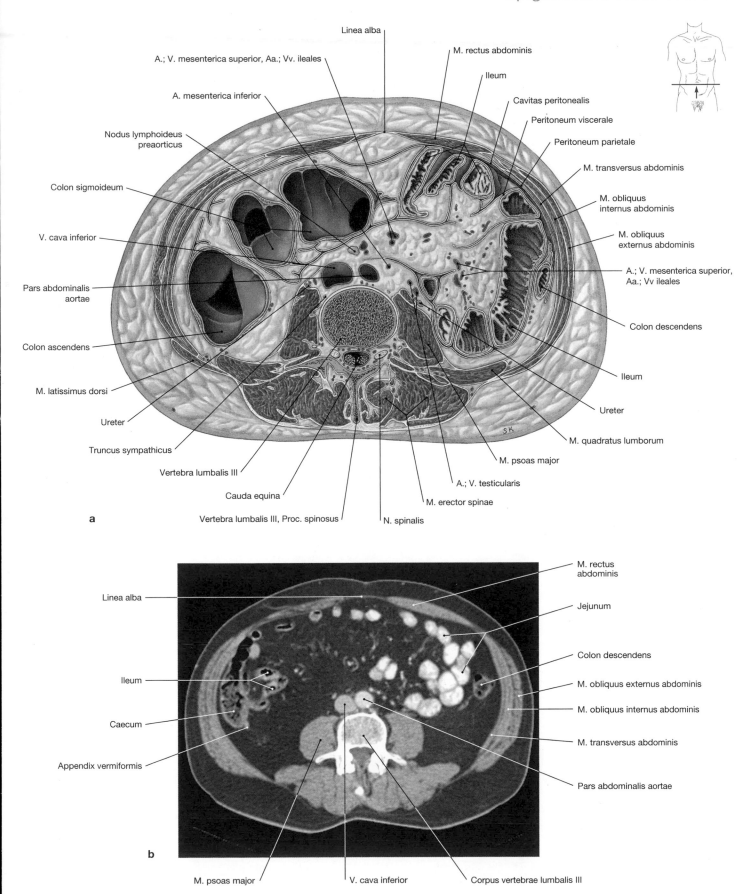

Linea alba

A.; V. mesenterica superior, Aa.; Vv. ileales

A. mesenterica inferior

Nodus lymphoideus preaorticus

Colon sigmoideum

V. cava inferior

Pars abdominalis aortae

Colon ascendens

M. latissimus dorsi

Ureter

Truncus sympathicus

Vertebra lumbalis III

Cauda equina

Vertebra lumbalis III, Proc. spinosus

N. spinalis

Vertebra lumbalis III, Proc. spinosus

M. rectus abdominis

Ileum

Cavitas peritonealis

Peritoneum viscerale

Peritoneum parietale

M. transversus abdominis

M. obliquus internus abdominis

M. obliquus externus abdominis

A.; V. mesenterica superior, Aa.; Vv ileales

Colon descendens

Ileum

Ureter

M. quadratus lumborum

M. psoas major

A.; V. testicularis

M. erector spinae

a

Linea alba

Ileum

Caecum

Appendix vermiformis

M. psoas major

V. cava inferior

Corpus vertebrae lumbalis III

M. rectus abdominis

Jejunum

Colon descendens

M. obliquus externus abdominis

M. obliquus internus abdominis

M. transversus abdominis

Pars abdominalis aortae

b

Fig. 6.155a and b Abdominal cavity, Cavitas abdominalis; caudal view.

a Cross-section at the level of the third lumbar vertebra. [S700-L238]
b Corresponding computed tomographic (CT) cross-section. [S700]

Epigastrium, cross-sections

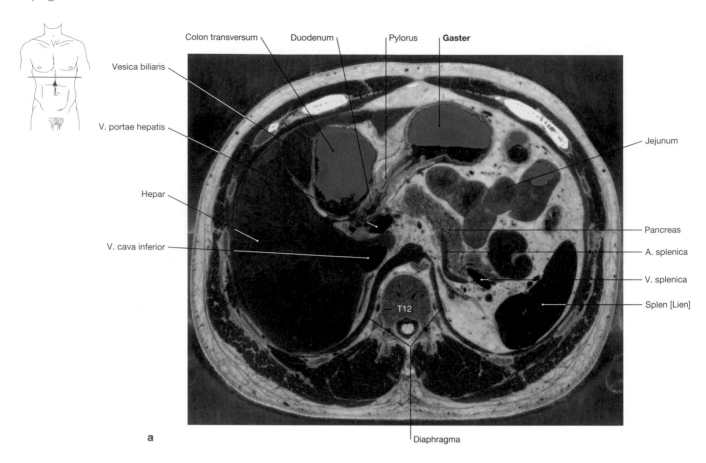

a

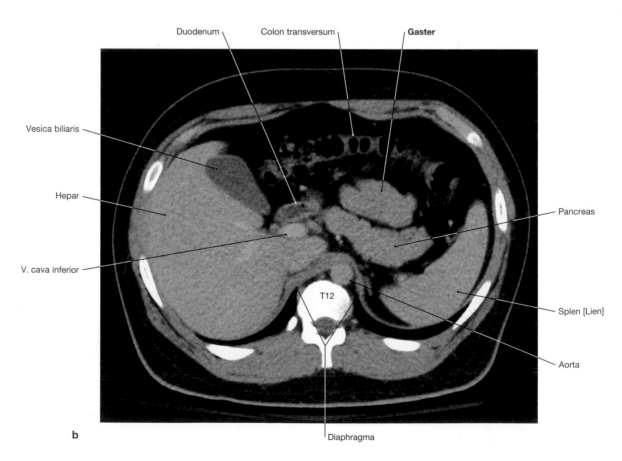

b

Fig. 6.156a and b Abdominal cavity, Cavitas abdominalis; caudal view. [X338]
a Cross-section at the level of the 12th thoracic vertebra.

b Corresponding computed tomographic (CT) cross-section.
The sectional image shows a section of the Pars pylorica of the stomach and the Pars superior of the duodenum.

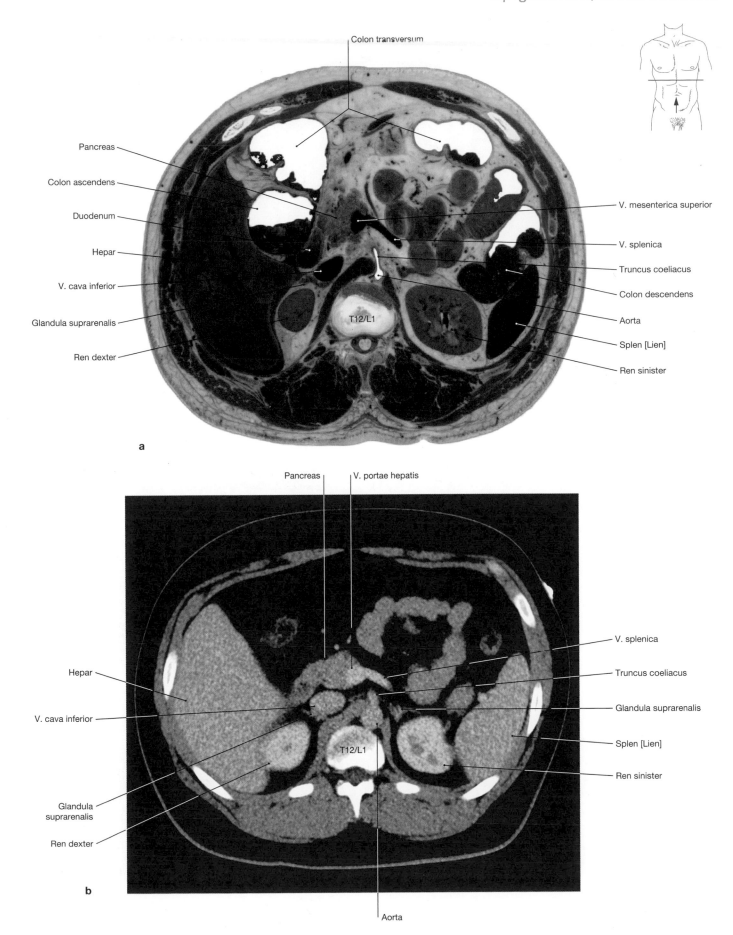

Colon transversum

Pancreas

Colon ascendens

Duodenum

Hepar

V. cava inferior

Glandula suprarenalis

Ren dexter

V. mesenterica superior

V. splenica

Truncus coeliacus

Colon descendens

Aorta

Splen [Lien]

Ren sinister

T12/L1

a

Pancreas | V. portae hepatis

Hepar

V. cava inferior

Glandula
suprarenalis

Ren dexter

V. splenica

Truncus coeliacus

Glandula suprarenalis

Splen [Lien]

Ren sinister

T12/L1

Aorta

b

Fig. 6.157a and b Abdominal cavity, Cavitas abdominalis; caudal view. [X338]
a Cross-section at the level of the transition between the 12th thoracic and the first lumbar vertebra.

b Corresponding computed tomographic (CT) cross-section.
The cross-sectional image shows the close proximity of the head of the pancreas to the hepatic portal vein, V. portae hepatis, with confluence of the V. splenica.

Epigastrium, cross-sections

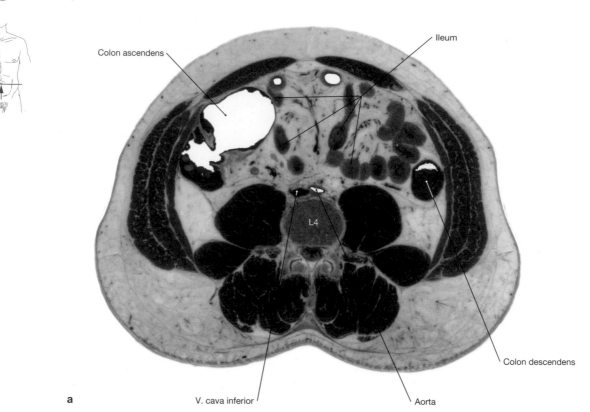

Colon ascendens

Ileum

V. cava inferior

Aorta

Colon descendens

a

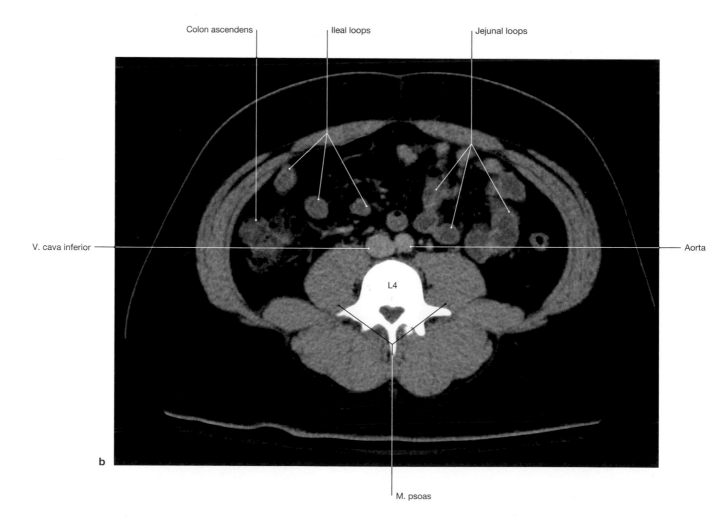

Colon ascendens

Ileal loops

Jejunal loops

V. cava inferior

Aorta

L4

M. psoas

b

Fig. 6.158a and b Abdominal cavity, Cavitas abdominalis; caudal view. [X338]
a Cross-section at the level of the fourth lumbar vertebra.
b Corresponding computed tomographic (CT) cross-section.

The sectional image shows small intestinal loops as well as the Colon ascendens and descendens. The section of the Pars abdominalis of the aorta is located above its bifurcation into the Aa. iliacae communes.

Sample exam questions

To check that you are completely familiar with the content of this chapter, sample questions from an oral anatomy exam are listed here.

Explain the significance of the relative positions of the individual abdominal organs.

Which peritoneal ligaments anchor the liver?

What is the relevance of the recess of the peritoneal cavity?

- Explain the structure of the Bursa omentalis in detail.

What is the structure of the Omentum majus and what are its functions?

How is the stomach (Gaster) structured?

Which vessels provide the stomach with blood?

- Show these and explain their origins.

Explain the stations of the stomach's lymphatic drainage on the dissection, along with its clinical importance.

Show the positional relationships of the individual intestinal segments on the dissection.

- Which projection points characterise the appendix and why are these necessary?

Where is the RIOLAN's arcade and what does it do?

Due to developmental changes, where do the areas supplied by neurovascular pathways switch between the individual intestinal sections?

Explain the anatomy and functional structure of the liver.

- What is meant by the segmental structure of the liver?

Which portocaval anastomoses do you know?

How is the liver supplied with blood?

Where is the portal vein and what does it originate from?

Explain the position, structure and projection of the pancreas, using the specimen.

How is the pancreatic duct system structured and how does it work?

Where is the spleen and where does it project onto the body surface?

What is the importance of the segmental structure of the spleen?

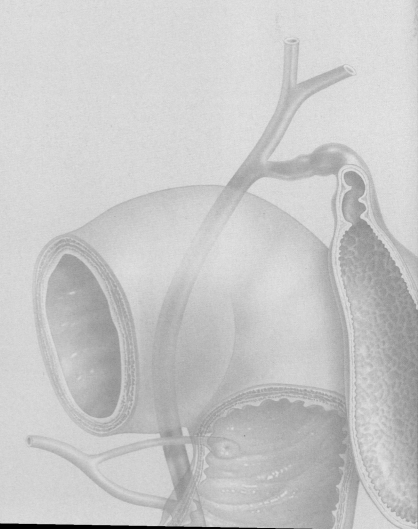

Retroperitoneal space and pelvic cavity

7

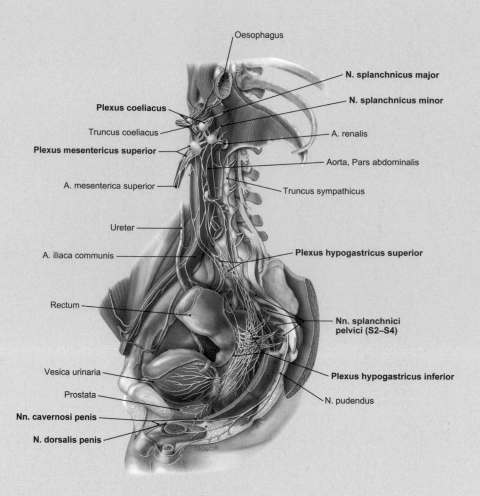

Oesophagus

N. splanchnicus major

N. splanchnicus minor

Plexus coeliacus

Truncus coeliacus

A. renalis

Plexus mesentericus superior

Aorta, Pars abdominalis

A. mesenterica superior

Truncus sympathicus

Ureter

A. iliaca communis

Plexus hypogastricus superior

Rectum

Nn. splanchnici
pelvici (S2–S4)

Vesica urinaria

Plexus hypogastricus inferior

Prostata

N. pudendus

Nn. cavernosi penis

N. dorsalis penis

Overview

There are good reasons to deal with the **retroperitoneal situs of the abdomen** (i. e. the organs which are not located in the peritoneal cavity, but at the dorsal wall) in combination with the pelvis. The kidneys, which are the major organs of the retroperitoneal space, initially develop in the pelvis and later ascend to a level just below the ribs. In contrast, the gonads, which are the testicles and ovaries, descend from the abdomen into the pelvis and, in men, even further down into the scrotum. Therefore, the subperitoneal connective tissue spaces of the pelvis and the retroperitoneal space form a continuum.

In the retroperitoneal space, a **kidney (Ren)** with a superior adjacent **adrenal gland (Glandula suprarenalis)** lies on each side. The **ureter** connects the kidney to the urinary bladder in the pelvis. The ureter runs on both sides of the major blood vessels, the aorta, and the inferior vena cava (V. cava inferior), and is accompanied by lymph vessels and autonomic nerves.

The **pelvis** is made up of three levels. Cranially, the **peritoneal cavity** extends from the abdominal cavity into the pelvis. The so-called **greater pelvis** lies between the wings of the ilium and essentially contains the intestinal loops and therewith the abdominal organs. Caudally it is joined by the conical **lesser pelvis,** which contains the actual pelvic organs. Here the parietal peritoneum marks the boundary of the **subperitoneal space** as the second level of the pelvis. This level is caudally bordered by the pelvic floor, which is connected to the **perineal region.** The pelvic organs include the internal genitalia, the urinary bladder (Vesica urinaria) and urethra as well as the rectum and anal canal (Canalis analis), as the distal portions of the large intestine.

Main topics

After working through this chapter, you should be able to:

Retroperitoneal space and pelvic cavity
- describe the structure of the retroperitoneal space and pelvic cavity, and to show their neurovascular pathways on a specimen;
- explain the neurovascular pathways of all organs, including their clinical relevance and organ-specific characteristics;

Kidney and adrenal glands
- demonstrate their vital importance based on their functions;
- explain the development and possible malformations;
- show their position and projection including the membranous sheath on a specimen;

Urinary system
- explain the structure of the urinary tract and its development;
- describe sections, constrictions and sphincter mechanisms in both sexes, as well as the basic processes during micturition;

Rectum and anal canal
- show the sections and topographical relationships of the rectum and anal canal on a specimen, and explain their development;
- explain the continence organ along with the functions of its different parts, and describe the key processes in defecation;

Genitalia
- explain the sections and positions of the internal and external male and female genitalia as well as their development and function;
- understand the membranous fasciae and content of the spermatic cord on a dissection;
- explain all the peritoneal duplications and ligaments of the internal genitalia along with their course and contents;
- explain the structure, innervation and function of the pelvic floor and the perineal muscles, and show the Fossa ischioanalis on a dissection.

Clinical relevance

In order not to lose touch with prospective everyday clinical life with so many anatomical details, the following describes a typical case that shows why the content of this chapter is so important.

Pelvic floor insufficiency

Case study
A 78-year-old female patient has an appointment with her gynaecologist because she increasingly passes urine when she coughs or sneezes. She has had these symptoms for a long time and has so far managed it well with pads, but now the involuntary passing of urine is becoming increasingly uncomfortable. The patient has four children, all born naturally (by vaginal delivery).

Result of examination
The physical examination is largely unremarkable. When her abdominal muscles contract (abdominal pressure), a mucus-coated enlargement prolapses into the vaginal orifice.

Diagnostic procedure
The vaginal examination (colposcopy) shows that the posterior wall of the urinary bladder has dropped (cystocele). When the intra-abdominal pressure increases, the anterior wall of the uterus also protrudes (uterine prolapse).

Diagnosis
Incontinence due to insufficiency of the pelvic floor, along with a cystocele and prolapse of the uterus (→ Fig. a). These issues are very common in elderly women and often caused by pregnancies. As the delivery mode apparently does not play an important role, caesarean sections would not significantly reduce the risk.

Treatment
The patient is advised to do pelvic floor exercises under the guidance of a physiotherapist. After two months the patient can increasingly better control the passing of urine.

Further developments
After five years, the incontinence gets worse again. The patient is admitted to the gynaecology ward for surgical treatment with so-called tension-free vaginal tapes (TVTs). After this, she is largely symptom-free.

Dissection lab
The **pelvic floor (Diaphragma pelvis)** and the adjacent **perineum (Regio perinealis)** are anatomically and clinically challenging regions. The pelvic floor can be easily dissected from the lesser pelvis once the pelvis has been split down the middle, and one half has been removed along with the bone. The Diaphragma pelvis is then visible as a striated muscle plate composed of three muscle parts.

 Across various dissections, compare the different thicknesses of the pelvic floor in men and women. As the majority of body donors are elderly, the pelvic floor is often in a very poor condition.

These parts are predominantly innervated by direct branches of the Plexus sacralis, and designated ventrally as **M. levator ani** (consisting of the M. pubococcygeus and M. iliococcygeus), and dorsally as **M. ischiococcygeus.** The term 'pelvic floor' (Diaphragma pelvis) was chosen because this muscle plate caudally closes off a body cavity, in the same way as the diaphragm closes off the lower opening of the thorax. The muscles of both sides leave an opening medially, the **Hiatus levatorius,** for the passage of the anal canal, urethra and, in women, the vagina. The name for these muscles largely reflects their route from the hip bone to the sacrum and coccyx. The M. iliococcygeus does not have a bony origin, and is only indirectly attached to the pelvic bones because it originates from a duplication of the fascia of the M. obturatorius internus **(Arcus tendineus m. levatoris ani).** This muscle can be easily identified due to the **Canalis obturatorius,** which penetrates the muscle and leads the **A./V. obturatoria** and the **N. obturatorius** from the pelvic cavity to the anterior aspect of the thigh. Caudally of the Arcus tendineus m. levatoris ani, it disappears below the pelvic floor,

 Here you can put your hand between the M. levator ani and the M. obturatorius internus to feel the different routes of the two muscles.

nestling against the lateral pelvic wall, where it is redirected at the ischium and then passes through the **Foramen ischiadicum minus** to the Trochanter major of the femur. This opening can be depicted better dorsally and caudally. To do this, the M. gluteus maximus must be detached medially from its origin in the dorsal gluteal region and folded back laterally. Then the M. piriformis becomes visible, as well as the **Lig. sacrotuberale** which bridges the Foramen ischiadicum minus. Through this opening, the **A./V. pudenda interna** and the **N. pudendus** pass caudally from the gluteal region into the **Fossa ischioanalis,** which occupies the posterior half of the perineal region on both sides of the anus. They are embedded here in another duplication of the fascia of the M. obturatorius **(Canalis pudendalis, ALCOCK's canal).**

 Once you have seen the dimensions of this space, you will understand how septic foci (abscesses) almost the size of a fist can form here, most of which spread from fistulas in the anal canal.

The Fossa ischioanalis is a pyramid-shaped space largely filled with adipose tissue, which at the top is limited medially by the lower surface of the M. levator ani and laterally by the M. obturatorius internus along with the ALCOCK's canal. It extends at the front up to the perineal musculature and forms very variable prolongations up to the **pubic symphysis (Symphysis pubica).**

Back in the clinic
The pelvic floor supports all the pelvic organs which lie on top of it. This explains why it is important for urinary and faecal continence, although it does not form a sphincter like the muscles of the perineum. In perineal operations, an aggravating factor for stabilising the pelvic floor is the fact that the patients are mostly in the supine 'lithotomy' position, which you have to keep in mind when visualising the anatomical relationships.

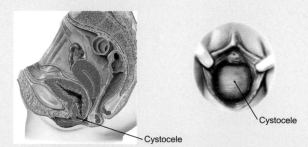
Cystocele
Cystocele

Fig. a On the left: pelvic floor insufficiency with a prolapse (ptosis) of the bladder (cystocele); view from the left side, sagittal section; **on the right:** cystocele; vaginal view. [S700-L266]

Topography

Surface anatomy

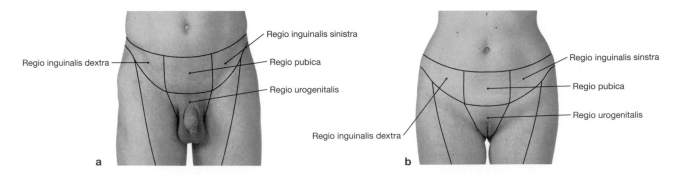

a

Regio inguinalis dextra

Regio inguinalis sinistra

Regio pubica

Regio urogenitalis

b

Regio inguinalis sinstra

Regio pubica

Regio urogenitalis

Regio inguinalis dextra

Fig. 7.1a and b Regions of the pelvic trunk, Pelvis; ventral view.
[S701-J803]

a Regions in the male.
b Regions in the female.

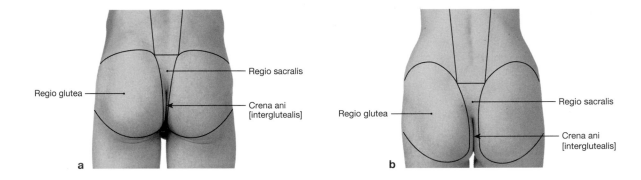

a

Regio glutea

Regio sacralis

Crena ani [interglutealis]

b

Regio glutea

Regio sacralis

Crena ani [interglutealis]

Fig. 7.2a and b Regions of the pelvic trunk, Pelvis; dorsal view.
[S701-J803]

a Regions in the male.
b Regions in the female.

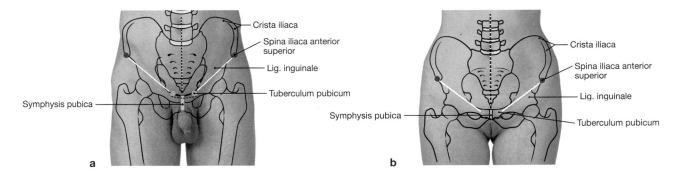

a

Crista iliaca

Spina iliaca anterior superior

Lig. inguinale

Tuberculum pubicum

Symphysis pubica

b

Crista iliaca

Spina iliaca anterior superior

Lig. inguinale

Tuberculum pubicum

Symphysis pubica

Fig. 7.3a and b Surface projections of the pelvic girdle, Cingulum pelvicum, and the bones of the thigh, Femora, and surface landmarks; ventral view. [S701-J803]

a Surface projections in the male.
b Surface projections in the female.

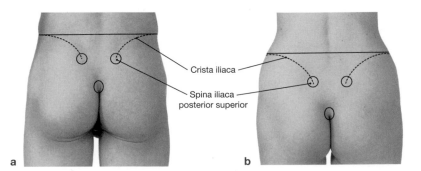

a

b

Crista iliaca

Spina iliaca posterior superior

Fig. 7.4a and b Surface projections of the pelvic girdle, Cingulum pelvicum, and the bones of the thigh, Femora, and surface landmarks; dorsal view. [S701-J803]

a Surface projections in the male.
b Surface projections in the female.

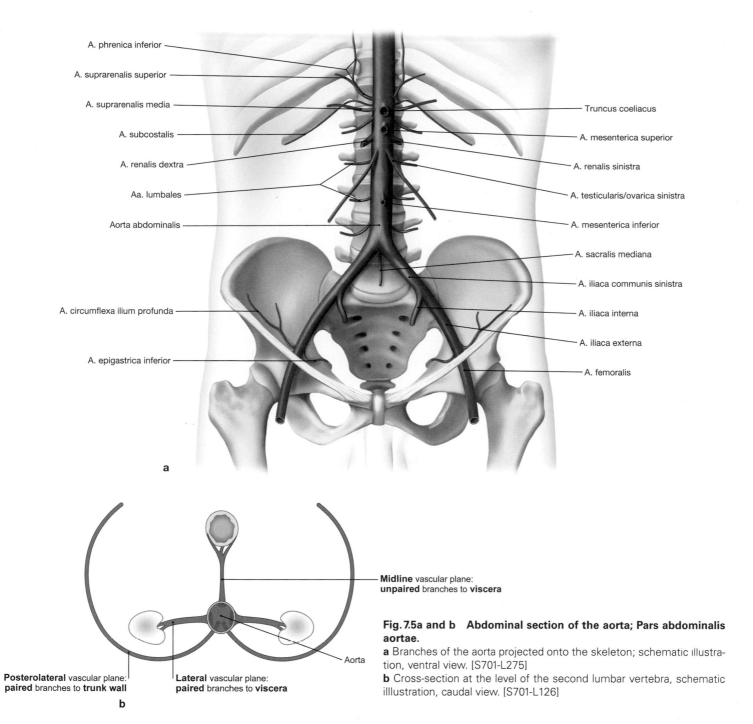

Fig. 7.5a and b   Abdominal section of the aorta; Pars abdominalis aortae.
a Branches of the aorta projected onto the skeleton; schematic illustration, ventral view. [S701-L275]
b Cross-section at the level of the second lumbar vertebra, schematic illlustration, caudal view. [S701-L126]

Branches of the abdominal aorta			
Branch	Vertebral level	Vessel position (→ Fig. 7.5b)	Area supplied
Truncus coeliacus	T12	Median, non-paired visceral	Stomach, small intestine, liver, gallbladder, pancreas, spleen
A. mesenterica superior	L1	Median, non-paired visceral	Pancreas, small and large intestines
A. mesenterica inferior	L3	Median, non-paired visceral	Large intestines
A. sacralis mediana	L4	Median, non-paired parietal terminal branch	Wall of the trunk, spinal cord
A. suprarenalis media	L1	Lateral, paired visceral	Adrenal gland
A. renalis	L2	Lateral, paired visceral	Kidney, adrenal gland
A. testicularis/ovarica	L2	Lateral, paired visceral	Testis and epididymis/ovary and FALLOPIAN tube
A. iliaca communis	L4	Lateral, paired terminal branches	Lower extremity
A. phrenica inferior	T12	Posterolateral, paired, parietal	Diaphragm
A. subcostalis	T12	Posterolateral, paired, parietal	Wall of the trunk
Aa. lumbales (4)	L1–L4	Posterolateral, paired, parietal	Wall of the trunk

Organs and vessels of the retroperitoneal space

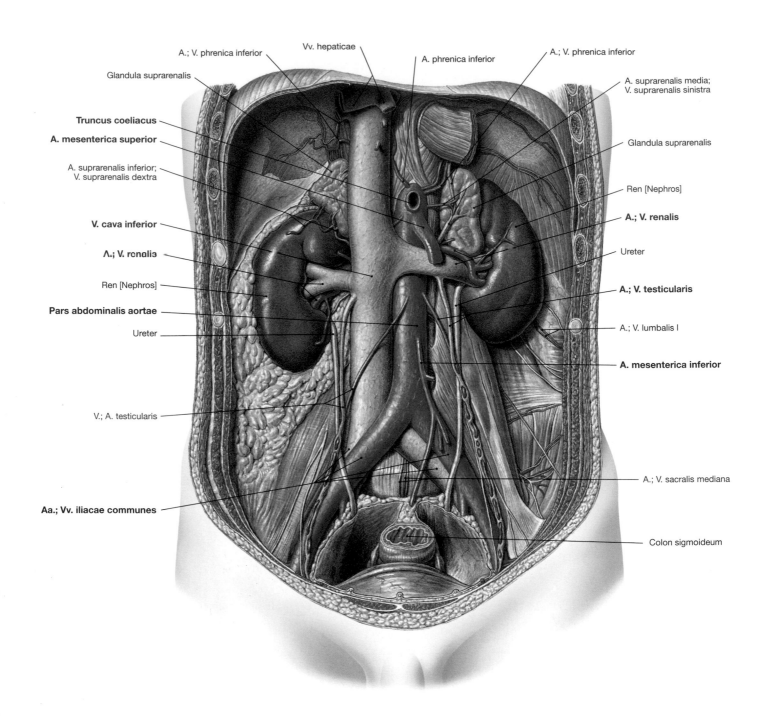

A.; V. phrenica inferior

Vv. hepaticae

A. phrenica inferior

A.; V. phrenica inferior

Glandula suprarenalis

A. suprarenalis media; V. suprarenalis sinistra

Truncus coeliacus

A. mesenterica superior

A. suprarenalis inferior; V. suprarenalis dextra

Glandula suprarenalis

Ren [Nephros]

V. cava inferior

A.; V. renalis

A.; V. renalis

Ureter

Ren [Nephros]

A.; V. testicularis

Pars abdominalis aortae

A.; V. lumbalis I

Ureter

A. mesenterica inferior

V.; A. testicularis

Aa.; Vv. iliacae communes

A.; V. sacralis mediana

Colon sigmoideum

Fig. 7.6 Organs and blood vessels of the retroperitoneal space; the intraperitoneal and secondary retroperitoneal abdominal organs have been removed, as well as the lymph vessels and autonomic nerves; ventral view. [S700]

The illustration shows a so-called **retroperitoneal situs,** i. e. the site of the organs and neurovascular pathways in the retroperitoneal space. This view is obtained in the dissection lab by removing all intraperitoneal and secondary retroperitoneal organs. As has occurred here, the organs can be removed all at once with the supplying structures. For this, it is necessary to cut the three **unpaired visceral branches (Truncus coeliacus, A. mesenterica superior, A. mesenterica inferior)** of the **aorta (Pars abdominalis aortae)** near their origin or in the case of the A. mesenterica inferior, more distally. As the veins of the removed

abdominal organs belong to the portal system, and thus are connected to the liver, they can be completely removed. Only the **hepatic veins (Vv. hepaticae)** were cut close to their opening into the **inferior vena cava (V. cava inferior).**

This dissection has been selected to present the neurovascular pathways of the retroperitoneal space and the organs located within it: **kidney (Ren)** with **ureter** and the **adrenal gland (Glandula suprarenalis).** After its passage through the diaphragm, the **aorta** continues as the **Pars abdominalis aortae,** and is located in the retroperitoneal space on the left side of the V. cava inferior in front of the spine. The **inferior vena cava (V. cava inferior)** emerges on the right side of the aorta at the level of the fifth lumbar vertebra, where the two Vv. iliacae communes unite.

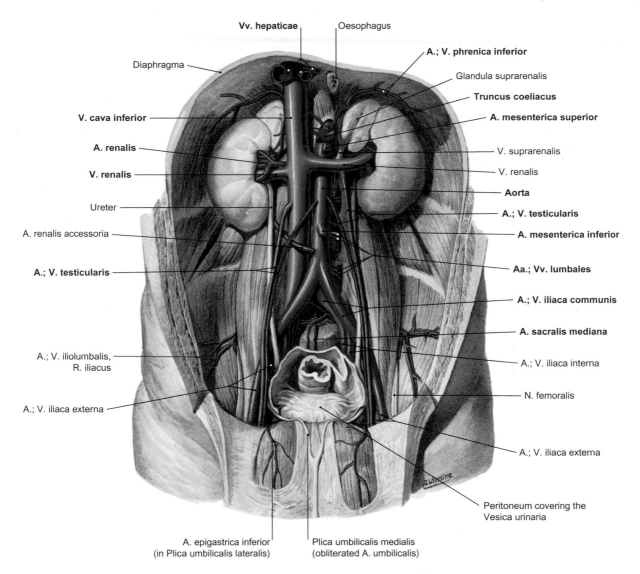

Vv. hepaticae — Oesophagus

Diaphragma —

A.; V. phrenica inferior

Glandula suprarenalis

Truncus coeliacus

A. mesenterica superior

V. cava inferior —

A. renalis —

V. renalis —

V. suprarenalis

V. renalis

Aorta

Ureter —

A. renalis accessoria —

A.; V. testicularis

A. mesenterica inferior

A.; V. testicularis —

Aa.; Vv. lumbales

A.; V. iliaca communis

A. sacralis mediana

A.; V. iliaca interna

A.; V. iliolumbalis, R. iliacus

N. femoralis

A.; V. iliaca externa —

A.; V. iliaca externa

Peritoneum covering the Vesica urinaria

A. epigastrica inferior (in Plica umbilicalis lateralis)

Plica umbilicalis medialis (obliterated A. umbilicalis)

Fig. 7.7 Blood vessels of the retroperitoneal space; the blood vessels are highlighted in colour, in order to categorise the arterial and venous systems; ventral view. [G1066-O1109]

The branches of the **Pars abdominalis aortae** are listed in the table. They can be divided into **parietal branches** for the abdominal wall, **visceral branches** for the organs and **terminal branches.**

Apart from the unpaired visceral branches – as these veins drain into the portal vein – the tributaries of the **V. cava inferior** largely correspond to the arterial branches of the aorta. It should be noted, however, that the three bilateral veins flowing directly into the V. cava on the right side are connected to the V. renalis on the left side of the body:

- V. phrenica inferior
- V. suprarenalis
- V. testicularis/ovarica.

Tributaries of the V. cava inferior

- Vv. iliacae communes
- V. sacralis mediana
- Vv. lumbales
- V. phrenica inferior dextra, flowing into the V. renalis on the left
- V. testicularis/ovarica dextra, flowing into the V. renalis on the left
- V. suprarenalis dextra, flowing into the V. renalis on the left
- Vv. renales dextra and sinistra
- Three Vv. hepaticae (Vv. hepaticae dextra, intermedia and sinistra)

Branches of the Pars abdominalis aortae [Aorta abdominalis]	
Branches	**Individual arteries**
Parietal branches for the abdominal wall	• A. phrenica inferior: underneath the diaphragm, provides the A. suprarenalis superior to the adrenal gland • Aa. lumbales: four pairs directly branching off the aorta, the fifth pair originates from the A. sacralis mediana
Visceral branches for the viscera	• Truncus coeliacus: unpaired, originates directly beneath the Hiatus aorticus and supplies the viscera of the epigastrium (→ Fig. 6.24) • A. suprarenalis media: supplies the adrenal gland • A. renalis: to the kidney, also provides the A. suprarenalis inferior to the adrenal gland • A. mesenterica superior: unpaired, supplies parts of the pancreas, the entire small intestine and the large intestine up to the left colonic flexure (→ Fig. 6.27) • A. testicularis/ovarica: supplies the testis and epididymis in men and the ovary in women • A. mesenterica inferior: unpaired, supplies the Colon descendens, the Colon sigmoideum and the upper rectum (→ Fig. 6.29)
Terminal branches	• A. iliaca communis: for the pelvis and leg • A. sacralis mediana: descends to the sacrum

Lymph vessels of the retroperitoneal space

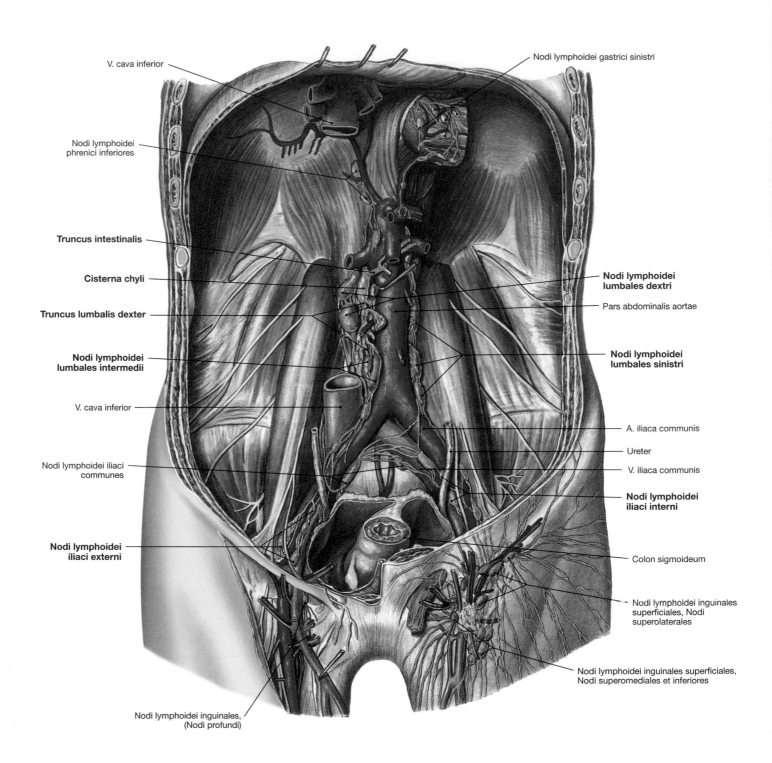

V. cava inferior

Nodi lymphoidei gastrici sinistri

Nodi lymphoidei phrenici inferiores

Truncus intestinalis

Cisterna chyli

Truncus lumbalis dexter

Nodi lymphoidei lumbales intermedii

V. cava inferior

Nodi lymphoidei iliaci communes

Nodi lymphoidei iliaci externi

Nodi lymphoidei inguinales, (Nodi profundi)

Nodi lymphoidei lumbales dextri

Pars abdominalis aortae

Nodi lymphoidei lumbales sinistri

A. iliaca communis

Ureter

V. iliaca communis

Nodi lymphoidei iliaci interni

Colon sigmoideum

Nodi lymphoidei inguinales superficiales, Nodi superolaterales

Nodi lymphoidei inguinales superficiales, Nodi superomediales et inferiores

Fig. 7.8 Lymph vessels and lymph nodes of the retroperitoneal space; ventral view. [S700]
Via the Nodi lymphoidei iliaci communes, the lymph from the pelvis is drained into the parietal lymph nodes of the retroperitoneal space, summarised as **Nodi lymphoidei lumbales.** These form three chains as the Nodi lymphoidei lumbales sinistri, located around the aorta, as Nodi lymphoidei lumbales dextri to both sides of the V. cava inferior, and as Nodi lymphoidei lumbales intermedii in between both blood vessels. The lumbar lymph nodes do not only represent the collecting lymph nodes of the lower limbs, the pelvic viscera and the Colon descendens, but also the regional lymph nodes of the kidneys, adrenal glands and testicles/ovaries.

From the efferent lymph vessels of the lumbar lymph nodes, the **Trunci lumbales** emerge on both sides, uniting in the Cisterna chyli with the **Truncus intestinalis** (collecting the lymph of the visceral lymph nodes in the abdominal cavity), and continue as the **Ductus thoracicus.** Thereby the Ductus thoracicus contains the entire lymph of the lower half of the body below the diaphragm.

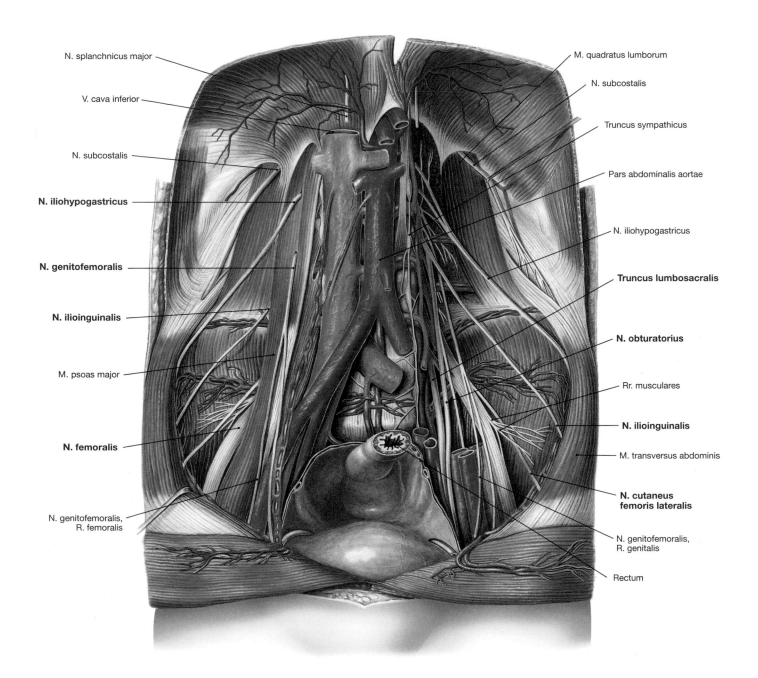

N. splanchnicus major

V. cava inferior

N. subcostalis

N. iliohypogastricus

N. genitofemoralis

N. ilioinguinalis

M. psoas major

N. femoralis

N. genitofemoralis, R. femoralis

M. quadratus lumborum

N. subcostalis

Truncus sympathicus

Pars abdominalis aortae

N. iliohypogastricus

Truncus lumbosacralis

N. obturatorius

Rr. musculares

N. ilioinguinalis

M. transversus abdominis

N. cutaneus femoris lateralis

N. genitofemoralis, R. genitalis

Rectum

Fig. 7.9 Somatic nerves of the retroperitoneal space; after removal of the M. psoas major on the left side, the pathway of the nerves of the Plexus lumbalis is more clearly visible; ventral view. [S700]

In addition to the blood and lymph vessels, the nerves of the **Plexus lumbalis,** which provide the innervation of the inguinal region and the anterior aspect of the bone, also pass through the retroperitoneal space (→ Fig. 4.146, Volume 1). The **Truncus lumbosacralis** is connected to the Plexus sacralis (→ Fig. 7.12) in the lesser pelvis, so that the two nerve plexuses are united in the **Plexus lumbosacralis** (→ Fig. 4.142, Volume 1).

Branches of the Plexus lumbalis (T12–L4):
* Motor branches to the M. iliopsoas and the M. quadratus lumborum (T12–L4)
* N. iliohypogastricus (T12, L1)
* N. ilioinguinalis (T12, L1)
* N. genitofemoralis (L1, L2)
* N. cutaneus femoris lateralis (L2, L3)
* N. femoralis (L2, L4)
* N. obturatorius (L2, L4).

→ T 42

Autonomic nerves of the retroperitoneal space

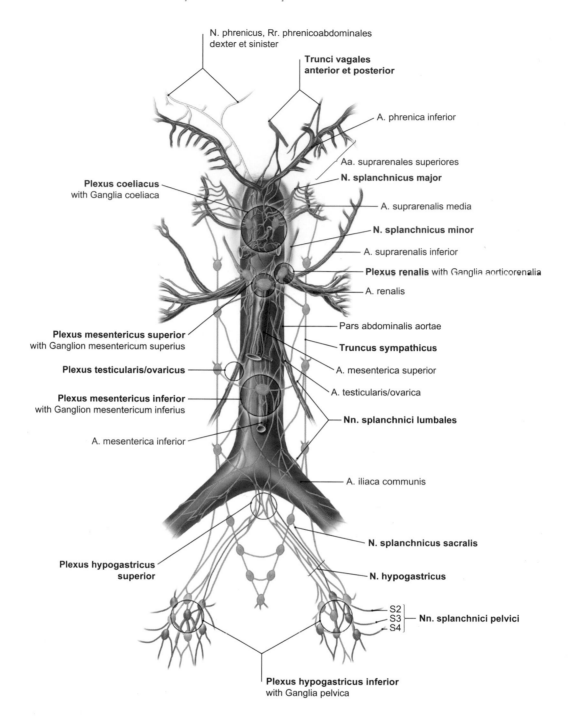

N. phrenicus, Rr. phrenicoabdominales dexter et sinister

Trunci vagales anterior et posterior

A. phrenica inferior

Aa. suprarenales superiores

N. splanchnicus major

A. suprarenalis media

N. splanchnicus minor

A. suprarenalis inferior

Plexus renalis with Ganglia aorticorenalia

A. renalis

Pars abdominalis aortae

Truncus sympathicus

A. mesenterica superior

A. testicularis/ovarica

Nn. splanchnici lumbales

A. iliaca communis

N. splanchnicus sacralis

N. hypogastricus

S2
S3   **Nn. splanchnici pelvici**
S4

Plexus coeliacus with Ganglia coeliaca

Plexus mesentericus superior with Ganglion mesentericum superius

Plexus testicularis/ovaricus

Plexus mesentericus inferior with Ganglion mesentericum inferius

A. mesenterica inferior

Plexus hypogastricus superior

Plexus hypogastricus inferior with Ganglia pelvica

Fig. 7.10   Plexus aorticus abdominalis and Plexus hypogastricus inferior; schematic illustration, ventral view. [S702-L238]
In front of the aorta, the autonomic sympathetic and parasympathetic nerve fibres form a plexus **(Plexus aorticus abdominalis),** which provides the vessels branching off from the aorta with their own plexuses, and these nerve fibres accompany the respective vessels to their target organs. These plexuses are located at the bifurcations of the three unpaired visceral branches of the aorta: the **Plexus coeliacus, and the Plexus mesenterici superior and inferior** (→ Fig. 6.84). Caudally, the nerve plexuses continue bilaterally from the Plexus hypogastricus superior via a bundle of nerve fibres, referred to as **N. hypogastricus,** to the **Plexus hypogastricus inferior** in the lesser pelvis, which innervates the pelvic viscera.
The preganglionic neurons of the **sympathicus** are located in the lateral horns of the spinal cord, and when reaching the **sympathetic trunk (Truncus sympathicus),** they continue without synaptic switching via the Nn. splanchnici major and minor to the aortic plexuses, where they become synaptically interconnected with postganglionic neurons (the axons of which accompany the branches of the respective arteries to

their target organs) in various ganglia (Ganglia coeliaca, Ganglia mesenterica superius and inferius, Ganglia aorticorenalia, Ganglia pelvica of the Plexus hypogastricus inferior).
The preganglionic parasympathetic neurons of the **Nn. vagi [X]** descend along the oesophagus as **Trunci vagales anterior and posterior,** and continue through the diaphragm to the autonomic nerve plexuses around the abdominal aorta; however, they pass through these plexuses without synapsing until they reach their target organs, where the postganglionic neurons are located in the wall or nearby. The area supplied by the N. vagus [X] ends in the Plexus mesentericus superior and thus, in the area of the left colonic flexure (splenic flexure or CANNON-BÖHM point). By contrast, the **Colon descendens** is supplied by the **sacral part of the parasympathicus;** its preganglionic neurons are located within the spinal cord (S2–S4), emerge with the spinal nerves as **Nn. splanchnici pelvici,** and then are interlinked to postganglionic neurons in the **Plexus hypogastricus inferior** in the rectal area. The postganglionic nerve fibres ascend to the Colon descendens and Colon sigmoideum.

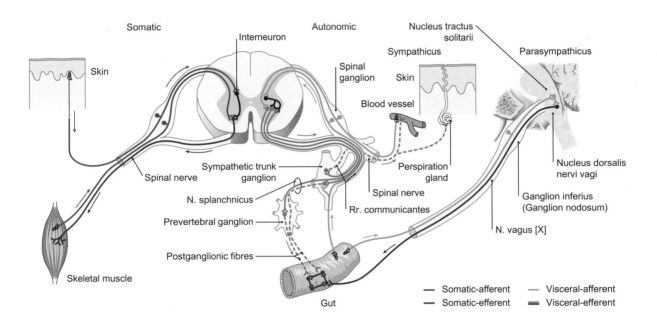

Somatic
Interneuron
Autonomic
Nucleus tractus solitarii
Skin
Sympathicus
Parasympathicus
Spinal ganglion
Skin
Blood vessel
Spinal nerve
Sympathetic trunk ganglion
N. splanchnicus
Perspiration gland
Nucleus dorsalis nervi vagi
Prevertebral ganglion
Spinal nerve
Rr. communicantes
Ganglion inferius (Ganglion nodosum)
Postganglionic fibres
N. vagus [X]
Skeletal muscle
Gut

— Somatic-afferent — Visceral-afferent
— Somatic-efferent — Visceral-efferent

Fig. 7.11 Organisation of the autonomic nervous system compared to the somatic nervous system; schematic illustration of the pathway and synaptic interconnection of a spinal cord segment. [S702-L127]/[G1076]

In contrast to the somatic nervous system, two **visceral-efferent neurons** in the autonomic nervous system are interconnected by synapses in a series on their way from the central nervous system to the target organ. The preganglionic neurons of the **sympathetic system (sympathicus)** are located in the lateral horns of the spinal cord and enter the spinal nerves together with somatic-efferent fibres via the ventral root. Via the **Rami communicantes** they reach the **sympathetic trunk (Truncus sympathicus)** and turn back as postganglionic neurons after their synaptic interconnection. These neurons run with the somatic nerves into the periphery, where they produce a narrowing (vasoconstriction) of the blood vessels **(vasomotor effect)**, activation of the sweat glands **(sudomotor effect)** and raise the lanugo (downy hair) on the body **(pilomotor effect,** not shown here). Postganglionic neurons also pass from the sympathetic trunk to the organs in the neck region and thoracic cavity, such as the heart and lungs. In contrast, the neurons to the abdominal organs are not synapsed in the sympathetic trunk, but pass via the **Nn. splanchnici major and minor** to the aortic plexuses, where they are synapsed with postganglionic neurons in various prevertebral ganglia; the axons of these neurons reach their target organs together with the branches of the respective arteries.

The preganglionic parasympathetic neurons, however, run with the **Nn. vagi [X]** without being synapsed through the autonomic nerve plexuses of the abdominal aorta, and only synapse to short postganglionic neurons in the wall or surrounding area of the target organs.

Visceral-afferent neurons also reach the central nervous system via the sympathetic trunk or the N. vagus [X].

Autonomic nerves of the retroperitoneal space

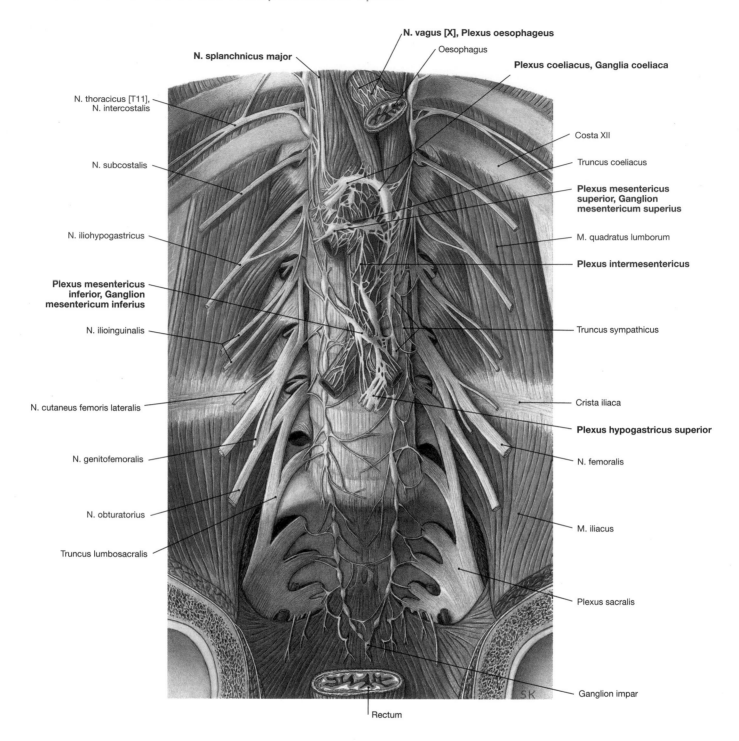

N. vagus [X], Plexus oesophageus

Oesophagus

N. splanchnicus major

Plexus coeliacus, Ganglia coeliaca

N. thoracicus [T11], N. intercostalis

Costa XII

Truncus coeliacus

N. subcostalis

Plexus mesentericus superior, Ganglion mesentericum superius

M. quadratus lumborum

N. iliohypogastricus

Plexus intermesentericus

Plexus mesentericus inferior, Ganglion mesentericum inferius

N. ilioinguinalis

Truncus sympathicus

N. cutaneus femoris lateralis

Crista iliaca

Plexus hypogastricus superior

N. femoralis

N. genitofemoralis

N. obturatorius

M. iliacus

Truncus lumbosacralis

Plexus sacralis

Ganglion impar

Rectum

Fig. 7.12 Somatic and autonomic nerves of the retroperitoneal space; ventral view; after removal of the viscera. [S700-L238]
The illustration shows the autonomic nerves around the aorta **(Plexus aorticus abdominalis).** Somatic nerves are depicted as well in order to provide topographical orientation.
The plexus consists of the sympathetic and parasympathetic neurons, which reach it in different ways and also show different synaptic interlinks within the nerve plexus.
The preganglionic **sympathetic neurons** pass from the sympathetic trunk (Truncus sympathicus) via the **Nn. splanchnici major and minor** to the aortic plexuses, where they are synapsed to postganglionic neurons in various ganglia (Ganglia coeliaca, Ganglia mesenterica superius and inferius, Ganglia aorticorenalia). This means that the ganglia in the plexuses, which are located around the bifurcations of the three un-

paired visceral branches of the aorta **(Plexus coeliacus, Plexus mesenterici superior and inferior)** are sympathetic ganglia. In contrast, the preganglionic parasympathetic neurons of the **Nn. vagi [X]** pass along the oesophagus as **Trunci vagales anterior and posterior** to the Plexus aorticus abdominalis.
The preganglionic sympathetic nerve fibres descend from the Plexus aorticus abdominalis into the lesser pelvis up to the **Plexus hypogastricus inferior** via which they supply the pelvic viscera. The parasympathetic neurons, on the other hand, only reach the Plexus mesentericus superior. In contrast, the pelvic organs are innervated by the **sacral part of the parasympathetic system (parasympathicus),** whereby the preganglionic nerve fibres leave the spinal cord as **Nn. splanchnici pelvici,** and then become synapsed in the Plexus hypogastricus inferior.

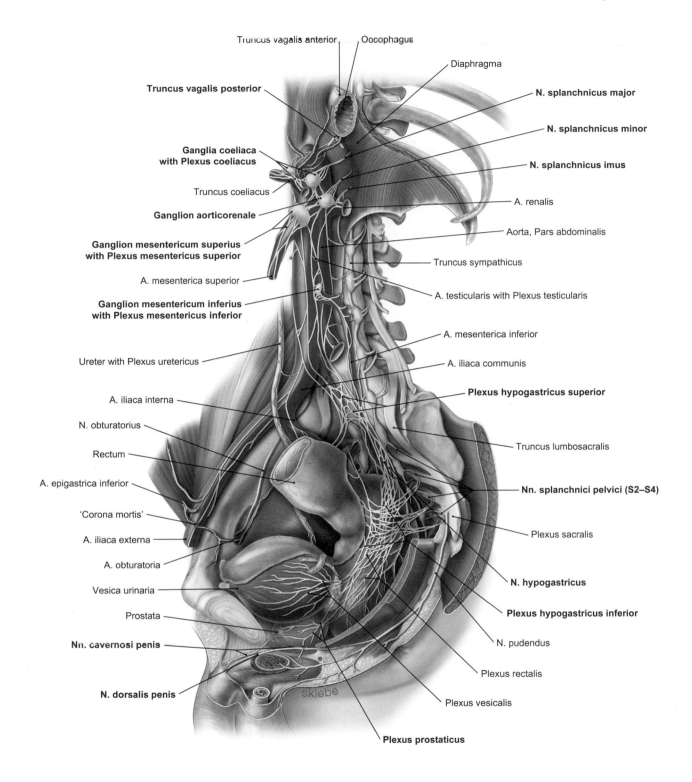

Truncus vagalis anterior
Oocophagus
Diaphragma
Truncus vagalis posterior
N. splanchnicus major
N. splanchnicus minor
Ganglia coeliaca with Plexus coeliacus
N. splanchnicus imus
Truncus coeliacus
A. renalis
Ganglion aorticorenale
Aorta, Pars abdominalis
Ganglion mesentericum superius with Plexus mesentericus superior
Truncus sympathicus
A. mesenterica superior
A. testicularis with Plexus testicularis
Ganglion mesentericum inferius with Plexus mesentericus inferior
A. mesenterica inferior
A. iliaca communis
Ureter with Plexus uretericus
Plexus hypogastricus superior
A. iliaca interna
N. obturatorius
Truncus lumbosacralis
Rectum
A. epigastrica inferior
Nn. splanchnici pelvici (S2–S4)
'Corona mortis'
Plexus sacralis
A. iliaca externa
A. obturatoria
Vesica urinaria
N. hypogastricus
Prostata
Plexus hypogastricus inferior
Nn. cavernosi penis
N. pudendus
Plexus rectalis
N. dorsalis penis
Plexus vesicalis
Plexus prostaticus

Fig. 7.13 Autonomic nerves of the pelvic cavity; semi-schematic illustration after removal of the retroperitoneal organs as well as of the veins and lymph vessels; ventral view. [S702-L238]
The illustration shows the pathway of the autonomic neurons in the pelvis. The sympathetic neurons descend from the Plexus aorticus abdominalis into the lesser pelvis, where they are switched synaptically in the **Plexus hypogastricus inferior** and reach the pelvic organs. The Plexus hypogastricus inferior forms smaller local plexuses around the pelvic organs, such as the Plexus rectalis, Plexus vesicalis and Plexus prostaticus (or the Plexus uterovaginalis in women).
In contrast, the parasympathetic neurons reach the plexus via the **Nn. splanchnici pelvici.** After switching, they reach the pelvic organs

and the left-sided colon up to the left colonic flexure via their own nerve branches.
It should be noted that the pathway of the parasympathetic neurons to the cavernous bodies of the penis is similar to the pathway they use to reach the cavernous bodies of the female genitalia. The neurons form the **Nn. cavernosi penis,** which pass along the prostate gland through the pelvic floor and perineal muscles into the Corpora cavernosa of the penis. The longer branches join the somatic N. dorsalis penis, which represents the terminal branch of the N. pudendus, and together with it enter the cavernous bodies. These neurons facilitate the erection of the penis by dilating the vessels in the cavernous bodies.

A. iliaca interna

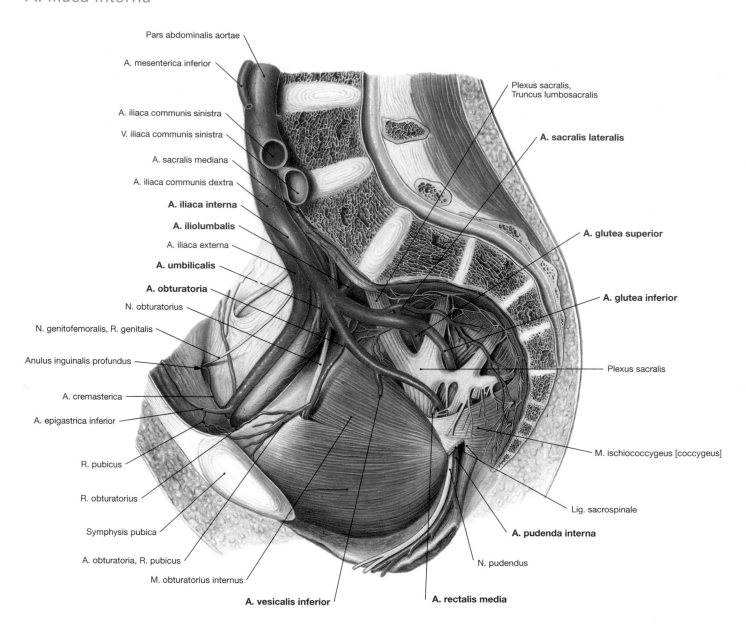

Pars abdominalis aortae
A. mesenterica inferior
A. iliaca communis sinistra
V. iliaca communis sinistra
A. sacralis mediana
A. iliaca communis dextra
A. iliaca interna
A. iliolumbalis
A. iliaca externa
A. umbilicalis
A. obturatoria
N. obturatorius
N. genitofemoralis, R. genitalis
Anulus inguinalis profundus
A. cremasterica
A. epigastrica inferior
R. pubicus
R. obturatorius
Symphysis pubica
A. obturatoria, R. pubicus
M. obturatorius internus
A. vesicalis inferior

Plexus sacralis, Truncus lumbosacralis
A. sacralis lateralis
A. glutea superior
A. glutea inferior
Plexus sacralis
M. ischiococcygeus [coccygeus]
Lig. sacrospinale
A. pudenda interna
N. pudendus
A. rectalis media

Fig. 7.14 A. iliaca interna; lateral view from the left side. [S700] Mostly (in 60 % of all cases), the A. iliaca interna divides into an anterior and a posterior trunk. Because they branch off in a rather variable sequence, the arterial branches are categorised according to their perfusion area as **parietal branches** for the pelvic wall and the external genitalia, and as **visceral branches** for the pelvic viscera. While the parietal branches are the same in both sexes, the visceral branches differ, since they supply the sexual organs. The parietal veins correspond to the arterial branches and accompany them.

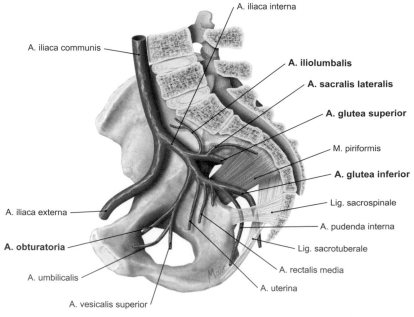

A. iliaca interna
A. iliaca communis
A. iliolumbalis
A. sacralis lateralis
A. glutea superior
M. piriformis
A. glutea inferior
Lig. sacrospinale
A. pudenda interna
Lig. sacrotuberale
A. rectalis media
A. uterina
A. iliaca externa
A. obturatoria
A. umbilicalis
A. vesicalis superior

Fig. 7.15 Parietal branches of the A. iliaca interna. [S700-L127]

- A. iliolumbalis: supplies the Fossa iliaca and the lumbar region
- Aa. sacrales laterales: supply the sacral canal
- A. obturatoria: passes through the Canalis obturatorius
- A. glutea superior: passes through the Foramen suprapiriforme into the gluteal region
- A. glutea inferior: passes through the Foramen infrapiriforme into the gluteal area

In up to 20 %, the A. obturatoria does not originate from the A. iliaca interna, but is a descending branch of the A. epigastrica inferior from the circulatory region of the A. iliaca externa.

For the visceral branches (different in men and women), → Fig. 7.16 and → Fig. 7.17.

Retroperitoneal space and pelvic cavity

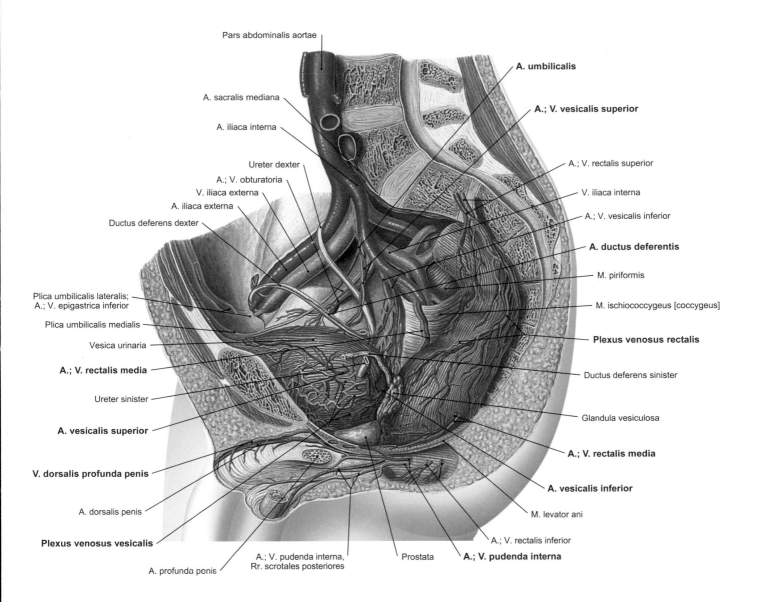

Pars abdominalis aortae

A. sacralis mediana

A. iliaca interna

Ureter dexter

A.; V. obturatoria

V. iliaca externa

A. iliaca externa

Ductus deferens dexter

Plica umbilicalis lateralis;
A.; V. epigastrica inferior

Plica umbilicalis medialis

Vesica urinaria

A.; V. rectalis media

Ureter sinister

A. vesicalis superior

V. dorsalis profunda penis

A. dorsalis penis

Plexus venosus vesicalis

A. profunda penis

A.; V. pudenda interna,
Rr. scrotales posteriores

Prostata

A. umbilicalis

A.; V. vesicalis superior

A.; V. rectalis superior

V. iliaca interna

A.; V. vesicalis inferior

A. ductus deferentis

M. piriformis

M. ischiococcygeus [coccygeus]

Plexus venosus rectalis

Ductus deferens sinister

Glandula vesiculosa

A.; V. rectalis media

A. vesicalis inferior

M. levator ani

A.; V. rectalis inferior

A.; V. pudenda interna

Fig. 7.16 Blood supply of the pelvic viscera in men; lateral view from the left side. [S700]

The pelvic viscera are supplied by the **visceral branches** of the A. iliaca interna. The **parietal branches** for the pelvic wall are identical in both sexes (→ Fig. 7.15).

Visceral branches of the A. iliaca interna in men:
- **A. umbilicalis:** provides the A. vesicalis superior to the urinary bladder, and usually (not here) the A. ductus deferentis to the spermatic duct (Ductus deferens), before its obliterated part (Lig. umbilicale mediale) forms the Plica umbilicalis medialis
- **A. vesicalis inferior:** supplies the urinary bladder, prostate and seminal vesicle, and occasionally (as shown here) provides the A. ductus deferentis
- **A. rectalis media:** above the pelvic floor to the rectum
- **A. pudenda interna:** passes through the Foramen infrapiriforme and the Foramen ischiadicum minus into the lateral wall of the Fossa ischioanalis (Canalis pudendalis, ALCOCK's canal). Here, the A. rectalis inferior branches off to the lower anal canal, before the A. pudenda divides into its superficial and deep terminal branches to supply the external genitalia. The superficial A. perinealis supplies the

perineum and sends the Rr. scrotales posteriores to the scrotum. The deep branches supply the penis and its spongy tissue (A. bulbi penis, A. dorsalis penis, A. profunda penis).

The venous blood from the pelvic viscera flows to the **V. iliaca interna,** forming venous plexuses (Plexus venosi) with its afferent branches around the individual organs, all of which are connected with each other. Most of these plexuses have to be removed during dissection to display the arteries and nerves of the pelvis:
- **Plexus venosus rectalis:** it is connected via the V. rectalis superior to the portal vein system and via the Vv. rectales media and inferior to the drainage area of the V. cava inferior (portocaval anastomosis).
- **Plexus venosus vesicalis:** located at the fundus of the bladder, also collects the venous blood of the accessory sex glands
- **Plexus venosus prostaticus (SANTORINI):** collects the blood of the prostate, and of the cavernous bodies of the penis (V. dorsalis profunda penis). Connections to the venous plexuses of the spine explain in part why prostate cancer is often associated with spinal metastases. The V. iliaca interna also collects blood from the parietal veins that correspond to the parietal arterial branches.

Vessels of the female pelvis

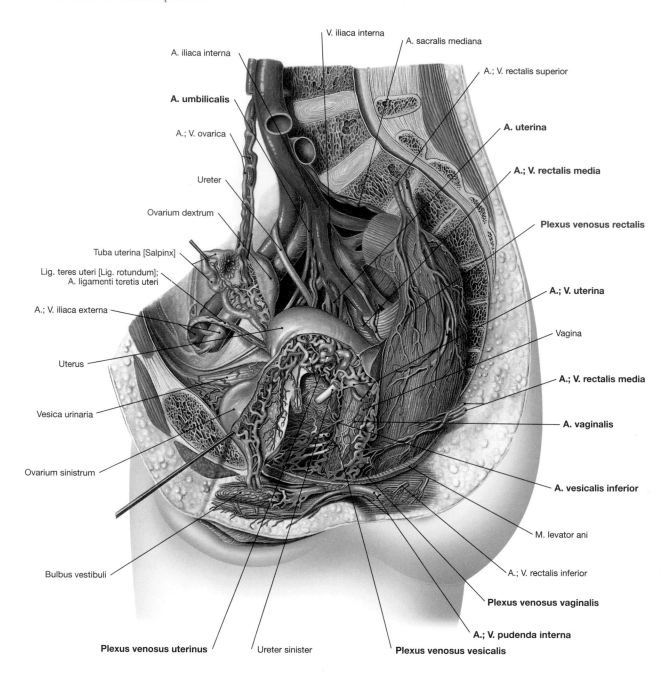

V. iliaca interna

A. sacralis mediana

A. iliaca interna

A.; V. rectalis superior

A. umbilicalis

A. uterina

A.; V. ovarica

A.; V. rectalis media

Ureter

Plexus venosus rectalis

Ovarium dextrum

Tuba uterina [Salpinx]

Lig. teres uteri [Lig. rotundum];
A. ligamenti teretis uteri

A.; V. uterina

A.; V. iliaca externa

Vagina

Uterus

A.; V. rectalis media

Vesica urinaria

A. vaginalis

Ovarium sinistrum

A. vesicalis inferior

M. levator ani

A.; V. rectalis inferior

Bulbus vestibuli

Plexus venosus vaginalis

A.; V. pudenda interna

Plexus venosus uterinus

Ureter sinister

Plexus venosus vesicalis

Fig. 7.17   Blood supply of the pelvic viscera in women; lateral view from the left side. [S700]

The pelvic viscera are supplied by the **visceral branches** of the A. iliaca interna. The **parietal branches** for the pelvic wall are identical in both sexes (→ Fig. 7.15).

Visceral branches of the A. iliaca interna in women:

- **A. umbilicalis:** provides the A. vesicalis superior to the urinary bladder before its obliterated part (Lig. umbilicale mediale) forms the Plica umbilicalis medialis
- **A. vesicalis inferior:** supplies the urinary bladder and the vagina, may be absent and is then replaced by the A. vaginalis
- **A. uterina:** supplies the uterus and with its own branches to Tuba uterina, ovary and vagina
- **A. vaginalis:** sometimes replaces the A. vesicalis inferior
- **A. rectalis media:** above the pelvic floor to the rectum
- **A. pudenda interna:** passes through the Foramen infrapiriforme and the Foramen ischiadicum minus into the lateral wall of the Fossa ischioanalis (Canalis pudendalis, ALCOCK's canal). Here, the A. rectalis inferior branches off to the lower anal canal, before the A. pu-

denda divides into its superficial and deep terminal branches to supply the external genitalia. The superficial A. perinealis supplies the perineum and sends the Rr. labiales posteriores to the labia. The deep branches supply the clitoris with its cavernous body and the vestibular erectile tissue in the Labia majora (A. bulbi vestibuli, A. dorsalis clitoridis, A. profunda clitoridis).

The venous blood from the pelvic viscera flows to the **V. iliaca interna,** forming venous plexuses (Plexus venosi) with its afferent branches around the individual organs, all of which are connected with each other. Most of these plexuses have to be removed during dissection to display the arteries and nerves of the pelvis:

- **Plexus venosus rectalis:** via the V. rectalis superior it is connected to the portal vein system and via the Vv. rectales media and inferior to the drainage area of the V. cava inferior (portocaval anastomosis)
- **Plexus venosus vesicalis:** located at the fundus of the urinary bladder, also collects the blood of the cavernous bodies (V. dorsalis profunda clitoridis)
- **Plexus venosi uterinus and vaginalis:** collect the blood of the uterus and vagina.

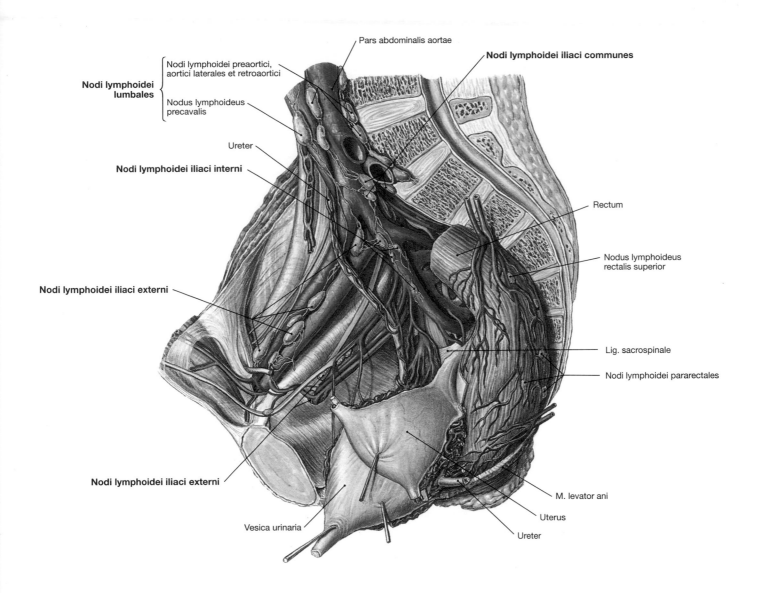

Pars abdominalis aortae

Nodi lymphoidei preaortici,
aortici laterales et retroaortici

**Nodi lymphoidei
lumbales**

Nodus lymphoideus
precavalis

Ureter

Nodi lymphoidei iliaci interni

Nodi lymphoidei iliaci communes

Rectum

Nodus lymphoideus
rectalis superior

Nodi lymphoidei iliaci externi

Lig. sacrospinale

Nodi lymphoidei pararectales

Nodi lymphoidei iliaci externi

M. levator ani

Uterus

Vesica urinaria

Ureter

Fig. 7.18 Lymph nodes and lymph vessels of the pelvis (shown here in a woman); lateral view from the left side. [S700]
In the pelvis, the Nodi lymphoidei iliaci interni and externi are located along the respective blood vessels, and the Nodi lymphoidei sacrales on the ventral side of the sacrum. Due to their close proximity, a strict separation between parietal lymph nodes in the pelvic wall and visceral lymph nodes around the pelvic viscera is not possible. Thus, the pelvic viscera (rectum, urinary bladder, pelvic part of the ureter and internal genitalia) are connected to all the groups of lymph nodes.
The lymph of the upper **rectum** is drained via the Nodi lymphoidei rectales superiores to the Nodi lymphoidei mesenterici inferiores in the retroperitoneal space, and to the Nodi lymphoidei iliaci interni in the pelvis. In contrast, the lymph of the lower rectum is drained to the Nodi lymphoidei inguinales superficiales. This explains why the lymph node

metastases of proximal rectal carcinomas are found in the retroperitoneal space and in the pelvis, but those of distal rectal carcinomas are found in the inguinal region.
The regional lymph nodes of the **urinary bladder** are predominantly the Nodi lymphoidei iliaci interni.
The lymphatic drainage of the **female genitalia** (→ Fig. 7.143, → Fig. 7.144, → Fig. 7.145) and the **male genitalia** (→ Fig. 7.104, → Fig. 7.105) is described in detail in the context of the respective organs.
Via the Nodi lymphoidei iliaci communes, the lymph finally drains into the parietal lymph nodes of the retroperitoneal space, which are summarised as Nodi lymphoidei lumbales on both sides of the aorta and the V. cava inferior.

Clinical remarks

A **pelvic lymph node dissection** performed in the case of malignancies in pelvic organs usually includes an extensive removal of all lymph nodes up to the bifurcation of the A. Iliaca communis. A care-

ful exposure of the neurovascular structures of the obturator canal (A./V. obturatoria and N. obturatorius) helps to prevent injury to those structures during the surgery.

Retroperitoneal space and pelvic cavity

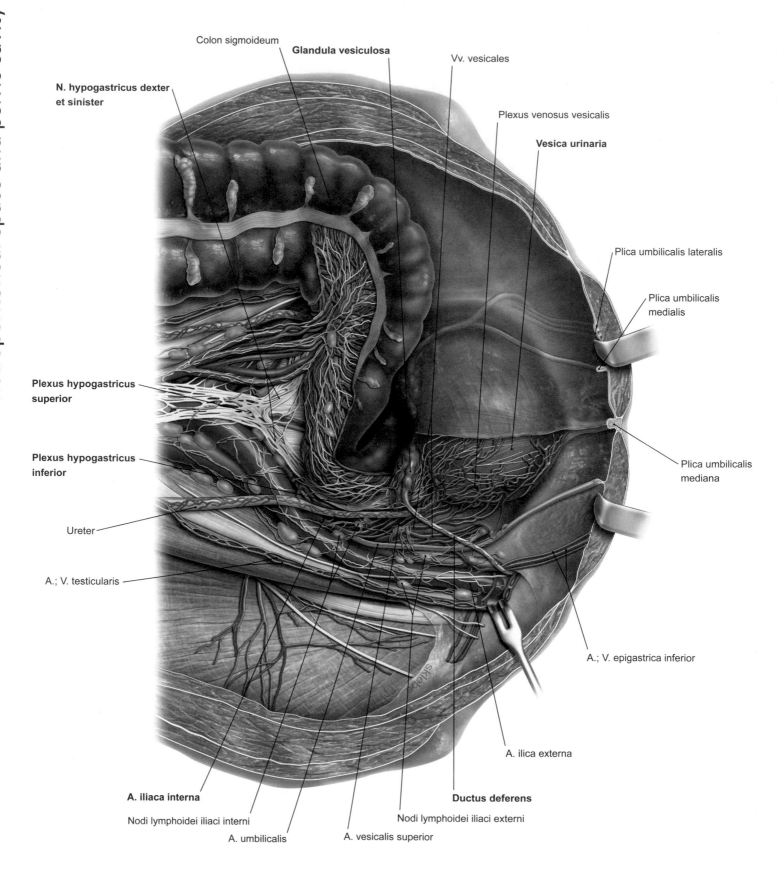

Colon sigmoideum

Glandula vesiculosa

Vv. vesicales

N. hypogastricus dexter et sinister

Plexus venosus vesicalis

Vesica urinaria

Plica umbilicalis lateralis

Plica umbilicalis medialis

Plexus hypogastricus superior

Plexus hypogastricus inferior

Plica umbilicalis mediana

Ureter

A.; V. testicularis

A.; V. epigastrica inferior

A. ilica externa

A. iliaca interna

Ductus deferens

Nodi lymphoidei iliaci interni

Nodi lymphoidei iliaci externi

A. umbilicalis

A. vesicalis superior

Fig. 7.19 **Pelvic viscera in the male;** cranial view. [S700-L238]/[Q300] The illustration shows the autonomic nervous system in the pelvis. The **Plexus hypogastricus superior** continues on both sides via a strand of nerve fibres that are referred to as **N. hypogastricus dexter and sinister,** up to the **Plexus hypogastricus inferior** in the fascia of the small pelvis (shown here on the right side).

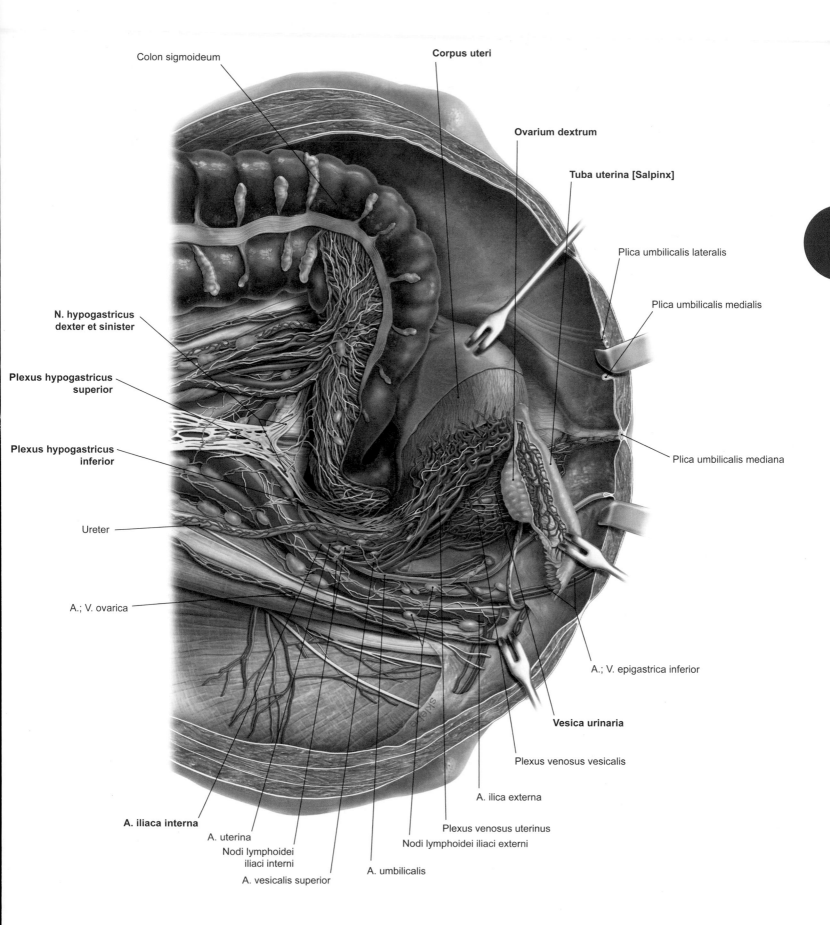

Colon sigmoideum

Corpus uteri

Ovarium dextrum

Tuba uterina [Salpinx]

Plica umbilicalis lateralis

Plica umbilicalis medialis

N. hypogastricus
dexter et sinister

Plexus hypogastricus
superior

Plexus hypogastricus
inferior

Plica umbilicalis mediana

Ureter

A.; V. ovarica

A.; V. epigastrica inferior

Vesica urinaria

Plexus venosus vesicalis

A. ilica externa

A. iliaca interna

A. uterina

Nodi lymphoidei
iliaci interni

Plexus venosus uterinus

Nodi lymphoidei iliaci externi

A. umbilicalis

A. vesicalis superior

Fig. 7.20 Pelvic viscera with neurovascular structures in the female;
cranial view. [S700-L238]/[Q300]
The illustration shows the autonomic nervous system in the pelvis. The
Plexus hypogastricus superior continues on both sides as a strand of

nerve fibres, that are referred to as **N. hypogastricus dexter and sinister,** up to the **Plexus hypogastricus inferior** in the fascia of the small pelvis (shown here on the right side).

Structure of the urinary system

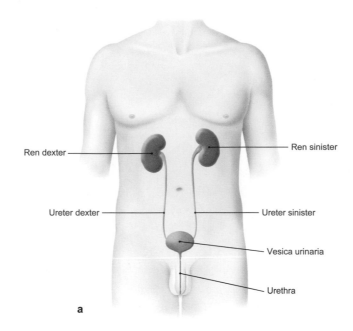

Ren dexter

Ren sinister

Ureter dexter

Ureter sinister

Vesica urinaria

Urethra

a

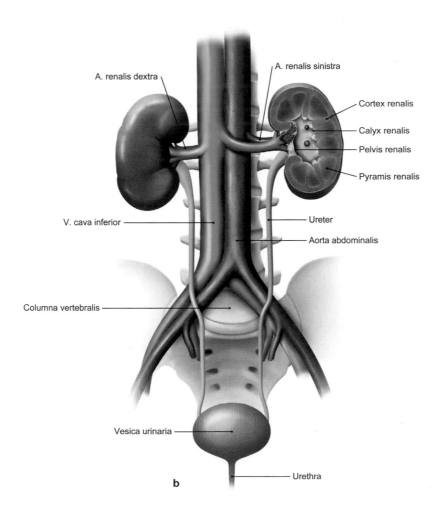

A. renalis dextra

A. renalis sinistra

Cortex renalis

Calyx renalis

Pelvis renalis

Pyramis renalis

V. cava inferior

Ureter

Aorta abdominalis

Columna vertebralis

Vesica urinaria

Urethra

b

Fig. 7.21a and b Structure of the urinary system; ventral view [S701-L275]
a Projection onto the surface of the body.
b Projection onto the skeleton, showing the A./V. renalis.
The **urinary system** comprises the paired **kidneys (Ren [Nephros])** which produce the urine, and the **urinary tract components** which drain the urine. These include:
- renal pelvis (Pelvis renalis)
- ureter

- urinary bladder (Vesica urinaria)
- urethra.

The **suprarenal glands** are endocrine glands → Fig. 7.22 and do not belong to the urinary system.
With the exception of the urethra, the urinary system is identically formed in both sexes. In a man, the urethra is a **tube for urine and semen** in the penis, as it also serves to transport the ejaculate, and is thereby part of the external male genitalia.

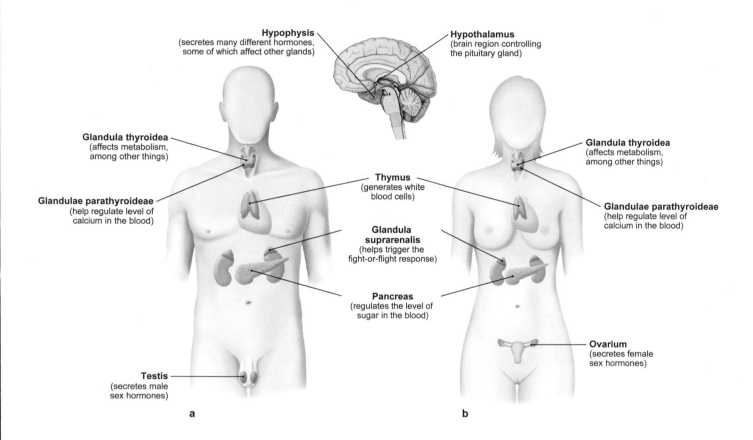

Fig. 7.22a and b Endocrine organs in men and women; ventral view. [S701-L275]

a Endocrine organs in the male.

b Endocrine organs in the female.

The **adrenal gland (Glandula suprarenalis)** is not part of the urinary organs, but part of the hormone-producing glands which are endocrine organs and defined as the endocrine system.

Since the adrenal glands adhere to the kidneys and are partly supplied by the same neurovascular pathways, the adrenal glands will be dealt with in conjunction with the kidneys.

Nevertheless, a brief introductory overview of the **endocrine system** is necessary to explain the function and regulation of the adrenal gland. Due to their development, the adrenal glands consist of two different parts (→ Fig. 7.43): the external layer (cortex) and the medulla, which produce different types of hormones and secrete them into the blood. The release of the hormones is also regulated in different ways in both parts. The cortex produces vital **steroid hormones,** such as aldosterone (mineralocorticoid) and cortisol (glucocorticoid), whereas the **medulla** produces **catecholamines** (adrenaline and noradrenaline). The release of cortisol, a stress hormone for the supply of energy, for example by breaking down sugars (glycogen) stored in the liver, is controlled by the **hypothalamic-pituitary axis.** The hypothalamus is part of the diencephalon and produces regulatory hormones (e. g. CRH, corticotro-

pin-releasing hormone) which induce the release of other hormones in the pituitary gland. These in turn control the peripheral hormone glands. In this way, CRH acts on the anterior lobe of the pituitary gland (adenohypophysis) and stimulates the release of corticotropin (ACTH, adrenocorticotropic hormone), which induces the release of cortisol in the adrenal cortex. The production of regulatory hormones in the hypothalamus and pituitary gland is inhibited by cortisol in a regulatory circuit. This principle is referred to as **negative feedback.** It is of great importance for medical diagnostics, as measuring the concentrations of individual hormones and of their regulatory hormones allows conclusions on the causes of hormone production disorders. In contrast, the release of aldosterone to increase blood pressure is controlled independently from the pituitary gland by a different regulatory system involving enzymes and hormones of the kidneys and the liver **(renin-angiotensin-aldosterone system, RAAS),** with the kidney functioning as a sensor for the blood pressure. The distinct endocrine regulatory systems are a topic for the area of microscopic anatomy.

Catecholamines produced in the medulla of the adrenal glands also increase blood pressure. However, their release is activated by the **sympathetic nervous system.** Since the adrenal medulla corresponds to a sympathetic ganglion in developmental terms, the preganglionic neurons end directly at the hormone-producing cells (→ Fig. 7.48).

Projection of kidney and adrenal gland

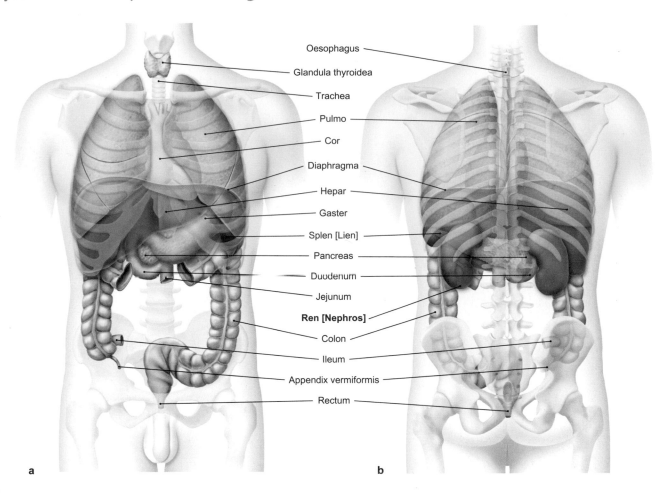

Oesophagus

Glandula thyroidea

Trachea

Pulmo

Cor

Diaphragma

Hepar

Gaster

Splen [Lien]

Pancreas

Duodenum

Jejunum

Ren [Nephros]

Colon

Ileum

Appendix vermiformis

Rectum

a

b

Fig. 7.23a and b   Projection of internal organs onto the body surface.
[S700-L275]
a Ventral view.
b Dorsal view.

Kidneys and adrenal glands are located in the retroperitoneal space. The adrenal glands adhere to the upper pole of the kidneys, and both structures share a common encasing system (→ Fig. 7.31).

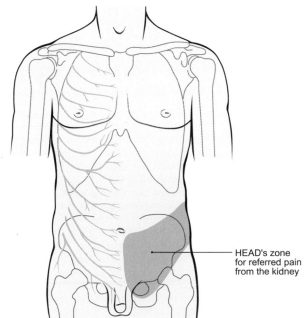

HEAD's zone
for referred pain
from the kidney

Fig. 7.24   HEAD's zone of the kidney, Ren [Nephros]; ventral view.
[S700-L126]/[G1071]
The organ-related area for referred pain or the **HEAD's zone** of the kidney are the cutaneous areas (dermatomes) T10–L1. Renal diseases can therefore lead to pain perceived in these cutaneous areas (referred pain). This is because the visceral-afferent neurons from the kidney converge in the spinal cord segments T10–L1 along with the somatic-afferent neurons from the surface of the body, so that the cause cannot be precisely determined.

Clinical remarks

Examining the kidneys for pain sensitivity is performed with a well-judged punch in the lumbar region (at the back of the trunk and at the level of the kidney, just below the ribs). However, the patient should not be alerted, as otherwise the punch would be attenuated too effectively by the anticipatory tensing of the back muscles. In the case of an inflammation of the renal pelvis (pyelonephritis), the patient will report considerable pain in response to the punch.

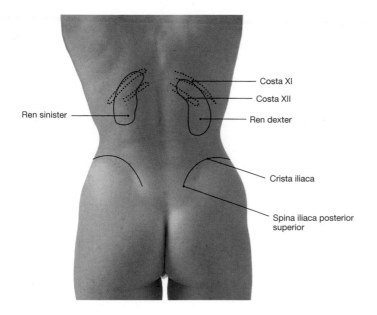

Costa XI
Costa XII
Ren dexter
Ren sinister
Crista iliaca
Spina iliaca posterior superior

Fig. 7.25   Projection of the kidney onto the dorsal wall of the trunk. [S700]

Projections of the left kidney only:
* superior pole: 12th thoracic vertebra (T12), rib 6
* hilum: second lumbar vertebra (L2)
* inferior pole: third lumbar vertebra (L3).

Due to the size of the liver, the right kidney is located about half a vertebra deeper (caudally). Hence its superior pole projects just below rib 6 on the right side.

Due to their proximity to the diaphragm, the position of the kidneys varies with breathing, so that they can both descend up to 3 cm during inhalation.

The adrenal glands project onto the neck of the 11th and 12th ribs.

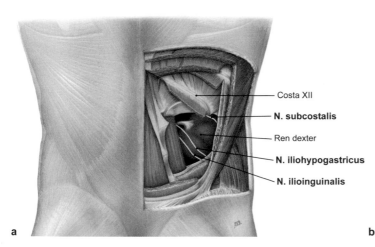

Costa XII
N. subcostalis
Ren dexter
N. iliohypogastricus
N. ilioinguinalis

a

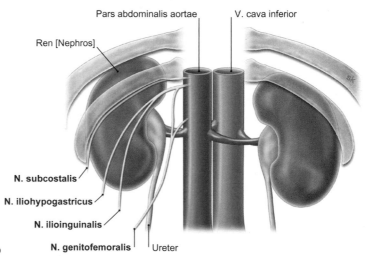

Pars abdominalis aortae   V. cava inferior
Ren [Nephros]
N. subcostalis
N. iliohypogastricus
N. ilioinguinalis
N. genitofemoralis   Ureter

b

Fig. 7.26a and b   Position of the kidneys in relation to the nerves of the Plexus lumbalis.
a Pathway of the nerves of the Plexus lumbalis in relation to the kidney; dorsal view. [S701-L285]
b Pathway of the nerves of the Plexus lumbalis in relation to the kidney, semi-schematic illustration after removal of muscles, dorsal view. [S702-L238]/[B500]
Between the renal fascia surrounding the lower pole of the kidney and the dorsal muscles of the trunk, the **N. iliohypogastricus** and **N. ilioin-**

guinalis from the Plexus lumbalis run between the renal fascia in the area of the inferior pole of the kidney and the muscles of the dorsal abdominal wall, and provide, among other things, sensory innervation to the inguinal region. Further cranially on the dorsal side of the kidneys and just below the two lowest ribs, the 11th and 12th intercostal nerves are found (12th intercostal nerve = **N. subcostalis**). The **N. genitofemoralis** descends further caudally and therefore has no contact with the kidney, only the ureter.

Clinical remarks

The close proximity of the kidney to the N. iliohypogastricus and N. ilioinguinalis explains why renal diseases such as inflammation of the renal pelvis (pyelonephritis) or entrapped kidney stones or renal calculi (nephrolithiasis) may cause **pain radiating into the inguinal region.**
[S702-L126]

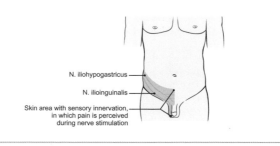

N. iliohypogastricus
N. ilioinguinalis
Skin area with sensory innervation, in which pain is perceived during nerve stimulation

Development of the kidney

Fig. 7.27 Development of the kidneys in week 5. [S700-L126]/ [B500/E107]

The kidneys and the efferent urinary tract derive from the mesoderm which initially, on both sides of the somites, forms **nephrogenic cell clusters or strands.** From these the kidneys develop successively **over three generations and in a cranial to caudal sequence:**

- The first generation is the **pronephros,** an immature form which completely regresses.
- The **mesonephros** is a kidney with temporary excretory function, but which also regresses, with the exception of its primitive ureter (WOLFFIAN duct). In men, a part of the small ducts is generated between the testes and epididymides.
- Beginning in week 5, the **metanephros** develops after induction by the ureteric bud from the WOLFFIAN duct into the parenchyma of the definitive kidney (nephrons).

The collecting ducts and the proximal parts of the efferent urinary tract (renal pelvis and ureter) develop directly from the ureteric bud.

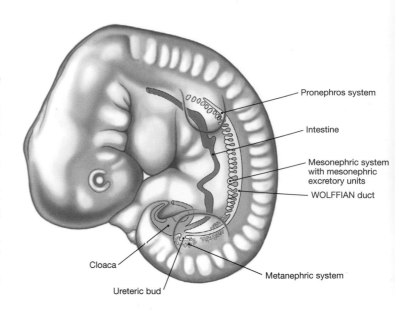

Fig. 7.28a–d Ascensus of the kidneys. [S700-L126]/[(B500~M282/ L132)/G322]

The metanephros develops at the level of the first to fourth sacral vertebrae and **(a)** ascends during weeks 6 to 9 of the development (ascensus, **b).** This is actually a relative ascent as the part located caudally to the inferior pole of the kidneys develops more quickly. In the absence of

this ascensus, a **pelvic kidney** will develop **(c).** If both kidneys are too close together during their ascent, they may fuse to form a horseshoe kidney **(d)** (incidence 1 in 400). This deformity usually does not reach the definitive position because its ascensus is impeded by the A. mesenterica inferior.

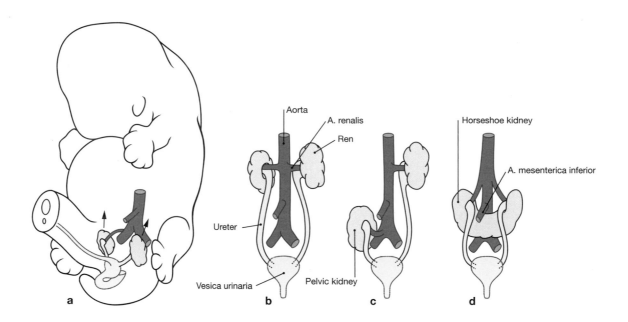

--- Clinical remarks ---

Pelvic kidneys (→ Fig. 7.28c) and **horseshoe kidneys** (→ Fig. 7.28d) are usually accidental findings and have no clinical relevance, if the ureter is not compromised. Displacement of the ureter, however, can cause a urinary stasis, which may result in renal damage due to the increased pressure and ascending infections.

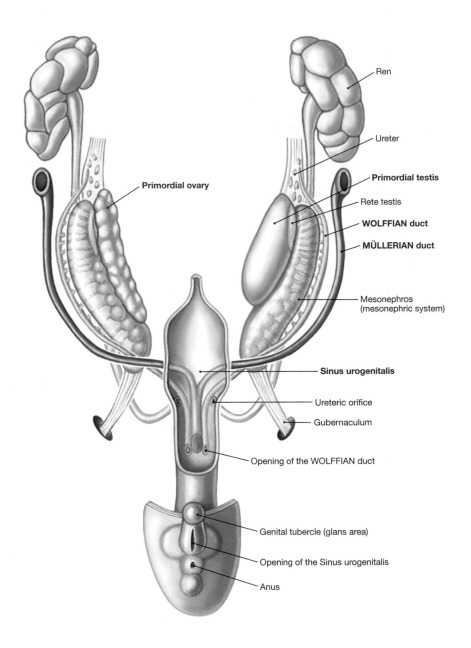

Ren

Ureter

Primordial testis

Rete testis

WOLFFIAN duct

MÜLLERIAN duct

Primordial ovary

Mesonephros
(mesonephric system)

Sinus urogenitalis

Ureteric orifice

Gubernaculum

Opening of the WOLFFIAN duct

Genital tubercle (glans area)

Opening of the Sinus urogenitalis

Anus

Fig. 7.29 Development of the urinary organs and early development of the internal genital organs in both sexes in week 8. [B500-L238]/[H233-001]

The kidneys develop from the metanephros and the ureteric bud which arises from the WOLFFIAN duct. The ureteric bud gives rise to the proximal efferent urinary tract (renal pelvis and ureter), whereas the urinary bladder and urethra develop from the Sinus urogenitalis (ventral part of the cloaca of the hindgut).

The internal genitalia develop in both sexes in the same way until week 7 (sexually indifferent gonadal stage). Besides the gonad which has not yet differentiated to testicle or ovary, there are two parallel pairs of ducts: the Ductus mesonephricus or **WOLFFIAN duct** and the Ductus paramesonephricus or **MÜLLERIAN duct.** In contrast to the WOLFFIAN duct, the distal ends of the MÜLLERIAN duct fuse prior to entering the Sinus urogenitalis. At the end of week 7, the indifferent gonad develops into the male testis or the female ovary. The testicular hormones (testosterone and anti-MÜLLERIAN hormone) induce the differentiation of the WOLFFIAN ducts to the male internal genitalia (→ Fig. 7.91) and suppress the further development of the MÜLLERIAN ducts. If both hormones are lacking, female internal genitalia will develop (→ Fig. 7.121).

Kidney and adrenal gland

Topography of the kidney and adrenal gland

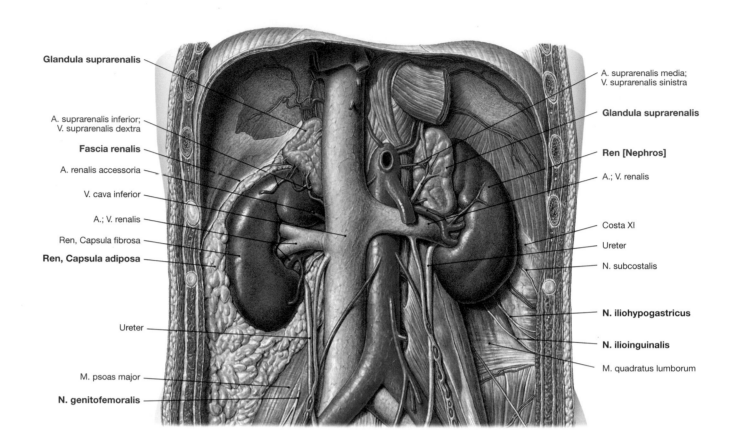

Glandula suprarenalis

A. suprarenalis inferior;
V. suprarenalis dextra

Fascia renalis

A. renalis accessoria

V. cava inferior

A.; V. renalis

Ren, Capsula fibrosa

Ren, Capsula adiposa

Ureter

M. psoas major

N. genitofemoralis

A. suprarenalis media;
V. suprarenalis sinistra

Glandula suprarenalis

Ren [Nephros]

A.; V. renalis

Costa XI

Ureter

N. subcostalis

N. iliohypogastricus

N. ilioinguinalis

M. quadratus lumborum

Fig. 7.30   Position of the kidney, Ren [Nephros], and adrenal gland, Glandula suprarenalis, in the retroperitoneal space; ventral view. [S700]

The kidney and adrenal gland are located in the retroperitoneal space ventrally of the M. psoas major and the M. quadratus lumborum. The kidney and the adrenal gland are embedded in a capsule of adipose tissue (Capsula adiposa), which is surrounded by a sheath of connective tissue (Fascia renalis, GEROTA's fascia). On the dorsal side of the renal fascia, the M. psoas major is located medially and the M. quadratus lumborum, as a muscle of the dorsal abdominal wall, is located laterally. Positioned between the renal fascia and the muscles, the N. iliohypogastricus and the N. ilioinguinalis from the Plexus lumbalis provide sensory innervation to the inguinal region, among others.

Clinical remarks

The retroperitoneal position of the kidneys determines the **surgical access** routes. The anterior approach through the abdominal peritoneal cavity always bears the risk of peritoneal infection **(Peritonitis)** with subsequent adhesions of intestinal loops to the parietal peritoneum. Therefore, the **transperitoneal** surgical approach to the kidney is chosen only when the removal of a renal or adrenal carcinoma requires procedural space. To access the kidney for benign diseases, such as the removal of kidney stones from the renal pelvis (nephrolithiasis), a **retroperitoneal** approach is chosen. This way, access is from dorsal through the Fascia thoracolumbalis (→ Fig. 7.33) or lateral thereof, demonstrating the importance of this fascia for spatial orientation.

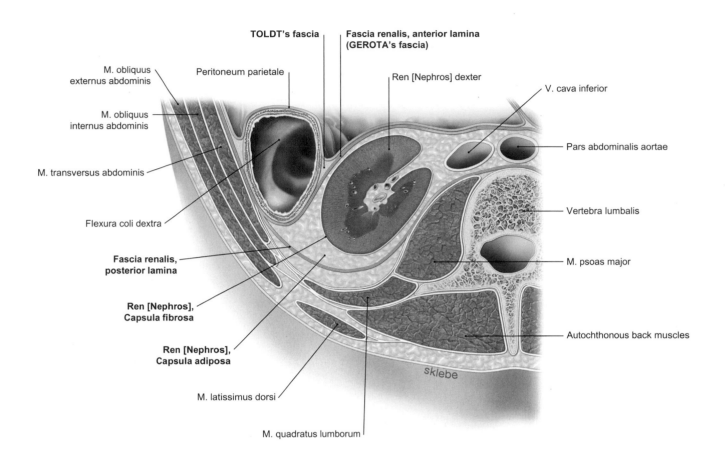

M. obliquus
externus abdominis

M. obliquus
internus abdominis

M. transversus abdominis

Flexura coli dextra

**Fascia renalis,
posterior lamina**

**Ren [Nephros],
Capsula fibrosa**

**Ren [Nephros],
Capsula adiposa**

M. latissimus dorsi

M. quadratus lumborum

TOLDT's fascia

Peritoneum parietale

**Fascia renalis, anterior lamina
(GEROTA's fascia)**

Ren [Nephros] dexter

V. cava inferior

Pars abdominalis aortae

Vertebra lumbalis

M. psoas major

Autochthonous back muscles

sklebe

**Fig. 7.31   Fascial systems of the kidney, Ren [Nephros], in the re-
troperitoneal space;** horizontal section at the level of the third lumbar
vertebra; caudal view. [S702-L238]/[B500-M580]
The kidney and adrenal gland are located in the retroperitoneal space
ventral of the M. psoas major and the M. quadratus lumborum.
The surface of the kidney is covered by a fibrous **capsule** of dense
connective tissue **(Capsula fibrosa).** Together with the adrenal gland,
the kidney is enclosed in a **capsule of adipose tissue (Capsula adiposa).** This capsule is surrounded by a **fascial sheath (Fascia renalis)**
which opens in the medial-inferior direction to allow the passage of the
neurovascular pathways and the ureter. The **anterior lamina of the renal fascia** is referred to by clinicians as **GEROTA's fascia.**

The illustration shows the topographical relationships of the **Colon
ascendens.** As with the **Colon descendens,** it shifted to the dorsal
body wall during development of the lower abdominal situs and transi-
tioned into a **secondary retroperitoneal position.** This means that
only its ventral surface is covered by parietal peritoneum. With the fusing of the embryonic mesocolon with the embryonic peritoneal coating
of the posterior abdominal wall, the so-called **TOLDT's fascia** was
formed. This fascia merged with the anterior layer of the Fascia renalis
(GEROTA's fascia). The reflection lines lateral of the Colon ascendens
and Colon descendens are visible as the 'white lines' of TOLDT in the
non-preserved body.

Clinical remarks

The fascial systems and topographical relationships of the kidneys
are clinically relevant. In cases of **malignant tumours,** the kidney is

always removed together with the adrenal gland, as well as the
GEROTA's fascia (nephrectomy).

Topography and fascial systems of the kidney

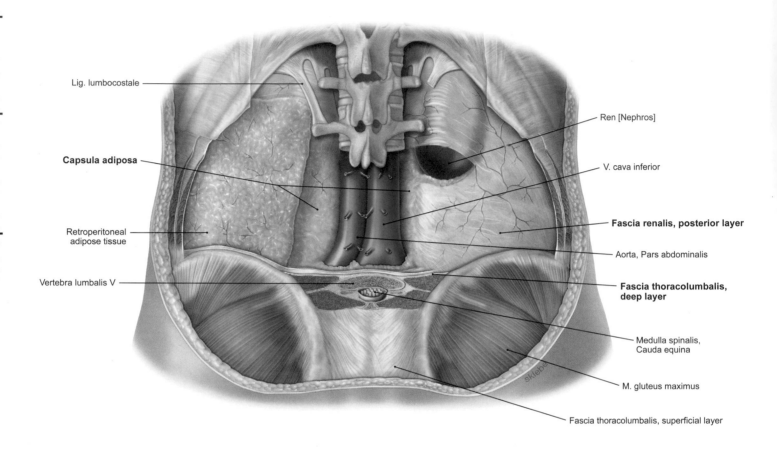

Lig. lumbocostale

Capsula adiposa

Retroperitoneal adipose tissue

Vertebra lumbalis V

Ren [Nephros]

V. cava inferior

Fascia renalis, posterior layer

Aorta, Pars abdominalis

Fascia thoracolumbalis, deep layer

Medulla spinalis, Cauda equina

M. gluteus maximus

Fascia thoracolumbalis, superficial layer

Fig. 7.32 Fascial systems of the kidney, Ren [Nephros], in the retroperitoneal space; after removal of the posterior wall of the trunk inferior to the ribs, the muscles of the back and the posterior aspects of the abdominal muscles, as well as most of the posterior neurovascular structures. The retroperitoneal adipose tissue **(Corpus adiposum pararenale)** was also removed on the right side to illustrate the renal fascia (Fascia renalis). Dorsal view. [S700-L238]/[G1079]

The deep layer of the **Fascia thoracolumbaris** envelops the intrinsic muscles of the back. A layer of retroperitoneal adipose tissue extends with variable thickness **(Corpus adiposum pararenale)** between the deep layer of the thoracolumbar fascia and the dorsal layer of the **kidney fascia (Fascia renalis).** The cranial extension of the Fascia thoracolumbalis to the 12th rib is also referred to as Lig. lumbocostale. The renal fascia is open medially and caudally (not shown here) for the passage of neurovascular structures and the ureter. Within the fascial sack, the kidney and adrenal glands are embedded within the **adipose capsule (Capsula adiposa).**

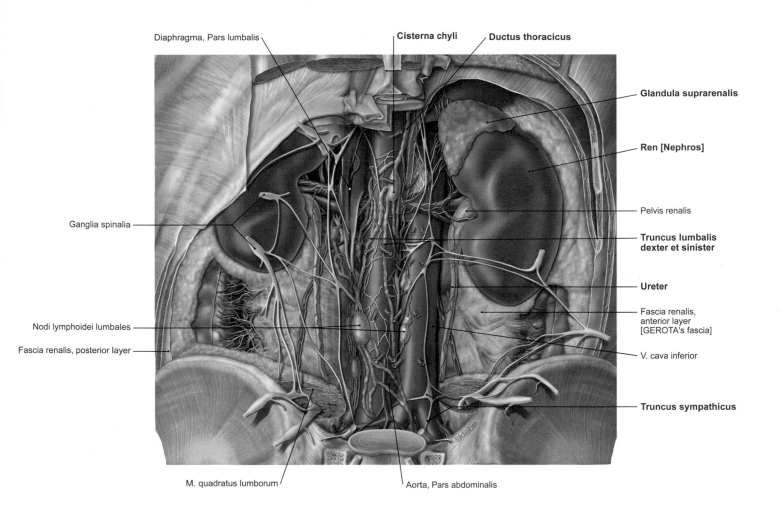

Diaphragma, Pars lumbalis

Cisterna chyli

Ductus thoracicus

Glandula suprarenalis

Ren [Nephros]

Pelvis renalis

Truncus lumbalis dexter et sinister

Ureter

Fascia renalis, anterior layer [GEROTA's fascia]

V. cava inferior

Truncus sympathicus

Ganglia spinalia

Nodi lymphoidei lumbales

Fascia renalis, posterior layer

M. quadratus lumborum

Aorta, Pars abdominalis

Fig. 7.33 Fascial systems of the kidney, Ren [Nephros], in the retroperitoneal space; after removal of the posterior wall of the trunk inferior to the ribs, including the Fascia renalis, the muscles of the back and the posterior aspects of the abdominal muscles and the M. psoas major. The vertebrae and the spinal cord are removed and the dorsal root ganglia are folded back laterally; dorsal view. [S700-L238]/[Q300]
As the liver occupies a large space in the right epigastrium, the right kidney is positioned half a vertebra lower and is visible here with the adjacent adrenal gland. Medially, the **ureter** descends from the renal pelvis in the retroperitoneal space to the urinary bladder in the lesser pelvis. Ventral of the adipose capsule **(Capsula adiposa),** the anterior

layer of the kidney fascia (Fascia renalis), clinically referred to as **GEROTA's fascia,** is visible. This thin connective tissue layer directly transitions into the **TOLDT's fascia,** which develops from the fusion of the Colon ascendens and Colon descendens, along with their mesenteries, with the dorsal wall of the trunk.
This illustration also shows the pathway of the lumbar lymphatics **(Trunci lumbales)** and their common lymphatic dilation **(Cisterna chyli)** to the Ductus thoracicus. It also illustrates the chain of ganglia of the sympathetic nervous system **(Truncus sympathicus).**

Structure of the kidney

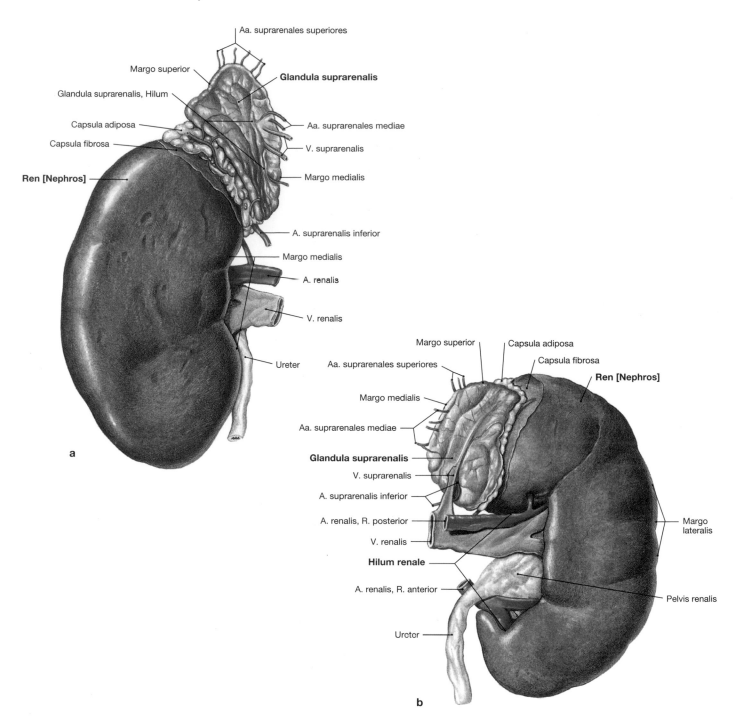

Aa. suprarenales superiores

Margo superior

Glandula suprarenalis

Glandula suprarenalis, Hilum

Capsula adiposa

Aa. suprarenales mediae

Capsula fibrosa

V. suprarenalis

Ren [Nephros]

Margo medialis

A. suprarenalis inferior

Margo medialis

A. renalis

V. renalis

Ureter

a

Margo superior

Capsula adiposa

Capsula fibrosa

Aa. suprarenales superiores

Ren [Nephros]

Margo medialis

Aa. suprarenales mediae

Glandula suprarenalis

V. suprarenalis

A. suprarenalis inferior

A. renalis, R. posterior

Margo lateralis

V. renalis

Hilum renale

A. renalis, R. anterior

Pelvis renalis

Ureter

b

Fig. 7.34a and b Kidney, Ren [Nephros], and adrenal gland, Glandula suprarenalis; ventral view. [S700]
a Right kidney and adrenal gland.
b Left kidney and adrenal gland.
The kidney is 'kidney-shaped' and 10–12 cm long, 5–6 cm wide and 4 cm thick. Its average weight is 150 g (120–200 g). It has a superior and an inferior pole with the medially oriented **hilum of the kidney (Hilum renale)** in between, which represents the access to an internal cavity **(Sinus renalis).** This is an opening for the passage of blood vessels and ureter entering or leaving the kidney.
The flat basis of the **adrenal gland** adheres to the kidney. Sometimes the entrance of the blood vessels at the medial margin is also referred to as the **hilum.**

Clinical remarks

The evaluation of the renal volume is clinically of great importance as it has prognostic relevance for the outcome of diseases. The **normal renal volume** is **120–200 ml,** when determined by ultrasound. In **polycystic kidney disease,** the volume can exceed 1,500 ml. With volumes exceeding 1,000 ml, a reduction of the renal function is to be expected. Autosomal dominant polycystic kidney disease (ADPKD) occurs with a frequency of 1:500–1:1,000 live births and is one of the most common genetic disorders.

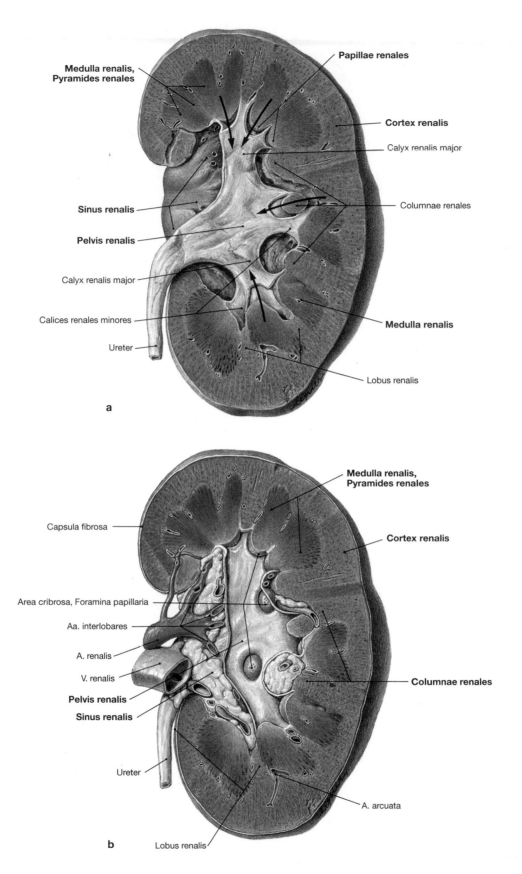

Medulla renalis, Pyramides renales

Papillae renales

Cortex renalis

Calyx renalis major

Sinus renalis

Columnae renales

Pelvis renalis

Calyx renalis major

Calices renales minores

Medulla renalis

Ureter

Lobus renalis

a

Medulla renalis, Pyramides renales

Capsula fibrosa

Cortex renalis

Area cribrosa, Foramina papillaria

Aa. interlobares

A. renalis

V. renalis

Columnae renales

Pelvis renalis

Sinus renalis

Ureter

A. arcuata

b Lobus renalis

Fig. 7.35a and b Kidney, Ren [Nephros], left side; ventral view. [S700].
a Sagittal section.
b Sagittal section with exposed renal pelvis.
The kidney is divided into the **cortex (Cortex renalis)** and **medulla (Medulla renalis).** The medulla has different sections, designated according to their shape as **medullary pyramids** (Pyramides renales). Between the pyramids are cortical parts, called the renal columns (Co-

lumnae renales). A pyramid with adjoining renal columns is called a **renal lobe** (Lobus renalis). In general, the border between the approx. 14 lobes is not visible on the surface of an adult human kidney. The tips of the pyramids (Papillae renales) open into the **renal calices (Calices renales majores and minores)** to release the urine (arrows). Together with adipose tissue and renal blood vessels, the **renal pelvis (Pelvis renalis)** is located in a deep indentation or sinus of the parenchyma of the kidney (Sinus renalis).

Structure of the kidney

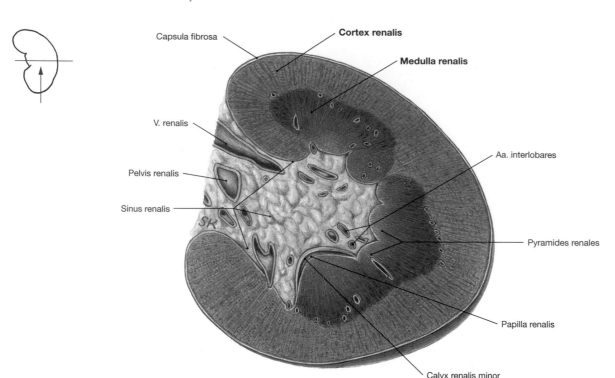

Capsula fibrosa
Cortex renalis
Medulla renalis
V. renalis
Pelvis renalis
Sinus renalis
SK
Aa. interlobares
Pyramides renales
Papilla renalis
Calyx renalis minor

Fig. 7.36   Kidney, Ren [Nephros]; cross-section through the renal sinus (Sinus renalis); caudal view. [S700-L238]

The parenchyma of the kidney is divided into the **cortex (Cortex renalis)** and the **medulla (Medulla renalis).**

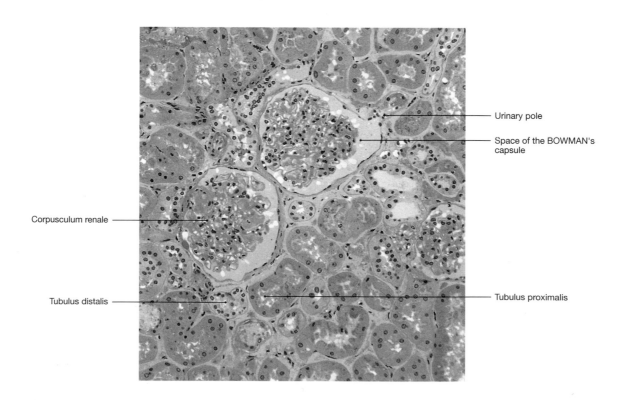

Urinary pole
Space of the BOWMAN's capsule
Corpusculum renale
Tubulus distalis
Tubulus proximalis

Fig. 7.37   Renal cortex, Cortex renalis; microscopic image, 100-fold. [R252]
The entire parenchyma of the kidney consists of **nephrons** and **collecting ducts.** The nephrons consist of the **renal corpuscles** and a **tubular system.** In contrast to the medulla, the cortex harbours renal corpuscles (Corpuscula renalia). The **convoluted capillaries (Glomerulus)** of the renal corpuscles filter the primary urine from the blood into the

space of the BOWMAN's capsule (170 l/day). From here the urine enters the proximal tubule (Tubulus proximalis) at the urinary pole of the glomerulus. In the tubular system and collecting ducts, the major part of the primary urine is reabsorbed, and its composition is additionally altered through secretion, before the final urine is released into the renal pelvis at the renal papillae (1.7 l/day).

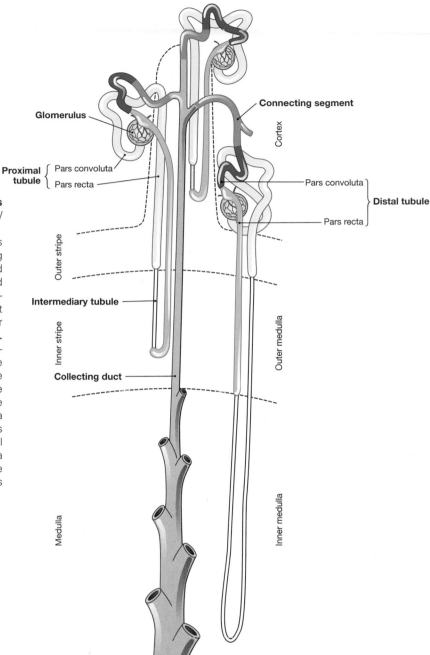

Fig. 7.38 Pathway of arteries (red), veins (blue), and nephrons (grey) in the renal parenchyma; schematic illustration. [S700-L126]/[B500-M580]

The **A.** and **V. renalis** bifurcate in the area of the hilum and ascend as the **A.** and **V. interlobaris** along the edge of the pyramids, arching along the cortical-medullary border of the pyramids as **A.** and **V. arcuata,** and leaving them at the base as **A.** and **V. corticalis radiata,** which ascend to the capsule. These sections are still macroscopically visible. In contrast to the veins, the arteries do not form closed vascular arches, but are instead terminal arteries. Therefore, an occlusion of the arteries, for example by a protracted blood clot (embolus), leads to **renal infarction.** To understand the renal function, the following microlevels of the vascular system are also important: the small arterioles derived from the A. corticalis radiata (Vasa afferentia) form the capillary convolutes of the **glomerulus of** the renal corpuscles. In the glomeruli, the primary urine is filtered from the blood into the tubular system of the nephrons. The capillary vessels then continue via a second system of arterioles (Vasa efferentia) into the peritubular capillaries and finally, into the venous Vasa recta, which have descending and ascending parts in the renal medulla. These vessels are ultimately connected to the veins. The Vasa recta, which are accompanied by arterial vessels in the medulla, are important for the exchange of electrolytes and water in the tubular parts of the nephron and in the collecting duct.

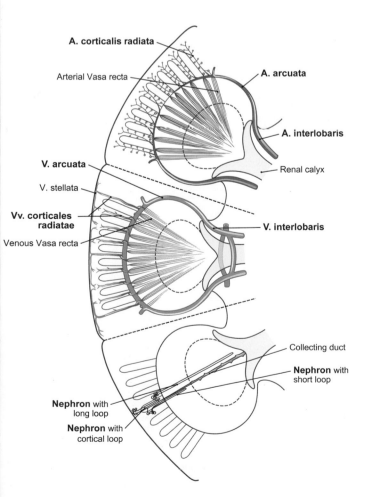

Fig. 7.39 Organisation of the nephron and collecting duct; schematic illustration. [S700-L126]/[B500-M580]

At the **renal corpuscle,** where the primary urine is produced, the **proximal tubule** begins with a convoluted part (Pars convoluta) and a consecutive straight part (Pars recta). This continues into the **intermediate tubule with** a descending (Pars descendens) and an ascending limb (Pars ascendens), which continues as the **distal tubule** (again with Pars recta and Pars convoluta). The **connecting or collecting tubule** is the transition to the **collecting duct,** from which the final urine passes into the renal pelvis.

Segments and topographical relationships of the kidney

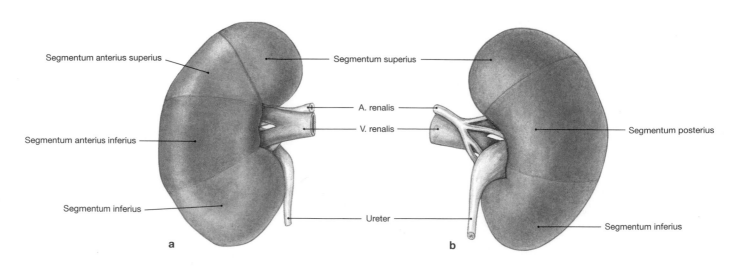

Segmentum anterius superius
Segmentum superius
A. renalis
V. renalis
Segmentum posterius
Segmentum anterius inferius
Segmentum inferius
Ureter
Segmentum inferius

a   **b**

Fig. 7.40a and b Kidney (renal) segments, Segmenta renalia, right side. [S700]
a Ventral view.
b Dorsal view.
The branching of the arterial vessels determines the kidney division into **segments** (Segmenta renalia). These segmental arteries do not interconnect and are therefore terminal arteries. If branches of the A. renalis

are occluded, the size and extension of **renal infarctions** correspond to the boundaries of the affected segments. However, the branching patterns are highly variable.
The renal artery (A. renalis) bifurcates in the area of the hilum into a R. principalis anterior, supplying with its different branches the superior, the two anterior and the inferior segments, and a R. principalis posterior for the posterior segment.

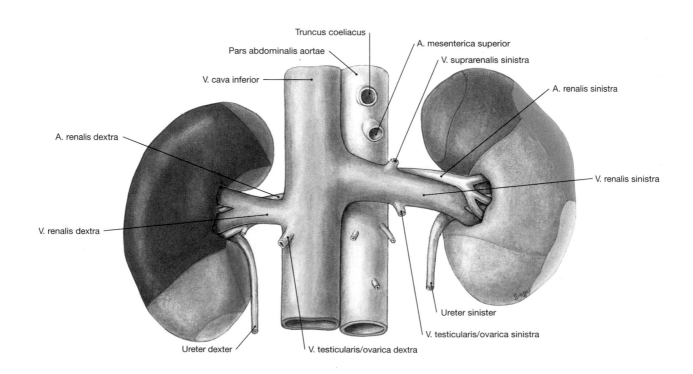

Truncus coeliacus
Pars abdominalis aortae
A. mesenterica superior
V. cava inferior
V. suprarenalis sinistra
A. renalis sinistra
A. renalis dextra
V. renalis sinistra
V. renalis dextra
Ureter sinister
Ureter dexter
V. testicularis/ovarica sinistra
V. testicularis/ovarica dextra

Fig. 7.41 Surfaces of the kidney, Ren [Nephros], in contact with adjacent organs; ventral view. [S700]
Whereas the dorsal side of the kidney is adjacent to the posterior abdominal wall, its ventral side has contact with various other organs. To-

gether with the adrenal glands, the kidneys are separated from the other abdominal organs by the Peritoneum parietale, the renal fascia, and the adipose capsule, so that these surfaces have no clinical relevance.

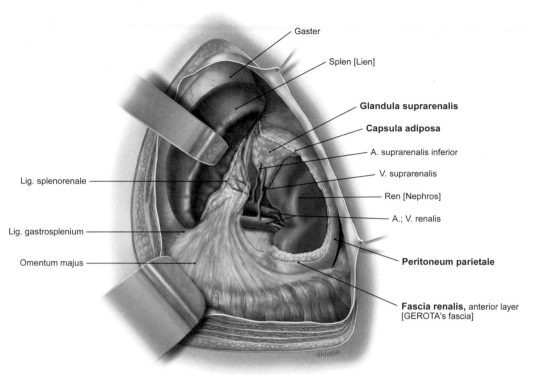

Fig. 7.42 Adrenal gland (Glandula suprarenalis) in situ; the spleen has been mobilised and reflected medially and the renal fascia has been partially resected, ventral view. [S700-L238]

The adrenal glands on both sides are positioned over the superior poles of the kidney and share their fasciae. The parietal peritoneum is directly adjacent to the anterior layer of the renal fascia **(Fascia renalis),** known clinically as **GEROTA's fascia.** Below the GEROTA's fascia, the **Capsula adiposa** surrounds the kidney and adrenal gland.

Gaster

Splen [Lien]

Glandula suprarenalis

Capsula adiposa

A. suprarenalis inferior

V. suprarenalis

Ren [Nephros]

A.; V. renalis

Peritoneum parietale

Fascia renalis, anterior layer [GEROTA's fascia]

Lig. splenorenale

Lig. gastrosplenium

Omentum majus

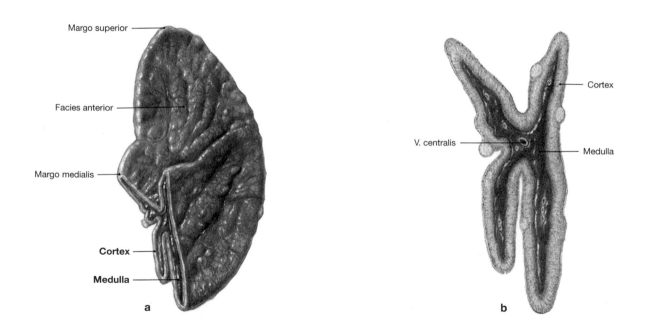

Margo superior

Facies anterior

Margo medialis

Cortex

Medulla

a

Cortex

V. centralis

Medulla

b

Fig. 7.43a and b Adrenal gland, Glandula suprarenalis, right side. [S700]
a Ventral view.
b Sagittal section, lateral view.

The adrenal gland is a vital endocrine gland. There are two parts with different developmental origins: the cortex and the medulla. The cortex develops from the mesoderm of the coelomic cavity (Coelomic epithelium), and the medulla is derived from the neuroectoderm of the neural crest and corresponds to a modified sympathetic ganglion. The **cortex**

produces **steroid hormones** (mineralocorticoids, glucocorticoids, androgens) and the **medulla** produces **catecholamines** (adrenaline and noradrenaline) which regulate the metabolism and blood pressure. Macroscopically, a distinction is made between its medial and superior margins **(Margo medialis and Margo superior),** which confine the anterior and posterior surfaces **(Facies anterior and Facies posterior),** as well as a basis **(Facies renalis).** At the medial margin, the **hilum** marks the entrance and exit of neurovascular pathways.

Clinical remarks

If both adrenal glands have to be removed in the case of disease, a therapeutic substitution of mineralocorticoids and glucocorticoids is essential, otherwise **life-threatening conditions** can cause low blood sugar levels (hypoglycaemia) and a decrease in blood pressure (hypotension). This may also be the case with insufficiency of the adrenal glands (ADDISON's disease).

Vessels of the kidney and adrenal gland

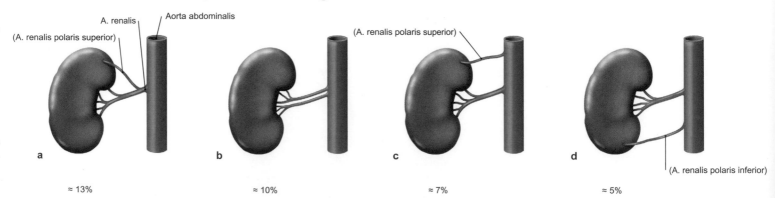

(A. renalis polaris superior)
A. renalis
Aorta abdominalis
(A. renalis polaris superior)
(A. renalis polaris inferior)

a ≈ 13%   b ≈ 10%   c ≈ 7%   d ≈ 5%

Fig. 7.44a–d Renal artery, A. renalis, with variants; ventral view. [S700-L275]
a A. renalis with a superior polar artery.
b Two Aa. renales to the hilum of the kidney.
c Accessory superior polar artery.
d Accessory inferior polar artery.

In 70 % of all cases there is only one renal artery, while accessory renal arteries exist in 30 %. In general, the **renal artery (A. renalis)** originates on both sides from the aorta and passes through the hilum into the kidney. The **polar arteries** of the kidneys do not enter via the hilum, but pass directly into the renal parenchyma. **Accessory arteries,** however, arise independently from the aorta.

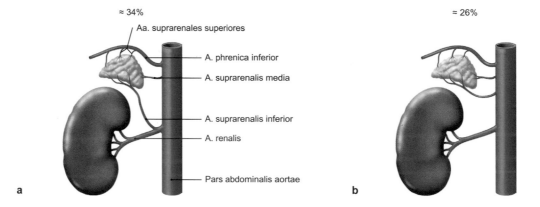

≈ 34%
Aa. suprarenales superiores
A. phrenica inferior
A. suprarenalis media
A. suprarenalis inferior
A. renalis
Pars abdominalis aortae
a

≈ 26%
b

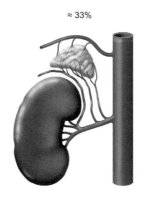
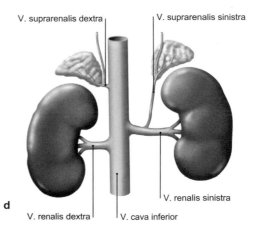

≈ 33%
c

V. suprarenalis dextra
V. suprarenalis sinistra
V. renalis sinistra
d
V. renalis dextra
V. cava inferior

Fig. 7.45a–d Suprarenal arteries, Aa. suprarenales, with variants, renal vein, V. renalis, and suprarenal vein, V. suprarenalis; ventral view. [S700-L275]
There are usually **three adrenal gland arteries:**
- **A. suprarenalis superior:** originates from the A. phrenica inferior
- **A. suprarenalis media:** directly from the aorta
- **A. suprarenalis inferior:** branch of the A. renalis.

This 'luxury perfusion' or hyperperfusion prevents infarctions that could jeopardise this vital organ. However, all the arteries of the adrenal gland are present in only a third of the cases. The various arteries of the adrenal gland penetrate the cortex of the organ. From there, the blood flows to the medulla and is collected by the V. suprarenalis. The blood-flow

directed from the cortex to the medulla is functionally important because the hormones of the adrenal cortex regulate the differentiation and function of the cells in the medulla.
Variants of the arterial supply of the adrenal gland:
a Arterial supply via three arteries (textbook case).
b Arterial supply without inflow from the A. renalis.
c Arterial supply without a direct branch from the aorta.
The **V. renalis** of both sides flows to the V. cava inferior. Similarly, there is only one vein in each adrenal gland, the **V. suprarenalis,** which collects the blood and drains into the V. cava inferior on the right side and into the V. renalis on the left side **(d).**

Clinical remarks

As renal carcinomas often invade the renal veins, a tumour growth on the left side can cause a venous stasis in the V. testicularis in men, with convoluted and dilated veins in the scrotum **(varicocele).** In a left-sided varicocele a kidney tumour must therefore always be excluded!

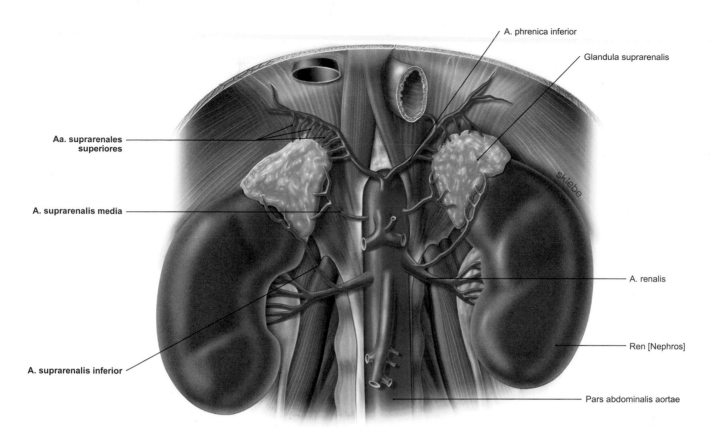

A. phrenica inferior

Glandula suprarenalis

Aa. suprarenales superiores

A. suprarenalis media

A. renalis

Ren [Nephros]

A. suprarenalis inferior

Pars abdominalis aortae

Fig. 7.46   Arterial blood supply of the kidney and adrenal gland; ventral view. With exception of the kidney and adrenal gland, all organs of the abdominal cavity together with veins, lymph vessels and nerves of the retroperitoneal space have been removed. [S702-L238]
The **A. renalis** originates bilaterally from the aorta and runs to the hilum of the kidney, where it divides very variably into several terminal branch-

es. Usually the **A. suprarenalis inferior** also branches off. In contrast, the A. suprarenalis superior arises in most cases with several smaller branches of the A. phrenica inferior. The **A. suprarenalis media** is an independent branch of the aorta, but just like the A. suprarenalis inferior, it is often missing (→ Fig. 7.6).

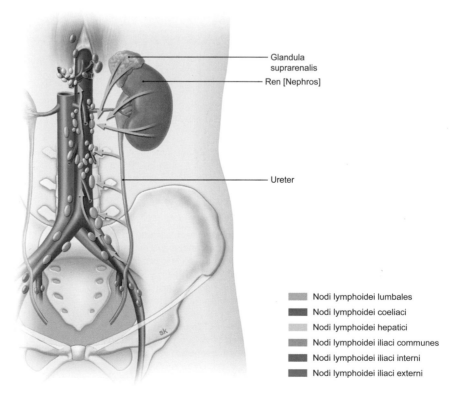

Glandula suprarenalis

Ren [Nephros]

Ureter

Fig. 7.47   Lymphatic drainage pathways of kidney and adrenal gland; ventral view. [S700-L238]
The regional lymph nodes of the kidney, the adrenal gland and the upper ureter are the **Nodi lymphoidei lumbales** on the respective side. From here the lymph drains through the Trunci lumbales to the **Ductus thoracicus.**
Only the pelvic part of the ureter is connected to the lymph nodes in the pelvis (→ Fig. 7.18).

▨ Nodi lymphoidei lumbales
▨ Nodi lymphoidei coeliaci
▨ Nodi lymphoidei hepatici
▨ Nodi lymphoidei iliaci communes
▨ Nodi lymphoidei iliaci interni
▨ Nodi lymphoidei iliaci externi

Clinical remarks

Carcinomas of the kidneys and adrenal glands can metastasise to the lumbar lymph nodes. Based on embryonic development, the lumbar lymph nodes are also sentinel nodes for the gonads (testis/ ovary). In the case of enlarged lumbar lymph nodes, a primary tumour of the internal genitalia also needs to be excluded.

Innervation of the kidney and adrenal gland

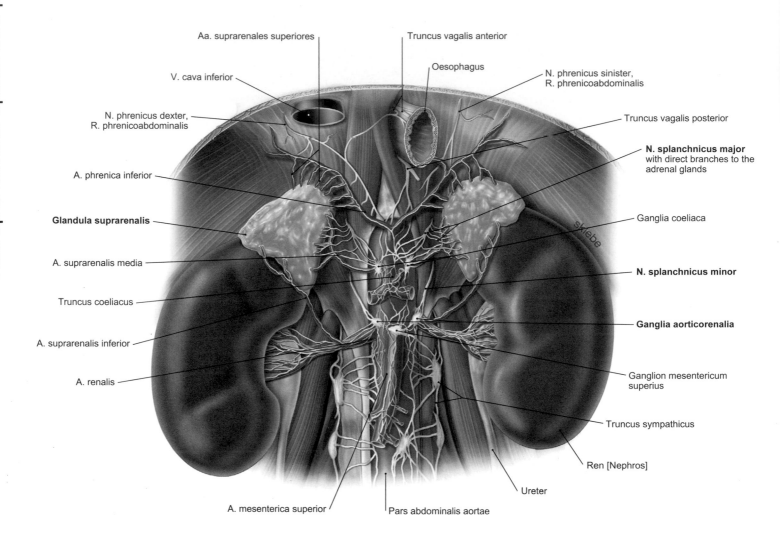

Aa. suprarenales superiores

V. cava inferior

N. phrenicus dexter,
R. phrenicoabdominalis

A. phrenica inferior

Glandula suprarenalis

A. suprarenalis media

Truncus coeliacus

A. suprarenalis inferior

A. renalis

A. mesenterica superior

Truncus vagalis anterior

Oesophagus

N. phrenicus sinister,
R. phrenicoabdominalis

Truncus vagalis posterior

N. splanchnicus major
with direct branches to the
adrenal glands

Ganglia coeliaca

N. splanchnicus minor

Ganglia aorticorenalia

Ganglion mesentericum
superius

Truncus sympathicus

Ren [Nephros]

Ureter

Pars abdominalis aortae

Fig. 7.48 Autonomic innervation of the kidney and adrenal gland; ventral view. With exception of the kidney and adrenal gland, all organs of the abdominal cavity as well as the veins and lymph vessels of the retroperitoneal space have been removed. [S702-L238]

The **autonomic innervation** of the kidney and adrenal gland is provided largely by the sympathetic system. But there are fundamental differences between both organs:

- The **kidney** is innervated by its own plexus **(Plexus renalis)** which extends along the A. renalis. The cell bodies of the **postganglionic** neurons are located in the **Ganglia aorticorenalia,** which lie near the outlets of the renal arteries from the aorta and therefore belong to the Plexus aorticus abdominalis.

- In contrast, the **adrenal gland** is supplied by **preganglionic** (!) sympathetic nerve fibres from the Nn. splanchnici. The nerve endings are located on medullary cells of the adrenal gland and induce the release of catecholamines. Thus the medulla of the adrenal gland corresponds to a modified sympathetic ganglion. The blood vessels in the adrenal medulla are also innervated by postganglionic sympathetic neurons.

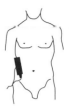

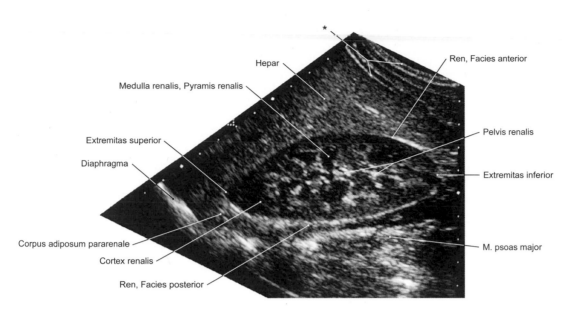

Fig. 7.49 Kidney, Ren [Nephros], right side; ultrasound image; lateral view; nearly vertical position of the transducer. [S700-T894]

* abdominal wall

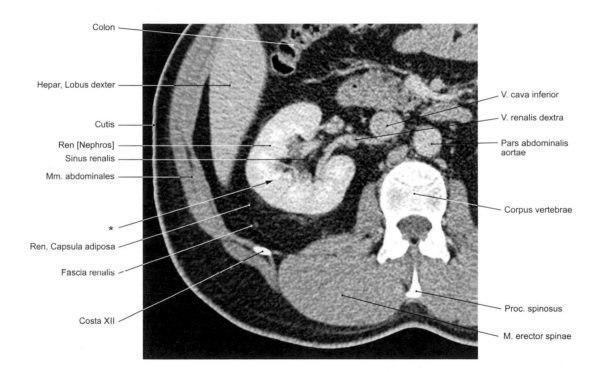

Fig. 7.50 Kidney, Ren [Nephros], right side; computed tomography (CT) scan; caudal view. [S700-T900]

It is also possible to perform a CT-guided biopsy, e.g. to assess functional disorders which are not clear.

* route of the needle for kidney biopsy

Clinical remarks

The **ultrasound** is a particularly suitable imaging technique for the kidneys. A mass, such as a cyst (→ figure) or tumour, can usually be detected easily. Where findings are inconclusive, **CT examination** is available, and with this, lymph node metastases to the lumbar lymph nodes and an invasion into the renal vein can be reliably identified. [S701-T975]

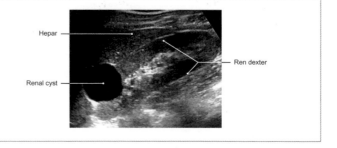

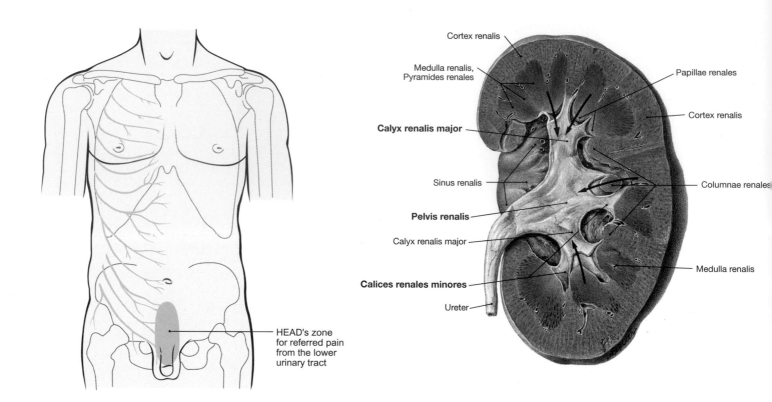

Cortex renalis

Medulla renalis, Pyramides renales

Calyx renalis major

Sinus renalis

Pelvis renalis

Calyx renalis major

Calices renales minores

Ureter

Papillae renales

Cortex renalis

Columnae renales

Medulla renalis

HEAD's zone for referred pain from the lower urinary tract

Fig. 7.51 HEAD's zone of the efferent urinary tracts; ventral view. [S700-L126]/[G1071]

The **efferent urinary system** includes:
- renal pelvis (Pelvis renalis)
- ureter
- urinary bladder (Vesica urinaria)
- urethra.

The organ-related area of referred pain or the **HEAD's zone** of the **renal pelvis** corresponds to that of the kidney and projects onto the **cutaneous areas (dermatomes) T10–L1;** the HEAD's zone of the **urinary bladder** projects medially onto the **dermatomes T11–L1.** Diseases like an inflammation of the renal pelvis (pyelonephritis) or a bladder inflammation (cystitis) can therefore lead to pain, which is perceived in these cutaneous areas (referred pain).

Fig. 7.52 Renal pelvis, Pelvis renalis, left side; ventral view. [S700]
After the urine has been separated from the blood as so-called primary urine in the renal corpuscles, it is concentrated in the tubular system of collecting ducts of the nephron and changes its composition through a process of exchanging electrolytes and water. This so-called final urine is passed at the tip of the **medullary pyramids (Pyramides renales),** the perforated areas of which are called **renal papillae (Papillae renales),** into the **renal calices** (Calices renales) of the **renal pelvis (Pelvis renalis)** (arrows).
For the neurovascular pathways of the urinary system in the pelvis → Fig. 7.13, → Fig. 7.16, → Fig. 7.17 and → Fig. 7.18.

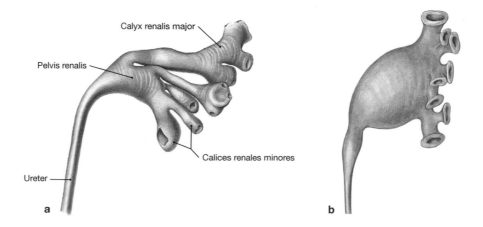

Calyx renalis major

Pelvis renalis

Calices renales minores

Ureter

a

b

Fig. 7.53a and b Renal pelvis, Pelvis renalis, left side; cast dissection, ventral view. [S700]
a Dendritic type of the renal pelvis.

b Ampullary type of the renal pelvis.
The dendritic and ampullary types of the renal pelvis are differentiated based on the width and the length of the renal calices.

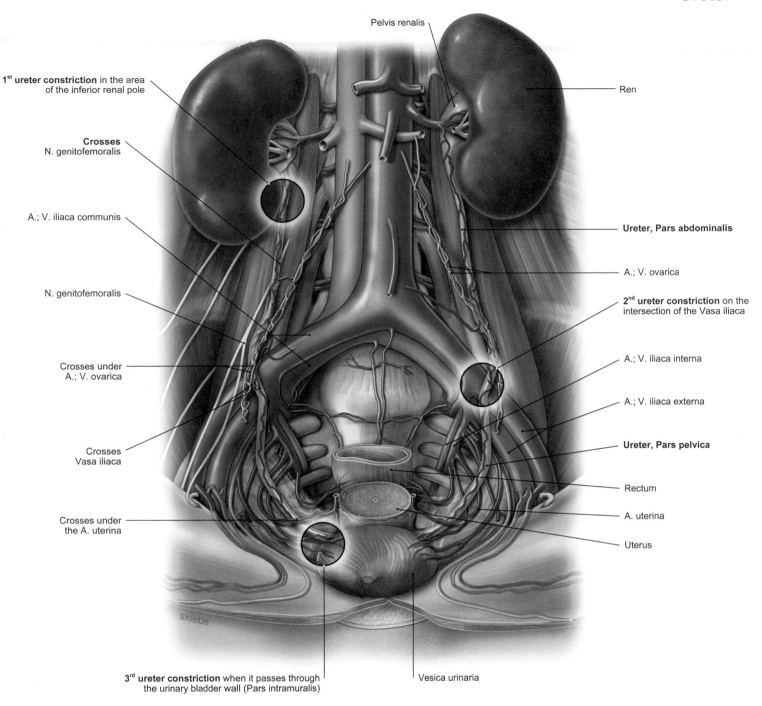

1st ureter constriction in the area of the inferior renal pole

Crosses N. genitofemoralis

A.; V. iliaca communis

N. genitofemoralis

Crosses under A.; V. ovarica

Crosses Vasa iliaca

Crosses under the A. uterina

Pelvis renalis

Ren

Ureter, Pars abdominalis

A.; V. ovarica

2nd ureter constriction on the intersection of the Vasa iliaca

A.; V. iliaca interna

A.; V. iliaca externa

Ureter, Pars pelvica

Rectum

A. uterina

Uterus

3rd ureter constriction when it passes through the urinary bladder wall (Pars intramuralis)

Vesica urinaria

Fig. 7.54 Parts, constrictions and pathway of the ureter; ventral view. [S702-L238]

From the renal pelvis the urine passes via the **ureter** into the **urinary bladder (Vesica urinaria).** After leaving the medulla of the kidney, the urine remains unchanged in its composition and in its volume. Transport through the ureter is carried out by peristaltic waves of smooth muscles in its wall. The ureter is divided into three parts and has three constrictions.

Parts:
* Pars abdominalis: in the retroperitoneal space
* Pars pelvica: in the lesser pelvis

* Pars intramuralis: traverses the wall of the urinary bladder.

Constrictions:
* at the exit from the renal pelvis
* at the intersection of the A. iliaca communis or A. iliaca externa
* at the passage through the wall of the urinary bladder (narrowest part).

The narrow urethral passage through the wall of the urinary bladder is a physiologically important constriction because it prevents a reflux of urine from the bladder.

Structure and function

Course of the ureter

Along its route, the ureter comes into contact with various structures. Its **Pars abdominalis** usually crosses over the genitofemoral nerve and crosses underneath the A./V. testicularis/ovarica. On the right side it is covered by the duodenum, the A. colica dextra and the mesenteric root (Radix mesenterii), and on the left side by the A./V. mesenterica inferior or the A. colica sinistra. At the transition to the

Pars pelvica the ureter crosses over the A./V. iliaca communis. In the male it crosses in the lesser pelvis under the vas deferens (Ductus deferens) and in the female the A. uterina.

'Over-under' rule: the ureter firstly passes **over** the N. genitofemoralis, crossing **under** the A. and V. testicularis/ovarica, then crosses **over** the A. and V. iliaca, and in men crosses **under** the Ductus deferens and in women the A. uterina.

Vessels of the ureter

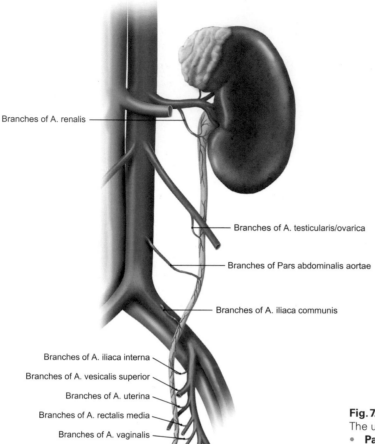

Branches of A. renalis

Branches of A. testicularis/ovarica

Branches of Pars abdominalis aortae

Branches of A. iliaca communis

Branches of A. iliaca interna

Branches of A. vesicalis superior

Branches of A. uterina

Branches of A. rectalis media

Branches of A. vaginalis

Branches of A. vesicalis inferior

Fig. 7.55 **Arteries of the ureter;** ventral view. [S701-L275]
The ureter is supplied by blood vessels from its suroundings:
* **Pars abdominalis:** A. renalis, A. testicularis/ovarica, Pars abdominalis of the aorta, A. iliaca communis
* **Pars pelvica:** A. Iliaca interna and its visceral branches.

Clinical remarks

As the renal pelvis and the ureter also develop from the ureteric bud (→ Fig. 7.27), they may be divided in the same way as the ureteric bud is split to form the individual renal calices and the collecting ducts. One thereby differentiates between the:
* Bifid renal pelvis (Pelvis renalis bifida; → Fig. a)
* Bifid ureter (Ureter fissus; → Fig. b)
* Duplicated ureter (Ureter duplex; → Fig. c).

Just as with the bifid renal pelvis (**Pelvis renalis bifida**), the **Ureter fissus** is usually discovered by accident and has no clinical relevance (→ Fig. 7.57b). However, the **Ureter duplex** (→ Fig. 7.57a) occurs unilaterally in 0.8 % and bilaterally in 0.125 % of all newborns and is frequently associated with problematic junctions in the urinary bladder, causing urinary reflux or urinary incontinence. Usually, both ureters cross each other (MEYER-WEIGERT-law), whereby the ureter arising from the higher positioned renal pelvis drains at a lower point into the urinary bladder or even further distally into the urethra, which can cause urinary incontinence. In contrast, the ureter from the lower renal pelvis has a shorter Pars intramuralis within the wall of the urinary bladder, which may cause urinary reflux. The reflux causes recurrent ascending infections which may cause permanent damage to the kidney parenchyma. [S701-L126]

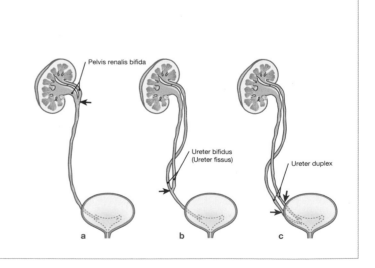

Pelvis renalis bifida

Ureter bifidus
(Ureter fissus)

Ureter duplex

a   b   c

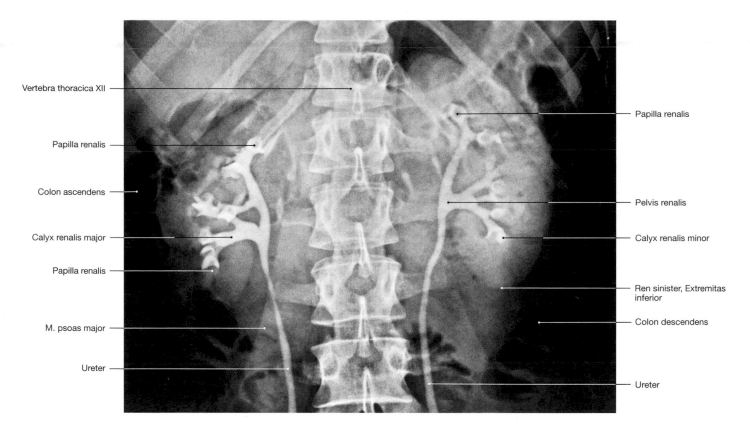

Vertebra thoracica XII

Papilla renalis

Colon ascendens

Calyx renalis major

Papilla renalis

M. psoas major

Ureter

Papilla renalis

Pelvis renalis

Calyx renalis minor

Ren sinister, Extremitas inferior

Colon descendens

Ureter

Fig. 7.56 Renal pelvis, Pelvis renalis, and ureter; X-ray in anteroposterior (AP) projection after retrograde injection of a contrast agent via both ureters; ventral view. [S700]

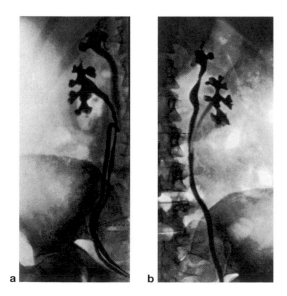

a   b

Fig. 7.57a and b Common variants of the ureter; X-rays in anteroposterior (AP) projection after retrograde injection of a contrast agent; ventral view. [S002-7]
a Double ureter (Ureter duplex).
b Split ureter (Ureter fissus).
In both cases two renal pelvises are present.

Clinical remarks

Descending **kidney stones** can remain stuck at the constrictions and cause very strong waves of pain (renal colic). The proximity of the ureter to the uterine artery has to be taken into account with the surgical **removal of the uterus** (hysterectomy) to avoid ligation of the ureter along with the artery. Urine retention would lead to irreversible damage to the kidney.

Efferent urinary tracts

Urinary bladder

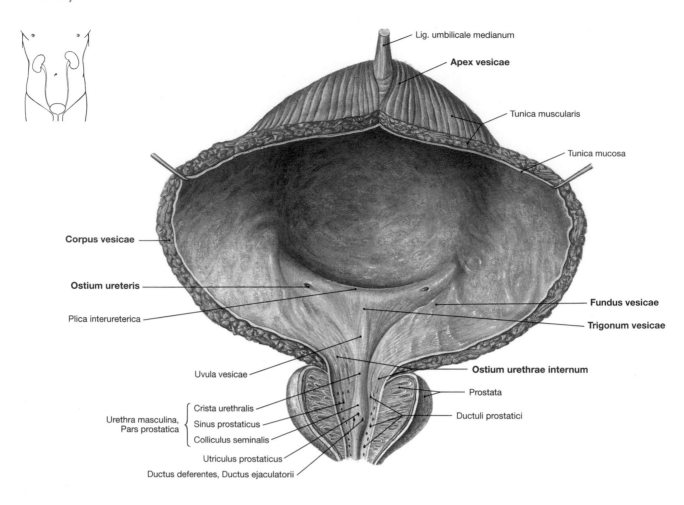

Lig. umbilicale medianum

Apex vesicae

Tunica muscularis

Tunica mucosa

Corpus vesicae

Ostium ureteris

Plica interureterica

Fundus vesicae

Trigonum vesicae

Uvula vesicae

Ostium urethrae internum

Prostata

Ductuli prostatici

Urethra masculina, Pars prostatica
- Crista urethralis
- Sinus prostaticus
- Colliculus seminalis

Utriculus prostaticus

Ductus deferentes, Ductus ejaculatorii

Fig. 7.58   Urinary bladder, Vesica urinaria, and internal urethal orifice, Urethra, in men; ventral view. [S700]
The urinary bladder is positioned **subperitoneally** and is divided into a **body (Corpus vesicae),** which drains upwards to the **apex (Apex vesicae)** and has a **bladder fundus (Fundus vesicae)** at the bottom. At the base, the internal urethral orifice (Ostium urethrae internum), along with the junction of the ureters located on both sides (Ostium ureteris), form the **trigone of the bladder (Trigonum vesicae).** The urinary bladder holds about 500–1500 ml of urine, although the urge to urinate starts when a volume of 250–500 ml is reached. The wall consists of an internal mucosal layer (Tunica mucosa), followed by three layers of smooth muscle with parasympathetic innervation **(Tunica muscularis = M. detrusor vesicae),** and the external Tunica adventitia or the cranial serous layer (peritoneum), respectively.
The urinary bladder is surrounded by paravesical adipose tissue and secured by various **ligaments.** From the top, the **Lig. umbilicale medianum** (containing the Urachus = a remnant of the passage of the allantois from the later Sinus urogenitalis into the umbilical cord) runs to the umbilicus. In women, the bilateral **Lig. pubovesicale** (→ Fig. 7.166), and in men the bilateral Lig. puboprostaticum (→ Fig. 7.165) ensures anchorage to the bony pelvis. In men, the prostate gland is directly under the fundus of the urinary bladder and is traversed by the urethra.

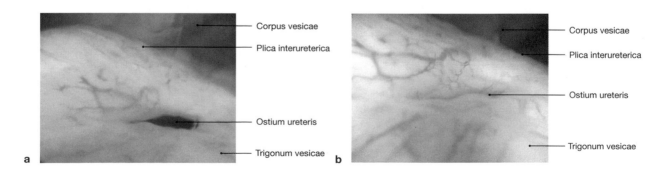

Corpus vesicae

Plica interureterica

Ostium ureteris

Trigonum vesicae

Corpus vesicae

Plica interureterica

Ostium ureteris

Trigonum vesicae

a   **b**

Fig. 7.59a and b   Urethral opening, Ostium ureteris; cystoscopy. [S700-T898]
a Urethral opening has opened, a peristaltic wave has transported urine into the bladder.

b Urethral opening has closed.
The valve-like shape of the urethral opening is crucial for avoiding urinary reflux, which may endanger the kidney due to ascending infections.

Fig. 7.60 Urinary bladder, Vesica urinaria, Vasa deferentes, Ductus deferentes, seminal vesicles, Glandulae vesiculosae, and prostate gland; dorsal view. [S700]

In men, the following paired anatomical structures are positioned posterior and adjacent to the urinary bladder, from **medial to lateral:**

* dilated part of the vas deferens (Ampulla ductus deferentis)
* seminal vesicle (Glandula vesiculosa)
* ureter.

The urinary bladder is positioned directly superior to the prostate gland.

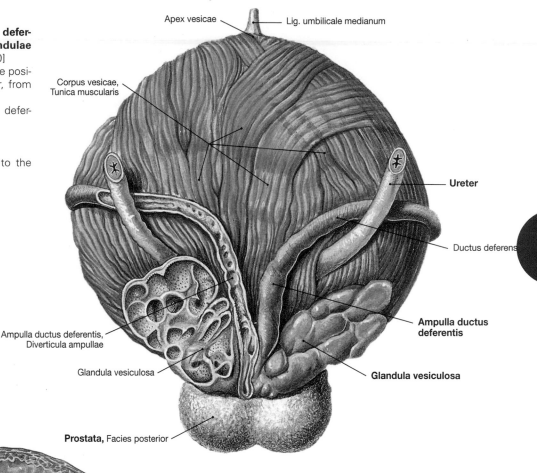

Apex vesicae

Lig. umbilicale medianum

Corpus vesicae, Tunica muscularis

Ureter

Ductus deferens

Ampulla ductus deferentis

Ampulla ductus deferentis, Diverticula ampullae

Glandula vesiculosa

Glandula vesiculosa

Prostata, Facies posterior

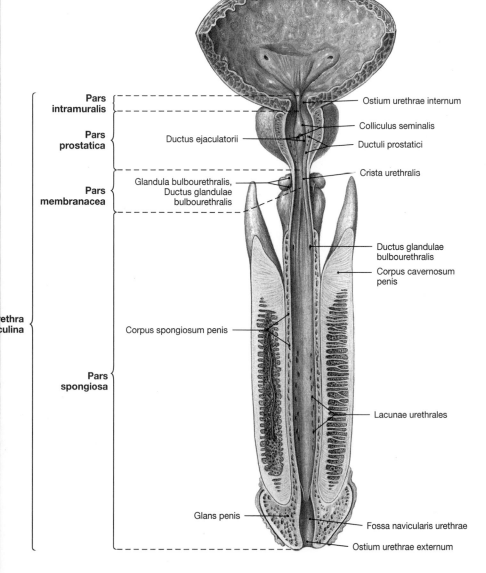

Pars intramuralis

Ostium urethrae internum

Pars prostatica

Ductus ejaculatorii

Colliculus seminalis

Ductuli prostatici

Crista urethralis

Glandula bulbourethralis, Ductus glandulae bulbourethralis

Pars membranacea

Urethra masculina

Ductus glandulae bulbourethralis

Corpus cavernosum penis

Corpus spongiosum penis

Pars spongiosa

Lacunae urethrales

Glans penis

Fossa navicularis urethrae

Ostium urethrae externum

Fig. 7.61 Urinary bladder, Vesica urinaria, and male urethra, Urethra masculina; ventral view; urinary bladder and urethra opened ventrally. [S700]

Parts of the urethra:

* **Pars intramuralis** (1 cm): within the wall of the urinary bladder
* **Pars prostatica** (3.5 cm): crosses the prostate gland. Here, the Ductus ejaculatorii (common duct of vas deferens and seminal vesicle) flow into the Colliculus seminalis and on both sides of the prostate gland.
* **Pars membranacea** (1–2 cm): crosses the pelvic floor.
* **Pars spongiosa** (15 cm): runs in the Corpus spongiosum of the penis up to the external urethral orifice (Ostium urethrae externum). The COWPER's glands (Glandulae bulbourethrales) and glands of LITTRÉ (Glandulae urethrales), which are only visible under the microscope, drain here. The terminal part extends to the Fossa navicularis.

The urethra has the following **constrictions:**

* Ostium urethrae internum
* Pars membranacea
* Ostium urethrae externum.

In comparison, the urethra is wide in the

* proximal Pars spongiosa ('Ampulla urethrae')
* Fossa navicularis.

Urethra in men

Retroperitoneal space and pelvic cavity

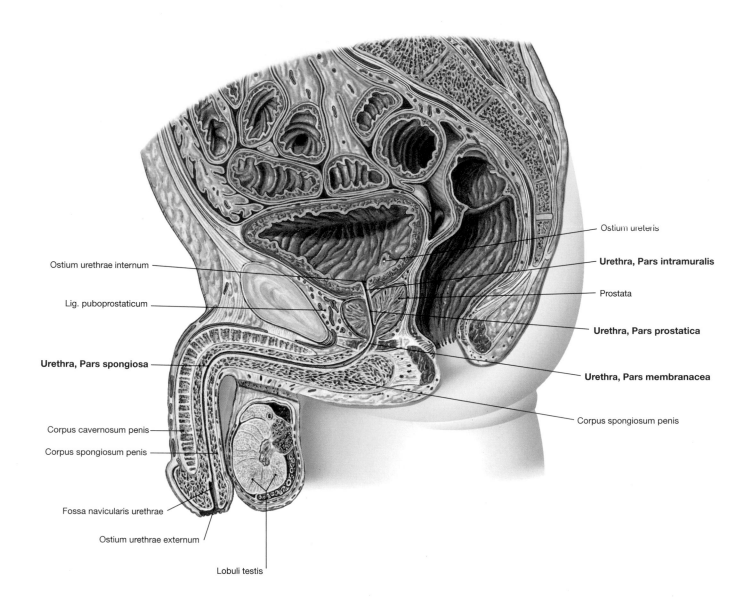

Ostium ureteris

Urethra, Pars intramuralis

Ostium urethrae internum

Prostata

Lig. puboprostaticum

Urethra, Pars prostatica

Urethra, Pars spongiosa

Urethra, Pars membranacea

Corpus spongiosum penis

Corpus cavernosum penis

Corpus spongiosum penis

Fossa navicularis urethrae

Ostium urethrae externum

Lobuli testis

Fig. 7.62 Pelvis of a man; median section; view from the left side. [S700]
The illustration shows the course and the parts of the male urethra (Urethra masculina):
- **Pars intramuralis:** within the wall of the urinary bladder
- **Pars prostatica:** crosses the prostate gland

- **Pars membranacea:** penetrates the pelvic floor
- **Pars spongiosa:** embedded in the Corpus spongiosum of the penis, exits at the Glans penis.

The urethra has two **angles:**
- at the transition of Pars membranacea and Pars spongiosa
- in the middle part of the Pars spongiosa.

Clinical remarks

The greater length and the exposed position are the reason that **injuries to the urethra** are more common in men than in women. The proximal Pars spongiosa within the bulb of the penis is the most common site of injury (straddle injuries). The distal Pars spongiosa may be affected with injuries to the penis or during transurethral catheterisation. Pelvic fractures may cause injuries to the Pars membranacea when the Ligg. puboprostatica are sheared off the pelvic bones with displacement of the urethra.

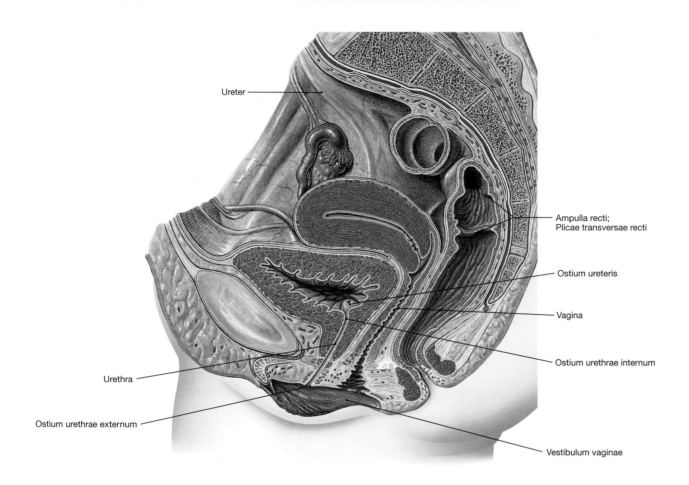

Ureter

Ampulla recti;
Plicae transversae recti

Ostium ureteris

Vagina

Ostium urethrae internum

Urethra

Vestibulum vaginae

Ostium urethrae externum

Fig. 7.63 **Pelvis of a woman;** median section; view from the left side. [S700]

The illustration shows the course and the external orifice of the female urethra. The female urethra is 3–5 cm long and opens directly in front of the vagina into the **vestibule of the vagina (Vestibulum vaginae).**

Clinical remarks

Because of the shorter length of the female urethra, **ascending infections** of the urinary bladder (cystitis) are more common in women than in men.

Inserting a catheter

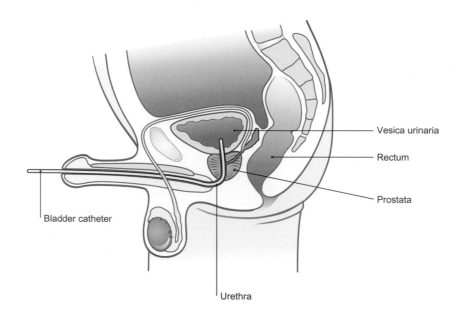

Fig. 7.64 **Catheterisation of the urinary bladder in men;** schematic illustration of a median section; view from the left side. [S700-L126]

For the procedure of catheterising the urinary bladder, the parts and curvatures of the urethra are significant.

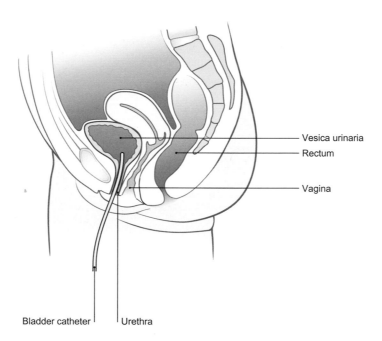

Fig. 7.65 **Catheterisation of the urinary bladder in women;** schematic illustration of a median section; view from the left side. [S700-L126]

In the catheterisation of the urinary bladder in women, it is important that the external urethral orifice lies ventrally to the opening of the vagina.

Clinical remarks

The inserting of a **bladder catheter** is one of the first procedures that one can perform as a medical student in nursing or clinical internship. In these situations it is very important to concentrate on working in a very sterile manner, and it is helpful if one has mastered the anatomical basics. Placing the bladder catheter in **men** is made more difficult by the length tract and the angles in the urethra. The angles in the urethra must therefore be compensated for by aligning the penis, to prevent perforations especially in the tissue of the prostate, which are painful and can lead to severe bleeding. First, the catheter is passed through the tip of the Glans penis into the urethra, where the penis of the supine patient is then straightened out (→ Fig. 7.64) to smooth out the angle of the urethra in the Pars spongiosa. This

allows the catheter to advance up to the second angle at the transition to the Pars membranacea. Now the penis is placed diagonally downwards between the legs, in order to avoid a perforation of the urethra in the Corpus spongiosum penis (→ Fig. 7.62). Then the catheter can be moved forwards into the bladder, while being careful in the Pars prostatica not to damage the surrounding prostate tissue, which can lead to scar constrictions.

Due to the straight course of the relatively short female urethra, the placing of a **bladder catheter is much easier in women.** However, one should consider that the external opening of the urethra is positioned **ventrally** to the opening of the vagina (Ostium vaginae) in the vestibule of the vagina.

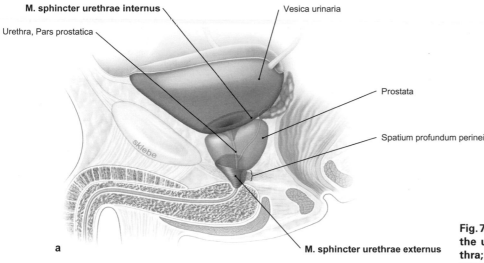

M. sphincter urethrae internus

Urethra, Pars prostatica

Vesica urinaria

Prostata

Spatium profundum perinei

a

M. sphincter urethrae externus

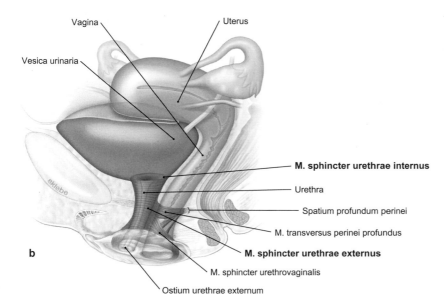

Vagina

Uterus

Vesica urinaria

M. sphincter urethrae internus

Urethra

Spatium profundum perinei

M. transversus perinei profundus

M. sphincter urethrae externus

M. sphincter urethrovaginalis

Ostium urethrae externum

b

Fig. 7.66a and b Sphincter mechanisms of the urinary bladder, Vesica urinaria, and urethra; median section; view from the left side. [S700-L238]
a In men.
b In women.
The sphincter mechanisms both involve contraction of smooth muscles in the wall of the urethra and by striated muscles in the perineal area:

- **smooth muscles** of the circular muscle layer of the **urethra** (M. sphincter urethrae internus): morphologically, a true sphincter muscle is not identified.
- **M. sphincter urethrae externus:** in men there is a separation of the M. transversus perinei profundus, but in women there is no independent muscle.

In addition, the shape of the **pelvic floor (Diaphragma pelvis)** is crucial for continence because it supports the bladder.
When **passing water (micturition),** the activated sacral parasympathetics lead to contraction of the smooth muscles in the wall of the urinary bladder (M. detrusor vesicae). At the same time, the relaxation of the striated muscles of the pelvic floor allow the bladder to descend and the sphincter muscles to relax, and urination to occur.

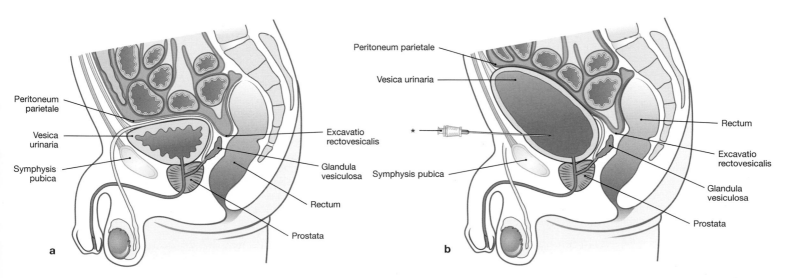

Peritoneum parietale

Vesica urinaria

Symphysis pubica

Excavatio rectovesicalis

Glandula vesiculosa

Rectum

Prostata

a

Peritoneum parietale

Vesica urinaria

*

Symphysis pubica

Rectum

Excavatio rectovesicalis

Glandula vesiculosa

Prostata

b

Fig. 7.67a and b   Urinary bladder, Vesica urinaria, schematic median section; view from the left side. [S700-L126]
a Almost empty.
b Urine-filled.

* puncture needle

The urinary bladder is positioned subperitoneally and is covered on the upper side with the Peritoneum parietale. The empty bladder is positioned behind the pubic symphysis (Symphysis pubica). However, when filled it rises above the pubic bone, giving transabdominal access to the bladder without having to open the peritoneal cavity (**suprapubic urinary catheter**).

Projection of the rectum and anal canal

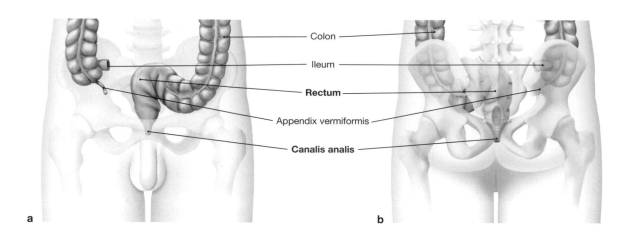

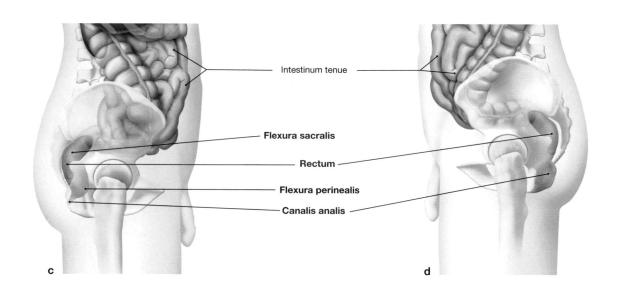

Fig. 7.68a–d Projection of the rectum and the anal canal, Canalis analis, onto the body surface. [S700-L275]
a Ventral view.
b Dorsal view.
c View from right lateral.
d View from left lateral.

The **rectum** and **anal canal (Canalis analis)** are the last two parts of the large intestine (Intestinum crassum). Since these two parts are situated in the lesser pelvis, there are certain characteristics in the topo-

graphical relationships and neurovascular pathways, so that it is sensible to treat them separately as pelvic organs. The rectum begins at the level of the second to third sacral vertebrae and ends at the pelvic floor through which the anal canal passes. In the sagittal plane, the rectum has two angles: the dorsally convex **Flexura sacralis** and the ventrally convex **Flexura perinealis.** The upper part of the rectum up to the Flexura sacralis is in a **secondary retroperitoneal position,** and the distal part and the anal canal are located in the **subperitoneal space.**

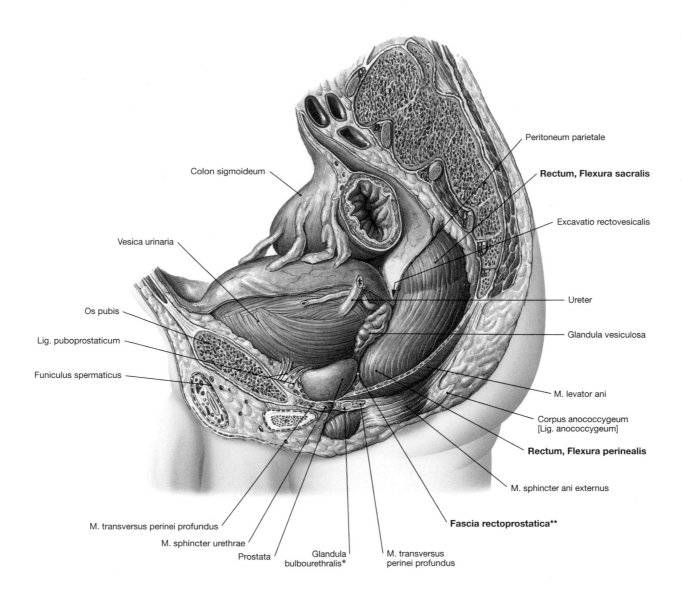

Peritoneum parietale

Rectum, Flexura sacralis

Excavatio rectovesicalis

Colon sigmoideum

Vesica urinaria

Ureter

Glandula vesiculosa

Os pubis

Lig. puboprostaticum

Funiculus spermaticus

M. levator ani

Corpus anococcygeum
[Lig. anococcygeum]

Rectum, Flexura perinealis

M. sphincter ani externus

Fascia rectoprostatica**

M. transversus perinei profundus

M. sphincter urethrae

Prostata

Glandula
bulbourethralis*

M. transversus
perinei profundus

Fig. 7.69   Rectum and anal canal, Canalis analis, in the male pelvis;
view from the left side. [S700]
The illustration shows the two angles of the rectum in the sagittal
plane. In the upper secondary retroperitoneal portion, the rectum adjusts to the curvature of the sacrum and displays the **dorsally convex
Flexura sacralis.** Then the rectum loses its parietal peritoneal covering
and enters the subperitoneal space. Here it turns back, thus forming
the **ventrally convex Flexura perinealis.** Passing through the pelvic
floor, the rectum continues into the anal canal. In men, it adheres to the

anterior aspect of the rectum, initially from the posterior wall of the
urinary bladder (Vesica urinaria) and the seminal vesicles (Glandulae vesiculosae) and further caudally to the prostate gland. Here, the rectum
is separated from the prostate gland only by the thin **Fascia rectoprostatica** (**clin.: DENONVILLIER's fascia). In women, the rectum is positioned in close relation to the posterior aspect of the vagina and is only
separated from it by the Fascia rectovaginalis (→ Fig. 7.166).

* clin.: COWPER's glands

Clinical remarks

The prostate gland is separated from the rectum only by the thin
Fascia rectoprostatica (DENONVILLIER's fascia) and can therefore
be assessed by **digital rectal examination (DRE).** Due to the high

incidence of benign prostatic hyperplasia (BPH) and prostatic carcinoma, the digital rectal examination should be part of a complete
physical examination in men over 50 years of age.

Position of the rectum in the mesorectum

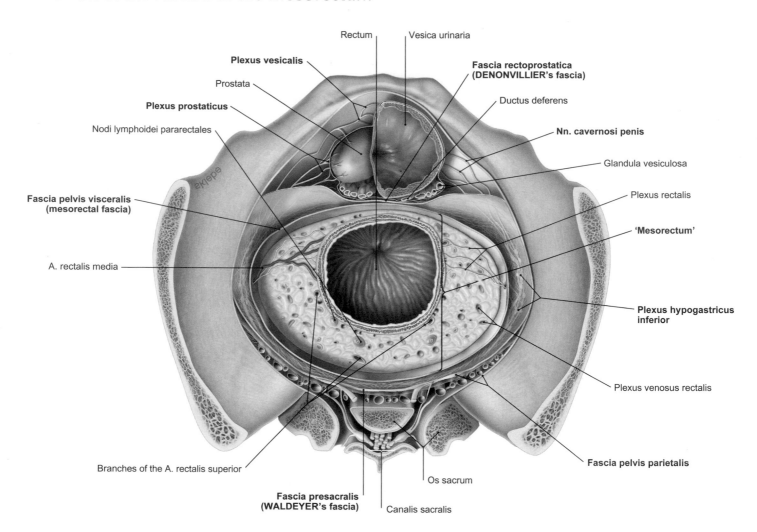

Rectum — Vesica urinaria

Plexus vesicalis

Fascia rectoprostatica (DENONVILLIER's fascia)

Prostata — Ductus deferens

Plexus prostaticus

Nodi lymphoidei pararectales — **Nn. cavernosi penis**

Glandula vesiculosa

Plexus rectalis

Fascia pelvis visceralis (mesorectal fascia)

'Mesorectum'

A. rectalis media

Plexus hypogastricus inferior

Plexus venosus rectalis

Fascia pelvis parietalis

Branches of the A. rectalis superior

Os sacrum

Fascia presacralis (WALDEYER's fascia)

Canalis sacralis

Fig. 7.70 Positional relationship of the rectum in the male pelvis; semi-schematic drawing; cranial view. [S700-L238]/[G1060-002]
The lesser pelvis contains connective tissue densifications at various points that are referred to as **fascia.** The pelvic fascia is of major clinical relevance, but unfortunately cannot be demonstrated in conventional, formalin-fixed bodies. Therefore, their arrangement as shown in this illustration needs to be explained.
The bony pelvis is covered on the inside with a **parietal fascia (Fascia pelvis parietalis)** that represents a continuation of the Fascia transversalis of the abdominal wall. The part covering the ventral surface of the sacrum is the **Fascia presacralis** (clin.: **WALDEYER's fascia**). In the pelvic cavity, each organ is covered by a **visceral fascia (Fascia pelvis visceralis).** The presacral fascia comprises several layers because the parietal fascia is joined by TOLDT's fascia that forms with the positional change of the rectum from an intraperitoneal to a subperitoneal position.

The visceral fascia (Fascia pelvis visceralis) around the rectum is called the **mesorectal fascia** and surrounds the rectum along with adipose tissue and the neurovascular structures. The space enclosed by the mesorectal fascia is clinically called the **mesorectum.** This term is based on newer studies that clearly associate the mesorectum with the most caudal peritoneal duplication of the mesentery, the most cranial part of which is the mesogastrium. Lateral to the mesorectum is the **Plexus hypogastricus inferior,** which is responsible for the autonomic innervation of all the pelvic organs. The nerve plexus is enveloped by the connective tissue of the parietal fascia.
Embedded in the mesorectum, the rectum is ventrally in contact with the posterior wall of the urinary bladder (Vesica urinaria), and the seminal vesicles in men (Glandulae vesiculosae). Caudal from here the rectum is only separated by a further thin **Fascia rectoprostatica** (clin.: **DENONVILLIER's fascia)** from the prostate gland.

Clinical remarks

The mesorectum plays a role in coloproctological surgery, as the mesorectal fascia forms a structural border in operations for **carcinoma of the rectum.** It enables resection of the rectum and its regional lymph nodes **(total mesorectal excision, TME)** with greatly reduced blood loss. The Plexus hypogastricus inferior is located outside the mesorectal fascia. It is required for urinary and faecal continence, and in men for erection and ejaculation; or in women for the function of the cavernous bodies and the BARTHOLIN's glands of the external genitalia. The Plexus hypogastricus inferior is usually not injured during rectal surgery, because it is integrated into the parietal fascia. [E393]

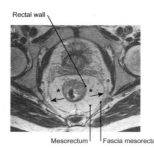

Rectal wall

Mesorectum | Fascia mesorectalis

T2-weighted magnetic resonance image (MRI). The mesorectum (stars) is the space inside the mesorectal fascia (arrows).

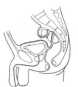

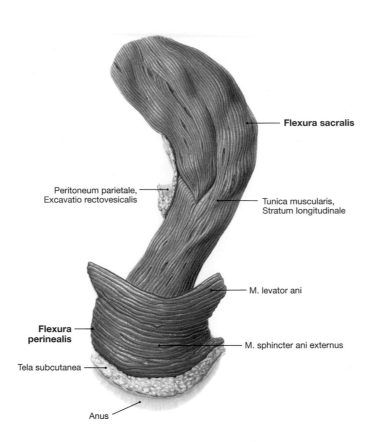

Fig. 7.71 Rectum; view from the left side. [S700]
The rectum cranially forms the dorsal convex Flexura sacralis and cau-dally passes through the M. levator ani of the pelvic floor, forming the ventrally convex Flexura perinealis.

Unlike the colon, the muscular layer (Tunica muscularis) of the rectum not only contains the circular layer (Stratum circulare) but also a contin-uous longitudinal layer (Stratum longitudinale).

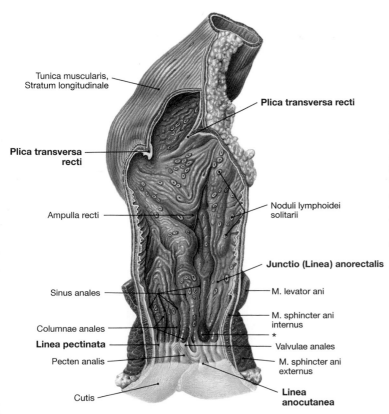

Fig. 7.72 Rectum and anal canal, Canalis analis; ventral view. [S700]
On the inner surface, the rectum has transverse folds, Plicae transver-sae recti. One of up to three folds is relatively reliably palpable at about 6–7 cm above the anus **(KOHLRAUSCH's fold).** Under this fold the rec-tum expands to the Ampulla recti. The Linea anorectalis forms the tran-sition to the anal canal. It is caused by the transition from the transverse folds of the rectum to the longitudinal folds of the anal canal and is therefore actually less of a line than a transition zone (Junctio anorecta-lis).

The **anal canal** itself is divided into **three segments:**
- **Zona columnaris:** contains longitudinal folds (Columnae anales) which are introduced by the Corpus cavernosum recti/ani.
- **Zona alba:** as a result of multi-layered non-cornified squamous epi-thelium, the mucous membrane has an off-white colour; the upper limit of this transition zone which is also referred to as the **Pecten analis,** is marked by the **Linea pectinata** (clin.: **Linea dentata**); its course is 'serrated', as the anal valves from the bottom here meet the whitish squamous epithelium running along the longitudinal folds from the top.
- **Zona cutanea:** external skin, which is bordered by the fuzzy Linea anocutanea.

* haemorrhoidal nodes

Anorectal continence organ

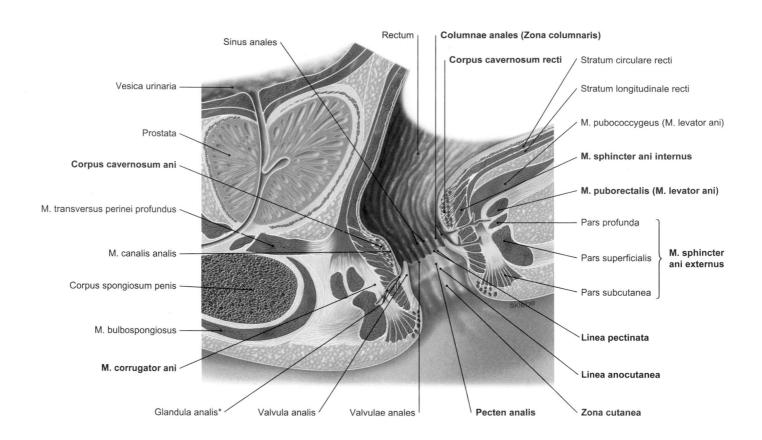

Fig. 7.73 Rectum and anal canal, Canalis analis, in men; median section; view from the left side. [S702-L238]/[B500/G1078]

The figure illustrates the different parts of the anal canal and the structure of the continence organ. The anal canal is divided into **three segments** (→ Fig. 7.72).

The pectinate line **(Linea pectinata)** is the developmental border between the hindgut and the proctodeum and marks the border between the Zona columnaris and the Pecten analis in the adult. Similar to the left colonic flexure, the pectinate line represents the watershed for several neurovascular structures and serves as a clinically important landmark in the anal canal. Therefore, the pectinate line is an important orientation line in the anal canal.

The anal canal possesses a **continence organ** controlled by the CNS which is composed of the anus, sphincter muscles and the Corpus cavernosum recti. Apart from defecation, the anus is closed by the permanent contractions of the internal anal sphincter muscles. The Corpus cavernosum is supplied by the A. rectalis superior and ensures a gastight closure.

The **sphincter muscles** include:
- **M. sphincter ani internus** (smooth muscle, involuntary sympathetic innervation): continuation of the circular muscular layer
- **M. corrugator ani** (smooth muscle): continuation of the longitudinal muscular layer
- **M. sphincter ani externus** (striated muscle, voluntary control via the N. pudendus): includes various parts (Partes subcutanea, superficialis and profunda)
- **M. puborectalis** (striated muscle, voluntary control via the N. pudendus and direct branches of the Plexus sacralis): part of the M. levator ani; forms a loop behind the rectum to pull it ventrally and creates the Flexura perinealis.

* proctodeal gland

→ T 22

Clinical remarks

As the rectum has transverse folds (Plicae transversae recti) and the anal canal has longitudinal folds (Columnae anales), gut portions bulging out from the anus (prolapse) allow one to determine with the naked eye whether a **prolapse is rectal or anal.** Both of these could result in faecal incontinence. Due to the change of the supplying neurovascular structures, the pectinate line is an important orientation line in **surgical interventions for carcinomas of the anal canal.** Proximal tumours metastasise to the pelvic lymph nodes, but distal carcinomas spread first to the inguinal lymph nodes. However, the classification currently depends on the distance between the tumours and the Linea anocutanea. Dilations of the Corpus cavernosum of the rectum are referred to as **haemorrhoids** (→ Fig. 7.79 and → Fig. 7.80). Behind the anal valves are the anal sinuses (Sinus anales), visible as indentations, from which the anal glands (Glandulae anales) arise. These can push through the sphincter muscles and in the case of an inflammation can lead to the formation of **fistulas,** which can spread into the ischioanal fossa.

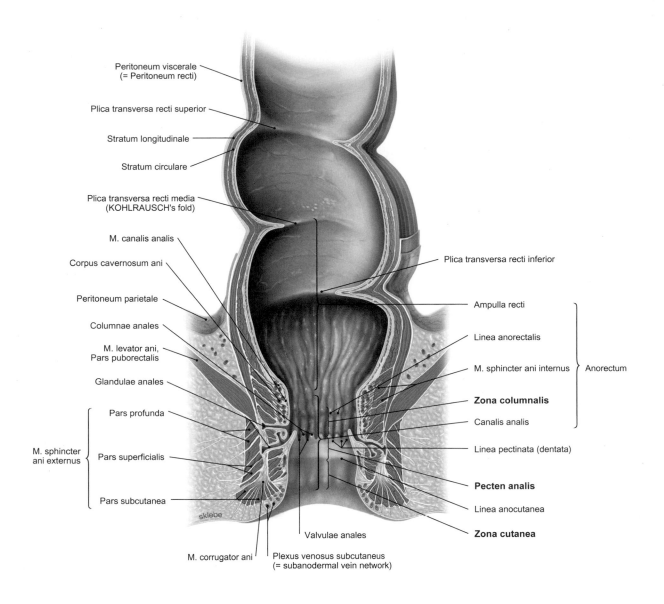

Peritoneum viscerale
(= Peritoneum recti)

Plica transversa recti superior

Stratum longitudinale

Stratum circulare

Plica transversa recti media
(KOHLRAUSCH's fold)

M. canalis analis

Corpus cavernosum ani

Peritoneum parietale

Columnae anales

M. levator ani,
Pars puborectalis

Glandulae anales

Pars profunda

M. sphincter
ani externus
Pars superficialis

Pars subcutanea

sklebe

M. corrugator ani

Plexus venosus subcutaneus
(= subanodermal vein network)

Valvulae anales

Plica transversa recti inferior

Ampulla recti

Linea anorectalis

M. sphincter ani internus   Anorectum

Zona columnalis

Canalis analis

Linea pectinata (dentata)

Pecten analis

Linea anocutanea

Zona cutanea

Fig. 7.74 Rectum and anal canal, Canalis analis, with continence organ; frontal section; ventral view. [S702-L238]

The **continence organ** extends from the Ampulla recti down to the anus. With filling of the ampulla via visceral-afferent and -efferent neurons in the Nn. splanchnici pelvici by short-term relaxation of the M. sphincter ani internus, an **anal-rectal relaxation reflex** is triggered, and this leads to an increase in tone of all the sphincter muscles. The voluntarily innervated muscles allow conscious control of faecal continence:

- **M. puborectalis:** this part of the M. levator ani is found in a state of permanent contraction.
- **M. sphincter ani externus:** has a regulatory function because it induces an increase in tone in the M. sphincter ani internus when defecation needs to be arbitrarily prevented.

Additionally, there are involuntarily innervated muscles that enable closure of the continence organ without conscious control:

- **M. sphincter ani internus:** in the resting state it ensures 70 % of the continence performance and is therefore the **centre of the continence organ.** Its fibres partially interlace with the Corpus cavernosum recti and are anchored in the mucosa of the anal canal. Hence they are separately highlighted as the **M. canalis analis.**
- **M. corrugator ani:** the longitudinal muscle fibres insert in the perianal skin and pull this inwards.

The sphincter muscles in their entirety may not provide complete closure of the anus. For this, the **cavernous body of the rectum (Corpus cavernosum recti/ani)** is necessary and is located under the mucous membrane; fed from the A. rectalis superior, it provides a gas-tight closure (another 10 % of the continence performance in the resting state). The cavernous bodies form, together with the interlacing muscle fibres of the M. canalis analis, an **angiomuscular closure apparatus.**

Arteries of the rectum and anal canal

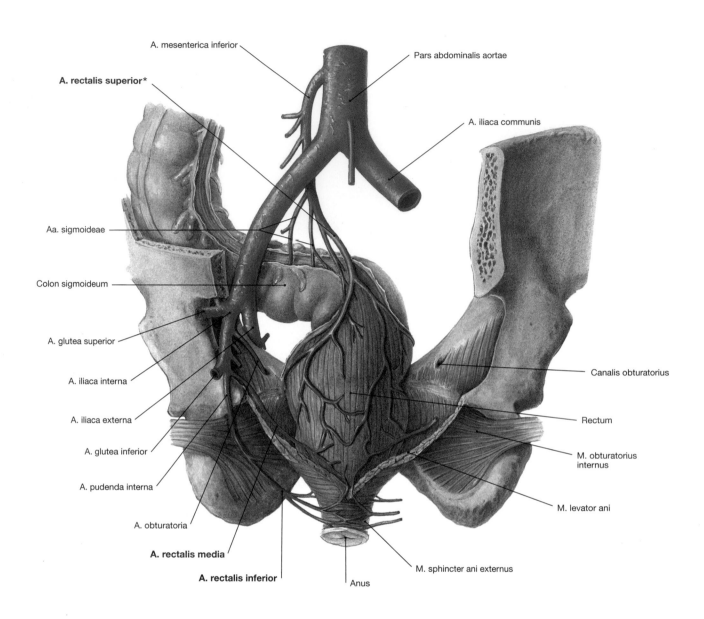

A. mesenterica inferior

A. rectalis superior*

Pars abdominalis aortae

A. iliaca communis

Aa. sigmoideae

Colon sigmoideum

A. glutea superior

A. iliaca interna

A. iliaca externa

A. glutea inferior

A. pudenda interna

A. obturatoria

A. rectalis media

A. rectalis inferior

Anus

M. sphincter ani externus

M. levator ani

M. obturatorius internus

Rectum

Canalis obturatorius

Fig. 7.75 **Rectal arteries, Aa. rectales;** dorsal view. [S700]
The rectum and anal canal are supplied by three arteries:

- **A. rectalis superior** (unpaired): from the A. mesenterica inferior. It supplies the major part of the rectum and the anal canal above the Linea pectinata, so it is vital for the filling of the **Corpus cavernosum recti/ani.**
- **A. rectalis media** (paired; although usually only on one side or completely missing): from the A. iliaca interna above the pelvic floor (M. levator ani). When present, it supplies only a small area of the lower rectum.
- **A. rectalis inferior** (paired): from the A. pudenda interna beneath the pelvic floor. The artery supplies the **sphincter muscles of the anal canal** from outside and the mucosa below the Linea pectinata.

The border between the area supplied by the A. mesenterica inferior and the area supplied by the A. iliaca interna is located in the area of the **Linea pectinata,** where numerous anastomoses usually exist between these arteries. The A. rectalis superior is the last branch of the A. mesenterica inferior and provides a branch for the anastomosis with the Aa. sigmoideae. From this point (*clin.: SUDECK's point), it is a terminal artery. The Corpus cavernosum recti is perfused from the A. rectalis superior. Therefore, bleeding from haemorrhoids, representing the dilated rectal cavernous bodies, is an arterial bleeding which can be identified by its bright red colour.

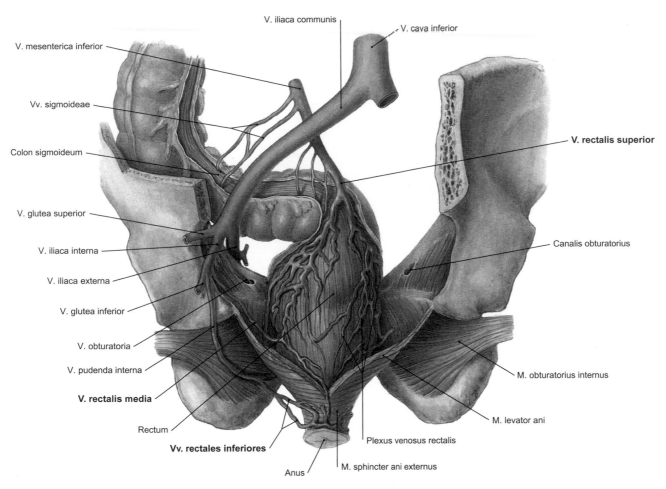

Fig. 7.76 **Rectal veins, Vv. rectales;** dorsal view. [S700]
Depending on the rectal arteries, the venous blood from the rectum
and anal canal flows through three veins:
* **V. rectalis superior** (unpaired): connection via the V. mesenterica
  inferior to the portal vein (V. portae hepatis)
* **V. rectalis media** (paired): connection via the V. iliaca interna to the
  V. cava inferior
* **V. rectalis inferior** (paired): connection via the V. pudenda interna
  and the V. iliaca interna to the V. cava inferior.
The border between the venous drainage of the V. portae hepatis and
the V. cava inferior is located in the area of the Linea pectinata. How-
ever, there are numerous anastomoses.

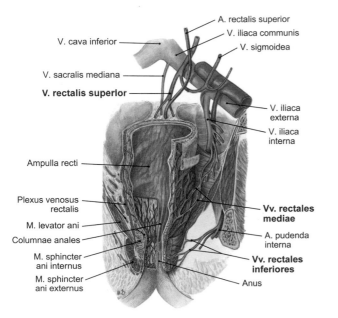

Fig. 7.77 **Venous drainage of the rectum and anal canal, Canalis
analis;** ventral view. Tributaries to the V. portae hepatis (purple) and to
the V. cava inferior (blue). [S700]
This illustration demonstrates that the venous drainage pathways to the
portal vein (V. rectalis superior) and to the inferior vena cava (V. rectalis
media and V. rectalis inferior) have formed numerous anastomoses.

Clinical remarks

With an increase in blood pressure in the portal system **(portal hypertension),** e. g. in cirrhosis of the liver, the venous blood can drain
via connections between the superior and inferior rectal veins **(portocaval anastomoses)** to the V. cava inferior. This does not cause
haemorrhoids and these anastomoses are therefore clinically insig-
nificant. It should be kept in mind that by administering rectal sup-
positories, the direct venous drainage of the lower rectal veins into
the V. cava inferior are used to bypass the metabolism in the liver.

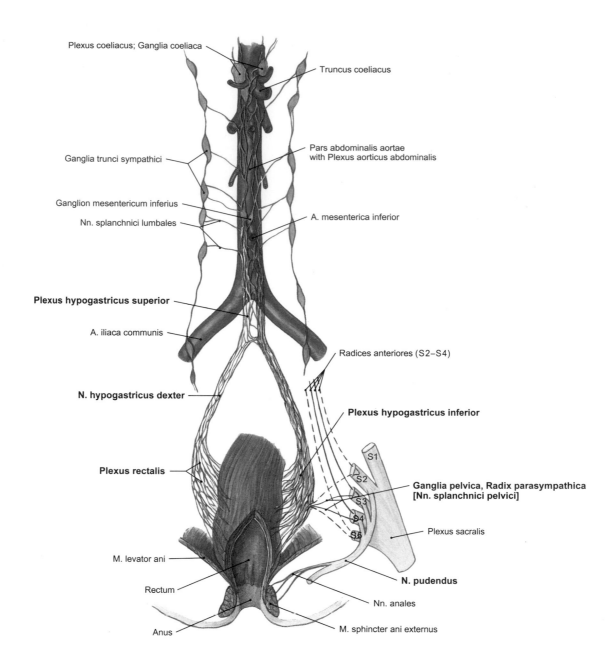

Plexus coeliacus; Ganglia coeliaca

Truncus coeliacus

Ganglia trunci sympathici

Pars abdominalis aortae
with Plexus aorticus abdominalis

Ganglion mesentericum inferius

Nn. splanchnici lumbales

A. mesenterica inferior

Plexus hypogastricus superior

A. iliaca communis

Radices anteriores (S2–S4)

N. hypogastricus dexter

Plexus hypogastricus inferior

S1

Plexus rectalis

S2

S3

**Ganglia pelvica, Radix parasympathica
[Nn. splanchnici pelvici]**

S4

S5

Plexus sacralis

M. levator ani

Rectum

N. pudendus

Nn. anales

Anus

M. sphincter ani externus

Fig. 7.78 Innervation of the rectum and anal canal, Canalis analis;
ventral view; schematic drawing. The Plexus rectalis contains sympathetic (green) and parasympathetic (purple) nerve fibres. [S700]
The Plexus rectalis is a continuation of the Plexus hypogastricus inferior. The preganglionic **sympathetic nerve fibres** (T10–L3) descend
from the Plexus aorticus abdominalis via the Plexus hypogastricus
superior and from the sacral ganglia of the sympathetic trunk (Truncus
sympathicus) via the Nn. splanchnici sacrales, to be synapsed to postganglionic neurons in the ganglia of the **Plexus hypogastricus inferior.**
As the **Plexus rectalis,** this serves the rectum and the anal canal. The
sympathetic fibres activate the sphincter muscles.
The preganglionic **parasympathetic nerve fibres** pass from the sacral
parasympathetic nervous system (S2–S4) through the **Nn. splanchnici**

pelvici into the ganglia of the **Plexus hypogastricus inferior.** They are
switched either here or in the vicinity of the intestine to postganglionic
fibres, which promote peristalsis and inhibit the sphincter muscles
(M. sphincter ani internus) to facilitate defecation.
Autonomic innervation ends approximately in the area of the Linea
pectinata. The inferior portion of the anal canal is innervated by the **N.
pudendus** with somatic sensory fibres. Thus, anal carcinomas inferior
to the Linea pectinata are extremely painful, whereas carcinomas located above the demarcation line are not.
The N. pudendus also provides motor innervation to the M. sphincter
ani externus and M. puborectalis, and allows voluntary closure of the
anus.

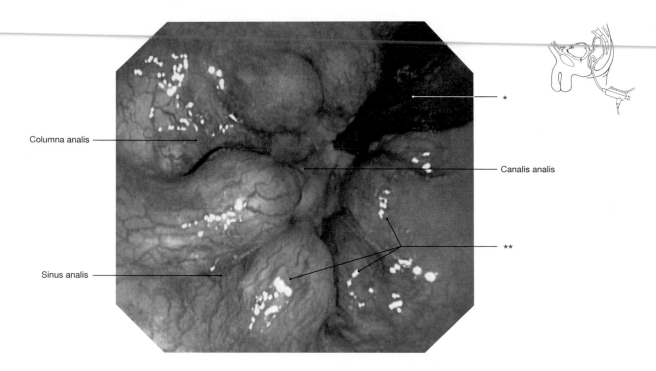

Fig. 7.79 Anal canal, Canalis analis; colonoscopy; cranial view. [S700-T901]
Six considerably larger nodes of the Corpus cavernosum recti (haemorrhoids) can be seen.

* colonoscope
** three haemorrhoidal nodes

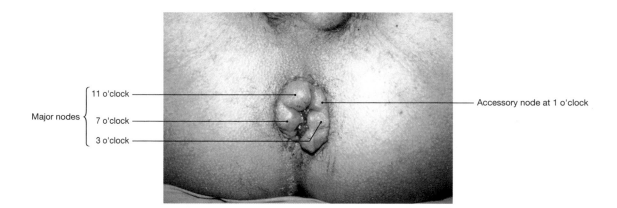

Fig. 7.80 Haemorrhoids stage IV; caudal view in the lithotomy position, when the patient is in a supine position and the examining person can see the perineum. [R234]
The position of each haemorrhoidal node is indicated using the face of a clock. Due to the branching pattern of the main branches of the

A. rectalis superior on entering the Corpus cavernosum recti, the major nodes are typically at three, seven and 11 o'clock. In addition, corresponding 'accessory nodes' may emerge from the smaller arterial branches. Here an 'accessory node' is shown at 1 o'clock.

Clinical remarks

Haemorrhoids are abnormal enlargements of the Corpus cavernosum recti and are common. The causes are unclear, but appear to be associated with nutritional habits in industrialised nations (too much fat, too little dietary fibre). Haemorrhoids occur in different **stages:**
* Stage I: only visible endoscopically
* Stage II: protrude during bearing down for defecation; afterwards retract into the anal canal.

* Stage III: protrude spontaneously, but can be repositioned manually.
* Stage IV: cannot be repositioned.
From stage II onwards they should be treated: either by sclerotherapy or rubber band ligation (stage II), or by surgical removal (stages III and IV).

Retroperitoneal space and pelvic cavity

External male genitalia

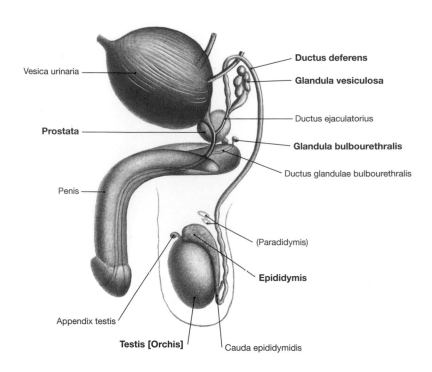

Fig. 7.81 External male genitalia, Organa genitalia masculina externa; schematic illustrations, ventral view. [S700]
In the male genitalia it is important to distinguish between the external genitalia (Organa genitalia masculina externa) and the internal genitalia (Organa genitalia masculina interna → Fig. 7.90).

The **external genitalia** include:
* penis
* Urethra masculina
* scrotum.
The external genitalia are the **sexual organs.** The penis is used for sexual intercourse.
The urethra is described along with the efferent urinary system (→ Fig. 7.61, → Fig. 7.62).

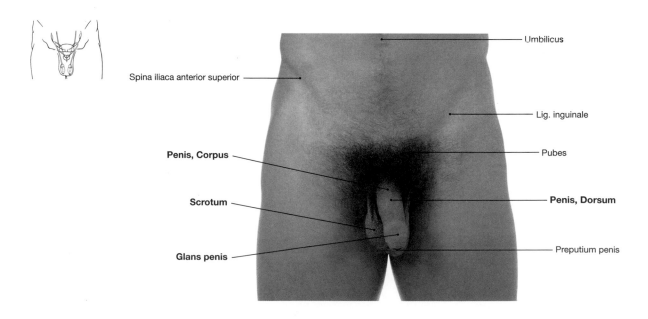

Fig. 7.82 External male genitalia, Organa genitalia masculina externa; ventral view. [S700]
The external male genitalia (Organa genitalia masculine externa) comprise the penis and the scrotum. The testes and epididymis are the parts of the internal male genitalia that are positioned outside of the pelvic cavity following their descensus during the development. These developmental differences are of clinical importance with respect to neurovascular structures and lymphatic drainage pathways.

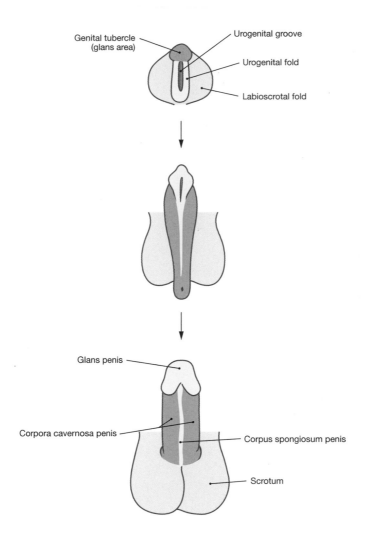

Fig. 7.83 Development of the external male genitalia, Organa genitalia masculina externa. [S700-L126]/[G1060-002]

The external genitalia develop from the caudal part of the Sinus urogenitalis. The Sinus urogenitalis develops from the cloaca of the hindgut and gives rise among other things to the urinary bladder and parts of the urethra (→ Fig. 7.29). In addition, there is also the ectoderm with the connective tissue (mesenchyme) beneath. Firstly, the external genitalia develop identically in both sexes (indifferent gonad). The anterior wall of the Sinus urogenitalis indents to form the **urethral groove** which is bordered on both sides by the **urethral folds.** Lateral of these are the **labioscrotal folds** and anterior to the groove is the **genital tubercle.** Subsequently, in men the **genital tubercle** develops into the **penis shaft** (Corpora cavernosa) due to the influence of the male sex hormone testosterone which is produced in the testes. The **genital folds** merge above the urethral groove to form the Corpus spongiosum and the **Glans penis.** This creates the Pars spongiosa of the **urethra.** The Pars prostatica and the Pars membranacea derive proximally from the Sinus urogenitalis. The **labioscrotal folds** enlarge and unite to become the **scrotum.**

Clinical remarks

If the fusion of the urethral folds is incomplete, the opening of the urethra is not located at the tip of the Glans penis but further proximally. In **hypospadias** (→ Fig. a), the urethra exits at the inferior side of the penis between the scrotum and the glans.

In **epispadias** (→ Fig. b), the urethra opens into a ridge at the dorsal side of the penis. In addition to problems with urination, this condition may involve a distortion of the penile body, requiring surgical correction within the first years of life. [S702-L266]

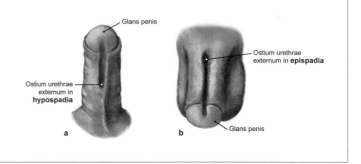

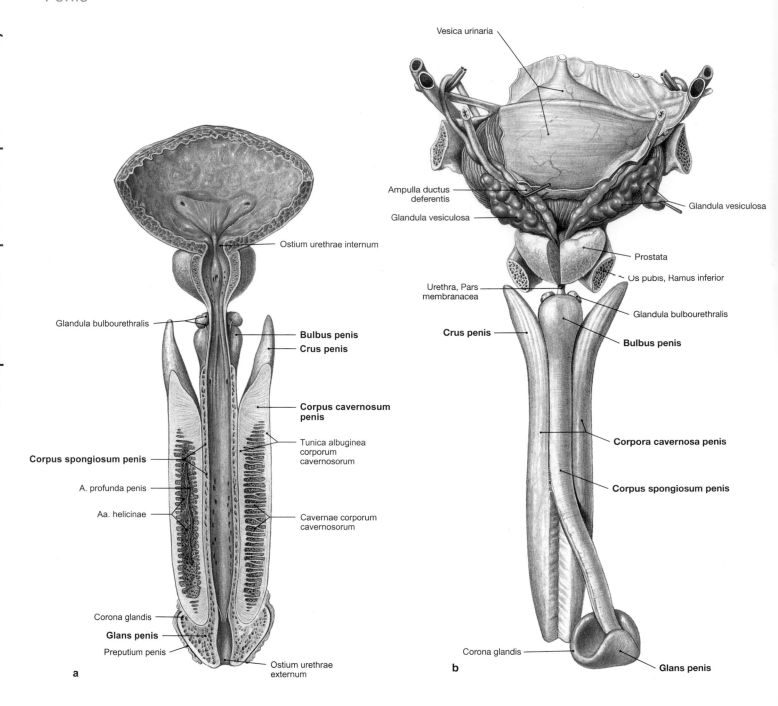

Fig. 7.84a and b   Urinary bladder, Vesica urinaria, prostate gland, Prostata, and penis, with exposed spongy tissue. [S700]
a Ventral view, urinary bladder and urethra opened.
b Dorsal view.
In a flaccid state, the penis is usually about 10 cm long and divided into the **Corpus penis, Glans penis** and the base or root **(Radix penis).** It comprises the paired **Corpora cavernosa** of the penis which are enclosed in a dense fibrous covering **(Tunica albuginea)** and separated by a Septum penis, and the **Corpus spongiosum** which surrounds the urethra. The proximal parts (Crura penis) of the Corpora cavernosa are fixed to the inferior Pubic rami. The Corpus spongiosum is enlarged proximally to the Bulbus penis and distally forms the Glans penis. Externally, all cavernous bodies are ensheathed as a whole by the **fascia of the penis (Fascia penis),** which was removed in this illustration.
For the structure of the male urethra (Urethra masculina) → Fig. 7.61 and → Fig. 7.62.

Clinical remarks

If the prepuce is too tight **(phimosis)** and cannot be pulled back, there may be problems with urination and infections may occur. Then the prepuce must be removed by circumcision.

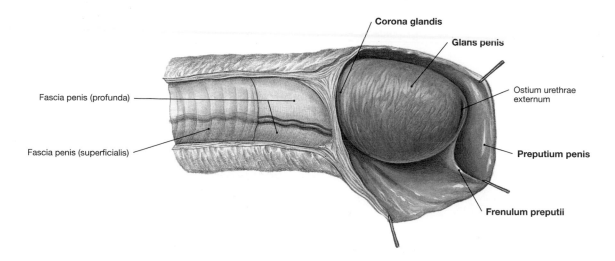

Corona glandis

Glans penis

Fascia penis (profunda)

Ostium urethrae externum

Preputium penis

Fascia penis (superficialis)

Frenulum preputii

Fig. 7.85 Penis, with glans, Glans penis, and prepuce, Preputium penis; view from the right side. [S700]
The distal end of the penis is enlarged to form the **Glans penis** and shows a ridge (Corona glandis) at its base. In the flaccid state of the

penis, the glans is covered by the **foreskin (Preputium penis),** which is attached at the bottom by a ribbon-like frenulum (Frenulum preputii).

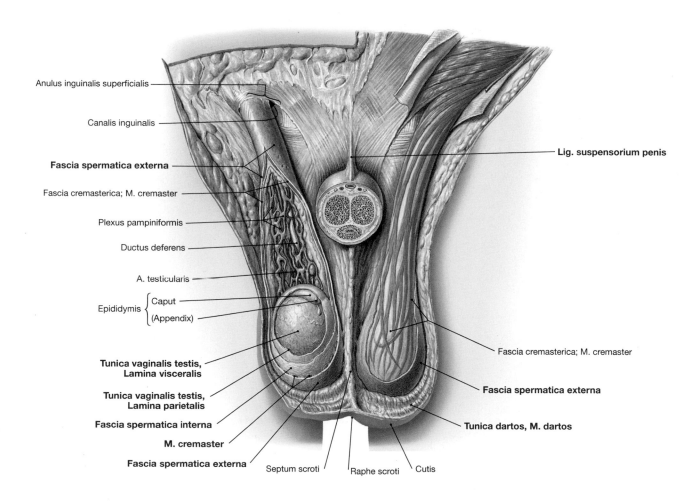

Anulus inguinalis superficialis

Canalis inguinalis

Fascia spermatica externa

Fascia cremasterica; M. cremaster

Plexus pampiniformis

Ductus deferens

A. testicularis

Epididymis { Caput
(Appendix)

Tunica vaginalis testis, Lamina visceralis

Tunica vaginalis testis, Lamina parietalis

Fascia spermatica interna

M. cremaster

Fascia spermatica externa

Septum scroti

Raphe scroti

Cutis

Lig. suspensorium penis

Fascia cremasterica; M. cremaster

Fascia spermatica externa

Tunica dartos, M. dartos

Fig. 7.86 Scrotum; ventral view; the scrotum is opened and the penis is cut through frontally. [S700]
The root of the penis is attached to the anterior body wall by the superficial **Lig. fundiforme penis** and, underneath it, the deep **Lig. suspensorium penis.** The scrotum is divided internally by a septum which externally resembles a seam (Raphe scroti).
Testes and **spermatic cord** have the following **coverings:**
* scrotal skin
* Tunica dartos: subcutaneous layer with smooth muscle cells

* Fascia spermatica externa: continuation of the superficial body fascia (Fascia abdominalis superficialis)
* M. cremaster with Fascia cremasterica
* Fascia spermatica interna: continuation of the Fascia transversalis.
The surface of the testes is also covered by the **Tunica vaginalis testis,** with an external Lamina parietalis (periorchium) outside and an internal Lamina visceralis (epiorchium), connected to each other by the mesorchium with the **Cavitas serosa scroti** between them.

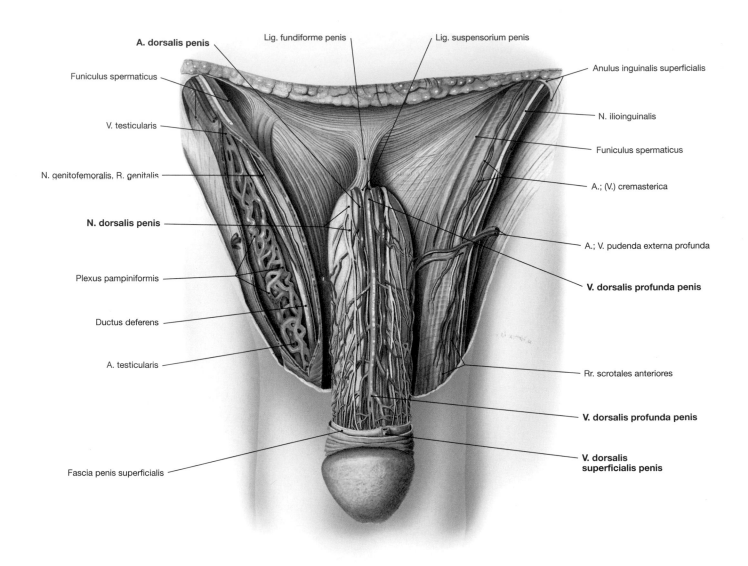

A. dorsalis penis

Funiculus spermaticus

V. testicularis

N. genitofemoralis, R. genitalis

N. dorsalis penis

Plexus pampiniformis

Ductus deferens

A. testicularis

Fascia penis superficialis

Lig. fundiforme penis

Lig. suspensorium penis

Anulus inguinalis superficialis

N. ilioinguinalis

Funiculus spermaticus

A.; (V.) cremasterica

A.; V. pudenda externa profunda

V. dorsalis profunda penis

Rr. scrotales anteriores

V. dorsalis profunda penis

V. dorsalis superficialis penis

Fig. 7.87 External male genitalia, Organa genitalia masculina externa, with neurovascular pathways; ventral view; after removal of the superficial fascia of the penis (COLLES' fascia) and the deep fascia of the penis (BUCK's fascia). [S700]

The penis is supplied by **three paired arteries** from the A. pudenda interna and **three venous systems** (→ Fig. 7.88). Here it is only the subfascially located blood vessels that are visible after the fascia of the penis (BUCK's fascia) has been removed.

The A. dorsalis penis is arranged in pairs and supplies the skin and the glans of the penis. Between the arteries of both sides runs the unpaired

V. dorsalis profunda penis, which drains the cavernous bodies into the Plexus venosus prostaticus.

The illustration shows the **nerves of the penis:**
- sensory: N. dorsalis penis (from the N. pudendus)
- autonomic: mainly parasympathetic Nn. cavernosi penis (from the Plexus hypogastricus inferior) pierce the pelvic floor and join the N. dorsalis penis (sympathetic stimulation causes vasoconstriction; parasympathetic stimulation causes vasodilation and consecutive erection).

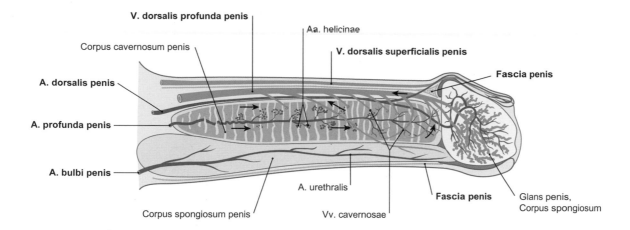

Fig. 7.88   Blood vessels of the penis; schematic illustration of a median section with presentation of the deep fascia of the penis (BUCK's fascia); view from the right side. [S702-L126]/[B500/O1107]
The position of the blood vessels in relation to the deep fascia of the penis (BUCK's fascia) is important.
The penis is supplied by **three paired arteries** from the A. pudenda interna:
* A. dorsalis penis: runs subfascially, supplies skin and glans of the penis
* A. profunda penis: in the Corpora cavernosa, responsible for filling them with blood

* A. bulbi penis: penetrates the bulb of the penis, supplies the Glandula bulbourethralis and continues, as the A. urethralis, to the urethra and Corpus spongiosum.
The venous blood is collected by **three venous systems:**
* V. dorsalis superficialis penis: paired or unpaired, epifascial, transfers blood from the penile skin to the V. pudenda externa
* V. dorsalis profunda penis: unpaired, subfascial, drains the cavernous bodies into the Plexus venosus prostaticus
* V. bulbi penis: paired, brings blood from the bulb of the penis to the V. dorsalis profunda penis.

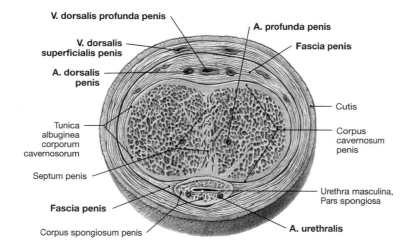

Fig. 7.89   Penis; cross-section in the area of the centre of the shaft; ventral view. [S700]
The Corpora cavernosa of the penis together with the deep blood vessels are enveloped by the deep fascia of the penis (Fascia penis; BUCK's fascia). The subcutaneous connective tissue condenses around the superficial veins and is also referred to as superficial fascia of the penis (COLLES' fascia).

The position of the blood vessels is important for the **erection** of the penis. Activated parasympathetically, the dilation of the **A. profunda penis** results in the engorgement of the Corpora cavernosa. This compresses the **V. dorsalis penis** under the tough fascia of the penis (Fascia penis), so that the blood cannot drain away. Due to additional contraction of the **Mm. ischiocavernosi** (innervated by the N. pudendus), this results in penile erection.

Clinical remarks

The parasympathetic nerve fibres release nitric oxide (NO). In the smooth muscle cells of the blood vessels, this NO leads to an increase of the second messenger cGMP, which inhibits the contraction of the smooth muscle cells. **Inhibitors of phosphodiesterase** (e.g. Viagra®) delay the degradation of cGMP, thus enhancing the **erection.**
With **injuries to the penis,** the distinct penile fasciae limit the spread of extravasated blood or urine. If the BUCK's fascia is intact, the

bleeding is confined to the body of the penis ('aubergine sign'). If the BUCK's fascia is injured, the haematoma spreads out in the shape of a butterfly and extends further into the scrotum and the superficial perineal region that is confined by COLLES' fascia. It may ascend to the anterior abdominal wall because COLLES' fascia forms a continuous membrane with the superficial fascia (SCARPA's) of the abdominal wall.

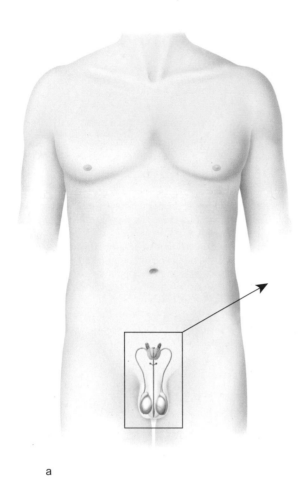

a

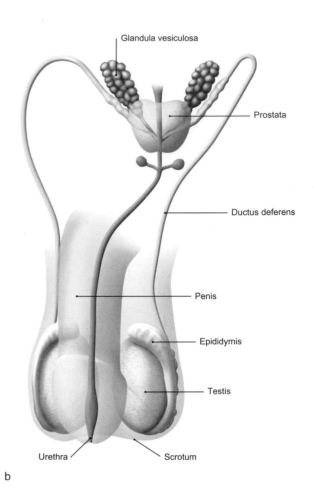

b

Fig. 7.90a and b Male urinary and reproductive organs, Organa urogenitalia masculina; view from the right side. [S701-L275]
The **internal male genitalia** include:
* testis
* epididymis
* spermatic duct (Ductus deferens)
* spermatic cord (Funiculus spermaticus)
* accessory sex glands:
  – prostate gland
  – seminal vesicle (Glandula vesiculosa), paired
  – COWPER's gland (Glandula bulbourethralis), paired.

The testis and epididymis belong to the internal genitalia because they were relocated during development together with a peritoneal sac (Cavitas serosa scroti) from the abdominal cavity into the scrotum.
The internal genitalia are **reproductive organs.** They serve the production, maturation, and transport of spermatozoa and the production of seminal fluid. The testes also produce male sex hormones (testosterone).

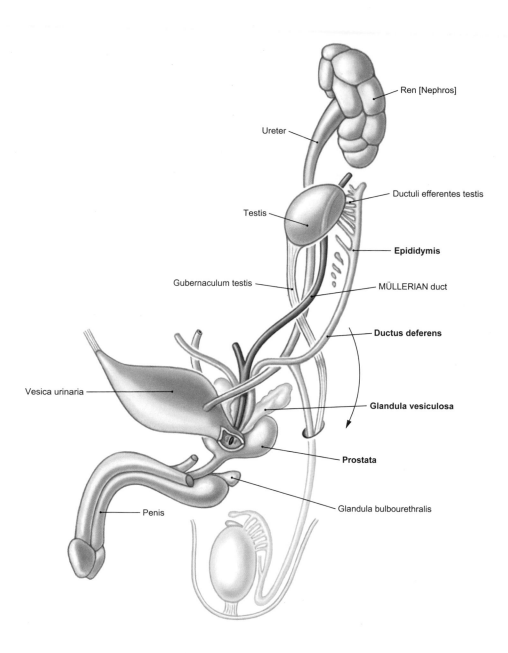

Ren [Nephros]

Ureter

Testis

Ductuli efferentes testis

Epididymis

Gubernaculum testis

MÜLLERIAN duct

Ductus deferens

Vesica urinaria

Glandula vesiculosa

Prostata

Penis

Glandula bulbourethralis

Fig. 7.91 Development of the internal male genitalia, Organa genitalia masculina interna. [B500-L238]/[H233-001]
The internal genitalia develop in both sexes in the same way until the seventh week (indifferent gonad → Fig. 7.29). In the male, the primordial gonad then develops into the testis. The testis develops in the lumbar region at the level of the mesonephros which contributes several canaliculi as a connection between the testis and the epididymis. As the body grows and develops, the testis then moves caudally **(Descensus testis)** accompanied by its neurovascular pathways. Along the inferior mesenchymal gubernaculum (Gubernaculum testis), a peritoneal space is formed (Proc. vaginalis peritonei) which reaches down to the future scrotum and serves in guiding the descent of the testis, a process normally completed at birth. At birth, the Proc. vaginalis peritonei closes in the area of the Funiculus spermaticus. The distal part of the Proc. vaginalis remains and forms a part of the testicular coverings (Tunica vaginalis testis).

The sex hormones of the testis (mainly testosterone) induce the final **differentiation of the WOLFFIAN ducts** to the internal male genitalia (epididymis, vas deferens), the seminal vesicles, and other accessory sex glands (prostate gland, COWPER's glands) from the Sinus urogenitalis. The anti-MÜLLERIAN hormone suppresses the differentiation of the MÜLLERIAN ducts in female genitalia.

Clinical remarks

The descent of the testis explains why the testicular blood vessels arise at the level of the kidneys and why their regional lymph nodes are positioned at this level in the retroperitoneal space. Hence it is here rather than in the groin where the sentinel lymph node metastases should be expected in **testicular cancer.** If the testes do not fully descend within the first years of life **(undescended testes, cryptorchidism),** this can lead to infertility. Cryptorchidism is associated with an increased risk of testicular cancer. More recent findings indicate that hormonal treatment or an operation in the first year of life can prevent infertility. However, the risk of cancer cannot be clearly influenced therapeutically. If the Proc. vaginalis fails to obliterate, accumulation of fluids may occur (even in adulthood) in the scrotum **(hydrocele testis)** (→ Fig. 7.96) or abdominal organs may prolapse into the scrotum **(congenital inguinal hernia).**
For inter- and transsexuality → Fig. 7.121.

Male genitalia

Organ-related cutaneous areas of the testis and epididymis

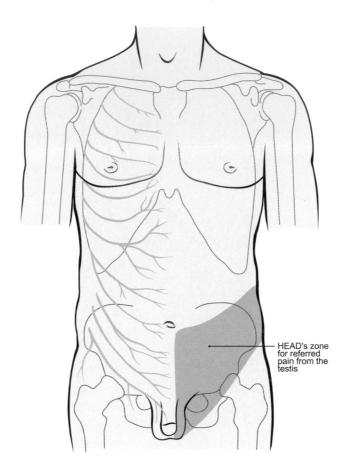

HEAD's zone
for referred
pain from the
testis

Fig. 7.92 HEAD's zone of the testis [Orchis]; ventral view. [S700-L126]/[G1071]
The organ-related area for referred pain **(HEAD's zone)** of the testis projects onto the **cutaneous areas (dermatomes) T10–L1** and thereby corresponds to that of the kidney. This localisation reflects the fact that the testis develops in the region that later becomes the lumbar region and when it descends (Descensus) into the scrotum, it takes with it the neurovascular pathways, including its autonomic innervation (Plexus testicularis). Diseases of the testis, such as an inflammation (orchitis) or a torsion of the testicular blood vessels (testicular torsion), can lead to severe pain which will be perceived in the dermatomes T10–L1 (referred pain).

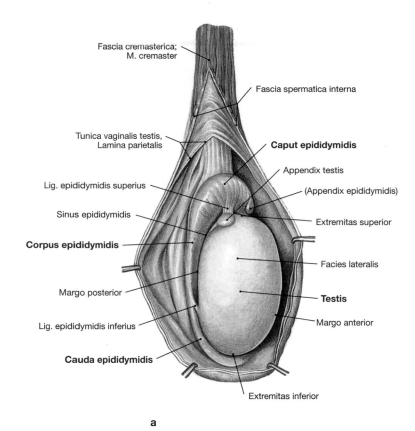

Fascia cremasterica;
M. cremaster

Fascia spermatica interna

Tunica vaginalis testis,
Lamina parietalis

Caput epididymidis

Appendix testis

Lig. epididymidis superius

(Appendix epididymidis)

Sinus epididymidis

Extremitas superior

Corpus epididymidis

Facies lateralis

Margo posterior

Testis

Lig. epididymidis inferius

Margo anterior

Cauda epididymidis

Extremitas inferior

a

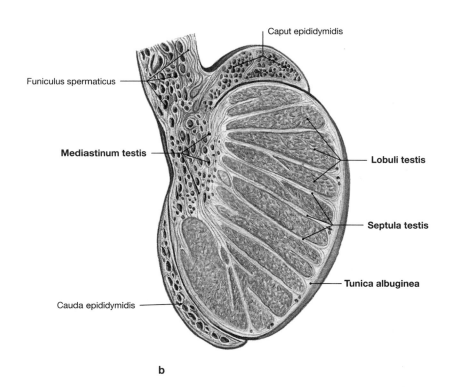

Caput epididymidis

Funiculus spermaticus

Mediastinum testis

Lobuli testis

Septula testis

Tunica albuginea

Cauda epididymidis

b

Fig. 7.93a and b   Testis [Orchis] and epididymis. [S700]
a View from the right side.
b Sagittal section; view from the right side.
The testis is egg-shaped and 4 × 3 cm in size (20–30 g). It has a **superior** and an **inferior pole** (Extremitas superior and inferior). The dense Tunica albuginea surrounding the testis sends septa into the parenchyma of the testis and thus subdivides it into 370 **lobules of testis (Lobuli testis).** Within the lobules, the sperm is produced in the **seminifer-** **ous tubules.** Between the tubules are testosterone-producing cells (LEYDIG's cells). The tubules are in the area of the **mediastinum testis,** where the neurovascular pathways enter and exit, connected to the head of the epididymis. The **epididymis** sits above and dorsal to the testis and is attached to it by an upper and a lower band (Ligg. epididymides superius and inferius). The epididymis is divided into the **head (Caput), body (Corpus), and tail (Cauda),** and continues into the spermatic duct (vas deferens).

Retroperitoneal space and pelvic cavity

Testis and epididymis

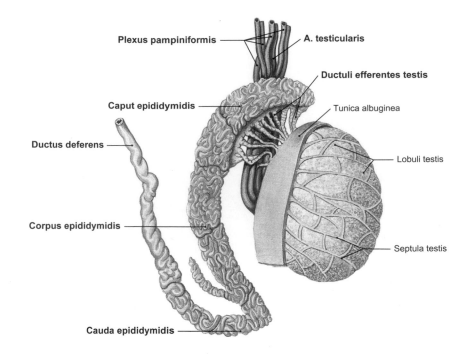

Fig. 7.94 Testis [Orchis] and epididymis, with blood vessels; view from the right side. [S700]
The **testis** is linked by fine tubules (Ductuli efferentes testis) with the head of the epididymis (Caput epididymidis). The **epididymis** itself con-

sists of a 6 m-long convoluted duct which continues as the **vas deferens (Ductus deferens)** at the tail of the epididymis.
Testis and epididymis are supplied by the **A. testicularis** and a plexus of veins **(Plexus pampiniformis)**.

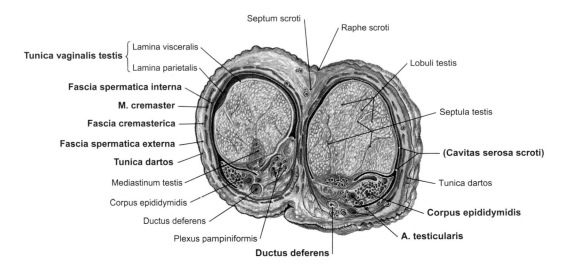

Fig. 7.95 Testis [Orchis] and epididymis; cross-section; cranial view. [S700]
In addition to the testicular coverings (→ Fig. 7.98), the neurovascular structures and the vas deferens (Ductus deferens) are sectioned. The

two serous layers of the **Tunica vaginalis testis** confine a serous cavity **(Cavitas serosa scroti)**.

Clinical remarks

If the Proc. vaginalis peritonei fails to obliterate after the testicular descent, fluid may collect in this cavity (Hydrocele testis), even in the adult (→ Fig. 7.91).
[S701-T975]

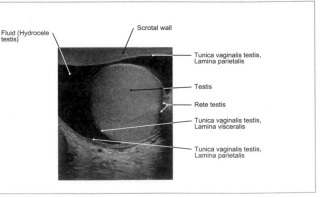

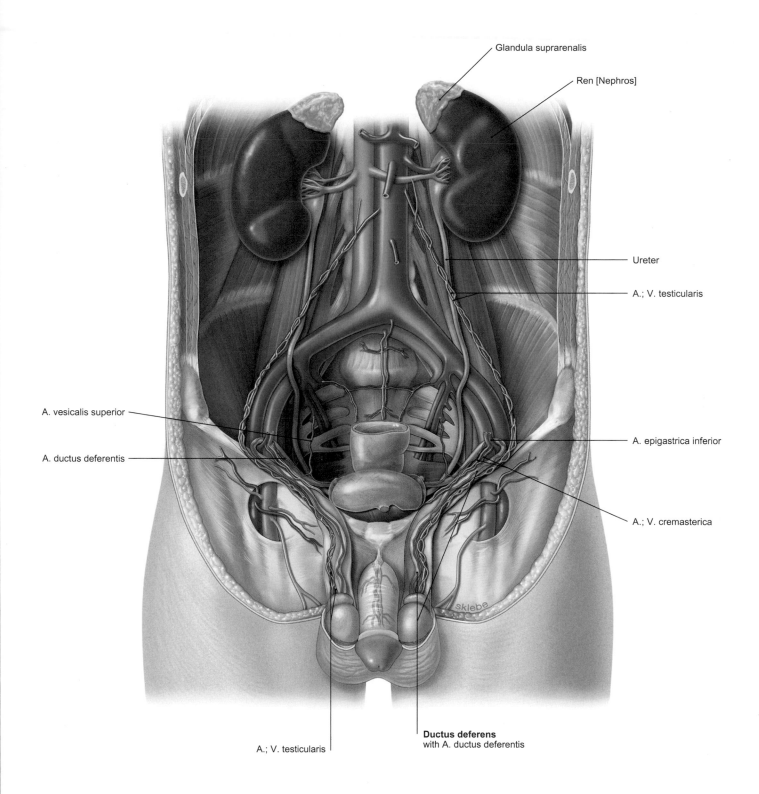

Glandula suprarenalis

Ren [Nephros]

Ureter

A.; V. testicularis

A. vesicalis superior

A. ductus deferentis

A. epigastrica inferior

A.; V. cremasterica

A.; V. testicularis

Ductus deferens
with A. ductus deferentis

Fig. 7.96 Parts and pathway of the vas deferens, Ductus deferens.
The abdominal wall and all intra- and secondary retroperitoneal organs have been removed; the vas deferens is opened down its length; ventral view. [S702-L238]

The **vas deferens (Ductus deferens)** is 35–40 cm long and has a diameter of 3 mm. It originates from the tail of the epididymis (Cauda epididymidis) and then ascends into the scrotum **(scrotal part),** before it continues into the Funiculus spermaticus **(funicular part).** The vas deferens goes through the inguinal canal **(inguinal part)** and then passes into the lesser pelvis **(pelvic part).**

In the lesser pelvis it crosses the ureters before adhering to the dorsal side of the urinary bladder. It extends here to the **Ampulla ductus deferentis** and combines with the duct of the seminal vesicle (Glandula vesiculosa) to the **Ductus ejaculatorius.** The latter traverses the prostate and exits at the Colliculus seminalis into the Pars prostatica of the urethra (→ Fig. 7.61 and → Fig. 7.62). Here spermatozoa are released by emission into the urethra. The vas deferens therefore has a very strong layer of smooth muscle (→ Fig. 7.97).

Retroperitoneal space and pelvic cavity

Spermatic cord

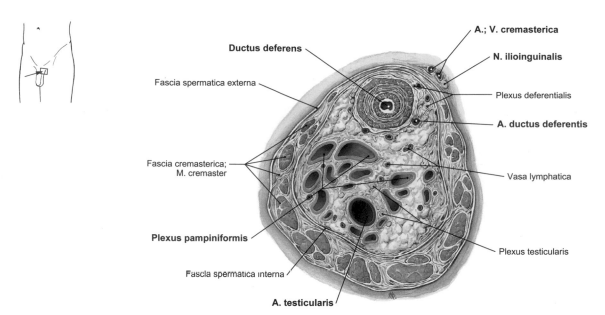

Fig. 7.97 Spermatic cord, Funiculus spermaticus, left side; frontal section; ventral view, magnification 2.5-fold. [B500-L240]
The spermatic cord contains the following:
* vas deferens (Ductus deferens) with A. ductus deferentis (from the A. umbilicalis)
* A. testicularis from the abdominal aorta and, as the Plexus pampiniformis, the accompanying veins

* N. genitofemoralis, R. genitalis (→ Fig. 7.87)
* lymph vessels (Vasa lymphatica) to the lumbar lymph nodes
* autonomic nerve fibres (Plexus testicularis) from the aortic plexus.
Externally, the **N. ilioinguinalis** and the **A. and V. cremasterica** are adjacent to the spermatic cord (→ Fig. 7.87 and → Fig. 7.98).

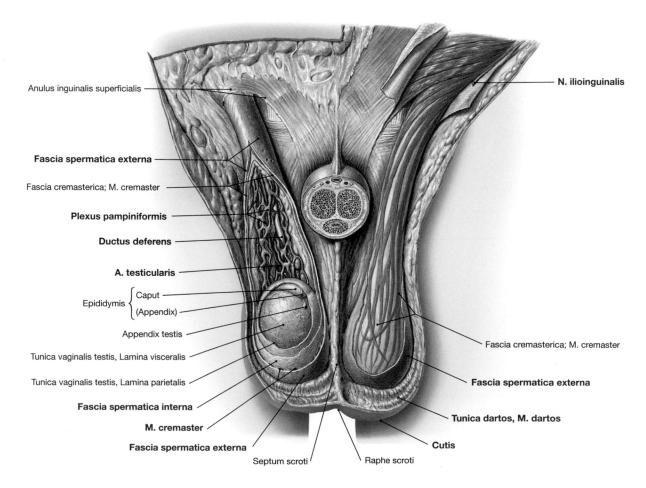

Fig. 7.98 Fasciae of the spermatic cord, Funiculus spermaticus, and the testis; ventral view; scrotum opened. [S700]
Testes and **spermatic cord** have the following **fasciae:**
* Fascia spermatica externa: continuation of the superficial body fascia (Fascia abdominalis superficialis)
* M. cremaster with Fascia cremasterica

* Fascia spermatica interna: continuation of the Fascia transversalis. In the area of the **scrotum,** two more layers join from the outside, enveloping the testes only:
* scrotal skin (cutis)
* Tunica dartos: subcutis with smooth muscle cells.

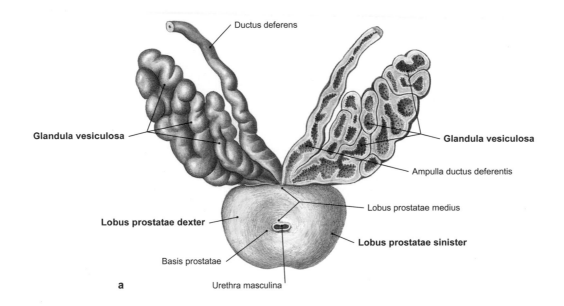

Ductus deferens

Glandula vesiculosa

Glandula vesiculosa

Ampulla ductus deferentis

Lobus prostatae medius

Lobus prostatae dexter

Lobus prostatae sinister

Basis prostatae

a

Urethra masculina

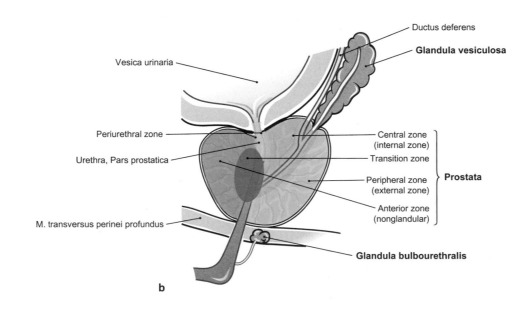

Ductus deferens

Glandula vesiculosa

Vesica urinaria

Periurethral zone

Central zone
(internal zone)

Urethra, Pars prostatica

Transition zone

Peripheral zone
(external zone)

Prostata

Anterior zone
(nonglandular)

M. transversus perinei profundus

Glandula bulbourethralis

b

Fig. 7.99a and b Seminal vesicles, Glandulae vesiculosae, and prostate gland, Prostata.
a Cranial view. [S700]
b View from the left side; median section. [S702-L126]
The internal male genitalia also include the **accessory sex glands.** They contribute to the formation of ejaculate and form secretions to moisten the female genitalia during sexual intercourse.
The **accessory sex glands** consist of:
- **Prostate gland:** unpaired gland below the base of the bladder. The prostate gland measures 4 × 3 × 2 cm (20 g) and has a superior base and an inferior apex. It has a right and a left lobe (Lobus dexter and sinister), which are separated by a shallow groove, as well as being divided into a middle lobe (Lobus medius). These lobes are tightly connected and cannot be separated during the dissection. The prostate gland discharges its secretion into the centrally traversing urethra (Pars prostatica). Histologically, the prostate is made up of 35–50 individual glands, all of which deliver their secretions via excreto-

ry ducts into the **Pars prostatica of the urethra.** The openings of the excretory ducts are on both sides of the Colliculus seminalis.
- **Seminal vesicle** (Glandula vesiculosa): paired gland at the dorsal aspect of the urinary bladder (→ Fig. 7.60). The seminal vesicles have an elongated oval shape (5 × 1 × 1 cm) and consist of a single winding pathway, approx. 15 cm in length. Each excretory duct combines with the vas deferens in the Ductus ejaculatorius and ends in the **Pars prostatica of the urethra** on the Colliculus seminalis.
- **COWPER's gland** (Glandula bulbourethralis): paired gland located within the perineal muscles (→ Fig. 7.61). The COWPER's glands are the size of lentils (up to approx. 1 cm) and drain with their 3 cm long excretory ducts into the **Pars spongiosa of the urethra.**
The seminal vesicles and the prostate form the liquid of the ejaculate, which serves the nutrition of the spermatozoa. The COWPER's glands emit their secretions as a lubricant before ejaculation.

Retroperitoneal space and pelvic cavity

Accessory male sex glands

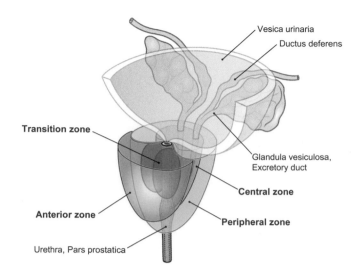

Vesica urinaria
Ductus deferens

Transition zone

Glandula vesiculosa, Excretory duct

Central zone

Anterior zone

Peripheral zone

Urethra, Pars prostatica

Fig. 7.100   Structure of the prostate gland; schematic illustration of the zones; view with the patient in supine position (as is usual in rectal examinations) from the left side. [S700-L126]
The **prostate gland,** in addition to its macroscopic structure dividing into a right and left as well as a median lobe, also presents a histological structure in **zones,** which are of major clinical significance:
- **central zone or internal zone** (25 % of the glandular tissue): wedge-shaped segment between Ductus ejaculatorii and urethra
- **peripheral zone or external zone** (70 % of the glandular tissue): it is coat-like and surrounds the inner zone on the dorsal side

- **periurethral zone:** narrow strip of tissue to the proximal urethra
- **transition zone** (5 % of the glandular tissue): lateral on both sides to the periurethral zone in the transition area to the internal zone
- **anterior zone:** nonglandular area ventral to the urethra, which contains only stroma of connective tissue and smooth muscles.
It should be noted that in former publications the only distinction made was between internal and external zones. Hence the transition zone is treated as part of the internal zone.

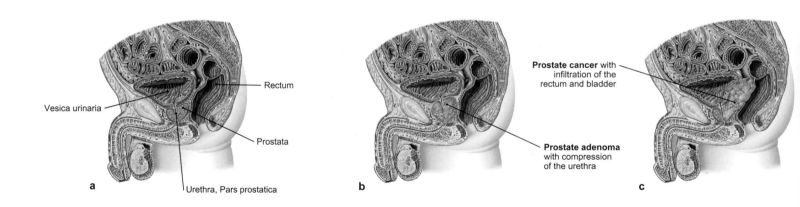

Vesica urinaria

Rectum

Prostata

Prostate cancer with infiltration of the rectum and bladder

Prostate adenoma with compression of the urethra

a   Urethra, Pars prostatica   **b**   **c**

Fig. 7.101a to c   Tumours of the prostate related to the zones of the prostate gland; sagittal section through a male pelvis, view from the left side. [S702-L266]
a Normal prostate.

b Prostate adenoma originating from the transition zone with compression of the urethra.
c Prostate cancer originating from the peripheral zone with infiltration of the rectum and bladder.

Clinical remarks

Benign prostatic hypertrophy or adenoma (BPH; hyperplasia) is a benign tumour of the prostate gland, causing it to enlarge up to a weight of 100 g, and occurring in almost all men over the age of 70. Since these adenomas usually originate from the **transition zone** (→ Fig. 7.101b) – which for several years now has been differentiated from the internal zone – problems arise here with urination and urinary retention at an early stage.
Prostate cancers are among the three most common malignant tumours in men. They usually develop from the **peripheral zone** of the

prostate gland (→ Fig. 7.101c), which can be detected under the microscope. Therefore, symptoms only arise later on. Because the prostate gland is separated from the rectum only by the thin Fascia rectoprostatica (DENONVILLIER's fascia; → Fig. 7.69), tumours are usually palpable through the rectum with a clinical examination. The digital rectal examination (DRE) should therefore be part of a complete physical examination in men over 50 years of age.

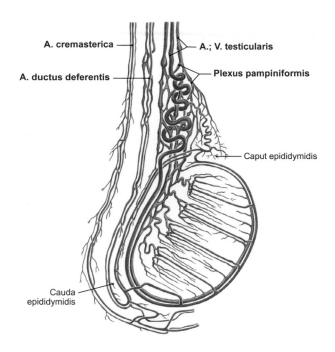

A. cremasterica

A. ductus deferentis

A.; V. testicularis

Plexus pampiniformis

Caput epididymidis

Cauda epididymidis

Fig. 7.102 Blood vessels of the internal male genitalia; view from the right side. [S700]

Testis and epididymis are supplied by the **A. and V. testicularis.** The V. testicularis is expanded distally to become a plexus (Plexus pampini-formis). The vas deferens is supplied by the **A. ductus deferentis** and the spermatic cord is supplied by the **A. cremasterica.**

Blood vessels of the internal genitalia		
Organ	**Arteries**	**Veins**
Testis and epididymis	A. testicularis (from the Pars abdominalis of the aorta)	Plexus pampiniformis: venous plexus, with its branches uniting to form the V. testi cularis, which on the right side enters the V. cava inferior, and on the left side the V. renalis sinistra
Vas deferens	A. ductus deferentis (mostly from the A. umbilicalis)	
Spermatic cord (M. cremaster)	A. cremasterica (from the A. epigastrica inferior)	
Accessory sex glands	A. vesicalis inferior and A. rectalis media (from the A. iliaca interna)	Plexus venosi vesicalis and prostaticus with connection to the V. iliaca interna

Clinical remarks

If the testis is not secured within the scrotum after descending, a torsion of the testis and spermatic cord **(testicular torsion)** may occur with physical activity. A testicular torsion always presents as a urological emergency because the ischaemia of the testis causes destruction of the parenchyma (→ figure).

Outflow obstructions at the junction in the V. renalis sinistra, or **renal cancers** growing in the renal vein, can cause a backflow of blood and thus a visual and tactile extension of the pampiniform plexus in the left scrotum **(varicocele).** Therefore, in a left-sided varicocele, a kidney tumour must be excluded. In addition, a persisteant varicocele can cause infertility.
[G724]

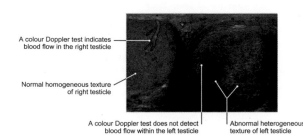

A colour Doppler test indicates blood flow in the right testicle

Normal homogeneous texture of right testicle

A colour Doppler test does not detect blood flow within the left testicle

Abnormal heterogeneous texture of left testicle

Vessels of the internal male genitalia

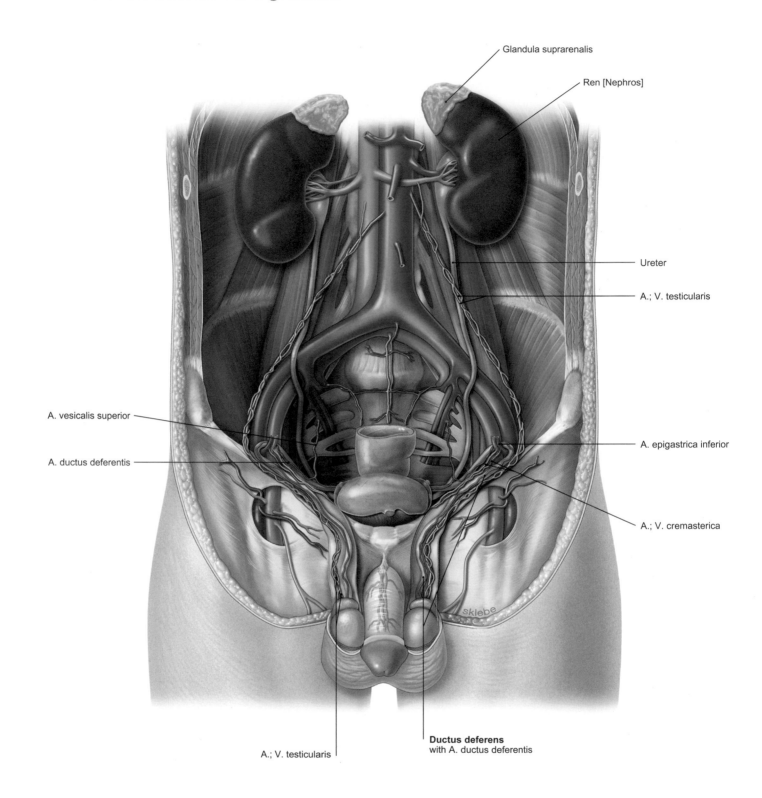

Glandula suprarenalis

Ren [Nephros]

Ureter

A.; V. testicularis

A. vesicalis superior

A. ductus deferentis

A. epigastrica inferior

A.; V. cremasterica

A.; V. testicularis

Ductus deferens
with A. ductus deferentis

Fig. 7.103 Blood vessels of the internal male genitalia. The abdominal wall and all intra- and secondary retroperitoneal organs have been removed; the spermatic cord is opened down its length; ventral view. [S702-L238]

Testis and epididymis are supplied by the **A. testicularis** that originates as a visceral branch of the abdominal aorta (Pars abdominalis aortae). It runs retroperitoneally up to the inguinal canal through which the spermatic cord enters the scrotum. The venous blood passes through the **V. testicularis** in the same way. This continues on the right into the V. cava inferior and on the left, on the other hand, into the V. renalis sinistra.

Along with the **A. ductus deferentis,** the **vas deferens** receives its own very fine artery originating either directly from the A. umbilicalis or

from the outgoing A. vesicalis superior. The A. ductus deferentis attaches directly to the vas deferens and accompanies it up to its origin in the epididymis.

The fasciae of the **spermatic cord** are supplied by the **A. cremasterica,** which originates as a branch of the A. epigastrica inferior from outside the spermatic cord, before it penetrates further along its pathway between its fasciae.

Not shown here are the **accessory sex glands,** which receive their blood supply from the **A. vesicalis inferior** and the **A. rectalis media,** branches of the A. iliaca interna. Only the COWPER's glands are supplied by the **A. pudenda interna,** which with its deep branches passes through the perineal space.

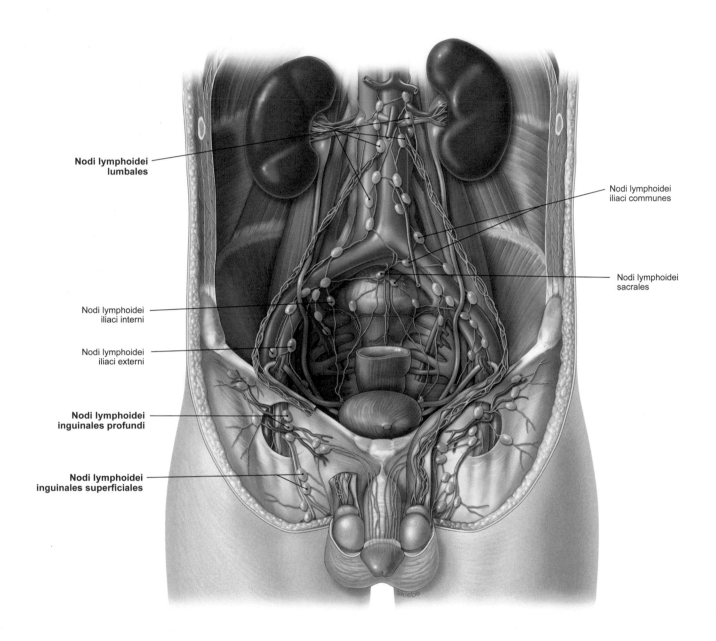

Nodi lymphoidei lumbales

Nodi lymphoidei iliaci communes

Nodi lymphoidei sacrales

Nodi lymphoidei iliaci interni

Nodi lymphoidei iliaci externi

Nodi lymphoidei inguinales profundi

Nodi lymphoidei inguinales superficiales

Fig. 7.104 Lymph vessels and lymph nodes of the external and internal male genitalia; ventral view. [S700-L238]
The regional lymph nodes for the external genitalia are the **inguinal lymph nodes (Nodi lymphoidei inguinales).** In contrast, the first re-

gional lymph nodes of the testis and epididymis are in a retroperitoneal position at the level of the kidneys **(Nodi lymphoidei lumbales).**

Clinical remarks

Due to the different lymphatic drainage pathways, the first **lymph node metastases** in penile carcinomas are found in the groin, whereas metastases of testicular tumours are found in the retroperitoneal space. Since the lymphatic drainage pathways of the internal and external genitalia do not communicate with each other, **no**

transscrotal biopsy can be made in the case of a suspected **testicular tumour,** because this can result in spreading of the tumour cells via the lymph vessels into the inguinal lymph nodes. The testicular biopsy must always be taken from the inguinal canal.

Male genitalia

Lymph vessels of the male genitalia

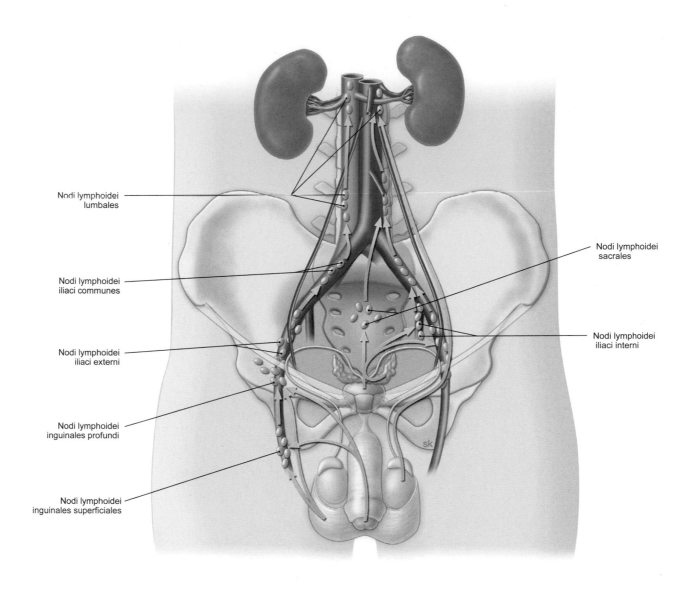

Nodi lymphoidei lumbales

Nodi lymphoidei iliaci communes

Nodi lymphoidei iliaci externi

Nodi lymphoidei inguinales profundi

Nodi lymphoidei inguinales superficiales

Nodi lymphoidei sacrales

Nodi lymphoidei iliaci interni

Fig. 7.105 Lymphatic drainage pathways of the external and internal male genitalia; ventral view. [S700-L238]

External and internal genitalia in men have completely separate lymphatic pathways.

External genitalia:

- penis and scrotum: Nodi lymphoidei inguinales.

Internal genitalia:

- testes and epididymis: Nodi lymphoidei lumbales at the level of the kidneys
- vas deferens, spermatic cord and accessory sex glands: Nodi lymphoidei iliaci interni/externi and Nodi lymphoidei sacrales.

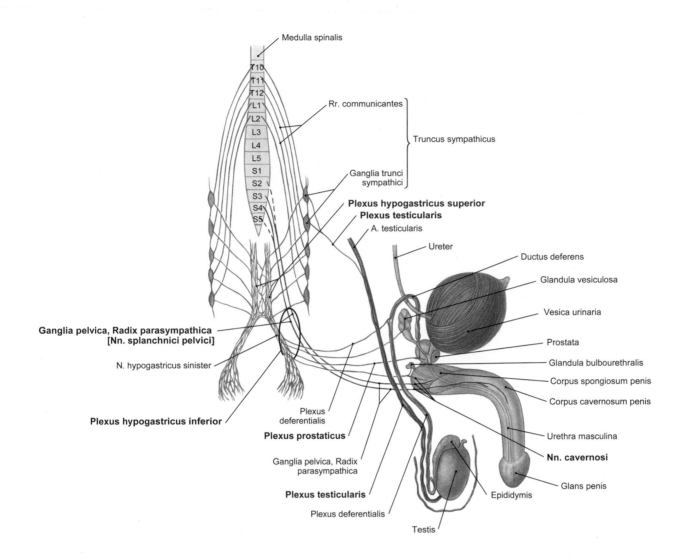

Fig. 7.106 Innervation of the male genitalia; ventral as well as lateral view; schematic illustration. The Plexus hypogastricus inferior contains sympathetic (green) and parasympathetic (purple) nerve fibres. [S700] Preganglionic **sympathetic nerve fibres** (T10–L2) descend from the Plexus aorticus abdominalis via the Plexus hypogastricus superior and from the sacral ganglia of the sympathetic trunk (Truncus sympathicus) via the Nn. splanchnici sacrales to be synapsed to postganglionic neurons in the ganglia of the **Plexus hypogastricus inferior.** These postganglionic fibres reach the pelvic viscera, including the accessory sex glands. Sympathetic fibres to the vas deferens **(Plexus deferentialis)** activate smooth muscle contractions for the **emission** of spermatozoa into the urethra. Some fibres also join the Nn. cavernosi and penetrate the pelvic floor to reach the Corpora cavernosa of the penis. The (predominantly) postganglionic sympathetic fibres to the testis and epididymis run within the **Plexus testicularis** alongside the A. testicularis after already being synapsed in the Ganglia aorticorenalia or the Plexus hypogastricus superior.

Preganglionic **parasympathetic nerve fibres** pass from the sacral parasympathicus (S2–S4) through the **Nn. splanchnici pelvici** into the ganglia of the **Plexus hypogastricus inferior.** They are synapsed either here or in the vicinity of the pelvic viscera (here: Ganglia pelvica) to postganglionic neurons which innervate the accessory glands. The **Nn. cavernosi penis** penetrate the pelvic floor and pass (partly in combination with the N. dorsalis penis) into the cavernous bodies, where they trigger the **erection.**

Somatic innervation via the **N. pudendus** conveys sensory innervation to the penis via the N. dorsalis penis and, along with the motor fibres of the Nn. perineales on the M. bulbospongiosus and the M. ischiocavernosus in the perineal area, it triggers the **ejaculation** of sperm from the urethra.

The **parasympathetic stimulation** induces the **erection,** the **sympathetic fibres** initiate the **emission,** and the **N. pudendus** causes the **ejaculation.**

Clinical remarks

During surgical resection of the para-aortal lymph nodes, e.g. with testicular or colon carcinomas in the area of the descending colon or in the case of operations on the aorta and the large iliac arteries, the sympathetic fibres can be injured. This may result in compromised emission and thereby ejaculation **(Impotentia generandi).** During

operations on the prostate gland, e.g. for prostate cancer or pronounced hyperplasia, the parasympathetic fibres to the penis may be severed, so that an erection is no longer possible **(Impotentia coeundi).**

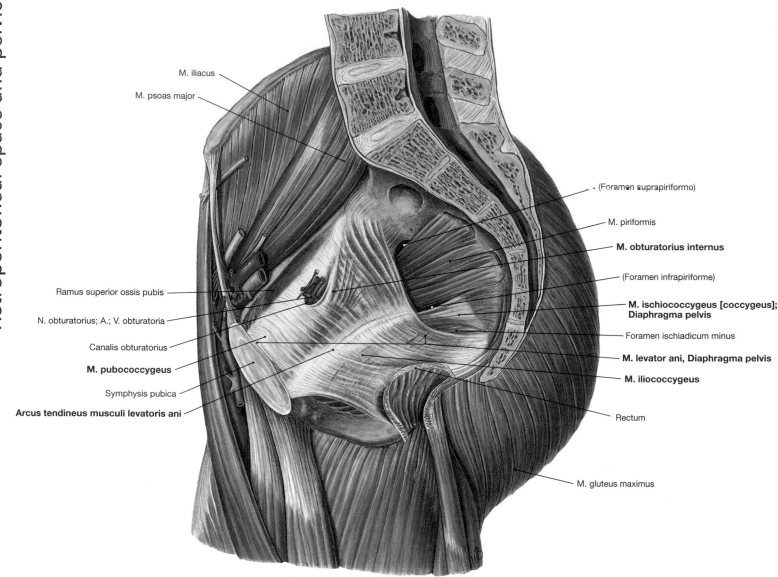

M. iliacus

M. psoas major

(Foramen suprapiriforme)

M. piriformis

M. obturatorius internus

(Foramen infrapiriforme)

Ramus superior ossis pubis

N. obturatorius; A.; V. obturatoria

M. ischiococcygeus [coccygeus]; Diaphragma pelvis

Canalis obturatorius

Foramen ischiadicum minus

M. pubococcygeus

M. levator ani, Diaphragma pelvis

Symphysis pubica

M. iliococcygeus

Arcus tendineus musculi levatoris ani

Rectum

M. gluteus maximus

Fig. 7.107 Muscles of the pelvic floor, Diaphragma pelvis, thigh and hip in men; view from the left side. [S700]
The pelvic floor closes the pelvic cavity caudally.
Structure:
- **M. levator ani,** comprising M. pubococcygeus, M. iliococcygeus, and M. puborectalis
- **M. ischiococcygeus.**

In contrast to the M. pubococcygeus and the M. ischiococcygeus, the M. iliococcygeus does not originate from the Os coxae but from the **Arcus tendineus musculi levatoris ani,** which strengthens the fascia of the M. obturatorius internus.
The muscles of both sides leave the levator hiatus (Hiatus levatorius) (→ Fig. 7.151) open between them. This gap is divided by the connective tissue of the perineal body (Centrum perinei) into a **Hiatus urogenitalis** (anterior) as a passage for the urethra and a **Hiatus analis** (posterior) for the rectum.
The pelvic floor is innervated by direct branches of the Plexus sacralis (S3–S4). Similar to the M. sphincter ani externus, the pelvic floor maintains a sustained resting tone.
Function: The pelvic floor stabilises the position of the pelvic organs and is thus essential for urinary and faecal continence. Pelvic floor weakness with incontinence is relatively rare in men, since potential injuries due to repetitive strain during childbirth is lacking.

→ T 22.1

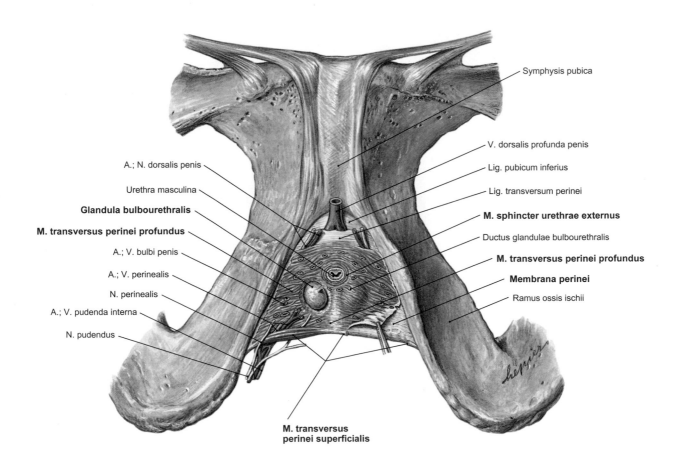

Symphysis pubica

V. dorsalis profunda penis

Lig. pubicum inferius

Lig. transversum perinei

M. sphincter urethrae externus

Ductus glandulae bulbourethralis

M. transversus perinei profundus

Membrana perinei

Ramus ossis ischii

A.; N. dorsalis penis

Urethra masculina

Glandula bulbourethralis

M. transversus perinei profundus

A.; V. bulbi penis

A.; V. perinealis

N. perinealis

A.; V. pudenda interna

N. pudendus

**M. transversus
perinei superficialis**

Fig. 7.108 Perineal musculature in men; caudal view; after removal of all other muscles. [S700]

In men, the levator hiatus (Hiatus levatorius) is almost entirely closed off by the connective tissue of the underlying perineal muscles, so that only the passage of the urethra (Urethra masculina) remains free.

The perineal muscles in men consist of a relatively strong **M. transversus perinei profundus,** located at the posterior margin of the thin **M. transversus perinei superficialis.** Since these muscles form a kind of muscle plate, the term 'Diaphragma urogenitale' was used to compare it to the Diaphragma pelvis of the pelvic floor. However, since there is no real diaphragm and a comparable muscle plate in women is not present, the term was dropped.

The M. transversus perinei profundus also forms the M. sphincter urethrae externus, which represents the voluntary sphincter of the urinary bladder.

On the top and underside, the M. transversus perinei profundus is covered by a fascia. On the bottom it is reinforced and here is referred to as the **Membrana perinei.**

The space between the two fasciae, which is almost completely filled by the M. transversus perinei profundus, is the **deep perineal space** (Spatium profundum perinei). In men, this contains the COWPER's glands (Glandulae bulbourethrales) next to the urethra which are traversed by the deep branches of the N. pudendus and the A. and V. pudenda interna on the way to the root of the penis.

The **superficial perineal space** (Spatium superficiale perinei) lies caudal to the Membrana perinei and contains amongst others the M. transversus perinei superficialis.

→ T 22.2

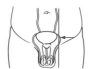

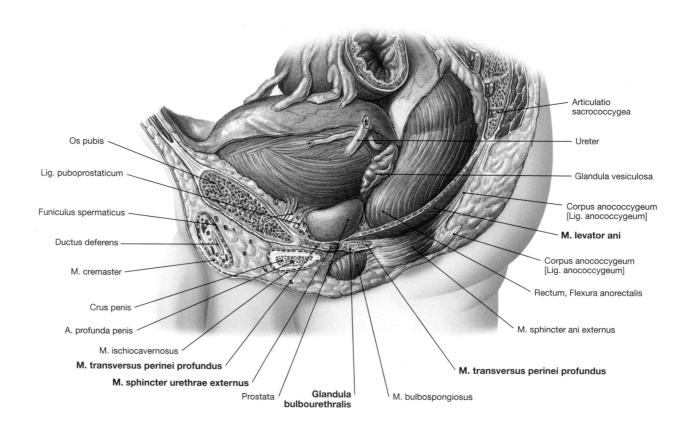

Os pubis

Lig. puboprostaticum

Funiculus spermaticus

Ductus deferens

M. cremaster

Crus penis

A. profunda penis

M. ischiocavernosus

M. transversus perinei profundus

M. sphincter urethrae externus

Prostata

Glandula bulbourethralis

M. bulbospongiosus

M. transversus perinei profundus

M. sphincter ani externus

Rectum, Flexura anorectalis

Corpus anococcygeum [Lig. anococcygeum]

M. levator ani

Corpus anococcygeum [Lig. anococcygeum]

Glandula vesiculosa

Ureter

Articulatio sacrococcygea

Fig. 7.109   Pelvic floor, Diaphragma pelvis, and perineal muscles in men; view from the left side. [S700]
At its anterior and posterior aspect, the pelvic floor consists of the **M. levator ani** and the **M. ischiococcygeus,** respectively. Below the pelvic floor is the **M. transversus perinei profundus** of the perineal muscle system, which also forms the **M. sphincter urethrae externus** as the sphincter for the urinary bladder. The COWPER's glands (Glandulae bulbourethrales) are embedded in the M. transversus perinei profundus.

→ T 22

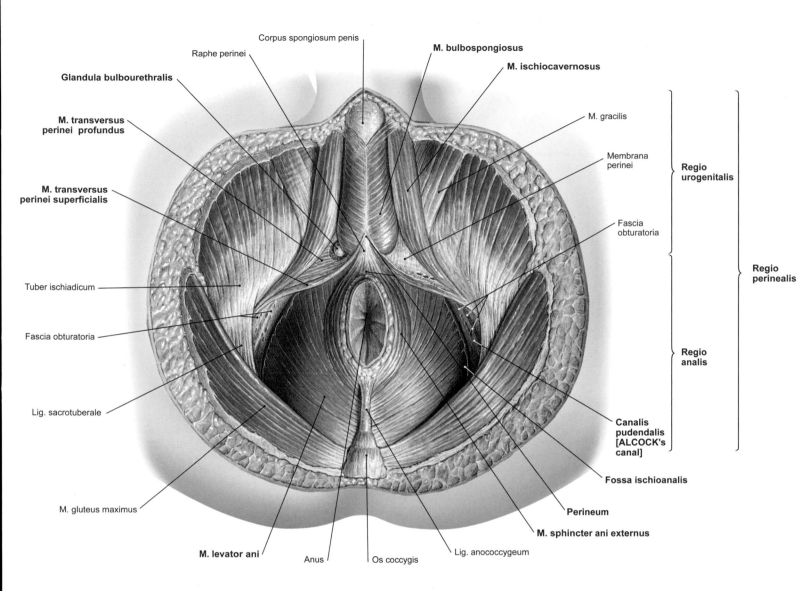

Corpus spongiosum penis

Raphe perinei

M. bulbospongiosus

M. ischiocavernosus

Glandula bulbourethralis

M. transversus perinei profundus

M. gracilis

Membrana perinei

Regio urogenitalis

M. transversus perinei superficialis

Fascia obturatoria

Tuber ischiadicum

Fascia obturatoria

Regio analis

Lig. sacrotuberale

Regio perinealis

Canalis pudendalis [ALCOCK's canal]

Fossa ischioanalis

M. gluteus maximus

Perineum

M. sphincter ani externus

M. levator ani

Anus

Os coccygis

Lig. anococcygeum

Fig. 7.110 Perineal region, Regio perinealis, in men; caudal view; after removal of all neurovascular pathways. [S700]
The **perineal region** extends from the inferior margin of the pubic symphysis (Symphysis pubica) to the tip of the coccyx (Os coccygis). The term **perineum** in men, however, exclusively describes the small connective tissue bridge between the root of the penis and the anus. The perineal region can be divided into a ventral **Regio urogenitalis** with external genitalia and urethra, and a dorsal **Regio analis** around the anus. Both areas include the following spaces:

• The Regio analis contains the **Fossa ischioanalis** (→ table), which constitutes a pyramid-shaped space on both sides of the anus. Cranially the space is delimited by the M. levator ani of the pelvic floor. The lateral wall encloses the fascial duplication of the M. obturatorius internus (Fascia obturatoria) and the pudendal canal (ALCOCK's canal). The A. and V. pudenda interna and the N. pudendus run inside it after passing through the Foramen ischiadicum minus from the gluteal region.

The Regio urogenitalis contains the two **perineal spaces:**

• The **deep perineal space** (Spatium profundum perinei) is occupied by the M. transversus perinei profundus and also contains the COWPER's glands (Glandulae bulbourethrales).
• In the **superficial perineal space** (Spatium superficiale perinei) there are the M. transversus perinei superficialis, the M. bulbospongiosus and the M. ischiocavernosus, which stabilise the cavernous bodies of the Radix penis and enable ejaculation.

Boundaries of the Fossa ischioanalis	
Orientation	**Confining structure**
Medial and cranial	M. sphincter ani externus and M. levator ani
Lateral	M. obturatorius internus
Dorsal	M. gluteus maximus and Lig. sacrotuberale
Ventral	Posterior margin of the superficial and the deep perineal spaces, anterior recesses extend up to the pubic symphysis
Caudal	Fascia and skin of the perineum

Neurovascular structures of the perineum in men

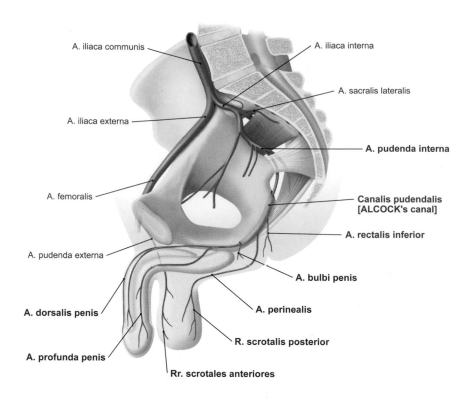

A. iliaca communis

A. iliaca externa

A. femoralis

A. pudenda externa

A. dorsalis penis

A. profunda penis

Rr. scrotales anteriores

A. iliaca interna

A. sacralis lateralis

A. pudenda interna

**Canalis pudendalis
[ALCOCK's canal]**

A. rectalis inferior

A. bulbi penis

A. perinealis

R. scrotalis posterior

Fig. 7.111   Arteries of the perineal region, Regio perinealis, in men; schematic illustration; left view. [S701-L275]
The perineum receives arterial blood from ventral through the **A. pudenda externa** (branch of the A. femoralis from the A. iliaca externa) and from dorsal through the **A. pudenda interna** (branch of the A. iliaca interna).
The **A. pudenda externa** branches off medially from the A. femoralis after its passage through the Lacuna vasorum beneath the inguinal ligament. The Rr. scrotales anteriores supply the anterior third of the perineum and the scrotum.
The **A. pudenda interna** leaves the pelvis along with its concomitant vein and the N. pudendus through the **Foramen infrapiriforme.** It loops around the Lig. sacrospinale and passes through the **Foramen ischiadicum minus** to enter the Fossa ischioanalis. Here the pudendal neurovascular structures are enveloped by the caudal fascia of the M. obturatorius internus in the **Canalis pudendalis (ALCOCK's canal).** After providing the A. rectalis inferior in the Fossa ischioanalis, the A. pudenda interna branches into superficial and deep terminal arteries in the perineum:

● The superficial **A. perinealis** supplies the posterior two-thirds of the perineum and provide Rr. scrotales posteriores to the posterior scrotum.
● The deep branches are formed by the **A. bulbi penis** to the proximal part of the Corpus spongiosum, as well as the **A. dorsalis penis** to the penis skin and the glans, and the **A. profunda penis** that supplies the Corpora cavernosa during erection (→ Fig. 7.89).

Fig. 7.112   Innervation of the male perineum; schematic illustration; view from the left. [S701-L275]
The perineum receives innervation from ventral by the **N. ilioinguinalis** (from the Plexus lumbalis; not shown here) and from dorsal by the **N. pudendus** (from the Plexus sacralis) and the N. cutaneus femoris posterior (Plexus sacralis; not shown here).
The **N. ilioinguinalis** runs adjacent to the spermatic cord and innervates the anterior third of the perineum and the scrotum through the Rr. scrotales anteriores.
The **N. pudendus** exits the pelvis together with the A./V. pudenda interna through the Foramen infrapiriforme, loops around the Lig. sacrospinale and reaches the Fossa ischioanalis through the the Foramen ischiadicum minus. Here the pudendal neurovascular structures are enclosed by the caudal fascia of the M. obturatorius internus forming the **Canalis pudendalis (ALCOCK's canal).** After providing the **N. rectalis inferior** in the Fossa ischioanalis, the N. pudendus branches into its terminal branches in the perineum:

● The **Nn. perineales** provide motor innervation to the perineal muscles and sensory innervation to the posterior two-thirds of the perineum and the scrotum with the Rr. scrotales posteriores.
● The **N. dorsalis penis** provides sensory innervation to the skin of the penis and the glans.

The **N. cutaneous femoris posterior** only innervates a small part of the lateral perineum (→ Fig. 7.115).

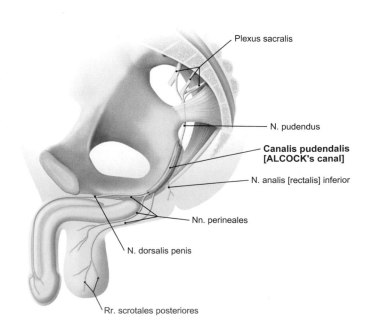

Plexus sacralis

N. pudendus

**Canalis pudendalis
[ALCOCK's canal]**

N. analis [rectalis] inferior

Nn. perineales

N. dorsalis penis

Rr. scrotales posteriores

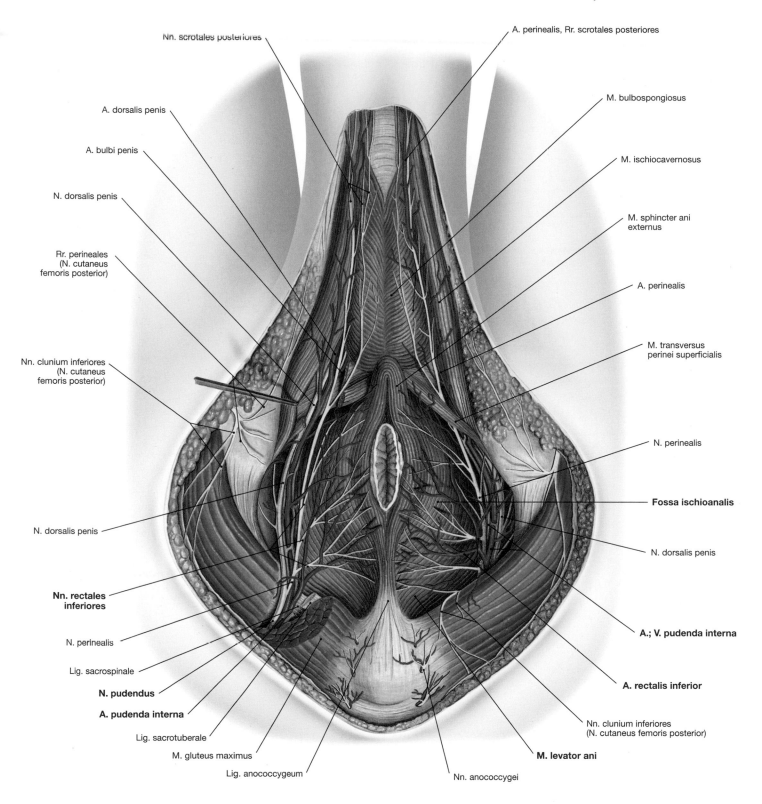

Nn. scrotales posteriores

A. perinealis, Rr. scrotales posteriores

A. dorsalis penis

A. bulbi penis

N. dorsalis penis

Rr. perineales
(N. cutaneus
femoris posterior)

Nn. clunium inferiores
(N. cutaneus
femoris posterior)

M. bulbospongiosus

M. ischiocavernosus

M. sphincter ani
externus

A. perinealis

M. transversus
perinei superficialis

N. perinealis

Fossa ischioanalis

N. dorsalis penis

N. dorsalis penis

**Nn. rectales
inferiores**

N. perinealis

Lig. sacrospinale

N. pudendus

A. pudenda interna

Lig. sacrotuberale

M. gluteus maximus

Lig. anococcygeum

A.; V. pudenda interna

A. rectalis inferior

Nn. clunium inferiores
(N. cutaneus femoris posterior)

M. levator ani

Nn. anococcygei

Fig. 7.113 Vessels and nerves of the perineal region, Regio perinealis, in men; caudal view. [S700]
The neurovascular pathways run dorsolaterally in the Canalis pudendalis (ALCOCK's canal), formed by a fascial duplication of the M. obturatorius internus, into the pyramid-shaped **Fossa ischioanalis** which is filled with fat. Next they form the branches to the anus and anal canal, and

traverse the space ventrally to pass through the two perineal spaces to the root of the penis.
Contents of the Fossa ischioanalis:
- A. and V. pudenda interna and N. pudendus: in the Canalis pudendalis (ALCOCK's canal)
- A., V. and N. rectalis inferior: to the anal canal.

Clinical remarks

The Fossa ischioanalis is clinically highly relevant because it extends on both sides of the anus. **Abscesses** (collections of pus), e.g. where there are fistulas from the anal canal, can extend throughout the Fossa ischioanalis up to the pubic symphysis. These kinds of abscesses do not only generate non-specific inflammatory signs but also cause intense pain in the perineal region.

Neurovascular structures of the perineum in men

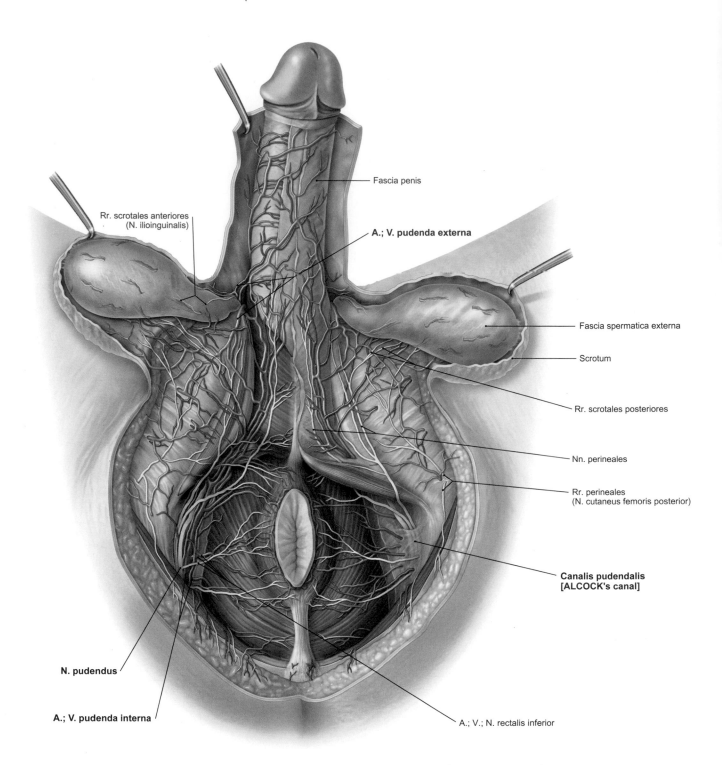

Rr. scrotales anteriores
(N. ilioinguinalis)

A.; V. pudenda externa

Fascia penis

Fascia spermatica externa

Scrotum

Rr. scrotales posteriores

Nn. perineales

Rr. perineales
(N. cutaneus femoris posterior)

**Canalis pudendalis
[ALCOCK's canal]**

N. pudendus

A.; V. pudenda interna

A.; V.; N. rectalis inferior

Fig. 7.114   Vessels and nerves of the perineal region, Regio perinealis, in men. The scrotum and the Canalis pudendalis on the right side have been opened out; caudal view. [S700-L238]/[Q300]
To supplement → Fig. 7.113, this illustration also shows the anterior neurovascular structures of the perineum. The anterior third of the perineum receives blood from the **A./V. pudenda externa,** which also branch off the Rr. scrotales to the scrotum. The **N. ilioinguinalis** provides corresponding innervation with the Rr. scrotales anteriores.
On the right side of the body and on the lateral wall of the **Fossa ischioanalis,** the image shows the exposed **Canalis pudendalis (ALCOCK's canal),** which is formed by the fascial duplication of the M. obturatorius internus. The A., V., and N. rectalis inferior to the anal canal are visible here.

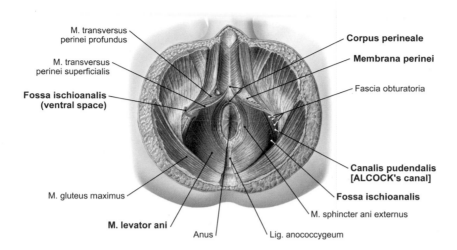

M. transversus perinei profundus
M. transversus perinei superficialis
Fossa ischioanalis (ventral space)
M. gluteus maximus
M. levator ani
Anus
Corpus perineale
Membrana perinei
Fascia obturatoria
Canalis pudendalis [ALCOCK's canal]
Fossa ischioanalis
M. sphincter ani externus
Lig. anococcygeum

Fig. 7.115   Perineal spaces in the male; caudal view.
The perineal spaces are located in the anterior part (Regio urogenitalis) of the perineum (Regio perinealis). [S700]
The **superficial perineal space** (Spatium superficiale perinei) extends between the Membrana perinei, attached to bottom of the M. transversus perinei, and the superficial body fascia (Fascia perinei).

The **deep perineal space** (Spatium profundum perinei) is almost completely occupied by the M. transversus perinei profundus between the fasciae of the muscles.

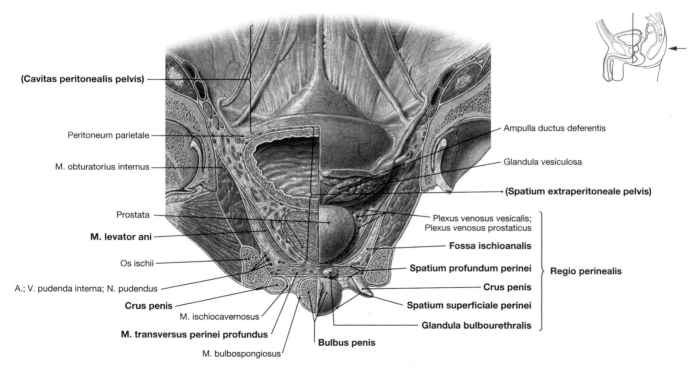

(Cavitas peritonealis pelvis)
Peritoneum parietale
M. obturatorius internus
Prostata
M. levator ani
Os ischii
A.; V. pudenda interna; N. pudendus
Crus penis
M. ischiocavernosus
M. transversus perinei profundus
M. bulbospongiosus
Bulbus penis
Ampulla ductus deferentis
Glandula vesiculosa
(Spatium extraperitoneale pelvis)
Plexus venosus vesicalis; Plexus venosus prostaticus
Fossa ischioanalis
Spatium profundum perinei
Crus penis
Spatium superficiale perinei
Glandula bulbourethralis
Regio perinealis

Fig. 7.116   Perineal spaces in men; on the left side; frontal section at the level of the femoral head; right side: dorsal view. (See also the section in the small sketch.) [S700]
The frontal section shows **three levels** of the male pelvis:
* **peritoneal cavity of the pelvis (Cavitas peritonealis pelvis),** which is caudally confined by the parietal peritoneum
* **subperitoneal space (Spatium extraperitonale pelvis)** which reaches down to the M. levator ani of the pelvic floor
* **perineal region (Regio perinealis)** below the pelvic floor; the anterior portion is generally taken up by the two perineal spaces; however it also still contains the very variable anterior recesses of the Fossa ischioanalis (shown here separately on the right and left).
The **deep perineal space** (Spatium profundum perinei) is almost completely filled by the M. transversus perinei profundus. It also contains the COWPER's glands (Glandulae bulbourethrales) and the passage of

the urethra. It is traversed by the deep branches of the N. pudendus (N. dorsalis penis), and of the A. and V. pudenda interna (A. bulbi penis, A. dorsalis penis, A. profunda penis) before reaching the root of the penis. The Nn. cavernosi penis pierce the perineum and enter the Corpora cavernosa of the penis.
The **superficial perineal space** (Spatium superficiale perinei) is located between the Membrana perinei at the underside of the M. transversus perinei profundus and the body fascia (Fascia perinei). In addition to the M. transversus perinei superficialis, it contains the proximal parts of the cavernous bodies of the penis. The Bulbus penis is surrounded by the M. bulbospongiosus, and the Crura penis is surrounded on both sides by the M. ischiocavernosus. The superficial branches (N. perinealis with Nn. scrotales posteriores) of the N. pudendus and the A. and V. pudenda interna (A. perinealis with Rr. scrotales posteriores) continue through this space to the scrotum.

External female genitalia

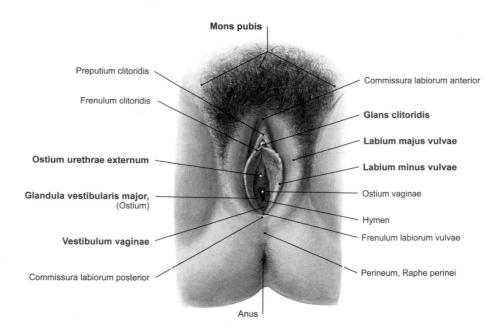

Fig. 7.117 **External female genitalia, Organa genitalia feminina externa;** caudal view. [S700]

With the female genitalia it is important to differentiate between the external genitalia (Organa genitalia feminina externa) and the internal genitalia (Organa genitalia feminina interna → Fig. 7.120).

The **external genitalia,** grouped together as the **vulva,** include the:
* Mons pubis
* Labia majora vulvae
* Labia minora vulvae
* clitoris
* Vestibulum vaginae
* Glandulae vestibulares majores (BARTHOLIN's glands) and minores.

The vaginal vestibule extends to the hymen, which borders the vaginal orifice (Ostium vaginae). Ventrally thereof is the external urethral orifice (Ostium urethrae externum).

The external genitalia are the **sex organs** and serve the purpose of intercourse.

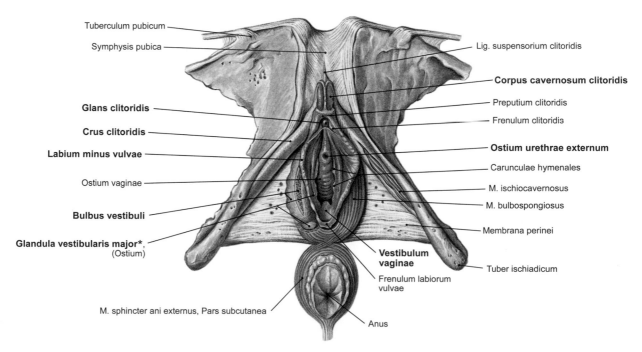

Fig. 7.118 **External female genitalia, Organa genitalia feminina externa;** caudal view, after removal of the body fascia and the neurovascular pathways. [S700]

The **Labia majora vulvae,** which have been removed here, contain the bulb of the vestibule (Bulbus vestibuli). Between these are the **Labia minora vulvae,** surrounding the **vaginal vestibule (Vestibulum vaginae),** into which the **vestibular glands (Glandulae vestibulares majores [BARTHOLIN's glands] and minores)** lead laterally. At the front, the labia minora pass with a ribbon of tissue (Frenulum clitoridis) to the glans of the clitoris (Glans clitoridis). The clitoris is the sensory organ for sexual arousal. The two cavernous bodies (Corpora cavernosa clitoridis)

form a short body (Corpus clitoridis), which caudally ends with the glans before separating into the Crura clitoridis which are anchored to the inferior ischiopubic rami. The crura are surrounded by the Mm. ischiocavernosi. The M. bulbospongiosus stabilises the **bulb of the vestibule (Bulbus vestibuli).**

Developmentally, there are some similarities between the structure of the clitoris, which also has a prepuce (Preputium clitoridis), and the structure of the penis. The filling mechanisms of the erectile tissue and erection are also similar in both sexes.

* clin.: BARTHOLIN's gland

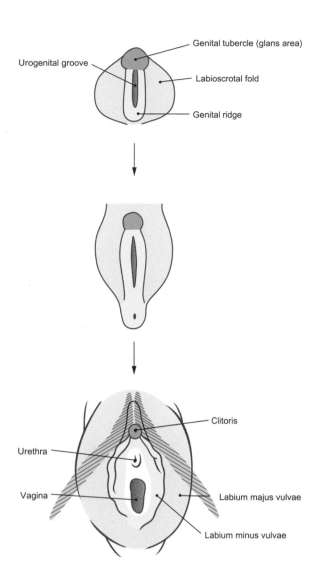

Genital tubercle (glans area)

Urogenital groove

Labioscrotal fold

Genital ridge

Clitoris

Urethra

Vagina

Labium majus vulvae

Labium minus vulvae

Fig. 7.119 Development of the external female genitalia, Organa genitalia feminina externa. [S700-L126]/[G1060-002]
The external genitalia develop from the caudal part of the Sinus urogenitalis. The urogenital sinus develops from the cloaca of the hindgut and forms the urinary bladder and parts of the urethra (→ Fig. 7.29). In addition, there is also the ectoderm with the lower connective tissue (mesenchyme) beneath. The first phase in the development of the external genitalia is identical in both sexes (indifferent gonad). The anterior wall of the Sinus urogenitalis indents to form the **urethral groove**

which is bordered on both sides by the **urethral folds.** Lateral of these are the **labioscrotal folds** and anterior is the **genital tubercle.**
Subsequently, the genital tubercle develops into the **clitoris** (Corpora cavernosa) under the influence of the female sex hormone, oestrogen, which is produced in the ovary. Unlike in men, the urethral folds and the labioscrotal folds do not close. The urethral folds become the **labia minora,** the labioscrotal folds form the **labia majora.** The short female urethra and the BARTHOLIN's glands develop from the **Sinus urogenitalis.**

Clinical remarks

The common developmental stages of the external genitalia in both sexes explain the occurrence of penis-like hyperplasias of the clitoris in cases of excessive production of male sex hormones, such as in

the **adrenogenital syndrome** (production of androgens in the cortex of the adrenal glands; → Fig. 7.121).

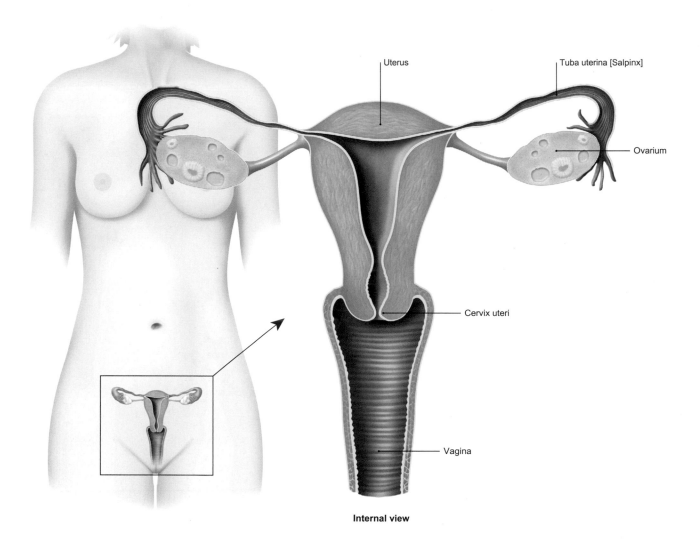

Uterus

Tuba uterina [Salpinx]

Ovarium

Cervix uteri

Vagina

Internal view

Fig. 7.120 Female urinary and genital organs, Organa urogenitalia feminina; ventral view. [S701-L275]
The **internal genitalia** include the:
* vagina
* uterus
* uterine tube (Tuba uterina)
* ovary.
Uterine tubes and ovaries are paired organs and are collectively regarded as uterine **adnexa.**

The internal genitalia in women are both **reproductive** and **sexual.** Functionally, the ovary serves to mature the follicles (with the ova) and to produce female sex hormones (oestrogens and progesterone). The uterine tubes are the location for insemination. They transport the ovum into the uterus, where the development of the child takes place during pregnancy. The vagina is used for sexual intercourse and is the birth canal.

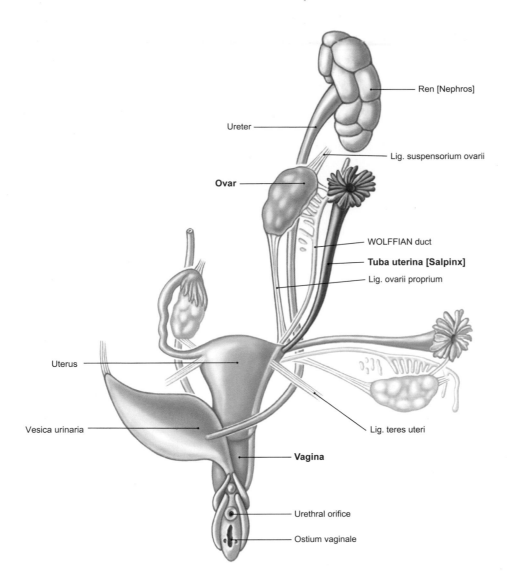

Ren [Nephros]

Ureter

Lig. suspensorium ovarii

Ovar

WOLFFIAN duct

Tuba uterina [Salpinx]

Lig. ovarii proprium

Uterus

Vesica urinaria

Lig. teres uteri

Vagina

Urethral orifice

Ostium vaginale

Fig. 7.121 Development of the internal female genitalia, Organa genitalia feminina interna. [B500-L238]/[H233-01]
The internal genitalia develop in both sexes in the same way until week 7 (indifferent gonad → Fig. 7.29). In the female, the primordium of the primitive gonad then develops into the ovary. Similar to the testis, the ovary also develops in the lumbar region at the level of the mesonephros. In the course of bodily growth and development, the ovary moves but only up to the lesser pelvis and it does not leave the peritoneal cavity. Hence the ovary and adnexa are **intraperitoneal.**
Without the suppressing effects of the anti-MÜLLERIAN hormone from the testis, the MÜLLERIAN ducts differentiate into female genitalia. From the 12th week, these form the uterine tubes and, in their distal fused area, the uterus and vagina. The lower part of the vagina develops from the urogenital sinus.

Clinical remarks

If the MÜLLERIAN ducts do not merge with each other, there may be **septation** of the lumen of the uterus (uterus septus or subseptus) or even a **double uterus** (uterus duplex).
The term **intersexuality** describes the biological situation in which sex chromosomes, genital organs or secondary sex characteristics do not conclusively match the male or female biology. The causes vary greatly and include genetic and hormonal factors. The intersex prevalence depends on the definition: if the chromosomal status does not clearly match a male or female phenotype, the prevalence is 0.02 %. **Hermaphroditismus verus** describes rare situations in which an ovary and a testicle are co-existent, but with the gonads usually lacking normal function. More commonly, a male or female **pseudohermaphroditism** is evident, with the presence of either ovaries or testicles, but without a clear sex association of the organs. Possible causes are defects in the enzymes which are required for testosterone- or AMH-production, or hormone receptor mutations. The highest prevalence is with female pseudohermaphroditism, caused by an **adrenogenital syndrome** with an enzyme defect, resulting in a reduced production of cortisol and an increased production of androgens in the adrenal cortex.
The term **transsexuality** describes the discrepancy between a person's chromosomal and phenotypical sex and their gender identity. A trans(gender) man is someone who was assigned to be a female at birth but has a male gender identity. A trans(gender) woman is a person who was assigned to be male at birth but has a female gender identity.

Structure and position

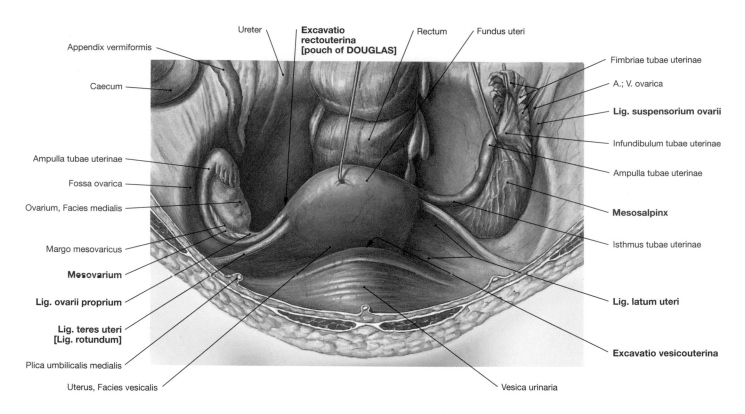

Appendix vermiformis

Caecum

Ampulla tubae uterinae

Fossa ovarica

Ovarium, Facies medialis

Margo mesovaricus

Mesovarium

Lig. ovarii proprium

Lig. teres uteri [Lig. rotundum]

Plica umbilicalis medialis

Uterus, Facies vesicalis

Ureter

Excavatio rectouterina [pouch of DOUGLAS]

Rectum

Fundus uteri

Fimbriae tubae uterinae

A.; V. ovarica

Lig. suspensorium ovarii

Infundibulum tubae uterinae

Ampulla tubae uterinae

Mesosalpinx

Isthmus tubae uterinae

Lig. latum uteri

Excavatio vesicouterina

Vesica urinaria

Fig. 7.122 Uterus, ovary, Ovarium, and uterine tube, Tuba uterina, with peritoneal duplication; ventral view. [S700]
The uterus, uterine tubes and ovaries are positioned intraperitoneally. Their peritoneal duplications (Lig. latum uteri, mesosalpinx, mesovarium) form a transverse fold in the lesser pelvis. The Lig. teres of the uterus passes from the angle of the uterine tubes to the front of the lateral pelvic wall and into the inguinal canal, to finally end in the connective tissue of the labia majora. The Lig. ovarii proprium also originates from the uterotubal junction and links the uterus and ovaries. The ovary nestles into an indentation, which is created by the branching of the A. and V. iliaca communis (Fossa ovarica). The Lig. suspensorium

ovarii ascends laterally. It is attached to the side of the pelvic wall and contains the A. and V. ovarica.
The close topographical relationships between the adnexa (ovary and Tuba uterina) and the vermiform appendix (Appendix vermiformis) of the colon explain why inflammations of the appendix (appendicitis) as well as those of the uterine tube (salpingitis) may cause similar pain in the right lower abdominal quadrant. Between the uterus and urinary bladder is the **Excavatio vesicouterina** as an enlargement of the abdominal cavity. The **Excavatio rectouterina** [pouch of DOUGLAS] behind the uterus is the most caudal extension of the peritoneal cavity in women and may collect fluids and pus in the case of inflammatory processes in the lower abdomen.

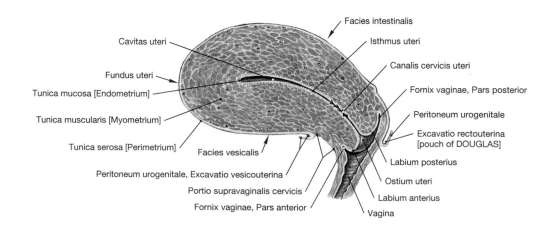

Cavitas uteri

Fundus uteri

Tunica mucosa [Endometrium]

Tunica muscularis [Myometrium]

Tunica serosa [Perimetrium]

Facies vesicalis

Peritoneum urogenitale, Excavatio vesicouterina

Portio supravaginalis cervicis

Fornix vaginae, Pars anterior

Facies intestinalis

Isthmus uteri

Canalis cervicis uteri

Fornix vaginae, Pars posterior

Peritoneum urogenitale

Excavatio rectouterina [pouch of DOUGLAS]

Labium posterius

Ostium uteri

Labium anterius

Vagina

Fig. 7.123 Layers of the wall of the uterus, sagittal section; view from the left side. [S700]
Internally, the wall of the uterus is made from a mucous membrane **(endometrium),** that changes in composition and thickness during the female menstrual cycle, in order to enable the implantation after fertilisation of an ovum. It is attached to a thick layer of **smooth muscles (myometrium),** of which the muscle fibres show different arrangements. On the outside is the peritoneal coating of visceral peritoneum

(perimetrium). Parts of the ligaments are referred to according to the nomenclature of the layers of the wall. The **Lig. latum uteri (mesometrium)** is the continuation of the peritoneal coating and forms a frontal abdominal peritoneal duplication from the intraperitoneally located body of the uterus to both sides of the lesser pelvis. The **Lig. cardinale (parametrium),** on the other hand, anchors the cervix of the uterus lying in a subperitoneal position on both sides on the pelvic bone.

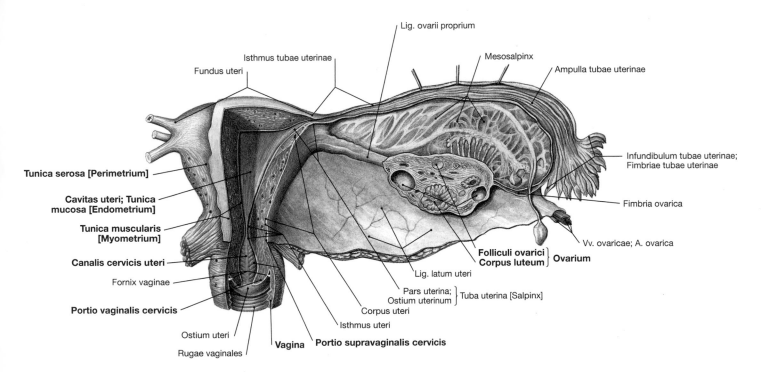

Lig. ovarii proprium

Isthmus tubae uterinae

Fundus uteri

Mesosalpinx

Ampulla tubae uterinae

Tunica serosa [Perimetrium]

Infundibulum tubae uterinae;
Fimbriae tubae uterinae

**Cavitas uteri; Tunica
mucosa [Endometrium]**

Fimbria ovarica

**Tunica muscularis
[Myometrium]**

Vv. ovaricae; A. ovarica

Canalis cervicis uteri

**Folliculi ovarici
Corpus luteum** } **Ovarium**

Fornix vaginae

Lig. latum uteri

Portio vaginalis cervicis

Pars uterina;
Ostium uterinum } Tuba uterina [Salpinx]

Corpus uteri

Ostium uteri

Isthmus uteri

Rugae vaginales

Vagina **Portio supravaginalis cervicis**

**Fig. 7.124   Uterus, vagina, ovary, Ovarium, and uterine tube, Tuba
uterina;** frontal section; dorsal view. [S700]
The uterus is 8 cm long, 5 cm wide and 2–3 cm thick. It comprises the
body (Corpus), the fundus (Fundus uteri) and the cervix (Cervix uteri).
The isthmus (Isthmus uteri) depicts the narrowing between the body
and the cervix. The lumen of the **uterus** is divided into the Cavitas uteri
in the body and the Canalis cervicis uteri in the cervix of the uterus. The
cervix opens with its lower portion into the vagina, and is therefore referred to as the Portio vaginalis cervicis. The upper portion is the Portio
supravaginalis cervicis. The **vagina** is a hollow muscular organ of about
10 cm in length in a **subperitoneal position.** Adjacent to the Portio vaginalis cervicis is the vaginal vault (Fornix vaginae). At the inner surface,

both the anterior and posterior walls of the vagina (Paries anterior and
Paries posterior) reveal transverse mucosal folds (Rugae vaginales).
The frontal section also shows the structure of the **uterine wall:** inside
lie the internal mucosal layer (Tunica mucosa, endometrium), then the
strong muscular layer (Tunica muscularis, myometrium) of smooth
muscles, and the outermost peritoneal lining (Tunica serosa, perimetrium).
The stroma of the **ovary** contains the follicles (Folliculi ovarici), which
contain the egg cells, and later in the female cycle turns into the yellow
body called the Corpus luteum. The follicles and the Corpora lutea produce the female sex hormones (oestrogen and progesterone) which
regulate the cycle-dependent differentiation of the endometrium.

Structure and suspensory ligaments

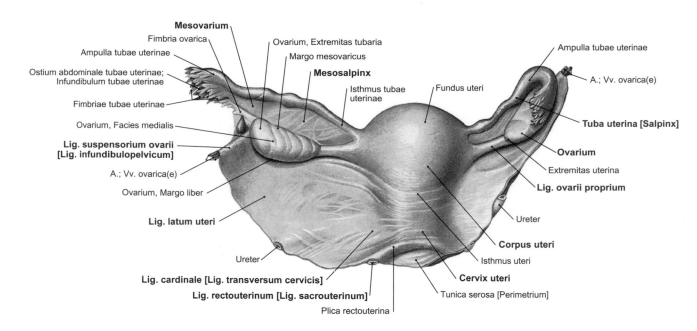

Fig. 7.125 Uterus, ovary, Ovarium, and uterine tube, Tuba uterina, with peritoneal duplication; dorsal view. [S700]
The uterine tubes (oviducts; Tuba uterina) are attached to the body of the uterus on both sides providing a connection to the ovary.
The **uterine tube** (Tuba uterina [Salpinx]) is 10–14 cm long and has several parts:
- **Infundibulum tubae uterinae:** 1–2 cm long, contains the opening to the abdominal cavity (Ostium abdominale tubae uterinae) and fringe-like appendages (Fimbriae tubae uterinae) for holding the ovum during ovulation
- **Ampulla tubae uterinae:** 7–8 cm long, crescent-shaped around the ovary
- **Isthmus tubae uterinae:** 3–6 cm long, constriction at the transition to the uterus
- **Pars tubae uterinae:** enters the uterus (Ostium uterinum).

The **ovary (Ovarium)** is 3 × 1.5 × 1 cm in size and oval-shaped. A distinction is made between an upper pole (Extremitas tubaria) and a lower pole (Extremitas uterina). At its anterior margin, the mesovarium is at-

tached (Margo mesovaricus), while the posterior margin remains free (Margo liber).
The uterus, uterine tubes and ovary are **intraperitoneal** and therefore have their own **peritoneal duplications** covered by a serous membrane; they also have additional **small ligaments,** which are of clinical relevance during gynaecological operations:
- **Lig. latum uteri:** frontally positioned peritoneal folds
- **mesovarium** and **mesosalpinx:** peritoneal duplications of the ovary and uterine tube to the Lig. latum
- **Lig. cardinale (Lig. transversum cervicis):** connective tissue attaching the cervix to the lateral pelvic wall
- **Lig. rectouterinum** (clin.: Lig. sacrouterinum): connective tissue attaching the cervix dorsally
- **Lig. teres uteri** (clin.: Lig. rotundum): the round ligament running from the uterotubal junction through the inguinal canal to the labia majora
- **Lig. ovarii proprium:** joins the ovary and uterus to each other
- **Lig. suspensorium ovarii** (clin.: Lig. infundibulopelvicum): attaches the ovary to the lateral pelvic wall, guides the A. and V. ovarica.

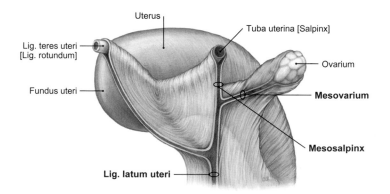

Fig. 7.126 Lig. latum uteri, mesovarium and mesosalpinx; right parasagittal section; schematic illustration; view from the right. [S701-L285]
The **Lig. latum uteri** is the continuation of the peritoneal lining of the Corpus uteri (perimetrium) and comprises a peritoneal duplication

which encloses the uterine neurovascular structures. The Lig. latum uteri continues as the **mesovarium** and **mesosalpinx** to the ovary and uterine tube, respectively.

Clinical remarks

Because of the close spatial relationships of the adnexa (ovary and uterine tube) on the right side of the body to the Appendix vermiformis of the large intestine, pain in women in the right lower abdo-

men always needs to be given a differential diagnosis of either inflammation of the appendix **(appendicitis)** or of the right uterine tube **(salpingitis),** and should be examined accordingly.

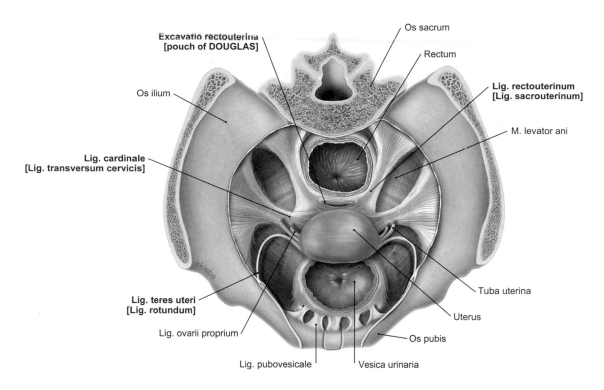

Os sacrum

Excavatio rectouterina
[pouch of DOUGLAS]

Rectum

Os ilium

Lig. rectouterinum
[Lig. sacrouterinum]

M. levator ani

Lig. cardinale
[Lig. transversum cervicis]

Tuba uterina

Uterus

Lig. teres uteri
[Lig. rotundum]

Os pubis

Lig. ovarii proprium

Vesica urinaria

Lig. pubovesicale

Fig. 7.127   Ligaments of the uterus; cross-section at the level of the cervix of the uterus; cranial view; semi-schematic illustration. [S702-L238]
In some positions, the connective tissue in the lesser pelvis is condensed into so-called ligaments. These ligaments serve for fixing the various sections of the uterus in place. The **Lig. transversum cervicis (Lig. cardinale)** fixes the Portio supravaginalis of the cervix on both sides to the pelvic bone. The **Lig. rectouterinum** (clin.: **Lig. sacrouterinum**) moves dorsally from the cervix and continues on both sides of the rectum to reach the inside of the sacrum. The **Lig. teres uteri,** however, is a remnant of the Gubernaculum and runs ventrally from the

uterotubal junction through the inguinal canal to the connective tissue above the labia majora. It is also accompanied by lymph vessels to the inguinal lymph nodes. The ligament is important for fixing the uterus in place, because it stabilises it in its anteversion in relation to the vagina and hence prevents the uterus from prolapsing as a result of an increase in intra-abdominal pressure, for example due to coughing and sneezing (→ Fig. 7.130).
The **pouch of DOUGLAS (Excavatio rectouterina)** is the deepest space of the peritoneal cavity, reaching into the connective tissue of the lesser pelvis.

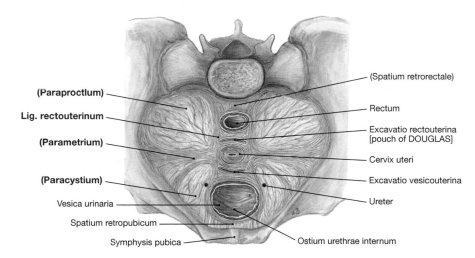

(Spatium retrorectale)

(Paraproctium)

Rectum

Lig. rectouterinum

Excavatio rectouterina
[pouch of DOUGLAS]

(Parametrium)

Cervix uteri

(Paracystium)

Excavatio vesicouterina

Vesica urinaria

Ureter

Spatium retropubicum

Symphysis pubica

Ostium urethrae internum

Fig. 7.128   Ligaments and connective tissue spaces of the uterus; cross-section at the level of the cervix of the uterus; cranial view; semi-schematic illustration. [S700]
The connective tissue in the lesser pelvis is clinically subdivided into the area of the individual organs; individual fibres are referred to as ligaments, even though such a distinction in anatomical terms cannot be definite.
* **Parametrium:** fibres attaching the cervix to the lateral pelvic wall (Lig. cardinale)
* **Paraproctium:** connective tissue around the rectum
* **paravesical space:** connective tissue around the bladder
* **Paracolpium:** connective tissue around the vagina.

Only the **Lig. rectouterinum** of the cervix is dorsally better delineated and is exposed during gynaecological operations, in order to spare the adjacent nerve fibres of the Plexus hypogastricus inferior.

Structure and position of uterus and vagina

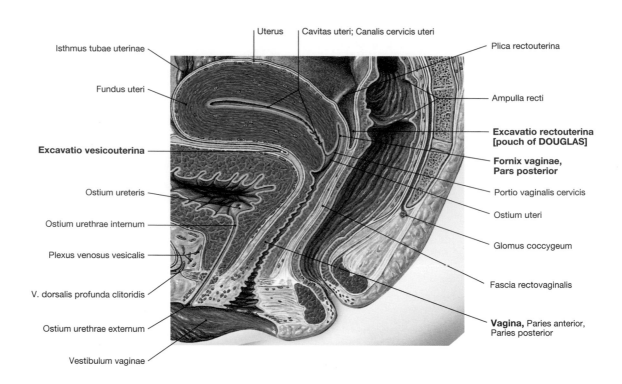

Isthmus tubae uterinae

Fundus uteri

Excavatio vesicouterina

Ostium ureteris

Ostium urethrae internum

Plexus venosus vesicalis

V. dorsalis profunda clitoridis

Ostium urethrae externum

Vestibulum vaginae

Uterus

Cavitas uteri; Canalis cervicis uteri

Plica rectouterina

Ampulla recti

Excavatio rectouterina [pouch of DOUGLAS]

Fornix vaginae, Pars posterior

Portio vaginalis cervicis

Ostium uteri

Glomus coccygeum

Fascia rectovaginalis

Vagina, Paries anterior, Paries posterior

Fig. 7.129 Vagina and uterus; median section; view from the left side. [S700]

The **neck of the uterus (Cervix uteri)** is divided into two parts: the inferior part (Portio vaginalis) extends into the vaginal vault and opens with its lumen (Canalis cervicis uteri) at the external cervical opening (Ostium uteri) into the vagina. The superior part (Portio supravaginalis) goes via a constriction (Isthmus) at the internal cervical opening (Ostium anatomicum uteri internum) into the uterine cavity (Cavitas uteri).

The **vagina** has anterior and posterior walls (Parietes anterior and posterior), both revealing transverse folds (Rugae vaginales). It culminates in the vestibule (Vestibulum vaginae), which is already regarded as one of the external genitalia. At the cranial end, the Portio vaginalis of the cervix surrounds the vagina with the vaginal vault (Fornix vaginae), which is divided into a frontal, posterior and anterior section. The posterior vaginal vault is in direct contact with the pouch of DOUGLAS, which represents a caudal enlargement of the peritoneal cavity.

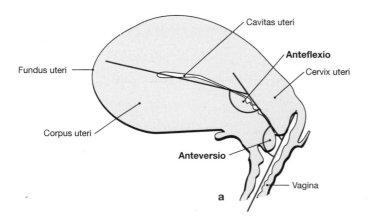

Fundus uteri

Corpus uteri

Cavitas uteri

Anteflexio

Cervix uteri

Anteversio

Vagina

a

Fig. 7.130a–d Position of the uterus and vagina; view from the right side. [S700]

a In the normal position, the uterus is angled in its ventral aspect in relation to the vagina **(anteversion)** and the body is tilted anteriorly in relation to the neck **(anteflexion).** This position acts as protection and prevents the uterus from bulging out through the vagina due to an increase in intraabdominal pressure (sneezing, coughing).

b Anteversion, anteflexion = normal position

c Anteversion, missing anteflexion

d Retroversion, retroflexion

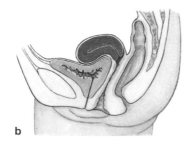

b

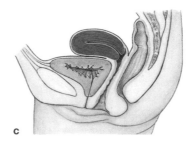

c

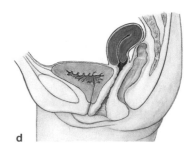

d

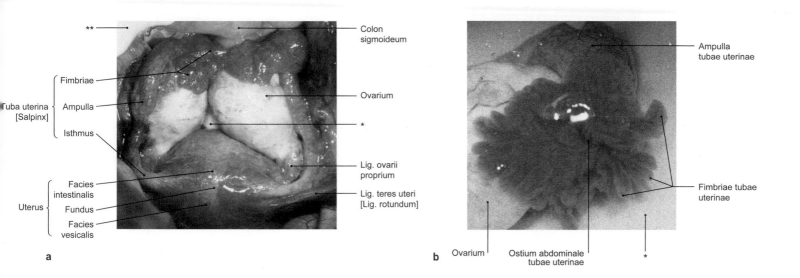

Tuba uterina [Salpinx]
- Fimbriae
- Ampulla
- Isthmus

Uterus
- Facies intestinalis
- Fundus
- Facies vesicalis

**

Colon sigmoideum

Ovarium

*

Lig. ovarii proprium

Lig. teres uteri [Lig. rotundum]

a

Ampulla tubae uterinae

Fimbriae tubae uterinae

b   Ovarium   Ostium abdominale tubae uterinae   *

Fig. 7.131a and b   Ovary, Ovarium, uterine tube, Tuba uterina, and uterus; surgical situs in a young woman. [S700-T911]
a The ovaries are pushed up medially by compresses (*); ventral view.
b For the representation of the tube funnel, the pelvic cavity was filled with saline; dorsal view.
The **tube funnel** at its abdominal end is open towards the abdominal cavity. The fimbriae, which are arranged around this opening, are in contact with the surface of the ovary and receive the ovulated ovum during ovulation. In the uterine tube, if applicable, fertilisation occurs. The ovum is then transported by the uterine tube motility to the uterus, where it is implanted if insemination has taken place. The size of the ovaries should be noted; this is typical in a young woman. Most other images in textbooks are mainly from dissections of elderly women, in whom the ovaries and uterus are often atrophied.

** swab

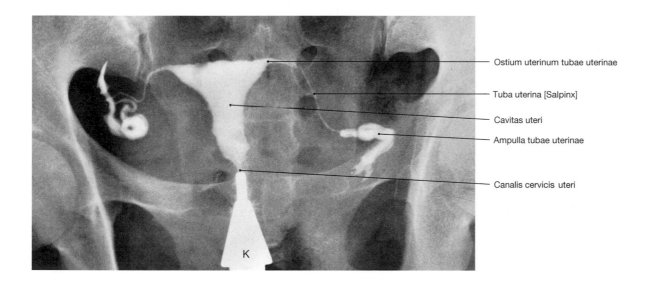

Ostium uterinum tubae uterinae

Tuba uterina [Salpinx]

Cavitas uteri

Ampulla tubae uterinae

Canalis cervicis uteri

K

Fig. 7.132   Uterus and uterine tube, Tuba uterina; X-ray imaging with contrast agent, ventral view. [S700]
The tubal patency can be checked with X-ray contrast imaging of the uterus and tubes **(hysterosalpingography),** in order to rule out stenosis of the uterine tubes in the case of infertility, which for example can result from inflammation. Today this procedure is usually carried out using ultrasound imaging in which a contrast agent is also used.

K = portio adapter of the injection probe for the contrast agent

Female genitalia

Structure and position

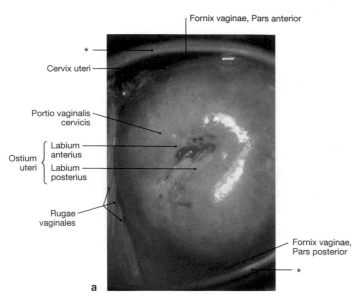

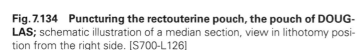

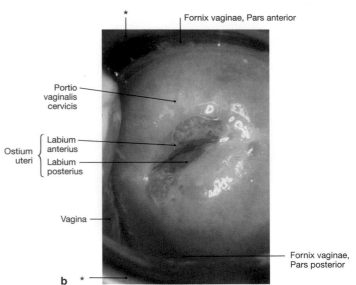

Fig. 7.133a and b Portio vaginalis cervicis; caudal view. [S700-T911]
a Portio vaginalis cervicis of a young woman who has not yet delivered a child (nullipara).
b Portio vaginalis cervicis of a young woman who has delivered two children.

To inspect the Portio vaginalis cervicis, the vagina is pulled wide open from the normally slit-shaped form by two specula.

* speculum

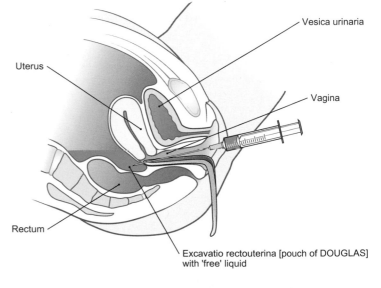

Fig. 7.134 Puncturing the rectouterine pouch, the pouch of DOUG-LAS; schematic illustration of a median section, view in lithotomy position from the right side. [S700-L126]
Due to the direct contact of the **Excavatio rectouterina [pouch of DOUGLAS]** with the posterior vaginal wall, it is possible to examine the peritoneal cavity from the vaginal perspective by using ultrasound or to even puncture the vaginal wall to sample free fluid in the pouch of DOUGLAS.

Clinical remarks

Inspection and smears of the cervix are part of the routine gynaecological exam in women. The examination should be carried out for early detection and removal of any degeneration as a precursor of a malignant tumour **(cervical cancer).** Cervical cancer is among the most common malignant tumours in women under the age of 40. As the cancer can be triggered by viruses of the Human Papilloma Virus (HPV) family, a vaccination has been developed that is recommended for girls in puberty. Vaccination can prevent infection with high certainty. However, due to limited experience to date, it is unclear how many cancers can actually be prevented, so the benefits of the vaccination are currently debated.

Since the rectouterine pouch represents the most inferior section of the peritoneal cavity in the upright position, the pouch of DOUGLAS may collect free fluid in patients with inflammation of the peritoneum **(peritonitis)** or the spread of tumour cells, e. g. from the ovary **(peritoneal cancer).** Also blood from a **ruptured spleen** can be detected by ultrasound. With advanced radiological imaging capabilities, a needle puncture of the pouch of DOUGLAS has lost significance. However, fluid sampled from the DOUGLAS pouch can be screened for white blood cells, bacteria and tumour cells.

Weakening of the cervical attachments or the removal of the uterus (hysterectomy) may cause a **prolapse of the vagina.** Surgical fixation of the Portio vaginalis to the Lig. sacrospinale or the Lig. longitudinale anterius (sacrocolpopexy) may be performed.

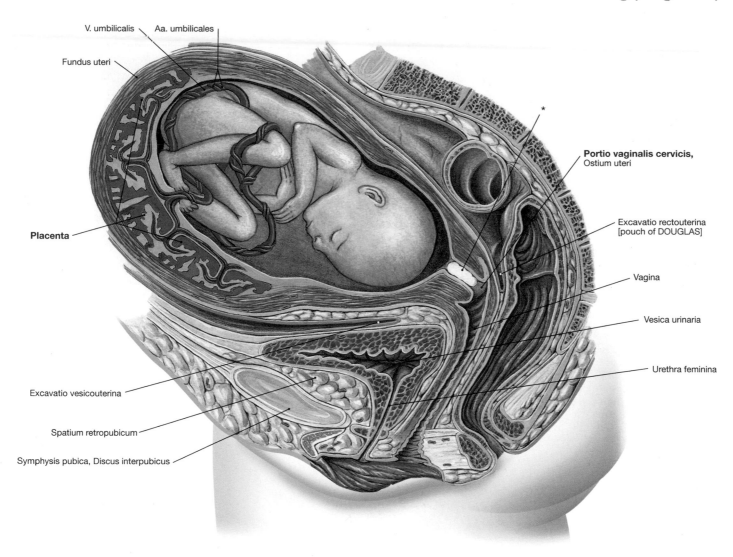

V. umbilicalis Aa. umbilicales

Fundus uteri

Placenta

Excavatio vesicouterina

Spatium retropubicum

Symphysis pubica, Discus interpubicus

*

Portio vaginalis cervicis,
Ostium uteri

Excavatio rectouterina
[pouch of DOUGLAS]

Vagina

Vesica urinaria

Urethra feminina

Fig. 7.135   Uterus with placenta and fetus; with the exception of the fetus median section of the pelvis; view from the left side. [S700]
The developing child in the uterus is nourished via the placenta which develops from maternal and fetal tissues after implantation. The cervix of the uterus is closed during pregnancy by the KRISTELLER's mucous plug (*).

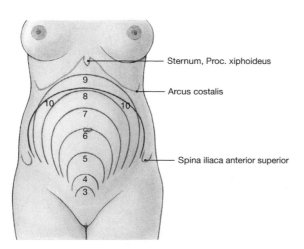

Sternum, Proc. xiphoideus

Arcus costalis

Spina iliaca anterior superior

Fig. 7.136   Level of the Fundus uteri during pregnancy; ventral view. [S700]
The numbers represent the end of the respective month of pregnancy. In the sixth month (24th week), the Fundus uteri is at the level of the umbilical region, and in the ninth month (36th week) at the costal arch. Up to parturition, the uterine volume increases 800–1,200 times and the uterine weight increases from 30–120 g to 1,000–1,500 g.

Placenta

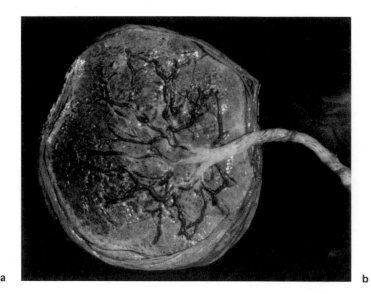

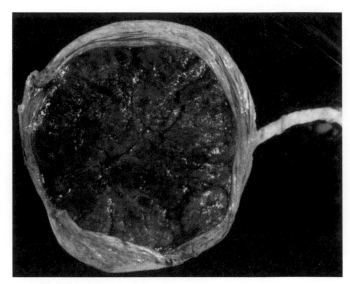

a **b**

Fig. 7.137a and b Placenta, and umbilical cord, Funiculus umbilicalis, after the birth. [S700]
a View from the fetal side.
b View from the maternal side.

The **placenta** is excreted following the birth of the child. In the child, the **umbilical cord (Funiculus umbilicalis)** is inserted onto the chorionic plate of the placenta. Here, the two umbilical cord arteries (Aa. umbilicales) originate from the internal iliac artery (A. iliaca interna) of the child and transport de-oxygenated and nutrient-poor blood to the placenta. After the gas and nutrient exchange, the blood is fed back through a single vein in the umbilical cord (V. umbilicalis) to the child. On the maternal side, the placenta is anchored in the mucous lining of the uterus. It can be seen in the image that the placenta is divided into 10–40 **functional folds (cotyledons).** After the birth, the placenta must be inspected to ensure it is complete, as any placental residues remaining in the uterus can lead to severe bleeding and infection.

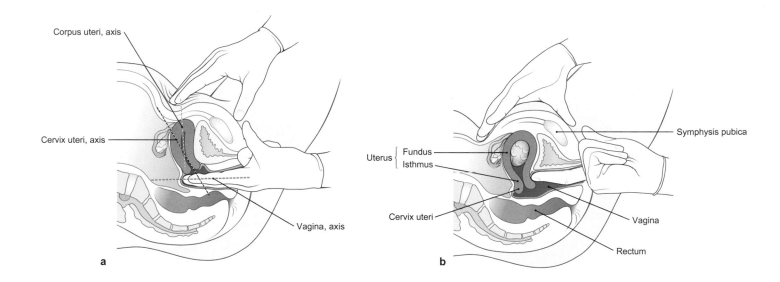

Corpus uteri, axis

Cervix uteri, axis

Vagina, axis

a

Uterus { Fundus
Isthmus

Symphysis pubica

Cervix uteri

Vagina

Rectum

b

Fig. 7.138a and b Manual palpation of the uterus; schematic illustration. [S701-L126]
a Bimanual palpation to determine the size and position of the uterus.

b Palpation to determine the softness of the cervix during pregnancy.

─Clinical anatomy─

Before the availability of current diagnostic measures, the bimanual investigation of the uterus during pregnancy was of great importance. To determine the size and position of the uterus by **bimanual palpation,** the index and middle finger of one hand are inserted into the posterior fornix of the vagina to push the uterus towards the anterior abdominal wall. The fundus of the uterus is palpated from the outside through the abdominal wall with the other hand. In addition, compressing the isthmus of the uterus from the anterior fornix of the vagina allows an assessment in the second and third months of an increased softening of the lower uterine segment as an indication of a pregnancy **(HEGAR sign).**

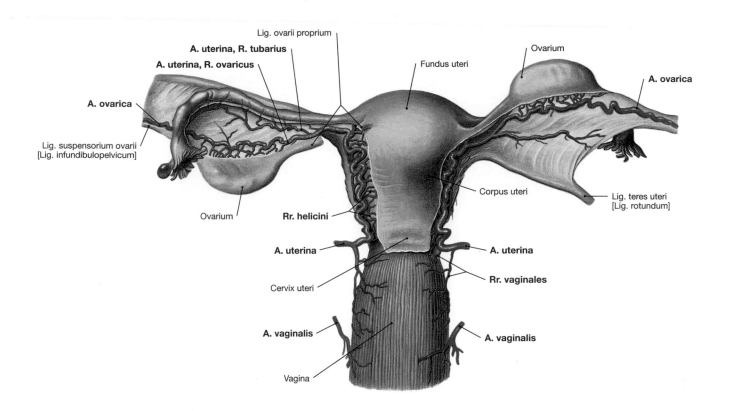

Fig. 7.139 Arteries of the internal female genitalia; dorsal view. [S700]
The internal female genitalia are supplied by **three paired arteries:**
* **uterus:** A. uterina (from the A. iliaca interna) with Rr. helicini
* **ovary:** A. ovarica (from the Pars abdominalis of the aorta) and A. uterina with R. ovaricus (ovarian branch)

* **Tuba uterina [Salpinx] (uterine tube):** A. uterina with R. tubarius and A. ovarica
* **vagina:** A. vaginalis (from A. iliaca interna) and A. uterina with Rr. vaginales.

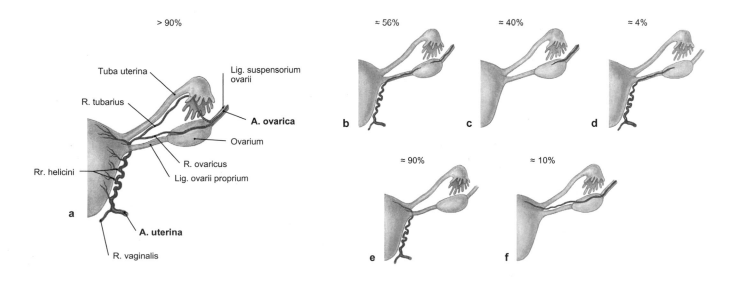

Fig. 7.140a–f Variants of the arterial supply of the internal female genitalia; dorsal view. [S700]
a Arterial supply of the uterus (textbook case).

b, c and **d** Arterial supply of the ovary (**b** textbook case).
e and **f** Arterial supply of the Fundus uteri (**e** textbook case).

Retroperitoneal space and pelvic cavity

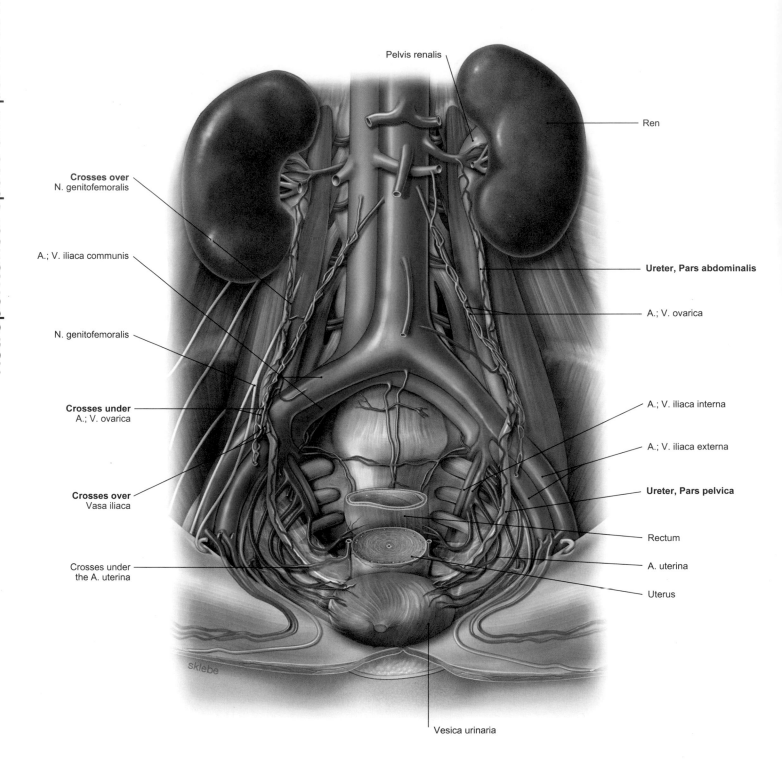

Pelvis renalis

Ren

Crosses over
N. genitofemoralis

A.; V. iliaca communis

Ureter, Pars abdominalis

A.; V. ovarica

N. genitofemoralis

Crosses under
A.; V. ovarica

A.; V. iliaca interna

A.; V. iliaca externa

Crosses over
Vasa iliaca

Ureter, Pars pelvica

Rectum

Crosses under
the A. uterina

A. uterina

Uterus

sklebe

Vesica urinaria

Fig. 7.141   Arteries of the internal female genitalia; ventral view. [S702-L238]
All internal female genitalia receive their blood supply via **three paired arteries.**
The **A. ovarica** originates from the Pars abdominalis of the aorta and descends first in the retroperitoneal space and then through the Lig. suspensorium ovarii into the lesser pelvis. As well as the ovary, it also

supplies the adjacent part of the uterine tube. The **A. uterina** is a visceral branch of the A. iliaca interna. It approaches in the Lig. latum uteri of the lower part of the Cervix uteri, where it passes across the ureter. Here it provides the **Rr. vaginales** to the vagina and then it ascends to the body of the uterus, which it supplies via the **Rr. helicini.** The uterine tube receives its own branch with the **R. tubarius** before the **R. ovaricus** anastomoses as a terminal branch with the A. ovarica.

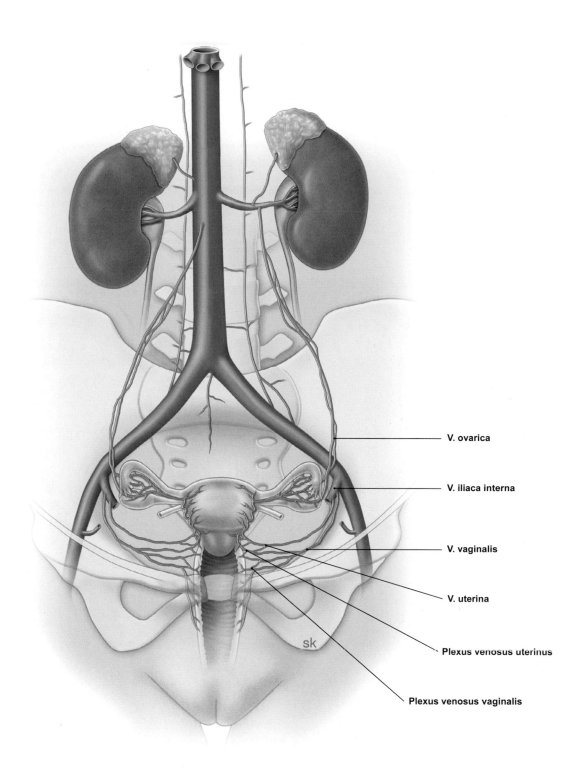

V. ovarica

V. iliaca interna

V. vaginalis

V. uterina

Plexus venosus uterinus

Plexus venosus vaginalis

sk

Fig. 7.142 Veins of the internal female genitalia; ventral view. [S701-L238]
Venous drainage takes place via **two venous systems:**

- the venous plexuses in the lesser pelvis **(Plexus venosi uterinus and vaginalis)** with connection to the V. iliaca interna
- **V. ovarica,** entering on the right into the V. cava inferior, and on the left into the V. renalis sinistra.

Lymph vessels of the female genitalia

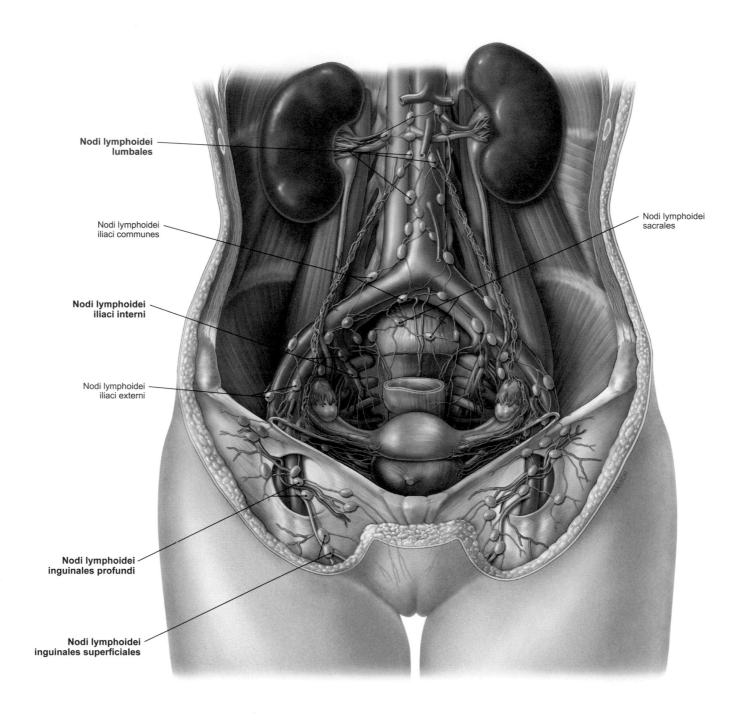

Nodi lymphoidei
lumbales

Nodi lymphoidei
iliaci communes

**Nodi lymphoidei
iliaci interni**

Nodi lymphoidei
iliaci externi

Nodi lymphoidei
sacrales

**Nodi lymphoidei
inguinales profundi**

**Nodi lymphoidei
inguinales superficiales**

Fig. 7.143 Lymph vessels and lymph nodes of the external and internal female genitalia; ventral view. [S700-L238]
The regional lymph nodes for the external female genitalia are the inguinal lymph nodes **(Nodi lymphoidei inguinales).** In contrast, the first regional lymph nodes of the ovary are located retroperitoneally at the level of the kidneys **(Nodi lymphoidei lumbales)** and the regional lymph nodes of the uterus are in the lesser pelvis **(Nodi lymphoidei iliaci interni).**

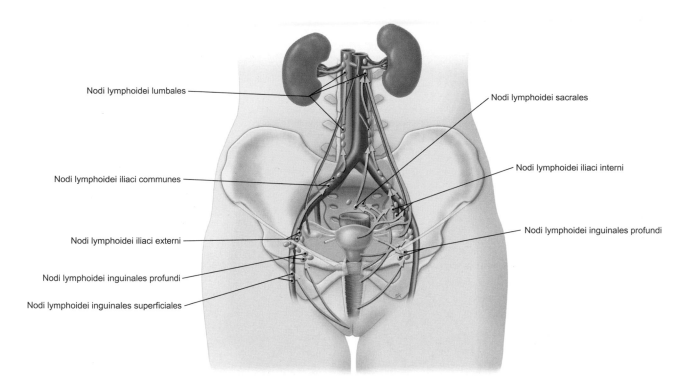

Fig. 7.144 Lymphatic drainage pathways of the external and internal female genitalia with projection to the skeleton; ventral view. [S700-L238]

Unlike with men, the lymphatic drainage pathways of the external and internal female genitalia are not completely separate, as parts of the lymph of the internal genitalia also drain into the inguinal lymph nodes. The lymph drains from the inguinal lymph nodes **(Nodi lymphoidei inguinales)** via the lymph nodes along the A. iliaca externa **(Nodi lymphoidei iliaci externi)** to the collecting lymph nodes of the pelvis **(Nodi lymphoidei iliaci communes).** The latter also collect lymph from along the A. iliaca interna **(Nodi lymphoidei iliaci interni)** and from the anterior sacrum **(Nodi lymphoidei sacrales).** The pelvic lymph nodes drain into the lumbar nodes **(Nodi lymphoidei lumbales)** that are located on both sides of the abdominal aorta and the inferior vena cava up to the level of the renal blood vessels. Here the lymph trunks **(Trunci lumbales)** originate, which merge beneath the diaphragm with the Trunci intestinalis to form the **Ductus thoracicus.**

Fig. 7.145 Lymphatic drainage pathways of the external and internal female genitalia; ventral view. [S701-L127]

Regional lymph nodes of the **external genitalia** of the vulva are the Nodi lymphoidei inguinales.

Regional lymph nodes of the **internal genitalia** are:

* **Nodi lymphoidei lumbales** at the level of the kidneys: ovaries, Tuba uterina, uterus (uterotubal junction), lymph vessels within the Lig. suspensorium ovarii (highlighted in **yellow)**
* **Nodi lymphoidei iliaci interni/externi** and **Nodi lymphoidei sacrales:** uterus, vagina, Tuba uterine (highlighted in **red)**
* **Nodi lymphoidei inguinales:** lower third of the vagina, uterus (uterotubal junction), lymph vessels within the Lig. teres uteri (highlighted in **blue).**

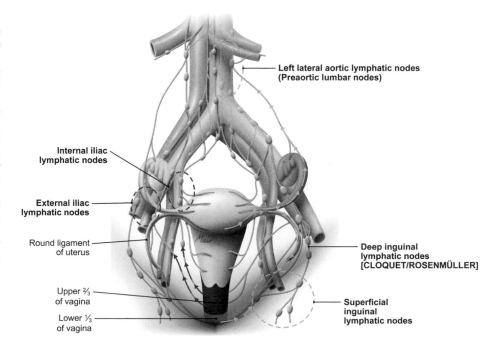

Clinical remarks

Due to the different lymphatic pathways, the first **lymph node metastases** of vulvar carcinomas occur in the groin. If the deep inguinal nodes **(CLOQUET's or ROSENMÜLLER's nodes)** are affected, metastasis to the pelvic nodes is assumed. In contrast, endometrial carcinoma of the uterus and cervical cancer metastases first occur in the lesser pelvis, and ovarian tumours first occur in the retroperitoneal space.

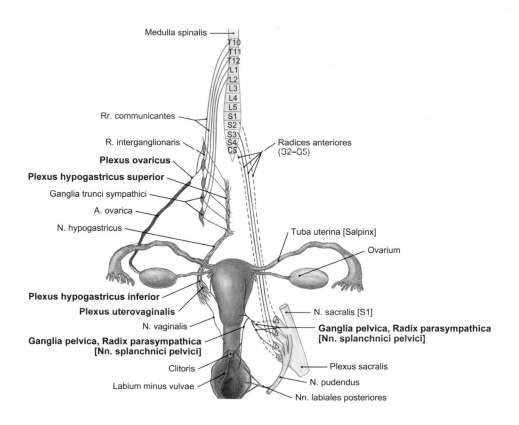

Medulla spinalis

T10
T11
T12
L1
L2
L3
L4
L5
S1
S2
S3
S4
C5

Rr. communicantes

R. interganglionaris

Plexus ovaricus

Plexus hypogastricus superior

Ganglia trunci sympathici

A. ovarica

N. hypogastricus

Radices anteriores (S2–S5)

Tuba uterina [Salpinx]

Ovarium

Plexus hypogastricus inferior

Plexus uterovaginalis

N. vaginalis

Ganglia pelvica, Radix parasympathica [Nn. splanchnici pelvici]

Clitoris

Labium minus vulvae

N. sacralis [S1]

Ganglia pelvica, Radix parasympathica [Nn. splanchnici pelvici]

Plexus sacralis

N. pudendus

Nn. labiales posteriores

Fig. 7.146 Innervation of the female genitalia; ventral view; schematic illustration. The Plexus hypogastricus inferior and Plexus uterovaginalis contain sympathetic (green) and parasympathetic (purple) nerve fibres. [S700]

Preganglionic **sympathetic nerve fibres** (T10–L2) descend from the Plexus aorticus abdominalis via the Plexus hypogastricus superior, and from the sacral ganglia of the sympathetic trunk (Truncus sympathicus) via the Nn. splanchnici sacrales, to be synapsed to postganglionic neurons in the ganglia of the **Plexus hypogastricus inferior.** Their axons reach the pelvic organs, and continue in the **Plexus uterovaginalis (FRANKENHÄUSER's plexus),** innervating the uterus, uterine tubes and vagina. The (mostly) postganglionic sympathetic fibres to the ovary pass through the Plexus ovaricus alongside the A. ovarica after being already synapsed in the Ganglia aorticorenalia or the Plexus hypogastricus superior.

Preganglionic **parasympathetic nerve fibres** pass from the sacral parasympathicus (S2–S4) via the Nn. splanchnici pelvici into the ganglia of the Plexus hypogastricus inferior. They are synapsed either here or in the vicinity of the pelvic viscera (Ganglia pelvica) to postganglionic neurons which innervate the uterus, uterine tubes and vagina.

Somatic innervation by the **pudendal nerve** conveys sensory innervation to the lower part of the vagina, the vaginal vestibule (Vestibulum vaginale) and the labia minora and majora via the Rr. labiales posteriores, and to the clitoris via the N. dorsalis clitoridis.

Clinical remarks

The **pelvic pain line** depicts a hypothetical separation of the pain afferents for the pelvic viscera.

Intraperitoneal viscera such as the Corpus uteri, ovary and uterine tube receive sympathetic innervation from the Plexus aorticus abdominalis. The Cervix uteri and the upper two-thirds of the vagina are innervated by parasympathetic neurons via the Plexus hypogastricus inferior. The lower third of the vagina receives somatic sensory innervation from the N. pudendus (→ figures).

There are several options for anaesthaesia during childbirth:

1. **Spinal anaesthesia:** anaesthetic is administered in the subarachnoid space at the level of L4/L5; blocks pain afferents from the lower extremities and the genital organs.
2. **Epidural anaesthesia:** anaesthetic is administered locally in the epidural space. a) At the level of L4/L5 (lumbar); blocks pain afferents from the lower extremities and the genital organs. b) At the sacral canal (caudal); anaesthetises S2–S4 visceral- and somatic-afferents from the lower birth canal, but allows for the perception of uterine contractions above the pelvic pain line.
3. **Pudendal nerve block:** anaesthetic is administered from the vagina near the ischial spine bilaterally to block somatic-afferents from the lower vagina and the perineum.

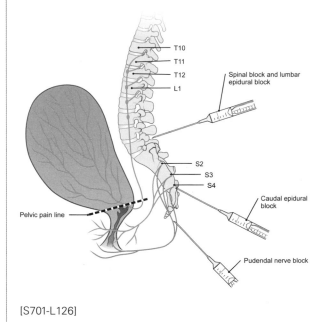

[S701-L126]

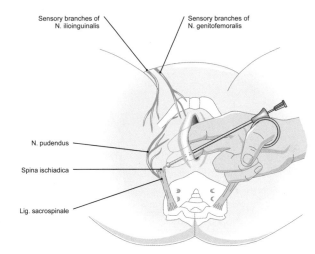

[R388-L157]

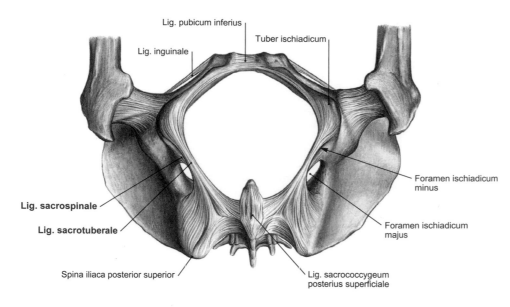

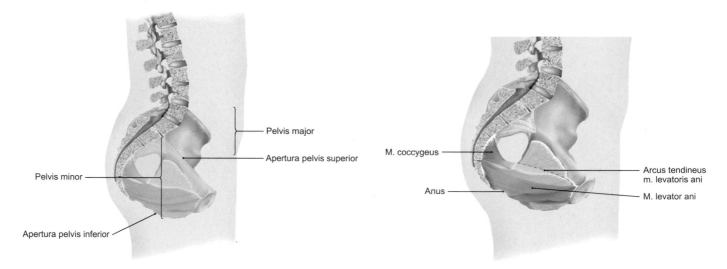

Fig. 7.147   Bones and ligaments of the pelvic outlet, Apertura pelvis inferior, in women; caudal view in lithotomy position. [S701]

The **pelvis outlet, Apertura pelvis inferior,** is defined by the following bones and ligaments:

* coccyx, Os coccygis, with Lig. sacrococcygeum posterius superficiale
* ischial tuberosity, Tuber ischiadicum, both sides, with Lig. sacrotuberale
* pubic symphysis, Symphysis pubica, with Lig. pubicum inferius.

Fig. 7.148   'True' or 'lesser' pelvis, Pelvis minor, in women; schematic illustration, view from the right side. [S701-L280]

The **lesser pelvis, Pelvis minor,** is separated from the greater pelvis, Pelvis major, at the **pelvic inlet, Apertura pelvis superior,** which is confined by the Linea terminalis (→ Fig. 4.5, Volume 1). The **Linea terminalis** extends ventrally from the pubic symphysis via the Pecten ossis pubis and dorsally via the Linea arcuata to the promontorium. The latter depicts the most ventrally positioned bony landmark of the Os sacrum.

Fig. 7.149   Pelvic floor, Diaphragma pelvis, in women; schematic illustration with a median pelvic section. The pelvic diaphragm is highlighted in green, view from the right side. [S701-L280]

The **pelvic floor, Diaphragma pelvis,** comprises **funnel-shaped striated muscles** and their fasciae which form the inferior confinement of the pelvic cavity. The pelvic floor is highlighted in green in this illustration.

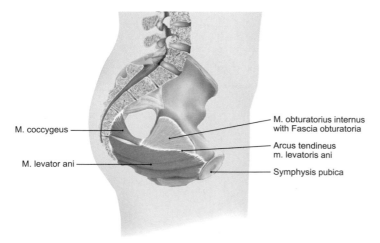

Fig. 7.150   Pelvic floor, Diaphragma pelvis, in women; schematic illustration with a median pelvic section. [S701-L280]

The pelvic floor comprises the **M. levator ani** and the **M. ischiococcygeus** and provides support for pelvic viscera through a sustained resting tone.

→ T 22.1

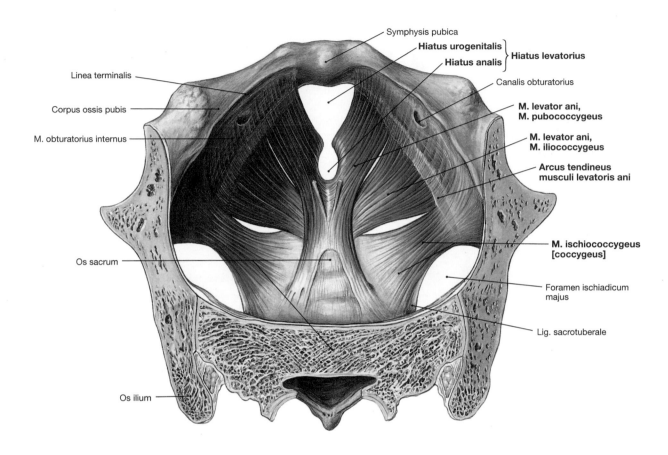

Symphysis pubica

Hiatus urogenitalis
Hiatus analis
} Hiatus levatorius

Canalis obturatorius

Linea terminalis

Corpus ossis pubis

M. obturatorius internus

M. levator ani,
M. pubococcygeus

M. levator ani,
M. iliococcygeus

Arcus tendineus
musculi levatoris ani

M. ischiococcygeus
[coccygeus]

Os sacrum

Foramen ischiadicum
majus

Lig. sacrotuberale

Os ilium

Fig. 7.151   Pelvic floor, Diaphragma pelvis, in women; cranial view.
[S700]
The pelvic floor of women is similar in its structure to the pelvic floor of
men and closes the pelvic cavity caudally.
Structure:
* **M. levator ani,** comprising M. pubococcygeus, M. iliococcygeus,
   and M. puborectalis
* **M. ischiococcygeus.**
In contrast to the M. pubococcygeus and the M. ischiococcygeus, the
M. iliococcygeus does not originate from the hip bone but from the Ar-
cus tendineus musculi levatoris ani, a reinforcement of the fascia of the
M. obturatorius internus.

The muscles of both sides leave the **levator hiatus (Hiatus levatorius)**
free between them. This muscular gap is subdivided by the connective
tissue of the perineum (Centrum perinei) to become the anterior **Hiatus
urogenitalis** for the passage of the urethra and vagina and the posteri-
or **Hiatus analis** for the passage of the rectum.
The pelvic floor is innervated by direct branches of the Plexus sacralis
(S3–S4) and shows a sustained resting tone, similar to the M. sphincter
ani externus.
Function: The pelvic floor stabilises the position of the pelvic organs
and is thus essential for urinary and faecal continence.

→ T 22.1

Clinical remarks

When giving birth, the extreme dilation of the pelvic floor muscles
and possible partial tearing off from the pelvic bones may lead to
pelvic floor insufficiency (→ Fig. 7.153) with the consequence of insufficient support of pelvic viscera.

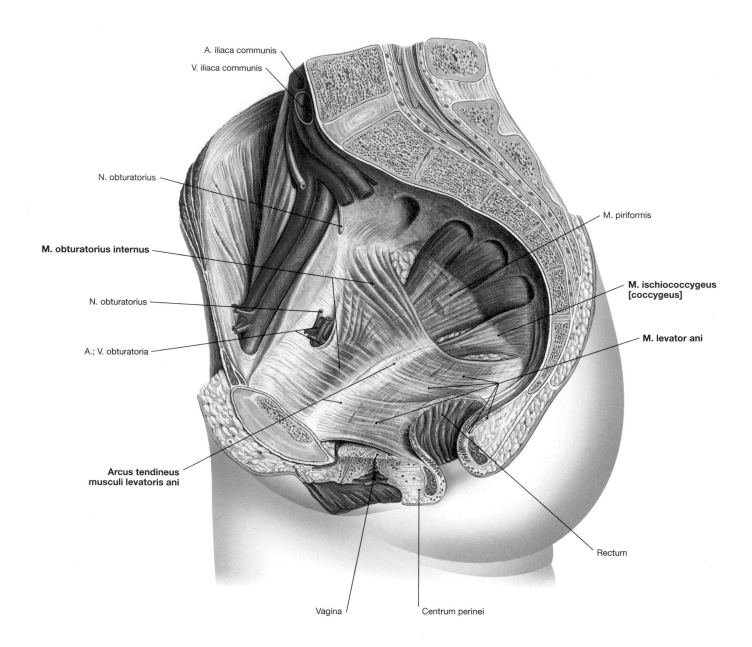

A. iliaca communis

V. iliaca communis

N. obturatorius

M. obturatorius internus

N. obturatorius

A.; V. obturatoria

Arcus tendineus musculi levatoris ani

M. piriformis

M. ischiococcygeus [coccygeus]

M. levator ani

Rectum

Vagina

Centrum perinei

Fig. 7.152 Pelvic floor, Diaphragma pelvis, in women; view from the left side. [S700]
The pelvic floor consists of the **M. levator ani** and the **M. ischiococcygeus.** The M. iliococcygeus of the M. levator ani originates from the **Arcus tendineus musculi levatoris ani.** This is a reinforcement of the fascia of the M. obturatorius internus. The M. obturatorius internus originates at the front of the superior pubic ramus, where it is clearly iden-
tifiable because it is perforated by the Canalis obturatorius with the A. and V. obturatoria and the N. obturatorius. At the Arcus tendineus musculi levatoris ani, the M. obturatorius internus then turns laterally and exits the pelvis via the Foramen ischiadicum minus. The M. levator ani extends to the sacrum and the coccyx and closes the pelvic cavity caudally.

→ T 22.1

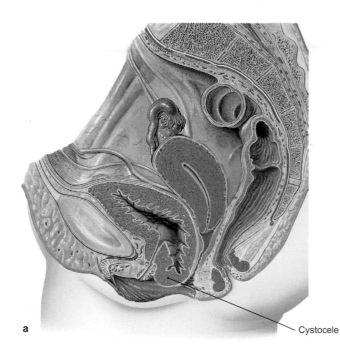

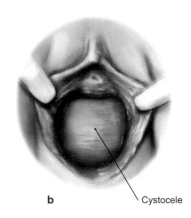

a   Cystocele   b   Cystocele

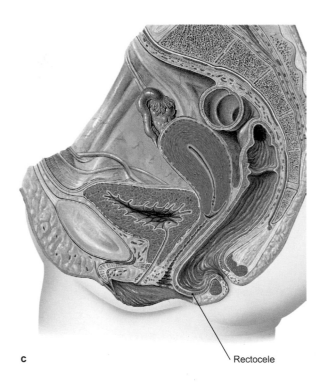

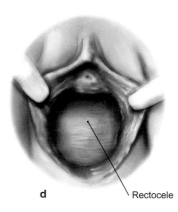

c   Rectocele   d   Rectocele

Fig. 7.153a–d Pelvic floor insufficiency in women; median section, view from the left side. [S702-L266]
a, b Cystocele.
c, d Rectocele.
If the stabilising function of the pelvic floor fails, this leads to pelvic floor insufficiency. In this case, the posterior wall of the urinary bladder **(a, b)** or the anterior wall of the rectum **(c, d)** can prolapse. Both the **cystocele (a)** and the **rectocele (c)** are visible as bulges from the vagina; from their appearance it is not always obvious to differentiate between them. The topographical relationships are highlighted here by a shadow which delineates the dorsal cystocele **(b)** and the ventral rectocele **(d)** of the prolapsed tissue.

Clinical remarks

In women, weakness of the pelvic floor **(pelvic floor insufficiency)** is much more frequent, because the pelvic floor is strained by vaginal births, where the levator hiatus is stretched significantly. As a result, a **drop** (Descensus) may occur, leading to **prolapse** of the uterus and vagina. Since the uterus is linked to the posterior wall of the urinary bladder and the vagina is linked to the anterior wall of the rectum, this is often accompanied by a prolapse of the urinary bladder (cystocele) and rectum (rectocele) and therefore associated with **urinary** and **faecal incontinence.**

Perineal musculature in women

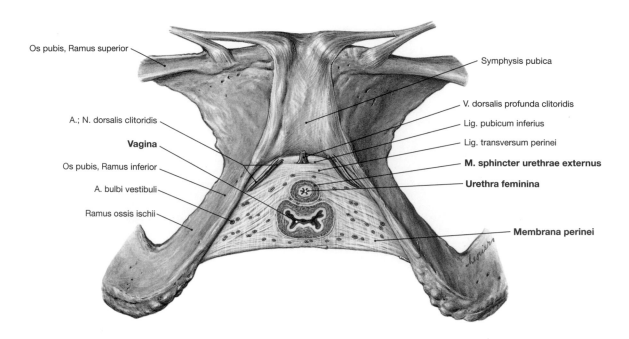

Os pubis, Ramus superior

Symphysis pubica

A.; N. dorsalis clitoridis

V. dorsalis profunda clitoridis

Lig. pubicum inferius

Vagina

Lig. transversum perinei

Os pubis, Ramus inferior

M. sphincter urethrae externus

A. bulbi vestibuli

Urethra feminina

Ramus ossis ischii

Membrana perinei

Fig. 7.154   Perineal muscles in women; caudal view; after the removal of all other muscles. [S700]

In women, the levator hiatus (Hiatus levatorius) is largely closed by connective tissue, so that only the passage of the vagina and urethra (Urethra feminina) remains open. Unlike in men, the perineal muscles in women are relatively weak (→ Fig. 7.108). Because the **M. transversus perinei profundus,** which only consists of single muscle fibres embedded within connective tissue (→ Fig. 7.155), and the thin **M. transversus perinei superficialis** do not constitute a muscle plate, the old term of 'Diaphragma urogenitale' has been dropped.

While in men the deep perineal space (Spatium profundum perinei) largely corresponds to the extension of the M. transversus perinei profundus, the delimitation of the perineal spaces is more difficult in women. The **deep perineal space** (Spatium profundum perinei) is however bordered inferiorly by the **Membrana perinei,** as in men (→ Fig. 7.162). In women this space also contains the vagina next to the urethra and is traversed by the deep branches of the N. pudendus and the A. and V. pudenda interna on their way to the vulva.

→ T 22.2

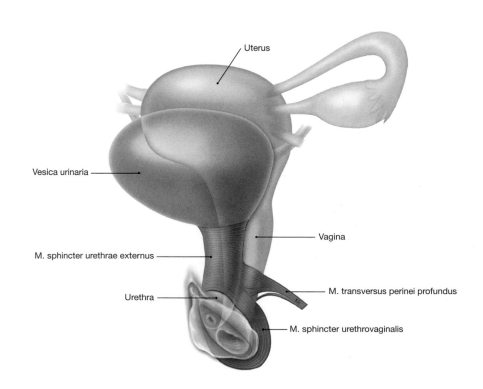

Uterus

Vesica urinaria

Vagina

M. sphincter urethrae externus

M. transversus perinei profundus

Urethra

M. sphincter urethrovaginalis

Fig. 7.155   Voluntary sphincter muscles of the urinary bladder. [S700-L238]

In women, the M. transversus perinei profundus does not form a solid muscle plate below the pelvic floor. Conversely, in the area of the urethra, individual striated muscle fibres form the **M. sphincter urethrae externus,** constituting the voluntary sphincter of the urinary bladder (→ Fig. 7.154). Some fibres continue to surround the distal vagina and are referred to as **M. sphincter urethrovaginalis.**

→ T 22.2

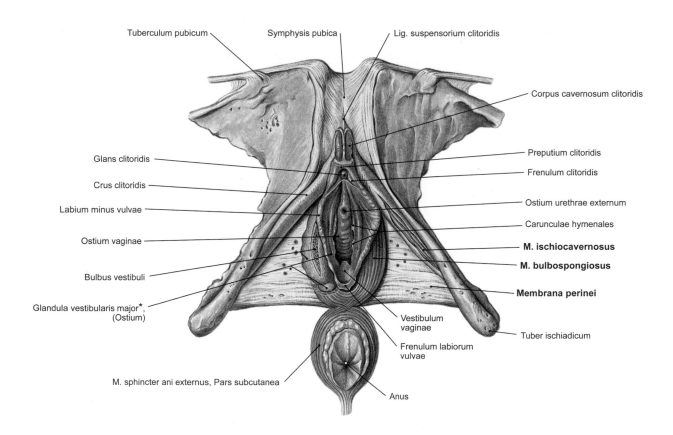

Tuberculum pubicum

Symphysis pubica

Lig. suspensorium clitoridis

Corpus cavernosum clitoridis

Preputium clitoridis

Frenulum clitoridis

Glans clitoridis

Crus clitoridis

Labium minus vulvae

Ostium vaginae

Bulbus vestibuli

Glandula vestibularis major*, (Ostium)

Ostium urethrae externum

Carunculae hymenales

M. ischiocavernosus

M. bulbospongiosus

Membrana perinei

Tuber ischiadicum

Vestibulum vaginae

Frenulum labiorum vulvae

M. sphincter ani externus, Pars subcutanea

Anus

Fig. 7.156 Superficial perineal muscles in women; caudal view. [S700]

The **Membrana perinei** borders the deep perineal space caudally. Below it joins with the **superficial perineal space (Spatium superficiale perinei)** (→ Fig. 7.162). This contains the M. transversus perinei superficialis and the external genitalia, the parts of which come together as the vulva. The two cavernous bodies of the vulva are also covered by the superficial perineal muscles: the crus of the clitoris is bilaterally ac-

companied by the **M. ischiocavernosus** on the inferior pubic ramus, and the bulb of the vestibule (Bulbus vestibuli) is covered by the **M. bulbospongiosus.**

* clin.: BARTHOLIN's gland

→ T 22.2

Retroperitoneal space and pelvic cavity

Perineal spaces in women

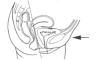

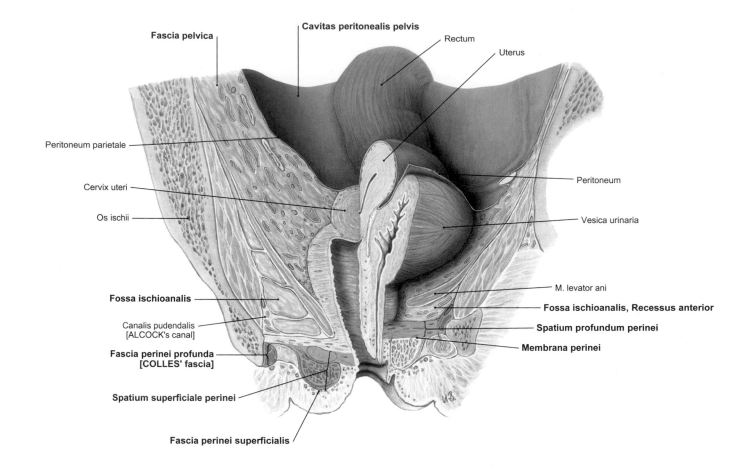

Fascia pelvica

Cavitas peritonealis pelvis

Rectum

Uterus

Peritoneum parietale

Peritoneum

Cervix uteri

Vesica urinaria

Os ischii

M. levator ani

Fossa ischioanalis

Fossa ischioanalis, Recessus anterior

Canalis pudendalis [ALCOCK's canal]

Spatium profundum perinei

Fascia perinei profunda [COLLES' fascia]

Membrana perinei

Spatium superficiale perinei

Fascia perinei superficialis

Fig. 7.157   Pelvic spaces in women; median section, and frontal section at the right side; ventral view. [S700].
The frontal section shows **three levels** of the female pelvic cavity:
* **peritoneal cavity of the pelvis (Cavitas peritonealis pelvis),** which is caudally confined by the parietal peritoneum

* **subperitoneal space (Spatium extraperitoneale pelvis),** which reaches down to the M. levator ani of the pelvic floor
* **perineal region (Regio perinealis)** below the pelvic floor.

Structure and function

The **deep perineal space** (Spatium profundum perinei) in women contains the following:
* vagina
* urethra
* deep branches of the N. pudendus (N. dorsalis clitoridis)

* deep branches of the A./V. pudenda interna (A. bulbi vestibuli, A. dorsalis clitoridis, A. profunda clitoridis)
* Nn. cavernosi clitoridis
* muscle fibres of the M. transversus perinei profundus, if present.

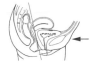

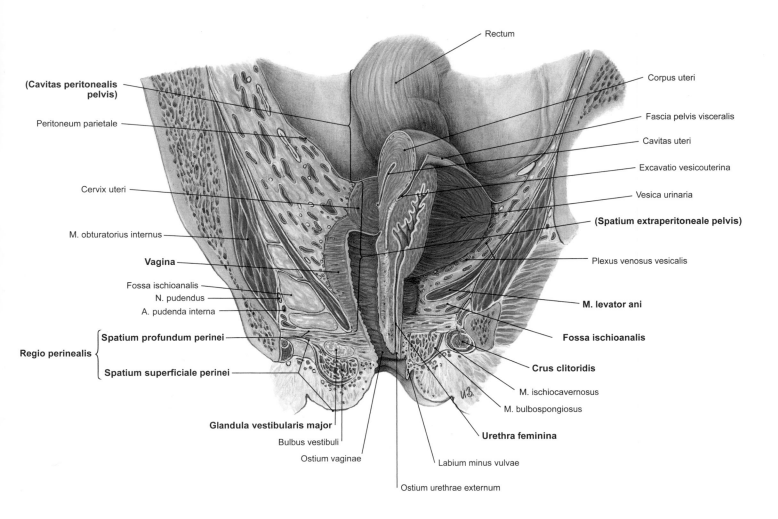

Fig. 7.158 **Perineal spaces in women;** median section, and frontal section at the right side; ventral view. See also the section in → Fig. 7.175b. [S700]

The front part of the perineal region, the Regio perinealis, is generally occupied by both of the perineal spaces, but additionally still contain the very variable anterior recesses of the Fossa ischioanalis (shown here on the right and left, differentiated).

The **deep perineal space (Spatium profundum perinei)** consists of the connective tissue and single muscle fibres of the M. transversus perinei profundus. It also contains the passage of the vagina and urethra. The deep perineal space is traversed by the deep branches of the N. pudendus (N. dorsalis clitoridis), and of the A. and V. pudenda interna (A. bulbi vestibuli, A. dorsalis clitoridis, A. profunda clitoridis) before

they reach the vulva. The Nn. cavernosi clitoridis pierce the perineum and enter the Corpora cavernosa of the clitoris.

The **superficial perineal space (Spatium superficiale perinei)** is located between the perineal membrane (Membrana perinei) and the body fascia (Fascia perinei). In addition to the M. transversus perinei superficialis and the proximal parts of the Corpora cavernosa clitoridis, it contains the Glandulae vestibulares majores (BARTHOLIN's glands) and the bulb of the vestibule (Bulbus vestibuli). The latter is surrounded on both sides by the M. bulbospongiosus, and the Crura clitoridis by the M. ischiocavernosus. The superficial branches of the N. pudendus (N. perinealis with Nn. labiales posteriores) and of the A. and V. pudenda interna (A. perinealis with Rr. labiales posteriores) continue through this space to the vulva.

Structure and function

The **superficial perineal space** (Spatium profundum perinei) in women contains the following:
- Glandulae vestibulares majores (BARTHOLIN's glands)
- Crura clitoridis
- bulb of the vestibule (Bulbus vestibularis)
- superficial branches of the N. pudendus (Nn. perineales with Nn. labiales posteriores)

- superficial branches of the A./V. pudenda interna (A./V. perineales with Rr. labiales posteriores)
- M. transversus perinei superficialis
- M. bulbospongiosus
- M. ischiocavernosus.

Perineal region in women

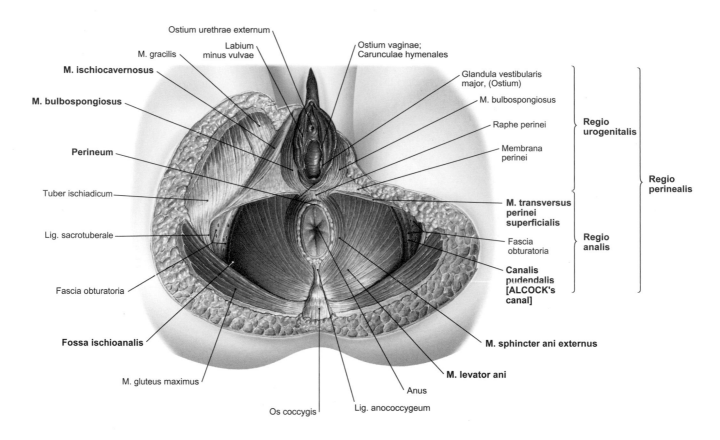

Ostium urethrae externum

Labium
minus vulvae

M. gracilis

Ostium vaginae;
Carunculae hymenales

M. ischiocavernosus

Glandula vestibularis
major, (Ostium)

M. bulbospongiosus

M. bulbospongiosus

Raphe perinei

Regio
urogenitalis

Perineum

Membrana
perinei

Regio
perinealis

Tuber ischiadicum

**M. transversus
perinei
superficialis**

Lig. sacrotuberale

Fascia
obturatoria

Regio
analis

Fascia obturatoria

**Canalis
pudendalis
[ALCOCK's
canal]**

Fossa ischioanalis

M. sphincter ani externus

M. levator ani

M. gluteus maximus

Anus

Os coccygis

Lig. anococcygeum

Fig. 7.159   Perineal region, Regio perinealis, in women; caudal view; after removal of all neurovascular pathways. [S700]

The **perineal region** extends from the inferior margin of the pubic symphysis (Symphysis pubica) to the tip of the coccyx (Os coccygis). The term **perineum** in women, however, describes exclusively the small connective tissue bridge between the posterior margin of the labia majora and the anus. The perineal region can be divided into an **anterior Regio urogenitalis** with external genitalia and urethra, and a **posterior Regio analis** around the anus. Both regions include spaces:

- The Regio analis contains the **Fossa ischioanalis** (→ table), which constitutes a pyramid-shaped space on both sides of the anus. The Fossa ischioanalis is similar in men and women. The lateral wall contains the Canalis pudendalis (ALCOCK's canal) in a fascial duplication of the M. obturatorius internus (Fascia obturatoria). In this canal, the A. and V. pudenda interna and the N. pudendus are arriving via the Foramen ischiadicum minus from the Regio glutealis.
- The **Regio urogenitalis** contains the two **perineal spaces:**
  - The **deep perineal space** (Spatium profundum perinei) is caudally confined by the Membrana perinei; and in women it contains the weak M. transversus perinei profundus and the M. sphincter urethrae externus.

- In the **superficial perineal space** (Spatium superficiale perinei) between the Membrana perinei and the body fascia (Fascia perinei), are the M. transversus perinei superficialis, the M. bulbospongiosus and the M. ischiocavernosus, which stabilise the cavernous bodies of the vestibule and clitoris as well as the Glandulae vestibulares majores (BARTHOLIN's glands).

Boundaries of the Fossa ischioanalis	
Orientation	**Confining structure**
Medial and cranial	M. sphincter ani externus and M. levator ani
Lateral	M. obturatorius internus
Dorsal	M. gluteus maximus and Lig. sacrotuberale
Ventral	Posterior margin of the superficial and the deep perineal spaces, anterior recesses reach up to the pubic symphysis
Caudal	Fascia and skin of the perineum

Clinical remarks

Childbirth can lead to uncontrolled tearing of the skin and muscles of the perineum, involving the sphincter muscles of the anus **(perineal tearing),** which in some cases can be prevented through targeted incision to the posterolateral side or in the median plane **(episiotomy).**

[S701-L126]

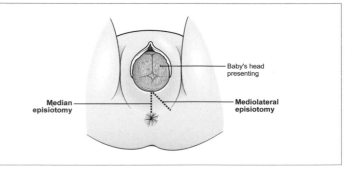

Baby's head
presenting

Median
episiotomy

Mediolateral
episiotomy

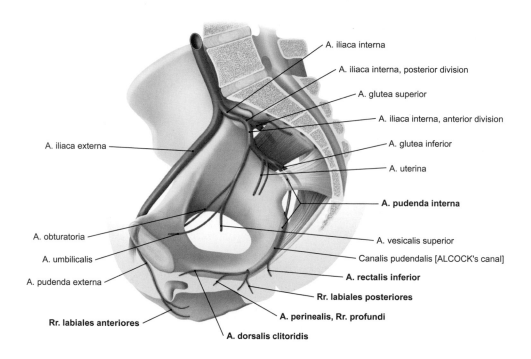

A. iliaca interna

A. iliaca interna, posterior division

A. glutea superior

A. iliaca interna, anterior division

A. glutea inferior

A. uterina

A. pudenda interna

A. vesicalis superior

Canalis pudendalis [ALCOCK's canal]

A. rectalis inferior

Rr. labiales posteriores

A. perinealis, Rr. profundi

A. dorsalis clitoridis

A. iliaca externa

A. obturatoria

A. umbilicalis

A. pudenda externa

Rr. labiales anteriores

Fig. 7.160 Arteries of the female perineum, Regio perinealis; schematic illustration; view from the left. [S701-L275]
The perineum receives arterial blood from ventral via the **A. pudenda externa** (branch of the A. femoralis from the A. iliaca externa) and from dorsal by the **A. pudenda interna** (branch of the A. ilica interna).
The **A. pudenda externa** branches off medially from the A. femoralis after its passage through the Lacuna vasorum beneath the inguinal ligament. The Rr. labiales anteriores supply the anterior third of the perineum and the labia majora.
The **A. pudenda interna** leaves the pelvis together with its concomitant vein and the N. pudendus through the **Foramen infrapiriforme.** It loops medially around the Lig. sacrospinale and passes through the **Foramen ischiadicum minus** to enter the Fossa ischioanalis. Here the

pudendal neurovascular structures are enclosed by the caudal fascia of the M. obturatorius internus, forming the **Canalis pudendalis (ALCOCK's canal).** After releasing the A. rectalis inferior in the Fossa ischioanalis, the A. pudenda interna branches into superficial and deep terminal arteries in the perineum:

- The superficial **A. perinealis** supplies the posterior two-thirds of the perineum and provides Rr. labiales posteriores to the posterior labia majora
- The deep branches which constitute the **A. bulbi vestibuli**
- the **A. dorsalis clitoridis** to the skin and the glans of the clitoris
- the **A. profunda clitoridis** supplies the Corpora cavernosa of the clitoris for sexual arousal.

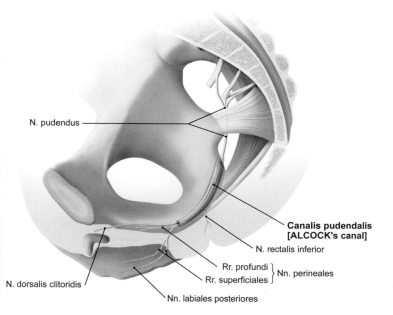

N. pudendus

Canalis pudendalis [ALCOCK's canal]

N. rectalis inferior

Rr. profundi
Rr. superficiales } Nn. perineales

N. dorsalis clitoridis

Nn. labiales posteriores

Fig. 7.161 Innervation of the female perineum; schematic illustration; view from the left. [S701-L275]
The perineum receives innervation from ventral via the **N. Ilioinguinalis** (from the Plexus lumbalis; not shown here) and from dorsal by the **N. pudendus** (from the Plexus sacralis) and the N. cutaneus femoris posterior (Plexus sacralis; not shown here).
The **N. ilioinguinalis** runs adjacent to the spermatic cord and innervates the anterior third of the perineum and the labia majora through the Rr. labiales anteriores.
The **N. pudendus** exits the pelvis together with the A./V. pudenda interna through the Foramen infrapiriforme, loops around the Lig. sacrospinale and reaches the Fossa ischioanalis through the **Foramen ischiadicum minus.** Here the pudendal neurovascular pathways are enclosed by the caudal fascia of the M. obturatorius internus forming the **Canalis pudendalis (ALCOCK's canal).** The **N. rectalis inferior** branches off in the Fossa ischioanalis, and bifurcates into its terminal branches in both of the perineal spaces:

- The **Nn. perineales** innervate the perineal musculature and supply the posterior two-thirds of the perineum, and the labia majora with the Rr. labiales posteriores.
- The **N. dorsalis clitoridis** provides sensory innervation to the glans of the clitoris.

The **N. cutaneous femoris posterior** only innervates a small part of the lateral perineum (→ Fig. 7.164).

Neurovascular structures of the perineum in women

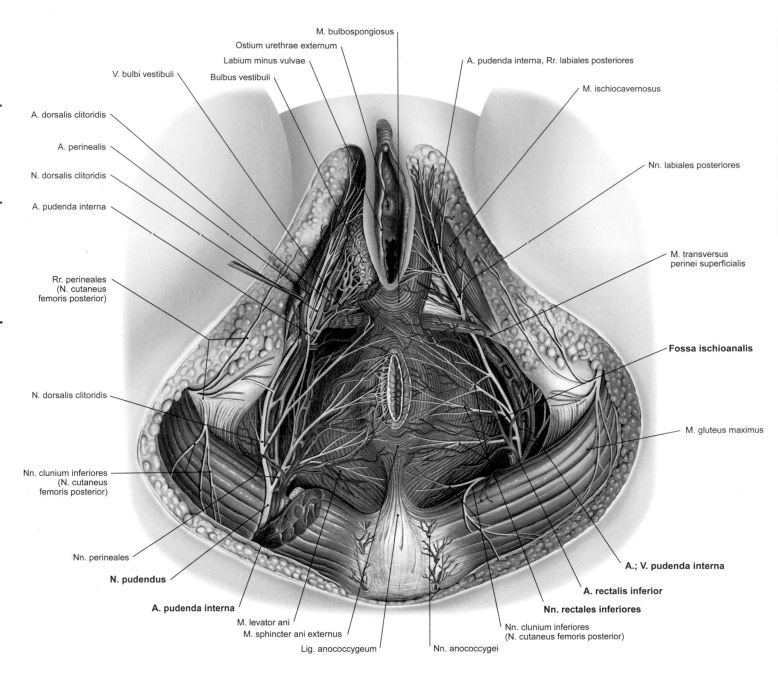

M. bulbospongiosus

Ostium urethrae externum

Labium minus vulvae

V. bulbi vestibuli

Bulbus vestibuli

A. dorsalis clitoridis

A. perinealis

N. dorsalis clitoridis

A. pudenda interna

Rr. perineales
(N. cutaneus
femoris posterior)

N. dorsalis clitoridis

Nn. clunium inferiores
(N. cutaneus
femoris posterior)

Nn. perineales

N. pudendus

A. pudenda interna

M. levator ani

M. sphincter ani externus

Lig. anococcygeum

A. pudenda interna, Rr. labiales posteriores

M. ischiocavernosus

Nn. labiales posteriores

M. transversus
perinei superficialis

Fossa ischioanalis

M. gluteus maximus

A.; V. pudenda interna

A. rectalis inferior

Nn. rectales inferiores

Nn. clunium inferiores
(N. cutaneus femoris posterior)

Nn. anococcygei

Fig. 7.162 Vessels and nerves of the perineal region, Regio perinealis, in women; caudal view. [S700]
The **Fossa ischioanalis** is similar in men and women. The neurovascular pathways run dorsolaterally in the Canalis pudendalis (ALCOCK's canal) formed by a fascial duplication of the M. obturatorius internus, into the pyramid-shaped Fossa ischioanalis which is filled with adipose tissue. They then provide branches to the anus and anal canal, and trav-

erse the Fossa ischioanalis ventrally to pass through both the perineal spaces to the vulva.
Contents of the Fossa ischioanalis:
- A. and V. pudenda interna and N. pudendus: in the Canalis pudendalis (ALCOCK's canal)
- A., V. and N. rectalis inferior: to the anal canal.

Clinical remarks

As in men, the Fossa ischioanalis is clinically highly relevant because of its expansion on both sides of the anus. **Abscesses** (collections of pus), e.g. where there are fistulas from the anal canal, can extend throughout the Fossa ischioanalis up to the front of the pubic symphysis. Not only do they generate non-specific inflammatory symptoms but also cause intense pain in the perineal region.

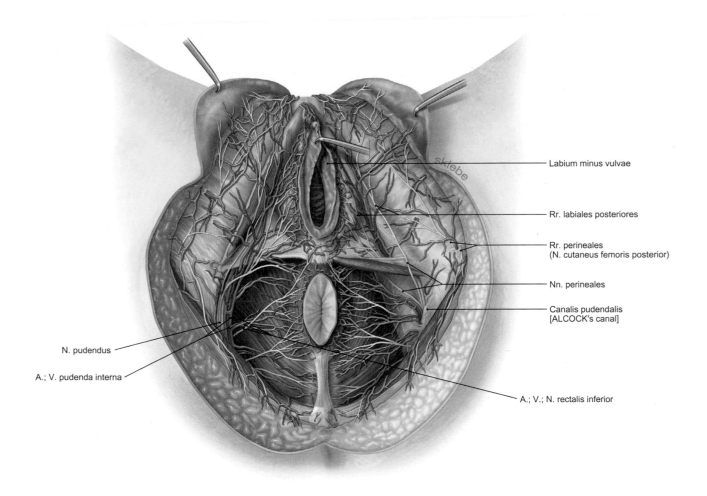

Labium minus vulvae

Rr. labiales posteriores

Rr. perineales
(N. cutaneus femoris posterior)

Nn. perineales

Canalis pudendalis
[ALCOCK's canal]

A.; V.; N. rectalis inferior

N. pudendus

A.; V. pudenda interna

Fig. 7.163 Neurovascular structures of the perineum, Regio perinealis, in women; the labia majora and the Canalis pudendalis on the right side are exposed; caudal view. [S700-L238]/[Q300]
To supplement → Fig. 7.163, this illustration also shows the anterior neurovascular pathways of the perineum. The anterior third of the perineum receives blood from the **A./V. pudenda externa** which also branch off the Rr. labiales anteriores to the labia. The **N. ilioinguinalis** provides corresponding innervation and also forms the Rr. labiales anteriores.

On the right side of the body and on the lateral wall of the **Fossa ischioanalis,** the image shows the exposed **Canalis pudendalis (ALCOCK's canal)** which is formed by the fascial duplication of the M. obturatorius internus. The A., V., and N. rectalis inferior to the anal canal are visible here.

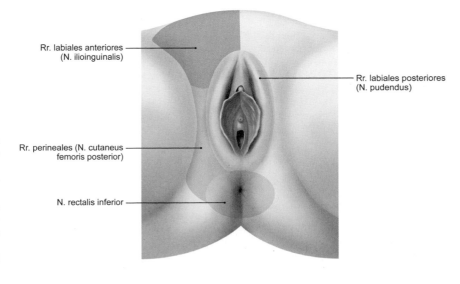

Rr. labiales anteriores
(N. ilioinguinalis)

Rr. labiales posteriores
(N. pudendus)

Rr. perineales (N. cutaneus
femoris posterior)

N. rectalis inferior

Fig. 7.164 Innervation of the perineum, Regio perinealis, in women; schematic illustration, caudal view in lithotomy position. [S701-L275]
The ventral third of the perineal region is innervated by the **N. ilioinguinalis** (Rr. labiales anteriores). The dorsal two-thirds receive sensory innervation from the **N. pudendus** (Rr. labiales posteriores) and laterally from the **N. cutaneus femoris posterior** (Rr. perinei).
The **N. rectalis inferior** innervates the perianal skin.

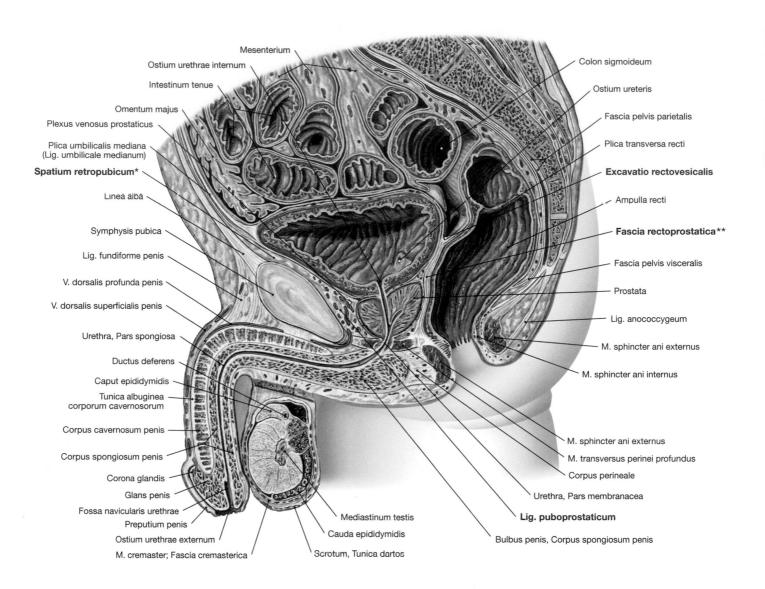

Mesenterium

Ostium urethrae internum

Intestinum tenue

Omentum majus

Plexus venosus prostaticus

Plica umbilicalis mediana
(Lig. umbilicale medianum)

Spatium retropubicum*

Linea alba

Symphysis pubica

Lig. fundiforme penis

V. dorsalis profunda penis

V. dorsalis superficialis penis

Urethra, Pars spongiosa

Ductus deferens

Caput epididymidis

Tunica albuginea
corporum cavernosorum

Corpus cavernosum penis

Corpus spongiosum penis

Corona glandis

Glans penis

Fossa navicularis urethrae

Preputium penis

Ostium urethrae externum

M. cremaster; Fascia cremasterica

Colon sigmoideum

Ostium ureteris

Fascia pelvis parietalis

Plica transversa recti

Excavatio rectovesicalis

Ampulla recti

Fascia rectoprostatica**

Fascia pelvis visceralis

Prostata

Lig. anococcygeum

M. sphincter ani externus

M. sphincter ani internus

M. sphincter ani externus

M. transversus perinei profundus

Corpus perineale

Urethra, Pars membranacea

Lig. puboprostaticum

Bulbus penis, Corpus spongiosum penis

Mediastinum testis

Cauda epididymidis

Scrotum, Tunica dartos

Fig. 7.165 Pelvis of a man; median section; view from the left side. [S700]

In men the most inferior pouch of the peritoneal cavity is the **Excavatio rectovesicalis.** This is laterally confined by the **Plica rectovesicalis** in which the Plexus hypogastricus inferior is found. Caudally, the **Fascia rectoprostatica** (**clin.: DENONVILLIER's fascia) follows in the subperitoneal space, separating the rectum and prostate. Behind the pubic symphysis lies a space filled with connective tissue **(Spatium retropubicum,** *clin.: cave of RETZIUS) in which the thin Lig. puboprostaticum attaches the prostate and the urinary bladder to the pelvic bone. In the inferior part of the Spatium retropubicum, the **V. dorsalis profunda penis** opens to drain the blood of the cavernous bodies of the penis into the **Plexus venosus prostaticus,** which is connected to the V. iliaca interna.

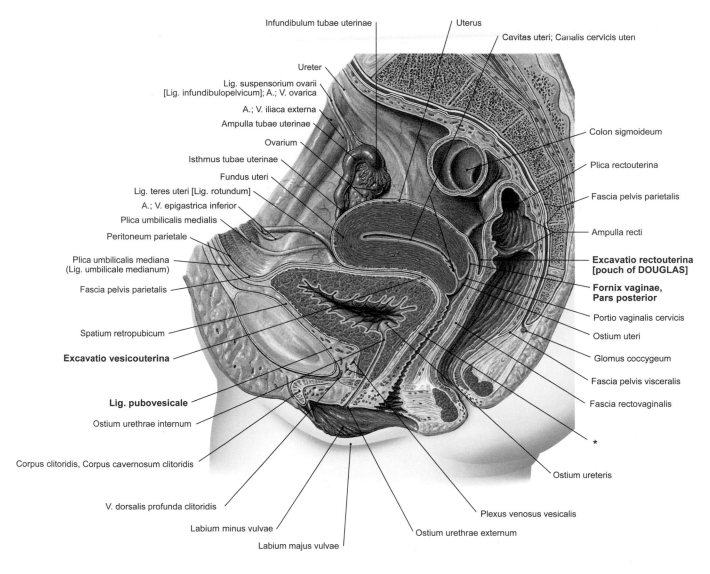

Infundibulum tubae uterinae

Uterus

Cavitas uteri; Canalis cervicis uteri

Ureter

Lig. suspensorium ovarii
[Lig. infundibulopelvicum]; A.; V. ovarica

A.; V. iliaca externa

Ampulla tubae uterinae

Ovarium

Isthmus tubae uterinae

Fundus uteri

Lig. teres uteri [Lig. rotundum]

A.; V. epigastrica inferior

Plica umbilicalis medialis

Peritoneum parietale

Plica umbilicalis mediana
(Lig. umbilicale medianum)

Fascia pelvis parietalis

Spatium retropubicum

Excavatio vesicouterina

Lig. pubovesicale

Ostium urethrae internum

Corpus clitoridis, Corpus cavernosum clitoridis

V. dorsalis profunda clitoridis

Labium minus vulvae

Labium majus vulvae

Colon sigmoideum

Plica rectouterina

Fascia pelvis parietalis

Ampulla recti

**Excavatio rectouterina
[pouch of DOUGLAS]**

**Fornix vaginae,
Pars posterior**

Portio vaginalis cervicis

Ostium uteri

Glomus coccygeum

Fascia pelvis visceralis

Fascia rectovaginalis

*

Ostium ureteris

Plexus venosus vesicalis

Ostium urethrae externum

Fig. 7.166 Pelvis of a woman; median section; view from the left side. [S700]

Because the uterus is slotted in between the urinary bladder and the rectum, the peritoneal cavity in women has two caudal pouches. The most caudal pouch is the **Excavatio rectouterina** (pouch of DOUG-LAS). It extends to the posterior vaginal vault (Fornix vaginae, Pars posterior). It is laterally confined by the **Plica rectouterina** in which the Plexus hypogastricus inferior is found. The **Fascia rectovaginalis** caudally follows in the subperitoneal space separating the rectum from the vagina. The **Excavatio vesicouterina** between the bladder and uterus is not as deep and covers the subperitoneal Septum vesicovaginale. Behind the pubic symphysis lies a space filled with connective tissue **(Spatium retropubicum),** in which the thin Lig. pubovesicale attaches the urinary bladder to the pelvic bone. In the inferior part of the Spatium retropubicum, the **V. dorsalis profunda clitoridis** opens, draining the blood of the cavernous bodies of the clitoris to the **Plexus venosus vesicalis,** which is connected to the V. iliaca interna.

* clin.: Septum vesicovaginale

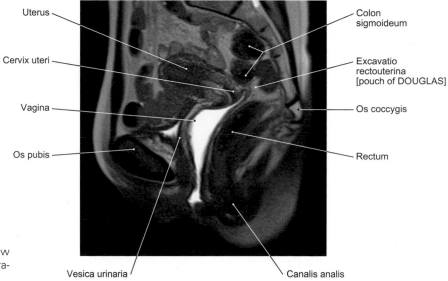

Uterus

Cervix uteri

Vagina

Os pubis

Vesica urinaria

Colon sigmoideum

Excavatio rectouterina [pouch of DOUGLAS]

Os coccygis

Rectum

Canalis analis

Fig. 7.167 Pelvis of a woman; sagittal section, T2w MRI sequence. The vagina has been filled with ultrasound gel to achieve a better contrast. [S700-T832]

Male pelvis, cross-sections

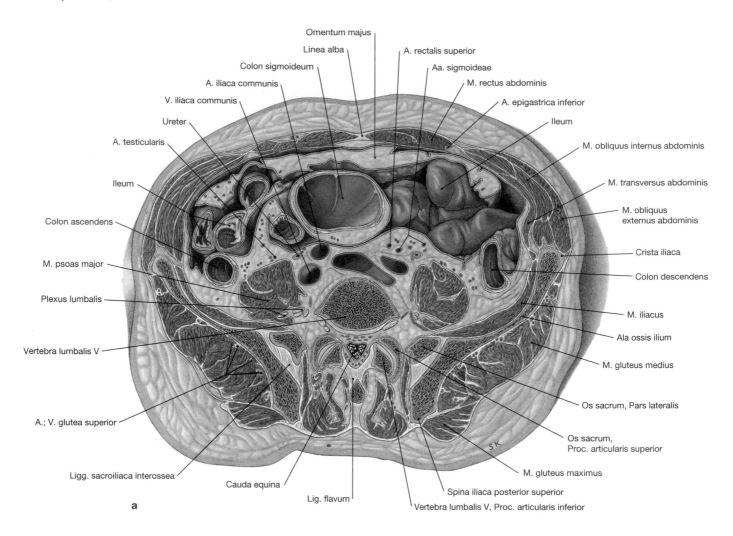

Omentum majus
Linea alba
Colon sigmoideum
A. iliaca communis
V. iliaca communis
Ureter
A. testicularis
Ileum
Colon ascendens
M. psoas major
Plexus lumbalis
Vertebra lumbalis V
A.; V. glutea superior
Ligg. sacroiliaca interossea
Cauda equina
Lig. flavum

A. rectalis superior
Aa. sigmoideae
M. rectus abdominis
A. epigastrica inferior
Ileum
M. obliquus internus abdominis
M. transversus abdominis
M. obliquus externus abdominis
Crista iliaca
Colon descendens
M. iliacus
Ala ossis ilium
M. gluteus medius
Os sacrum, Pars lateralis
Os sacrum, Proc. articularis superior
M. gluteus maximus
Spina iliaca posterior superior
Vertebra lumbalis V, Proc. articularis inferior

a

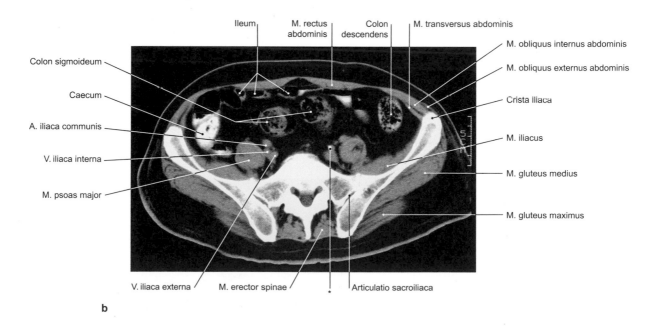

Ileum
M. rectus abdominis
Colon descendens
M. transversus abdominis
Colon sigmoideum
Caecum
A. iliaca communis
V. iliaca interna
M. psoas major
V. iliaca externa
M. erector spinae
Articulatio sacroiliaca

M. obliquus internus abdominis
M. obliquus externus abdominis
Crista Iliaca
M. iliacus
M. gluteus medius
M. gluteus maximus

b

Fig. 7.168a and b Pelvis of a man; cross-sections; caudal view.
a Cross-section at the level of the fifth lumbar vertebra. [S700-L238]
b Corresponding computed tomography (CT) scan. [S700-T893]
According to convention, CT scans are **always viewed from caudal.**
Since the section is at the level of the **greater pelvis,** the actual pelvic
organs cannot be seen. However, it is clear that the iliac bone (Os ili-

um), with its expansive pelvic bones (Alae ossis ilii), surrounds both the
small intestinal loops of the ileum and the Colon sigmoideum, which
continues its S-shaped loop in the median plane and then at the level of
the second to the third sacral vertebrae in the rectum.

* calcification in the wall of the A. iliaca communis

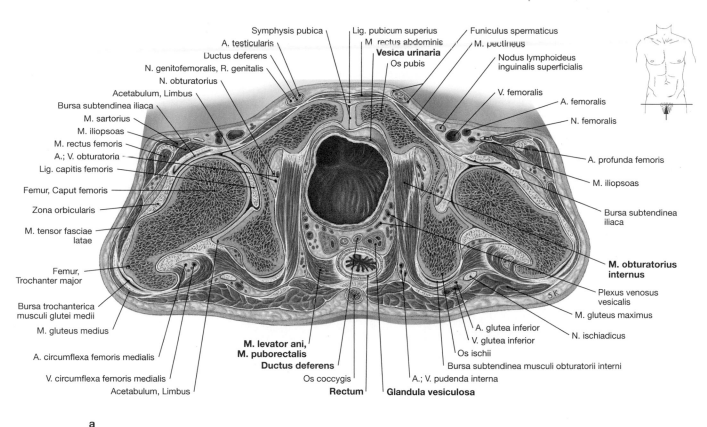

Symphysis pubica
A. testicularis
Ductus deferens
N. genitofemoralis, R. genitalis
N. obturatorius
Acetabulum, Limbus
Bursa subtendinea iliaca
M. sartorius
M. iliopsoas
M. rectus femoris
A.; V. obturatoria
Lig. capitis femoris
Femur, Caput femoris
Zona orbicularis
M. tensor fasciae latae
Femur, Trochanter major
Bursa trochanterica musculi glutei medii
M. gluteus medius
A. circumflexa femoris medialis
V. circumflexa femoris medialis
Acetabulum, Limbus

Lig. pubicum superius
M. rectus abdominis
Vesica urinaria
Os pubis

Funiculus spermaticus
M. pectineus
Nodus lymphoideus inguinalis superficialis
V. femoralis
A. femoralis
N. femoralis
A. profunda femoris
M. iliopsoas
Bursa subtendinea iliaca
M. obturatorius internus
Plexus venosus vesicalis
M. gluteus maximus
N. ischiadicus

M. levator ani, M. puborectalis
Ductus deferens
Os coccygis
Rectum

A. glutea inferior
V. glutea inferior
Os ischii
Bursa subtendinea musculi obturatorii interni
A.; V. pudenda interna
Glandula vesiculosa

a

A.; V. femoralis
M. pectineus
M. sartorius
M. tensor fasciae latea
M. gluteus medius
M. gluteus maximus

Vesica urinaria
Glandula vesiculosa
M. obturatorius internus
N. ischiadicus

M. rectus femoris
M. levator ani
Rectum

b

Fig. 7.169a and b   Pelvis of a man; cross-sections; caudal view.
a Cross-section at the level of the lesser pelvis. [S700-L238]
b Corresponding computed tomography (CT) scan of the male pelvis in portal venous phase. [S700-T832]
The cross-section makes it possible to show the course of several muscles. For instance, the M. puborectalis of the M. levator ani is shown, forming a loop behind the rectum and pulling it forwards. As a result,

this creates the Flexura perinealis in the rectum. This mechanism contributes to the closure of the rectum and is important for faecal continence. Furthermore, the complicated course of the M. obturatorius internus is very easy to understand: the muscle originates from the inner aspect of the pelvic bone and runs dorsally. It is then deflected by the Os ischii, which acts as a hypomochlion, and ends up on the inner aspect of the Trochanter major.

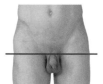

Retroperitoneal space and pelvic cavity

7

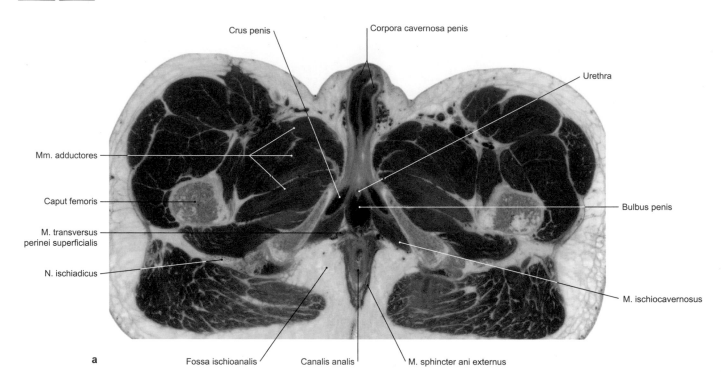

Crus penis

Corpora cavernosa penis

Urethra

Mm. adductores

Caput femoris

M. transversus
perinei superficialis

N. ischiadicus

Bulbus penis

M. ischiocavernosus

a

Fossa ischioanalis

Canalis analis

M. sphincter ani externus

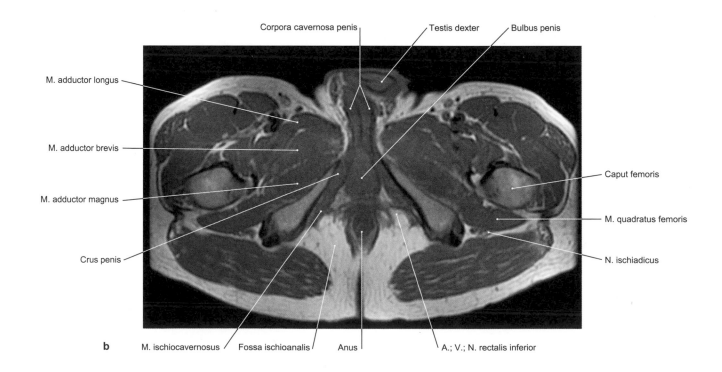

Corpora cavernosa penis

Testis dexter

Bulbus penis

M. adductor longus

M. adductor brevis

M. adductor magnus

Crus penis

Caput femoris

M. quadratus femoris

N. ischiadicus

b

M. ischiocavernosus

Fossa ischioanalis

Anus

A.; V.; N. rectalis inferior

Fig. 7.170a and b   Fossa ischioanalis and perineum in the male;
cross-sections; caudal view. [X338]

a Cross-section at the level of the Caput femoris.
b Magnetic resonance image (MRI) at the level of the Caput femoris.

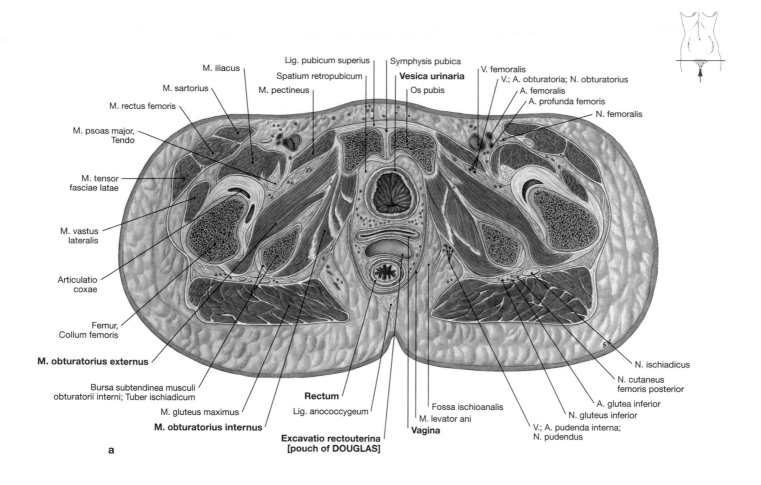

M. iliacus
Lig. pubicum superius
Symphysis pubica
V. femoralis
M. sartorius
Spatium retropubicum
Vesica urinaria
V.; A. obturatoria; N. obturatorius
M. rectus femoris
M. pectineus
Os pubis
A. femoralis
A. profunda femoris
M. psoas major, Tendo
N. femoralis

M. tensor fasciae latae

M. vastus lateralis

Articulatio coxae

Femur, Collum femoris

M. obturatorius externus
N. ischiadicus

Bursa subtendinea musculi obturatorii interni; Tuber ischiadicum
N. cutaneus femoris posterior
M. gluteus maximus
A. glutea inferior
Rectum
N. gluteus inferior
Lig. anococcygeum
Fossa ischioanalis
M. obturatorius internus
M. levator ani
V.; A. pudenda interna; N. pudendus
Excavatio rectouterina [pouch of DOUGLAS]
Vagina

a

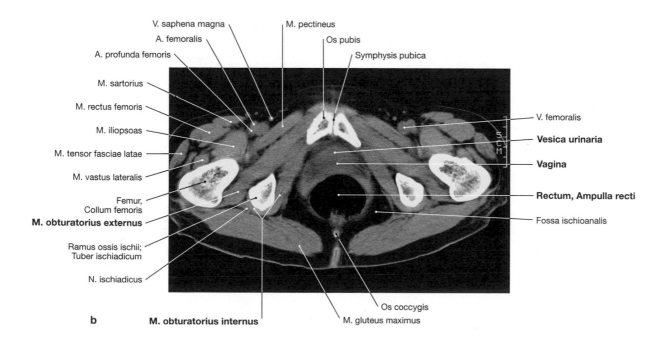

V. saphena magna
M. pectineus
A. femoralis
Os pubis
A. profunda femoris
Symphysis pubica
M. sartorius
M. rectus femoris
V. femoralis
M. iliopsoas
Vesica urinaria
M. tensor fasciae latae
Vagina
M. vastus lateralis
Femur, Collum femoris
Rectum, Ampulla recti
M. obturatorius externus
Fossa ischioanalis
Ramus ossis ischii; Tuber ischiadicum
N. ischiadicus
Os coccygis
b
M. obturatorius internus
M. gluteus maximus

Fig. 7.171a and b   Pelvis of a woman; cross-sections; caudal view.
a Cross-section at the level of the lesser pelvis. [S700-L238]
b Corresponding computed tomography (CT) scan. [S700-T893]
Of the pelvic viscera the following are recognisable: urinary bladder (Vesica urinaria), rectum, and between them the vagina and the Excava-

tio rectouterina [pouch of DOUGLAS] as the deepest part of the peritoneal cavity. Compared to the cross-section of the male pelvis (→ Fig. 7.168a), the cross-section here is further caudal. Therefore, in addition to the M. obturatorius internus, the M. obturatorius externus can also be seen at the front on the opposite side of the pelvic bone.

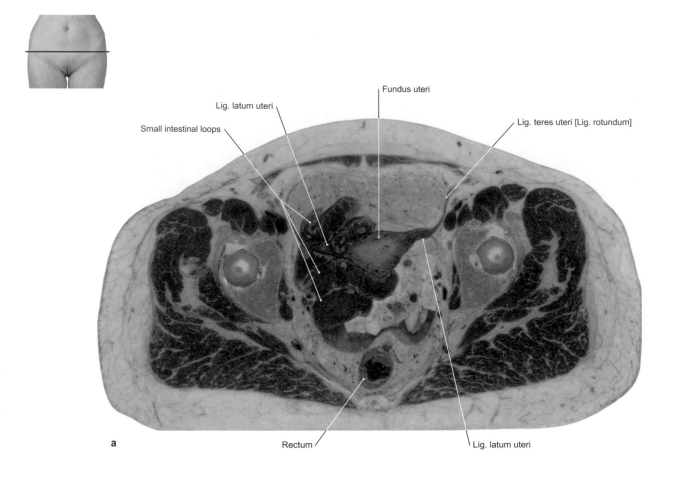

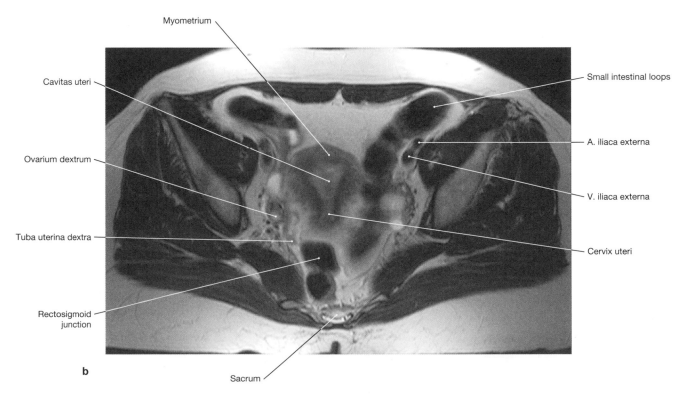

Fig. 7.172a and b   Cross-section of a female pelvis; cross-sections; caudal view. [X338]

a Cross-section at the level of the superior margin of the Caput femoris.
b Magnetic resonance image (MRI) of the female pelvis.

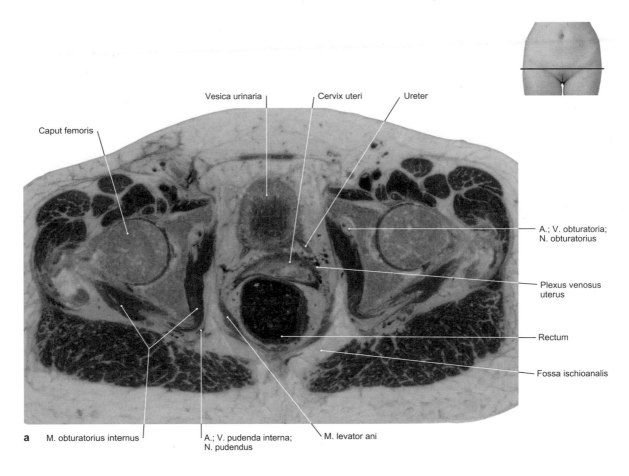

Vesica urinaria   Cervix uteri   Ureter

Caput femoris

A.; V. obturatoria;
N. obturatorius

Plexus venosus
uterus

Rectum

Fossa ischioanalis

a   M. obturatorius internus   A.; V. pudenda interna;   M. levator ani
N. pudendus

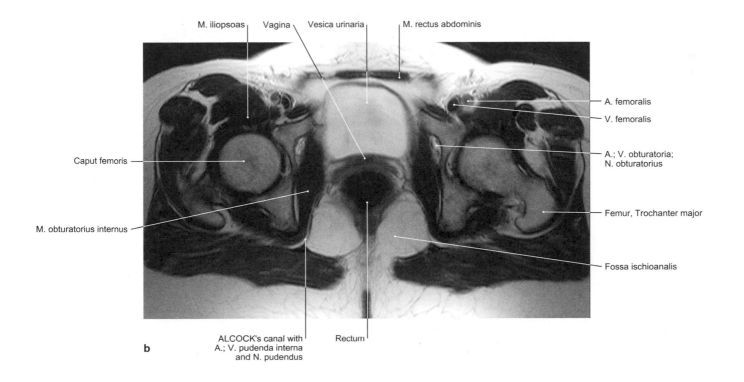

M. iliopsoas   Vagina   Vesica urinaria   M. rectus abdominis

A. femoralis

V. femoralis

A.; V. obturatoria;
N. obturatorius

Caput femoris

Femur, Trochanter major

M. obturatorius internus

Fossa ischioanalis

b   ALCOCK's canal with   Rectum
A.; V. pudenda interna
and N. pudendus

Fig. 7.173a and b Fossa ischioanalis in a woman; cross-sections; caudal view. [X338]
a Cross-section at the level of the hip joint.
b Magnetic resonance image (MRI) at the level of the hip joint.
The uterine cervix, Cervix uteri, with the Plexus venosis uterinus, and the junction of the distal ureter with the urinary bladder, Vesica uterina,

is visible. In addition, the neurovascular pathways in the Canalis obturatorius (A./V. obturatoria and N. obturatorius) and in the Canalis pudendalis (ALCOCK's canal) (A./V. pudenda interna and N. pudendus) are shown here.

Retroperitoneal space and pelvic cavity

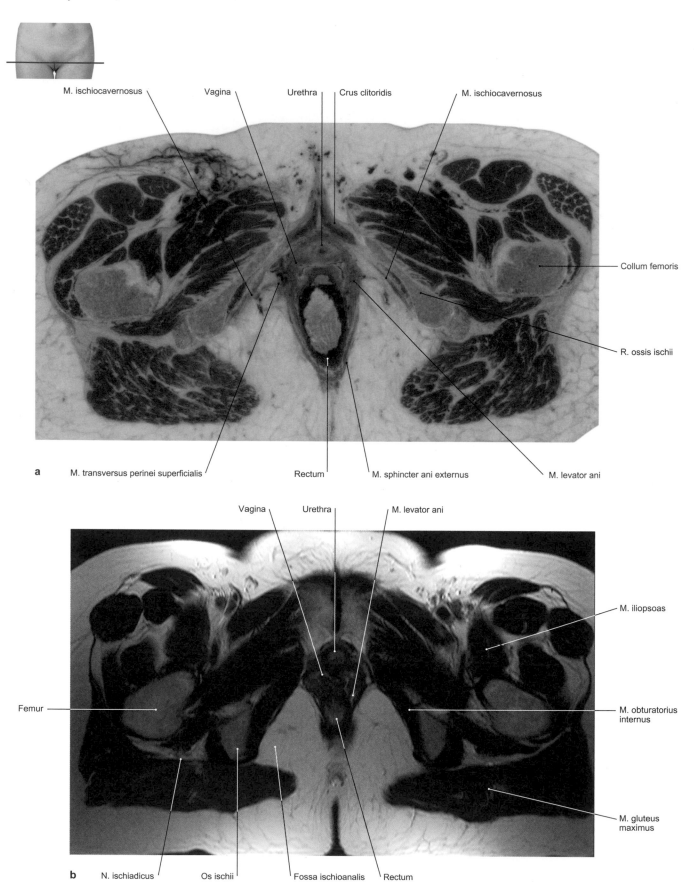

a

| M. ischiocavernosus | Vagina | Urethra | Crus clitoridis | M. ischiocavernosus |

Collum femoris

R. ossis ischii

M. transversus perinei superficialis   Rectum   M. sphincter ani externus   M. levator ani

Vagina   Urethra   M. levator ani

M. iliopsoas

Femur

M. obturatorius internus

M. gluteus maximus

b   N. ischiadicus   Os ischii   Fossa ischioanalis   Rectum

Fig. 7.174a and b   Fossa ischioanalis and superficial perineal space, Spatium perinei superficiale, in a woman; cross-sections; caudal view. [X338]

a Cross-section at the level of the Caput femoris. The M. ischiocavernosus and the M. transversus perinei superficialis on the right side are shown.
b Magnetic resonance image (MRI) of the female pelvis.

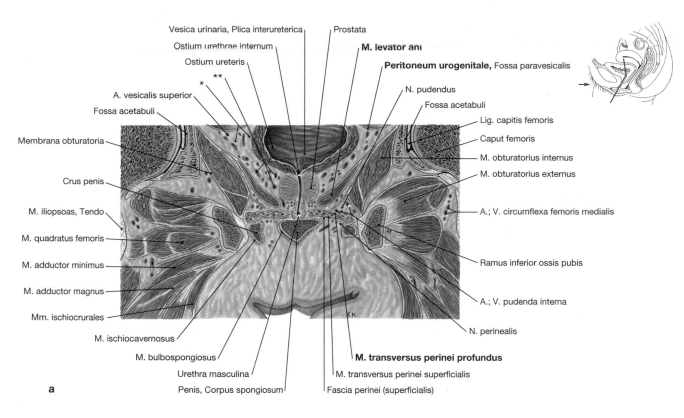

Vesica urinaria, Plica interureterica
Ostium urethrae internum
Ostium ureteris
* **
A. vesicalis superior
Fossa acetabuli
Membrana obturatoria
Crus penis
M. iliopsoas, Tendo
M. quadratus femoris
M. adductor minimus
M. adductor magnus
Mm. ischiocrurales
M. ischiocavernosus
M. bulbospongiosus
Urethra masculina
Penis, Corpus spongiosum

Prostata
M. levator ani
Peritoneum urogenitale, Fossa paravesicalis
N. pudendus
Fossa acetabuli
Lig. capitis femoris
Caput femoris
M. obturatorius internus
M. obturatorius externus
A.; V. circumflexa femoris medialis
Ramus inferior ossis pubis
A.; V. pudenda interna
N. perinealis
M. transversus perinei profundus
M. transversus perinei superficialis
Fascia perinei (superficialis)

a

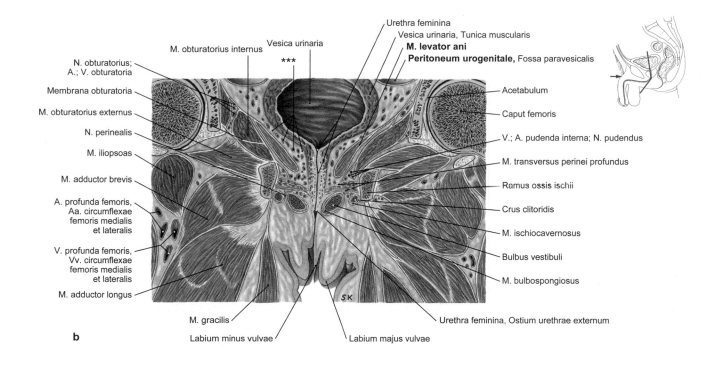

N. obturatorius;
A.; V. obturatoria
Membrana obturatoria
M. obturatorius externus
N. perinealis
M. iliopsoas
M. adductor brevis
A. profunda femoris,
Aa. circumflexae
femoris medialis
et lateralis
V. profunda femoris,
Vv. circumflexae
femoris medialis
et lateralis
M. adductor longus
M. gracilis
Labium minus vulvae

M. obturatorius internus
Vesica urinaria
***

Urethra feminina
Vesica urinaria, Tunica muscularis
M. levator ani
Peritoneum urogenitale, Fossa paravesicalis
Acetabulum
Caput femoris
V.; A. pudenda interna; N. pudendus
M. transversus perinei profundus
Ramus ossis ischii
Crus clitoridis
M. ischiocavernosus
Bulbus vestibuli
M. bulbospongiosus
Urethra feminina, Ostium urethrae externum
Labium majus vulvae

b

Fig. 7.175a and b Pelvis of a man and a woman; angled frontal section through the urinary bladder. [S700-L238]
a Angled frontal section through the pelvis of a man.
b Angled frontal section through the pelvis of a woman.
The section shows the pelvic floor and perineal musculature with the perineal spaces in a male (→ Fig. 7.116) and female (→ Fig. 7.159) pelvis. It shows the lower levels of the pelvic cavity clearly. Caudally of the **Peritoneum parietale** (here the Peritoneum urogenitale), the **subperitoneal space** expands up to the pelvic floor, formed here by the **M. levator ani.** Below, it connects with the **perineal region. In men,** the

M. transversus perinei profundus forms a solid muscle plate which fills the deep perineal space. Caudal to the Membrana perinei on the underside of the muscle is the superficial perineal space. **In women,** the perineal spaces are arranged in a similar way, but the M. transversus perinei profundus is predominantly permeated with connective tissue, so that there is usually no solid muscle plate present.

* clin.: paracystium
** clin.: Plexus venosus prostaticus
*** paracystium with venous plexus

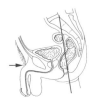

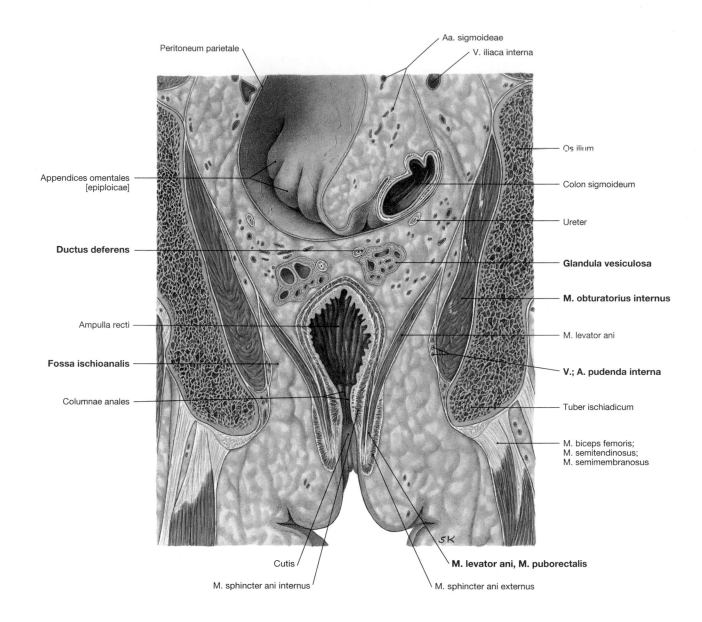

Peritoneum parietale

Aa. sigmoideae

V. iliaca interna

Appendices omentales [epiploicae]

Ductus deferens

Ampulla recti

Fossa ischioanalis

Columnae anales

Os ilium

Colon sigmoideum

Ureter

Glandula vesiculosa

M. obturatorius internus

M. levator ani

V.; A. pudenda interna

Tuber ischiadicum

M. biceps femoris; M. semitendinosus; M. semimembranosus

Cutis

M. sphincter ani internus

M. levator ani, M. puborectalis

M. sphincter ani externus

Fig. 7.176   Pelvis of a man; oblique frontal section through the lesser pelvis. [S700-L238]

The A. and V. pudenda interna run jointly with the N. pudendus in the fascial duplication of the M. obturatorius internus (clin.: ALCOCK's canal) in the Fossa ischioanalis.

Sample exam questions

To check that you are completely familiar with the content of this chapter, sample questions from an oral anatomy exam are listed here.

Which organs are in the retroperitoneal space (retroperitoneum)?

- Explain the **topographical relationships** of the pelvic viscera.

How do the kidneys develop and how are they structured?

What are the parts of the adrenal gland and what differentiates them in terms of functionality and regulation?

What functions do the kidneys have?

Which fascial systems surround them?

Which blood vessels supply the kidney and adrenal gland and which variants are you aware of?

Which parts does the urinary system have?

- From what do these develop?

What are the constrictions of the ureter?

How does the urinary bladder close itself?

How is the anal canal structured?

- Show the zones on the specimen.

How is the continence organ structured?

Which arteries supply the rectum and the anal canal?

Where are the regional lymph nodes for the individual parts?

How do the internal female genitalia develop and how do they differ from the male genitalia?

Explain the blood vessels of the penis on the specimen.

What are the fasciae of the spermatic cord?

Which neurovascular pathways supply the testes?

- Where are the regional lymph nodes?

What accessory sex glands are you aware of?

- Show these on the specimen.

Into which zones is the prostate divided?

Which ligaments fix the uterus in place?

Where is the pouch of DOUGLAS and what significance does it have?

How is the uterus supplied with blood?

Where are the regional lymph nodes of the ovary?

How is the pelvic floor structured?

- How is it innervated?

Show the perineal muscles.

- What function do they have?

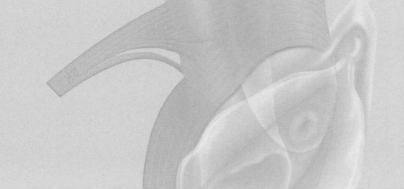

Appendix

Index

Page numbers are in **bold** when the corresponding entries on that page are also in bold.

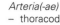

Index

Appendix

Index

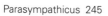

Appendix

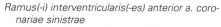

Index

Appendix